Infectious Diseases in the
Pediatric Intensive Care Unit

Simon Nadel (Ed.)

Infectious Diseases in the Pediatric Intensive Care Unit

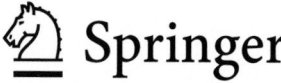 Springer

Simon Nadel, FRCP
St. Mary's Hospital
London
UK

British Library Cataloguing in Publication Data
Infectious diseases in the pediatric intensive care unit
  1. Communicable diseases in children   2. Pediatric intensive
  care
  I. Nadel, Simon
  618.9′29

Library of Congress Control Number: 2007928821

ISBN: 978-1-84628-916-3   e-ISBN: 978-1-84628-917-0

9 8 7 6 5 4 3 2 1

Springer Science+Business Media
springer.com

Foreword

Infectious diseases have always comprised an important component of the work of pediatric intensive care units. Historically, the need to provide respiratory support for children stricken by the epidemics of polio which affected many countries in the pre-vaccination era, led to the development of technology for ventilatory support. In the developed world, community-acquired infections, including septicaemia, severe pneumonia, meningitis and encephalitis remain important causes of intensive care admission in otherwise healthy children. In developing countries, malaria, septicaemia, and meningitis, and fulminant viral infections, such as Dengue, present major challenges to pediatricians working with limited resources. Of those patients admitted to pediatric intensive care units with noninfectious conditions, the development of hospital acquired opportunistic infections are an almost inevitable consequence of prolonged requirement for ventilatory support and vascular access. Patients undergoing intensive care for any length of time will invariably require investigation and treatment of nosocomial infections. With the specter of increasingly antibiotic resistant bacteria and fungi, all intensivists are faced daily with complex management problems of both primary and nosocomially acquired infections.

It is not surprising, in view of the importance of infectious diseases as causes of pediatric critical illness and death, that research on the mechanisms involved in life-threatening childhood infections has attracted the interest of pediatric intensivists, infectious diseases physicians, microbiologists, and basic scientists. Research on the inflammatory response triggered by microorganisms and the host response to infectious diseases has been one of the most exciting areas of medical research in the past three decades. Unraveling the role of innate immune mechanisms in the recognition of microbial pathogens, the cascade of events linking pattern recognition receptors to activation of host inflammatory pathways, and the production of cytokines, chemokines, and a myriad of inflammatory mediators responsible for tissue and organ damage have greatly improved the understanding not only of sepsis, but of the host response to trauma and inflammation.

Management of infection and infectious diseases in pediatric intensive care units usually requires multidisciplinary input from intensivists, infectious disease physicians, and microbiologists, as well as the hospital control of infection team. In view of the importance of infection as a problem in pediatric intensive care, there has been a need for a textbook that brings together information on the management of infectious diseases, as well as the scientific understanding underlying the interaction of infectious organisms and the host immune system, in a form which is accessible to those managing patients with infection in a pediatric intensive care setting. Simon Nadel, a pediatrician with dual training in pediatric intensive care and infectious diseases, has assembled a team of authors from Europe, Australia, and the United States representing the range of disciplines collaborating in the management of critically ill children with infection. This volume will provide those dealing with infection in critically ill children with up-to-date information not only on the diagnosis and management of infectious diseases, but on the immunological, genetic, and immunopathogenic mechanisms underlying the diseases in their patients. The book will be of great value to those training in pediatric intensive care and infectious diseases, as well as those seeking an understanding of the immuno-pathogenic processes causing critical illness in their patients.

In view of the rapid increase in scientific knowledge of the molecular and cellular processes involved in host pathogen interactions, and the rapidly changing spectrum of infectious diseases causing critical illness in children, we hope that this will be the first in a series which can be expanded and updated to provide those involved in the care of children with infections on intensive care units, with up-to-date information on the scientific basis underlying the management of infectious diseases in critically ill children.

Michael Levin
Professor of Paediatrics and International Child Health
Imperial College Faculty of Medicine
London, UK

Preface

This book is intended for all those working in the pediatric intensive care unit (PICU). Infectious diseases are some of the most common problems encountered in a PICU, either as a primary cause for admission or as a secondary complication in a patient admitted for another reason. Understanding the reasons behind such infectious complications, including their epidemiology, the susceptibility of children to infection, both as a primary cause of critical illness and as a secondary complication, the most common causes of infections in the critically ill child, aspects regarding prevention, and the exploration of new treatment modalities were the primary motives behind gathering together some world-renowned experts in aspects of pediatric infectious disease and critical care management. I hope that those who read this book will find useful information to help them in the management of children in their intensive care units, both in the developed and developing world.

In the pulling together of this book, I am extremely grateful to the authors of the chapters who have supplied such high quality contributions. I am also grateful to my wife Anne, and children, Sophie and Natasha, for their support and words of encouragement.

I hope the readers of this book learn some new information to help them in our goal of keeping children out of intensive care or keeping them in there for as short a time as possible and discharging them in the best possible condition.

Simon Nadel

Contents

Foreword *by Michael Levin* v
Preface vii
Contributors xi

1   The Immunology of Neonates and Children and Its Relation to
    Susceptibility to Infection 1
    E. Graham Davies

2   Infections in the Critically Ill Neonate 59
    Cheryl Jones

3   Fungal Infection in Critically Ill Children 97
    Alok Sharma

4   Toxin-Mediated Diseases and Toxic Shock Syndrome 113
    Andrew C. Steer and Nigel Curtis

5   Vaccines for the Prevention of Admission to the Pediatric
    Intensive Care Unit 143
    Shelley Segal, Matthew Snape, Dominic Kelly,
    and Andrew J. Pollard

6   Pathophysiology of Pediatric Sepsis 176
    Jan A. Hazelzet

7   The Epidemiology of Severe Infections in Children 194
    Mary E. Hartman, R. Scott Watson, Joseph A. Carcillo,
    and Derek C. Angus

8   Novel Challenges in Infection in the Pediatric Intensive Care
    Unit Setting 213
    Laura Jones and Mike Sharland

9   Host Genetic Susceptibility to Infection 225
    Shamez N. Ladhani and Robert Booy

10 Nosocomial Infections in the Pediatric Intensive Care Unit 312
    Xavier Sáez-Llorens and Octavio Ramilo

11 Infections in the Immunocompromised Patient in the Pediatric
    Intensive Care Unit 332
    Karyn Moshal, Olaf Neth, David Cubitt, and Nigel Klein

12 Infants and Children with Human Immunodeficiency Virus 350
    Steven B. Welch and E.G. Hermione Lyall

13 Life-Threatening Tropical Infections 370
    Kathryn Maitland and Bridget Wills

14 Cardiac Infections in the Pediatric Intensive Care Unit 438
    Laura M. Ibsen and Irving Shen

15 Pediatric Critical Care: Acute Central Nervous System Infection . 465
    Thomas Iolster and Robert C. Tasker

16 Respiratory Infection in Pediatric Intensive Care Unit 487
    D.R. O'Donnell and R.G. Branco

17 New Therapies for Sepsis 521
    Liz Whittaker and Simon Nadel

Index 559

Contributors

Derek C. Angus, MD, MPH
Department of Critical Care
  Medicine
University of Pittsburgh
Pittsburgh, PA, USA

Robert Booy, MBBS, MSc, MD,
  FRACP, FRCPCH
Academic Centre for Child Health
Institute of Community Health and
  Sciences
Queen Mary's School of Medicine
  and Dentistry
Royal London Hospital
London, UK

R.G. Branco, MD
Paediatric Intensive Care Unit
Addenbrooke's Hospital
Cambridge, UK

Joseph A. Carcillo, MD
Department of Critical Care
  Medicine
University of Pittsburgh
Pittsburgh, PA, USA

David Cubitt, MSc, PhD
Department of Host Defence
Hospital for Sick Children
Great Ormond Street
London, UK

Nigel Curtis, DCH, DTM&H, MRCP,
  MRCPCH, PhD
Department of Paediatrics
Royal Children's Hospital
Parkville, VIC, Australia

E. Graham Davies, MA, FRCP,
  FRCPCH
Department of Immunology
Great Ormond Street Hospital
London, UK

Mary E. Hartman, MD
Department of Critical Care
  Medicine
University of Pittsburgh
Pittsburgh, PA, USA

Jan A. Hazelzet, MD, PhD
Paediatric Intensive Care Unit
Erasmus MC-Sophia Children's
  Hospital
Rotterdam, The Netherlands

Laura M. Ibsen, MD
Department of Pediatrics
Oregon Health and Sciences
  University
Portland, OR, USA

Thomas Iolster, MD
Department of Paediatrics and
   Paediatric Intensive Care Unit
University of Cambridge Clinical
   School
Addenbrooke's Hospital
Cambridge, UK

Cheryl Jones, MBBS (Hons), PhD,
   FRACP
Discipline of Paediatrics and Child
   Health
University of Sydney
Parkville, Australia
Department of Allergy, Immunology
   and Infectious Diseases
The Children's Hospital at
   Westmead
Westmead, NSW, Australia

Laura Jones, MRCPCH
Paediatric Infectious Disease
St. George's Hospital
London, UK

Dominic Kelly, MRCPCH
Department of Paediatrics
University of Oxford
John Radcliffe Hospital
Oxford, Oxon, UK

Nigel Klein, BSc, MBBS, MRCP,
   PhD, FRCPCH
Paediatric Infectious Disease and
   Immunology
Institute of Child Health
London, UK

Shamez N. Ladhani, MRCPCH
Academic Centre for Child Health
Institute of Community Health and
   Sciences
Queen Mary's School of Medicine
   and Dentistry
Royal London Hospital
London, UK

E.G. Hermione Lyall, MBCHB Hons,
   MD, MRCPCH
Department of Paediatrics
St. Mary's Hospital
London, UK

Kathryn Maitland, MRCP, PhD
Department of Paediatrics
Imperial College London
London, UK
MRC-Clinical Trials Unit
KEMRI-Wellcome Trust Programme
Kilifi, Kenya

Karyn Moshal, MBChB, MRCP,
   MRCPCH, DTM&H
Paediatric Infectious Disease
Hospital for Sick Children
Great Ormond Street
London, UK

Simon Nadel, FRCP
St. Mary's Hospital
London, UK

Olaf Neth, MD, MRCPCH
Paediatric Infectious Disease and
   Immunology
Hospital for Sick Children
Great Ormond Street
London, UK

D.R. O'Donnell, MRCPCH, PhD
Paediatric Intensive Care Unit
Addenbrooke's Hospital
Cambridge, UK

Andrew J. Pollard, FRCPCH, PhD
Department of Paediatrics
University of Oxford
John Radcliffe Hospital
Oxford, Oxon, UK

Octavio Ramilo, MD
Department of Pediatrics
Division of Infectious Diseases
University of Texas Southwestern
   Medical Center at Dallas
Children's Medical Center Dallas
Dallas, TX, USA

Xavier Sáez-Llorens, MD
Department of Pediatrics
University of Panama School of
    Medicine
Department of Infectious Diseases
Hospital del Niño
Panama City, Panama

Shelley Segal, MBBcH
Department of Paediatrics
University of Oxford
John Radcliffe Hospital
Headington, Oxford
Oxfordshire, UK

Mike Sharland, MRCPCH
Paediatric Infectious Disease
St. George's Hospital
London, UK

Alok Sharma, MRCPCH
Torbay Hospital
Torquay, UK

Irving Shen, MD
Department of Surgery
Oregon Health and Sciences
    University
Portland, OR, USA

Matthew Snape, MBBS, FRACP
Department of Paediatrics
University of Oxford
John Radcliffe Hospital
Headington, Oxford
Oxfordshire, UK

Andrew C. Steer, MBBS, BMedSci
Department of Paediatrics
Royal Children's Hospital
Parkville, VIC, Australia

Robert C. Tasker, FRCP, PhD
Department of Paediatrics and
    Paediatric Intensive Care Unit
University of Cambridge Clinical
    School
Addenbrooke's Hospital
Cambridge, UK

R. Scott Watson, MD, MPH
Department of Critical Care
    Medicine
University of Pittsburgh
Pittsburgh, PA, USA

Steven B. Welch, BA (Hons), MSc,
    MBBS, MRCPCH
Department of Paediatrics
St. Mary's Hospital
London, UK

Liz Whittaker, MRCPCH
Department of Paediatrics
St. Mary's Hospital
London, UK

Bridget Wills, MRCP
Department of Pediatrics
Wellcome Trust Clinical Research
    Unit
Hospital for Tropical Diseases
Ho Chi Minh City, Vietnam

1
The Immunology of Neonates and Children and Its Relation to Susceptibility to Infection

E. Graham Davies

The young child is excessively susceptible to infections by virtue of immaturities in immune mechanisms and the lack of prior antigen exposure. This results in an increased frequency of infections that are often more severe than at older ages. Inherited primary deficiencies of the immune system may result in infections with common pathogens possibly manifesting in atypical fashion, and infections with opportunistic organisms. Genetic susceptibility to infections may also be associated with mutations or polymorphisms in the genes controlling immune and inflammatory responsiveness to microbial agents. Secondary immunodeficiency in childhood is seen in malnutrition, following infections particularly with HIV or after immunosuppressive treatments and chemotherapy.

The Immune System

The immune system comprises a number of innate mechanisms, which help the body deal with microbial invaders and a more sophisticated adaptive immune system. The latter is characterized by the possession of an almost infinite variety of unique antigen receptors that enable recognition of microbial antigens. Expansion of cells expressing such receptors allows maturation of immune responses (adaptation) and the development of immunologic memory. The innate and adaptive systems are functionally closely integrated particularly in the effector arm of immune function and some of the interactions are illustrated in Figure 1.1.

Innate Immune System

The innate immune system comprises humoral and cellular elements. Humoral factors include endogenous peptides and proteins present in the tissues and secretions, which have antimicrobial activity. Some of these factors are found in a wide range of multicellular organisms throughout plant and animal

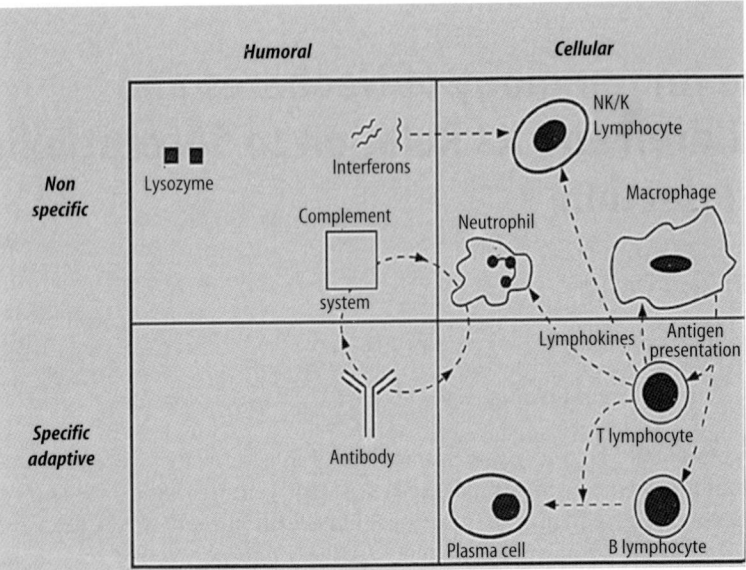

FIGURE 1.1. Non-specific (innate) and specific adaptive immune system. (Reproduced with permission from Cant AJ, et al—see Further Reading.)

kingdoms (1). Levels of these may become enhanced in the face of infection and inflammation. Examples include interferon-α, lysozyme, and iron sequestering proteins.

The complement system involves a sophisticated cascade of reactions resulting in deposition of complement on the surface of microorganisms. This is achieved either via the Classical pathway triggered when specific antibody binds the antigen, or by the Alternative pathway triggered directly by microbial antigens without the need for antibody or by the mannan-binding lectin system, which is again antibody independent but utilizes the classic pathway components (2). This is summarized in Figure 1.2.

The deposition of complement C3b acts as a powerful opsonin enabling cells of the immune system such as neutrophils to bind the organism prior to phagocytosis. In addition, the late complement components are involved in a lytic process, which can kill organisms directly. One other function of the complement system is to produce inflammatory and chemotactic signals (e.g., the anaphylotoxin, C5a), which enhance recruitment of immune effector mechanisms at the site of an infection.

The cells of the innate system comprise the myeloid series including neutrophils, macrophage/monocytes, and natural killer cells. Neutrophils are important in the phagocytosis of bacterial and fungal pathogens, a process facilitated by opsonization with antibody and complement components. Macrophages are responsible for the killing of intracellular pathogens, such as mycobacteria and certain fungi, and their ability to do this is greatly enhanced

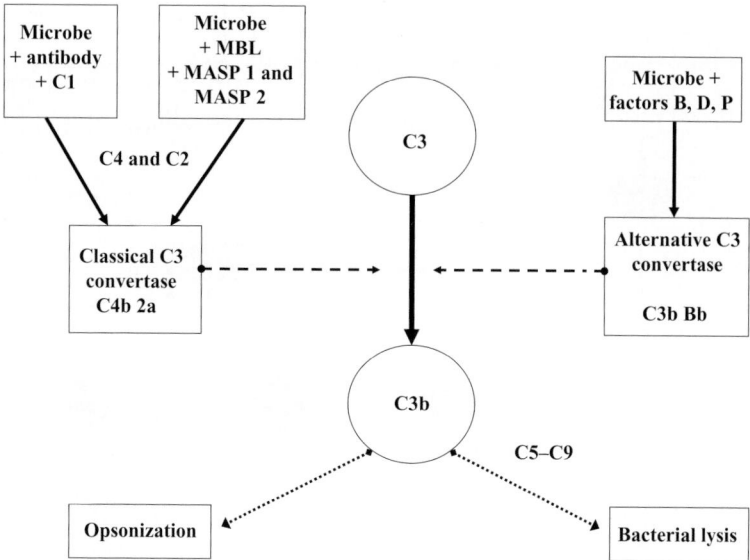

Figure 1.2. The complement system. C, complement component; MBL, mannan-binding lectin; MASP, MBL associated serine protease.

by interaction with the cell-mediated immune system through cytokines such as interferon-γ. The interferon-γ/interleukin-12 system is important in the handling of intracellular pathogens including mycobacteria, and *Salmonella* species (3) and is illustrated in Figure 1.3.

It has become increasingly recognized that cellular mechanisms particularly those involving the macrophages can respond directly to microbial components such as bacterial lipopolysaccharide to produce inflammatory responses. These are mediated through a series of cellular receptors called Toll-like receptors and

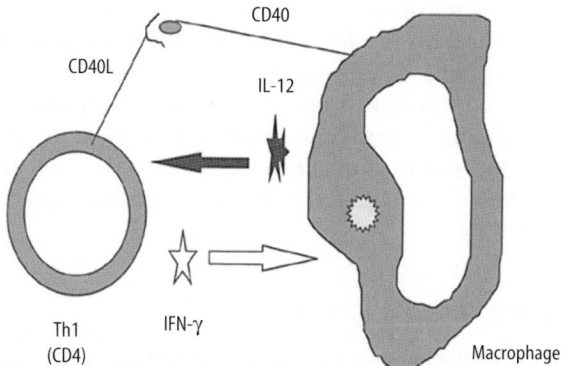

Figure 1.3. Interleukin-12 (IL-12)/interferon-γ (IFN-γ) loop. Macrophage IL-12 production by the infected macrophage stimulates IFN-γ production in a positive feedback loop. CD40 interaction with its ligand, CD40L, is a requirement for this interaction. (Reproduced with permission from Davies EG. Impaired Immunity in Children. Current Paediatrics 2006;16:16–28.)

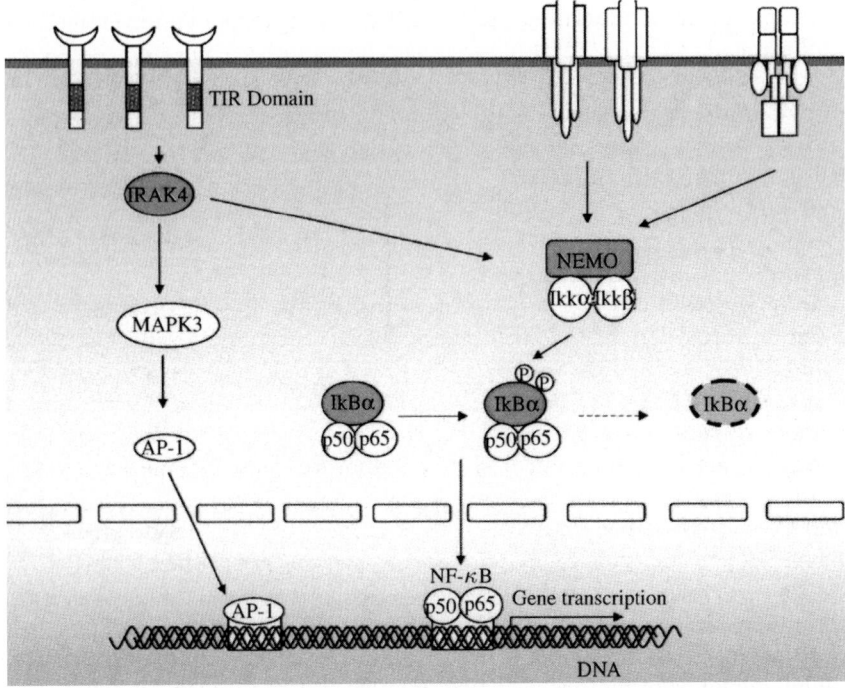

FIGURE 1.4. Signaling through Toll-like receptors. Abnormalities of three proteins (shaded) NEMO, IkBα, IRAK4 have been described as causing immunodeficiency (see page 17). MAPK, mitogen-activated protein kinase; NEMO, nuclear factor essential modulator; NF, nuclear factor; TIR, toll and interleukin-1 receptor; IRAK, interleukin-1 receptor-associated kinase. (Reproduced with permission from Reference 4.)

through other methods of recognizing a specific bacterial cell wall components such as muramyl dipeptide. The mechanisms are important in the early response to acute infections particularly with bacteria before the specific adaptive immune system can come into play (4) (Fig. 1.4).

Natural killer (NK) cells are large granular lymphocytes developing from lymphoid precursors but lacking specific antigen receptors. They have the ability to kill tumor cells and virus-infected cells, and are important in the early phases of virus infections before specific immunity has developed (5). They also have Fc receptors for immunoglobulin G (IgG) and when "armed" with bound antibody can kill target cells using a system called antibody-dependent cellular cytotoxicity (ADCC).

Specific Adaptive Immune System

This system involves the specific (T and B cell) lymphoid system. The process involved in the production of the antigen receptor involves the rearrangement of a number of genes (*V*, *D*, and *J* genes) coding for the variable (antigen-binding) part of the molecule, and then further rearrangement to bring this unique combination of genes to lie adjacent to a gene coding for the constant portion of the molecule. This is performed by excising loops of intervening DNA as illustrated in Figure 1.5. It involves a complex group of enzymes, including those that are part of the process of double-stranded DNA break repair (6).

Translation of the whole combination of genes then results in the receptor with a common constant portion and a unique variable region. Further diversification of the variable region may occur through a process of somatic hypermutation in the variable region genes and by the random addition of extra nucleotides through the action of the enzyme terminal deoxynucleotide transferase (TDT).

Different types of lymphocytes are recognized through their expression of different surface antigens, which can be detected using monoclonal antibody staining and fluorescence-activated cell sorting (FACS) analysis. B lymphocytes express immunoglobulin molecules on their surface, which act as the unique antigen receptor for individual cells. Leukocyte surface antigens have been given designated CD (cluster of differentiation) numbers. Table 1.1 lists the most important CD antigens.

B cells are so called because they are derived from the bone marrow in humans and express immunoglobulin molecules on their surface, which act as the specific antigen receptors for those cells. Following stimulation of the B cell through its antigen receptor, maturation occurs with immunoglobulin secretion. There is class switching from the initial antibody response of IgM to the other antibody classes during this process. This process mostly requires T-cell

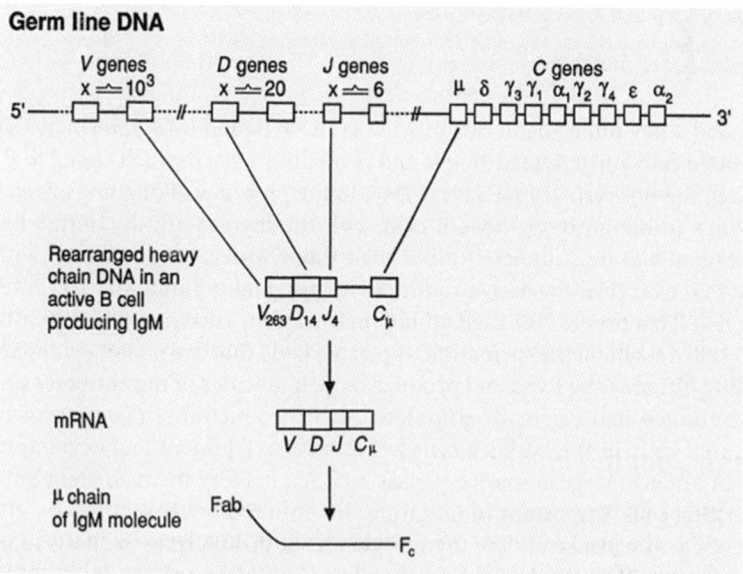

FIGURE 1.5. V, D, and J gene recombination. IgM, immunoglobulin M; mRNA, messenger RNA. (Reproduced with permission from Cant AJ, et al—see Further Reading.)

TABLE 1.1. Important leukocyte surface antigens

Antigen	Main cellular expression	Function where known
CD1 a,b,c	Thymocytes, Langerhans' cells	
CD3	All T cells	Part of T-cell receptor complex T-cell activation
CD4	Helper and regulatory T cells, monocytes	Part of antigen recognition with MHC-II, HIV receptor
CD5	T-cells, subset of B cells	Ligand for CD72
CD8	Cytotoxic and suppressor T cells, some NK cells	Part of antigen recognition with MHC-I
CD11 a,b,c	All leukocytes	Part of LFA-1 (β_2-integrin) adhesion (ligand—ICAM-1)
CD14	Monocytes	LPS receptor
CD15	Neutrophils	Selectin receptor
CD16	NK cells	IgG Fc receptor 3
CD18	All leukocytes	Part of LFA-1 (β_2-integrin) adhesion (ligand—ICAM-1)
CD19	B cells	
CD20	B cells	
CD21	B, dendritic cells	Complement receptor 2, EBV receptor
CD22	B cells	
CD25	Activated T cells	IL-2 receptor
CD40	B cells, macrophages, platelets, vascular endothelium	Co-stimulatory molecule for Ig class switching and macrophage activation
CD56	NK cells, some T cells (NK-T cells)	Adhesion molecule (N-CAM)
CD154	Activated T cells	Ligand for CD40
HLA class 1	All nucleated cells	Presentation of antigen to CD8 cells
HLA class 2 (DR)	Monocytes, B and activated T cells	Presentation of antigen to CD4 cells

EBV, Epstein-Barr virus; HLA, human leukocyte antigen; ICAM, intercellular adhesion molecule; LFA, leukocyte function antigen; LPS, lipopolysaccharide; MHC, major histocompatibility complex; N-CAM, nerve cell adhesion molecule; NK, natural killer.

help, and a key molecule in this process is CD40 ligand (also known as CD154) expressed only on activated T cells and providing a class switch signal to B cells through the cell surface molecule, CD40. In the presence of ongoing or repeated exposure to the antigen, those B cells with the highest affinity antibodies for the antigen will be stimulated more than those with a lower affinity, with the result that over time the body produces a higher quality (high-affinity) antibody response. This process is called affinity maturation. Terminal differentiation of the B cells results in the formation of plasma cells that are no longer capable of dividing but are long lived and produce large quantities of the antibody specific to the antigen that originally stimulated their production. In common with all nucleated cells in the body, B cells express class 1 human leukocyte antigens (HLAs) but also large amounts of class 2 HLAs, making them efficient antigen-presenting cells, important in initiating the immune response.

T cells are derived from the thymus gland, are produced in the bone marrow, and migrate to the thymus, where they become "educated" so that those with self-reactive specificity are induced to undergo apoptosis while cells with other specificities receive positive signals. Though the thymus is most active during fetal and early postnatal life, recent evidence suggests that thymopoiesis is important in maintaining circulating T-cell numbers well into the seventh decade of life (7). The T-cell receptor (TCR) comprises an anchoring β_2-microglobulin associated with two chains each with constant portions and highly variable portions, the latter forming the antigen recognition site. In normal health over 90% of T cells in the circulation express the $\alpha\beta$-TCR comprising the α and β chains. The remainder of the T cells express two different chains, γ and δ, which have a different pattern of antigen recognition. The $\gamma\delta$ T cells are thought to be important in certain aspects of gastrointestinal immunity and in responses to a limited range of cell wall products including those expressed on mycobacteria, *Listeria*, and *Escherichia coli* (8,9).

Stimulation of T cells by antigen is through presentation of processed peptides, derived from the antigen, in combination with major histocompatibility antigens. The main antigen-presenting cells are macrophages and dendritic cells, but B cells also have an important role in this respect. Major histocompatibility complex (MHC) class II presentation is particularly important in stimulating helper (CD4) T-cell responses, while CD8 T-cell responses are generally initiated by MHC class I presentation. Expansion of lymphocyte populations depends on stimulation, by cytokines, via cell surface receptors. Interleukin-2 is a good example. After engagement of the receptor, a process of signal transduction involving several intermediary steps results in the signal reaching the nucleus where transcription of relevant genes is induced to cause the cell to proliferate. This is illustrated in Figure 1.6.

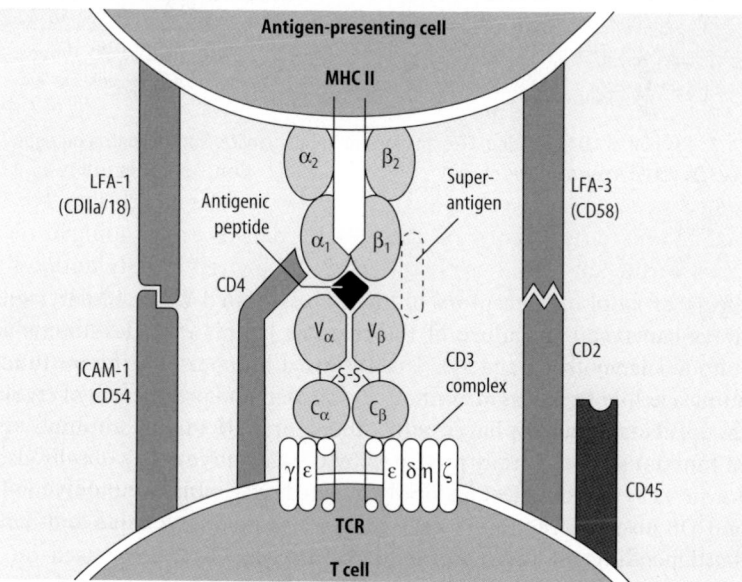

FIGURE 1.6. Signal transduction in lymphocytes. ICAM, intercellular adhesion molecule; LFA, leukocyte function antigen; MHC, major histocompatibility complex; TCR, T-cell receptor. (Reproduced with permission from Cant AJ, et al—see Further Reading.)

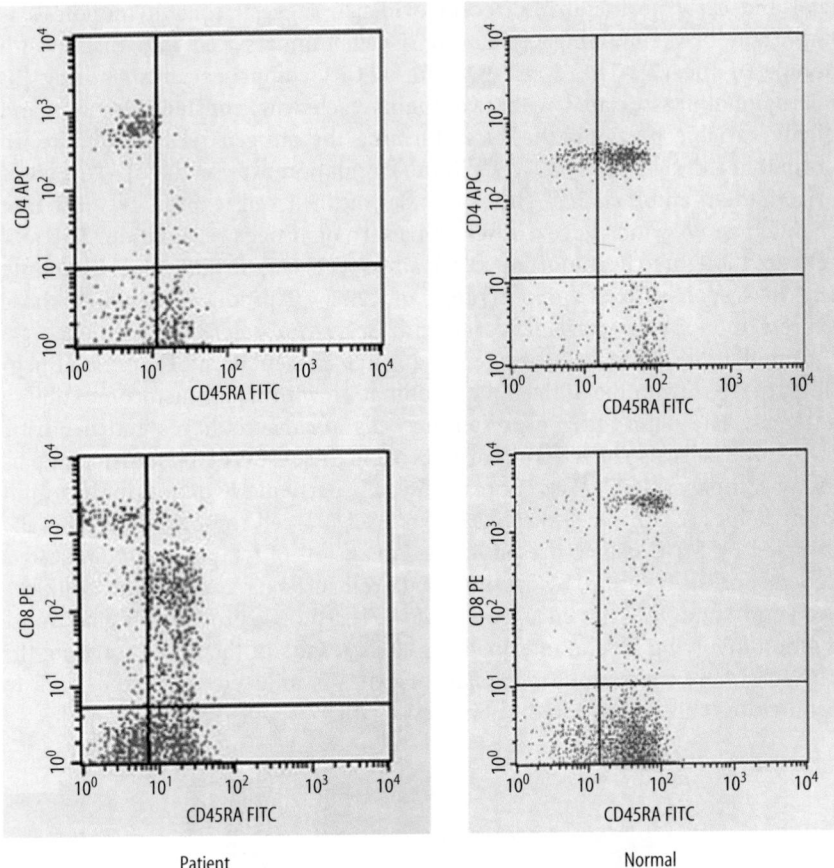

FIGURE 1.7. Fax plot of CD45 staining. FITC, fluorescein isothiocyanate. Normal control on right. Patient with low CD4 CD45RA cell numbers on left.

Defects of cytokine receptors or of the associated intracellular signaling pathways can result in failure of the relevant lymphocyte development and immunodeficiency (see page 33). T cells have a number of different functions including a helper function in antibody responses, and production of cytokines, which upregulate macrophages and other parts of innate immune system (these functions are generally mediated by CD4-positive cells). T cells also can exert a direct cytotoxic effect on virally infected cells, which is mainly mediated by the CD8 positive fraction. T cells can be classified into naive and memory T cells depending on the isoform of the antigen CD45 expressed on their surface. CD45 RA-positive cells are naive cells recently emigrated from the thymus, while CD45 R0 cells have undergone antigen exposure and/or activation (Fig. 1.7).

Developmental Aspects of Immunity

Prenatal

Elements of the adaptive immune system are detectable from as early as 10 weeks' gestation with the appearance of cells capable of responding to mitogens and to foreign histocompatibility antigens.

From early in the second trimester, T cells appear in the circulation, in numbers and subpopulation distribution similar to those found in postnatal life. This can facilitate second-trimester prenatal diagnosis of major immunodeficiency disorders by fetal blood sampling. B cells also appear in the circulation, retaining an immature phenotype until antigen exposure occurs after birth. Immunoglobulin production and B-cell maturation into plasma cells is dependent on this stimulation so that little is produced before birth. Transfer of maternal IgG across the placenta occurs late in pregnancy from around 30 weeks onwards to compensate for this and provide the newborn infant with some passively acquired immunity. This is an active process of transfer, and in full-term infants the levels of IgG often exceed those in the mother. However, even modest degrees of prematurity can result in significant reduction in IgG transfer. The other immunoglobulin isotypes do not cross the placenta. Figure 1.8 illustrates the kinetics of immunoglobulin transfer across the placenta (10).

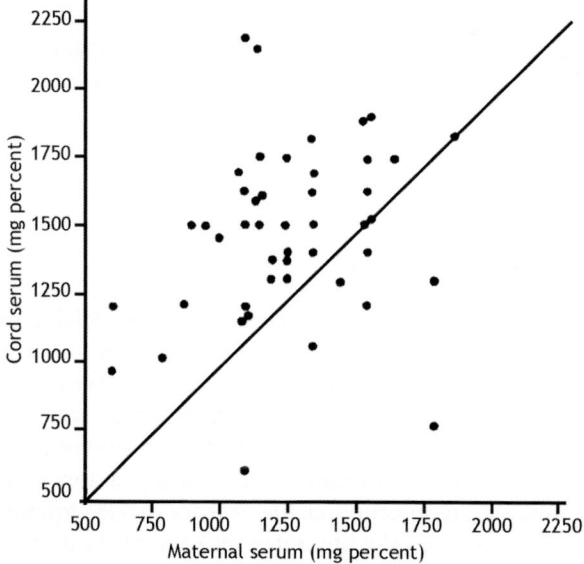

FIGURE 1.8. Immunoglobulin levels during fetal life. (Reproduced with permission from Reference 10.)

Neonatal Immune Status

At birth the neonate has good numbers of T cells, nearly all of which are anti-genically naive and express the RA isoform of CD45. These cells are relatively hyporesponsive to stimuli, resulting in reduced cytotoxic function, production of cytokines, such as interferon-γ, and poor ability to "help" B-cell responses. However, the system is able to respond sufficiently well to prevent opportunistic infections under normal circumstances.

B cells in the neonate are of an immature phenotype with a predominance of cells expressing the antigen CD5, producing polyreactive antibodies against self antigens such as DNA.

Lymph nodes lack germinal centers, but these develop soon after antigen exposure when the B-cell phenotype matures. Initial production of antibody is predominantly IgM and class switching to IgG begins to occur shortly after birth. The delay in class switching is partly due to an intrinsic immaturity in B cells and partly to a lack of T-cell help mediated through a lack of ability of the neonatal T cells to express CD40 ligand.

Though B cells expressing surface IgA are present at birth, development of adult circulating levels of this isotype of immunoglobulin is slow, taking until late childhood/adolescence to reach adult levels (11,12).

The innate system is also immature at birth. Neutrophil numbers increase during labor to normal levels shortly after birth, but bone marrow reserves are low so that in the face of sepsis the neutrophil count will often fall. Neonatal neutrophils show reduced functional capabilities in terms of phagocytosis and bacterial killing for reasons that are poorly understood. Complement levels are also relatively low at birth, being around two thirds of adult levels in a term infant but the significance of this is not known.

Premature delivery, even as early as 24 weeks, does not affect T-cell and B-cell numbers or responsiveness. Maternally transferred IgG, however, is markedly reduced before 33 weeks of gestation. Neutrophil function is further impaired in premature infants compared to full term.

Effect of Intrauterine Infection

When infected in utero the fetus can make some immunologic response, but the pattern of immunologic development may be altered.

Fetal immunoglobulin production is predominantly in the IgM class, though other isotypes can also be produced. Measurement of specific IgM in the newborn, therefore, may be used as a diagnostic tool for congenital infection but is not always produced, for example after congenital toxoplasmosis. Confirmation of intrauterine infection in the absence of IgM production can be achieved using assays of avidity of antitoxoplasma IgG to distinguish maternally transferred antibody from an infant generated response (13).

In the face of congenital infection, T cells are stimulated and a proportion change from the naive CD45RA phenotype to the activated/memory phenotype CD45RO (14).

After Birth

T-cell function, in terms of cytokine production, ability to express CD40 ligand, and cytotoxicity, matures over the early weeks of life. The ability to activate these cells in vitro with antigens and mitogens remains apparently low, but this is probably an artifact due to the fact that a high proportion of circulating T cells are still of the less easily activated naive phenotype. Young infants remain excessively prone to intracellular bacteria such as *Salmonella* spp. and *Mycobacterium tuberculosis*, indicating that immature immune responsiveness carries some clinical significance.

Maturation of B-cell function is slower than that of T cells. The ability to class switch to IgG occurs relatively early allowing, good IgG responses to protein and conjugate vaccine antigens from 2 months of age. The magnitude of the antibody response to tetanus toxoid is inversely related to the level of passively transferred maternal IgG, which means that in general antibody responses are lower the earlier the immunization program is started (15). Nevertheless, protective levels are achieved in the great majority of children immunized at 2, 3, or 4 months, and good immunologic memory is generated. Evidence in relation to hepatitis B vaccination suggests that infants are able to generate better immunologic memory than adults (16).

The ability to make antibodies against polysaccharide antigens develops more slowly. Though immunogenicity varies between different polysaccharides, as a generalization children under 2 years of age do not produce good antipolysaccharide responses. The development of such responses is dependent on the development of the marginal zone of the white pulp of the spleen occurring from around 2 to 3 years of age. The characteristic cells populating this zone (marginal zone B cells, MZBs) make up 20% to 30% of the B cells in the spleen, expressing IgM, IgD, and CD27, and high levels of CD21, the CR2 complement receptor. They are found exclusively in the circulation for the first 2 years of life (17).

Conjugation of certain polysaccharides to proteins or peptides, such as tetanus toxoid, can overcome this immaturity in responsiveness, resulting in protective antibodies to the polysaccharide component. One of the best examples of this is the conjugation of the capsular polysaccharide polyribosyl ribitol phosphate (PRP) of *Haemophilus influenzae* type b to produce the conjugate Hib vaccine, which is immunogenic from 2 months of age, enabling protective antibodies to be produced against the polysaccharide component from this age. Following its introduction to the infant vaccination schedule in the United Kingdom in 1992, meningitis caused by Hib fell from being the commonest cause of bacterial meningitis to being a rare disease. However, one study indicates that after a 2-, 3-, or 4-month schedule, antibody levels to conjugate vaccines are poorly sustained (18). Though immunologic memory results in good booster antibody responses, on subsequent exposure in some cases this may not occur quickly enough to prevent disease, and this is probably the basis of the Hib vaccine failures seen in the U.K. in recent years (19). The newly introduced (in the U.K.) booster dose of vaccine from the first birthday onward is likely to overcome this problem by inducing a more sustained antibody response. In the case of long incubation period infections, such as hepatitis B, the immunologic memory generated by infant vaccination is sufficient for long-term protection even if antibody levels wane, since the incubation period is sufficiently long to allow time for a booster response before disease occurs.

Similar developments have occurred with meningococcal C conjugate vaccine and conjugate pneumococcal vaccines. The problem with the latter organism is that there are multiple (about 80) disease-causing serotypes, each with its own capsular polysaccharide. Vaccine development has therefore depended on making multivalent polysaccharide vaccines covering the most common serotypes. The vaccine currently licensed in the U.K. is a seven valent, while nine- and 11-valent vaccines are being developed. The seven-valent vaccine covers about 80% of the disease-causing serotypes in Western countries, including those serotypes in which penicillin resistance is most commonly found. The higher valency vaccines also include serotypes found in poor countries. Seven-valent pneumococcal conjugate vaccine has recently been introduced in the UK to the routine infant schedule.

Another example of a physiologic delay in maturation of antibody response is that to *Moraxella catarrhalis*, a cause of sinopulmonary infections. Reliable specific antibody responses are not seen before 4 years of age despite the fact that the antibody is not directed against a polysaccharide antigen (20).

These observations go a long way to explaining why infants and young children are excessively susceptible to invasive bacterial disease particularly with polysaccharide encapsulated organisms.

Delayed Maturation of Immunity

Over and above the normal physiologic delay in development of immune mechanisms, a significant proportion of children suffer an additional delay in maturation of their immune responses. This can be seen particularly in the humoral immune system. In its most marked form there may be pan-hypogammaglobulinemia in the early years of life (transient hypogammaglobulinemia of infancy), but more frequently there is a delayed maturation in the ability to produce IgA and/or IgG2 subclass antibodies.

Transient Hypogammaglobulinemia of Infancy

In its full-blown form this is a relatively rare disorder. The underlying basis of the condition is poorly understood. Affected infants may be found incidentally with very low immunoglobulins or may be investigated because of a susceptibility to infections, usually of a relatively minor nature. Measurement of immunoglobulins in the blood shows low levels of immunoglobulins usually affecting all three of the major classes (21). The differential diagnosis may be x-linked agammaglobulinemia (see page 24), but enumeration of lymphocyte subsets shows normal circulating numbers of B cells, which excludes this diagnosis. Measurement of specific functional antibodies against vaccine antigens such as tetanus and Hib will often show normal responses, which is taken as a good prognostic sign and probably explains why affected children, even though they have profound hypogammaglobulinemia, suffer few infections and usually only those of a relatively minor nature. The name of this condition is misleading in that the hypogammaglobulinemia may persist beyond infancy for the first 2 to 3 years of life.

Other Forms of Delayed Humoral Maturation

The development of the IgA system in children is the slowest part of humoral immune development. Some children suffer an additional delay, with IgA levels not catching up to the normal range until 5 to 6 years of age. These children may present with recurrent respiratory tract and ear infections in early childhood, but serious invasive bacterial disease is uncommon. Typically, the IgG and IgM levels are found to be normal and the IgA level is low. Usually this is not a complete deficiency of IgA, and the level lies above the limit of detection (0.05 g/L) but below the age-related normal range. Roberton et al. (22) showed that in young children partial deficiency of IgA resolved in 80% of cases at 3-year follow-up, while complete IgA deficiency (less than 0.05 g/L) resolved in only 20% of cases. The former group of patients was more likely to have symptoms of recurrent infections than the latter. This finding suggests that the absolute level of IgA is not the crucial factor, but rather that the low level of IgA is a marker of generally immature humoral immune responses. Further investigation of this group of children will often reveal normal responses to Hib and tetanus vaccination but poor responses to polysaccharide vaccine immunization (for example, pneumococcal polysaccharide vaccine, Pneumovax) beyond the normal physiologic delay in the development of such responsiveness.

Immunodeficiency

Deficiencies of the immune system, which may be primary or secondary, result in an increased susceptibility to infection and are overrepresented in the population of children who require admission to intensive care units.

Significant primary (genetic) immunodeficiency disorders, excluding IgA deficiency, occur with an incidence of around 1 in 10,000 in Western populations (23,24). In populations where consanguinity is common, the incidence is much higher. As these are chronic conditions, the prevalence will be much higher. The molecular basis of many of the primary immunodeficiencies has now been elucidated and knowledge of the genes involved, and the mutations in those genes allows precise diagnosis, genetic counseling, and prenatal diagnosis. It has become clear that different mutations in the same gene may sometimes lead to different phenotypic variants of the disorder, sometimes, but not always, associated with preservation of some partial function of the gene.

For convenience, immune defenses can be classified into an innate system of resistance including humoral factors (such as the complement system) and cells (phagocytic and NK cells) and adaptive (T cell and antibody mediated) immunity in which immunologic memory develops. In practice, the two systems interact very closely.

Immunologic Function Tests: General Principles

Complex or unusual immunologic tests are always best performed after discussion with the laboratory. Lymphocyte subset analysis and functional tests and neutrophil function tests all have to be done on fresh blood. In all but exceptional circumstances, this should be on the day of venesection. While some proteins, such as immunoglobulins, are very stable in serum, others, such as some of the complement factors, are labile, and samples for testing need to be processed in the laboratory within 1 or 2 hours of the blood being collected. Administration of blood products to the patient will make interpretation of immunoglobulin and antibody measurements almost impossible for several weeks (the half-life of IgG is 21 days). It is therefore a good practice to collect and store a serum sample before administration of any of these products. In the case of white cell tests, this is less critical, particularly if the blood will be irradiated and filtered (as is good practice when immunodeficiency is suspected). Some of the commonly used tests for diagnosing immunodeficiency are tabulated in the relevant sections below.

Primary Disorders of the Innate Immune System

Complement Disorders

Deficiency of mannan-binding lectin is a common primary disorder predisposing to a broad range of infections. Deficiencies in the classic and alternate pathway components of the complement system are usually secondary or acquired as part of an inflammatory/infective processes. Primary deficiencies of individual components leading to excess infection susceptibility are rare but have been described for all the known components (25). Tests for deficiencies of the complement system are summarized in Table 1.2. These disorders are mostly inherited in an autosomal recessive fashion apart from properdin deficiency (X linked) and C1 inhibitor deficiency (autosomal dominant). Apart from C1 inhibitor deficiency they all lead to an excess susceptibility to infection. In addition to predisposing to an increased susceptibility to infection, many of these disorders can result in an increased susceptibility to the development of autoimmune disease such as atypical forms of systemic lupus erythematosus. Complement disorders can be classified into a number of groupings:

Early classical component deficiencies involve C1 QR and S, C2, and C4, and result in a predisposition to a broad variety of pyogenic bacterial infections.

TABLE **1.2.** Tests for complement disorders

Test	Type of test	Conditions tested for	Comments
C3, C4	Nephelometry	Low levels of C3 and C4 nearly always secondary to consumption due to renal or inflammatory disease	
Classical pathway components C 1 to C9	CH100 red cell lysis test involving sheep red cells sensitized with human antibody and incubated with test serum as a source of complement	Genetic defects of one of the complement cascade protein	May be low in consumptive hypocomplementemia
Complement alternative pathway	AP50 measures integrity of alternate pathway complement cascade in the absence of specific antibody	Genetic deficiencies of alternative pathway components	Falsely low results may result from secondary hypocomplementemia
Individual specific component measurements	ELISA or other serologic detection method	Individual complement component deficiencies	Only available in highly specialized laboratories if CH100 or AP50 screening tests are abnormal
C1 inhibitor assay	ELISA for detection of protein and functional assay	Hereditary angioedema; type 1 (low protein) and type 2 (functionally abnormal protein)	
Mannan binding Lectin	ELISA for measurement of levels; genotyping for the genetic polymorphisms associated with low levels	Mannan-binding lectin deficiency	

ELISA, enzyme-linked immunosorbent assay.

Affected individuals may suffer an excess of sinopulmonary infections as well as serious deep-seated life-threatening infections. C4 deficiency is usually secondary to consumption occurring in inflammation/infectious disorders or C1 inhibitor deficiency.

Alternative pathway component defects involve factors B, D, I, and H, as well as properdin, and all result in a greatly increased susceptibility to a broad variety of bacterial infections. In properdin deficiency there is a particular susceptibility to meningococcal disease.

C3 deficiency is mostly found as a secondary phenomenon in patients with nephritis or other autoimmune disease. Genetic defects affecting C3 production are extremely rare. As predicted from its central role in the complement system, affected individuals are profoundly immunodeficient, suffering a variety of pyogenic bacterial infections including pneumococcal and staphylococcal disease.

Late terminal complement component deficiencies involve factors C5 to C9 and result in impaired lysis of bacteria that have been opsonized with C3. This is particularly important in the handling of neisserial species (26). Deficiencies are relatively common in certain populations such as Japanese (C6 and C9), African Americans (C6), and Sephardic Jews (C7). There is a predisposition to meningococcal disease and to gonococcal disease. In the former there is a pre-dominance of rare serogroups such as W135, X, and Y (27). The increased sus-ceptibility to infection with C9 deficiency is relatively mild since this component is not essential for complement-mediated lysis.

Low levels of *mannan-binding lectin (MBL)* in the blood result in an increased susceptibly to a variety of different infections. These result from either struc-tural allelic variants or polymorphisms in the gene promoter or a combination of both. Very low levels of the lectin are found in approximately 5% of the general population. It is believed that this deficiency is particularly relevant to infection susceptibility in children under the age of 4 years whose humoral immune systemic will not have reached their full maturity. This has been reviewed recently (28). Other recent studies have shown that individuals with MBL deficiency are overrepresented among pediatric intensive care patients with systemic inflammatory response syndrome (SIRS) (29). Similarly, an excess of infections associated with chemotherapy-induced neutropenia was found in patients with MBL deficiency among a series of patients being treated for leukemia (30). Deficiency of MBL has also been associated with susceptibility to meningococcal disease (31).

Secondary Complement Deficiency

Deficiency of complement is most commonly encountered in an acquired form. C3 and C4 consumption occurs in sepsis and autoimmune/inflammatory condi-tions including glomerulonephritis. Such deficiency may contribute to infection susceptibility in seriously ill children.

Management of Complement Disorders Leading to Excess Infections

Children identified with complement disorders require long-term prophylaxis with antibiotics. Penicillin is the treatment of choice for the terminal component deficiencies, but for early component and severe MBL deficiency a broader spectrum agent such as a macrolide should be used. Immunity to meningococcus should be maximized through immunization with meningococcal C conjugate vaccine and then quadrivalent (A, C, Y, W135) meningococcal polysaccharide vaccine. When a quadrivalent conjugate vaccine becomes available, this should be used in preference. Pneumococcal conjugate vaccine followed by polysaccharide vaccines should be also be given. Transfusion of fresh frozen plasma provides complement factors in seriously ill children. Recombinant and purified human MBL preparations are under development and may have a role in treating severe deficiency in the future.

Deficiencies of Cytokines and Their Receptors

These deficiencies of innate immunity can affect all aspects of immune function (32). Some defects lead to deficiency of the specific adaptive system through effects on lymphoid development. For example, deficiency of the common γ chain forms part of a number of different interleukin receptors and results in deficiency of lymphocyte development, leading to severe combined immunodeficiency (see page 30). Defects of the interferon-γ/interleukin-12 system (illustrated in Fig. 1.3) result in a profound defect of cell-mediated immunity to mycobacteria (including environmental mycobacteria and bacille Calmette-Guérin [BCG]) as well as other intracellular pathogens such as *Salmonella* species.

Defects in Cellular Signaling Through Toll-Like Receptors

The toll-like receptors (TLR) on cells of the myeloid system recognize bacterial and viral components directly resulting in cellular activation and production of proinflammatory cytokines including tumour necrosis factor-α, interleukin-1 (IL-1), IL-6 as well as interferon-α and -γ. There are 10 different TLRs in humans recognizing different microbial components with some overlap. Polymorphisms in molecules involved in TLR signalling can be associated with an increased susceptibility to infection for example tuberculous meningitis (33). Mendelian defects in signaling pathways are also described including defects of IL-1 receptor–associated kinase 4 (IRAK4), resulting in an increased susceptibility to pyogenic bacterial infections (34) (see Fig. 1.4, page 4). The common final signaling molecule in many of these pathways is nuclear factor (NF) κB. Defects of signalling through this molecule have also been described, resulting in immunodeficiency. The most common of these defects affects nuclear factor essential modulator (NEMO), resulting in X-linked anhidrotic ectodermal dysplasia with immunodeficiency. Affected boys have a variable form of immunodeficiency often with a hyper IgM type picture (see below) and poor responses to polysaccharide encapsulated bacteria such as pneumococcus. Some carrier mothers suffer from incontinentia pigmenti. Defects of Toll-like receptor signaling have recently been reviewed (4).

Neutrophil Disorders

Neutropenia

A circulating neutrophil count below the normal range is most commonly found as a secondary effect of myelosuppressive influences such as drugs or radiation. This may be non–dose-related or idiosyncratic, often involving a form of hypersensitivity, as occurs when a drug induces myelosuppression in a non–dose-related fashion.

The mechanism in these cases is often one of hypersensitivity, for example to chloramphenicol or flucloxacillin. Dose-related myelosuppression occurs as a result of chemotherapeutic treatments and is usually present for a finite time before the marrow recovers. Secondary neutropenia may also occur when consumption/destruction of neutrophils exceeds production. This occurs as a result of sepsis in the neonatal period (where bone marrow reserves are low) and can occur at any age as a result of hypersplenism or as a consequence of an autoimmune process directed against the neutrophils. Primary neutropenias are much rarer and include severe congenital neutropenia, cyclical neutropenia, and multisystem syndromes in which bone marrow disturbance forms a part, such as Schwachman-Diamond syndrome (35).

Severe Congenital Neutropenia

In this condition there is an arrest in early myeloid differentiation, resulting in an absence of neutrophils and myelocytes. Both autosomal recessive and autosomal dominant forms of this condition are seen. The autosomal dominant form is associated with mutations in the gene-encoding neutrophil elastase (36). Similar mutations can also result in autosomal dominant cyclical neutropenia. The gene for the most common recessive form (Kostmann's syndrome) has recently been identified (37). Typically a child with congenital neutropenia presents in early life with recurrent infections of mucous membranes and skin, which may be accompanied by deep-seated invasive infections. Most frequently these are caused by *Staphylococcus aureus*, but other common pathogens include *Pseudomonas aeruginosa*, other gram-negative enteric bacilli, and fungi including *Candida* and *Aspergillus* species.

Cyclical Neutropenia

This is a familial condition usually inherited in an autosomal dominant fashion. Mutations in the gene encoding neutrophil elastase can be found in a majority (but not all) affected individuals (36). It is not understood why similar mutations in the same gene can result in a much more severe congenital neutropenia or in the more benign form of cyclical neutropenia. Affected individuals suffer periodic bouts of illness, often with mouth ulcers, fevers, and malaise; the bouts last for a few days only to recur in a regular cyclic fashion usually with a periodicity of 3 to 4 weeks. There is often a family history of one or other parent affected by similar symptoms.

Shwachman-Diamond Syndrome–Associated Neutropenia

This is a rare autosomal recessive condition. Skeletal abnormalities are associated with pancreatic exocrine insufficiency and bone marrow abnormalities leading to neutropenia, which can progress to aplastic anemia or to myeloid leukemia.

Investigation of Neutropenia

Further investigation is merited in those cases where a careful history does not reveal a cause of the problem. A bone marrow aspirate may reveal hypoplasia of the myeloid series or an arrest in myeloid maturation. Cytogenetic studies should also be performed since preleukemia or leukemia may complicate some of these disorders. In the consumptive form of neutropenia the marrow will be hypercellular in the myeloid series, while in cyclical neutropenia the appearances vary according to the stage of the cycle. The diagnosis of cyclical neutropenia can be confirmed by taking sequential blood counts twice a week for a period of 8 weeks and looking for evidence of cycling. In autoimmune neutropenia, antineutrophil antibodies can usually be detected by testing the serum against panels of neutrophils expressing known neutrophil specific antigens.

Treatment of Neutropenic Disorders

Careful attention to mouth hygiene and the prophylactic use of antifungal agents are helpful in all forms of neutropenia. In drug-induced neutropenia where the low counts are expected to be relatively short-lived, treatment should be expectant. Injections of granulocyte colony-stimulating factor (G-CSF) will shorten the period of neutropenia by accelerating myelopoiesis.

Granulocyte colony-stimulating factor is also useful in cases of primary neutropenia. Even in severe congenital neutropenia some cases will respond to high doses of this cytokine. In cyclical neutropenia, G-CSF works by shortening cycling time so that, although dips in the counts still occur, the period of neutropenia is reduced (38).

Most cases of autoimmune neutropenia in childhood run a benign course and are often self-limiting. In exceptional cases therapeutic interventions are necessary and these may include G-CSF injections or treatment with corticosteroids (39).

Neutrophil Function Disorders

Deficiency of neutrophil function is mostly found in patients with primary genetic defects. Occasional acquired neutrophil dysfunction can be found mainly in the adult population (e.g., acquired myeloperoxidase deficiency).

TABLE 1.3. Neutrophil function tests

Test	Type of test	Condition being tested for	Comments
Neutrophil adhesion markers	FACS analysis for CD11 and CD18	Leukocyte adhesion deficiency, type 1	
NBT test	Reduction of NBT on a slide and manual counting of numbers of cells showing reduction of the NBT*	Chronic granulomatous disease	Normal tests shows that all the cells reduced the NBT; a negative NBT test is therefore an abnormal finding
Oxidative burst	Measurement of reduction of dihydrorhodamine by neutrophil oxidative burst	CGD and other bacterial-killing defects	Alternative to NBT test
Neutrophil phagocytosis	Uptake of fluorescent label bacteria or zymosam granules analyzed by FACS	Defects of phagocytosis	See Fig 1.9
Neutrophil mobility	Measurement of distance migrated by neutrophil in response to a chemotactic stimulus	Defects of neutrophil migration	Tests relatively poorly reproducible

CGD, chronic granulomatous disease; FACS, fluorescence-activated cell sorting; NBT, nitroblue tetrazolium.
*See Figure 1.10.

Neutrophil handling of microbes involves a series of steps—chemotaxis, adherence, phagocytosis, and bacterial killing—and defects may occur at any stage. Tests for these aspects of neutrophil function are summarized in Table 1.3.

Defects of Neutrophil Chemotaxis/Adhesion: Leukocyte Adhesion Deficiency

Migration of neutrophils to the site of infection involves expression of a series of surface molecules (ligands) to enable the cells to egress from the circulation by a process of diapedesis. This process has been well described elsewhere (40). Briefly, the initial steps involve expression of selectins on the neutrophils and their receptors on vascular endothelium. "Loose" (low-affinity) attraction between these ligand/receptor pairs causes neutrophils to slow down in the circulation by a process of "rolling" adherence, along the endothelium. At sites of inflammation and infection, chemokine and cytokine signaling causes further activation of the neutrophil and endothelial cell, resulting in downregulation of selectin expression and upregulation of adherence molecules (β-integrins) on the neutrophils and their receptors on the endothelium. There are a whole series of these molecules (41), but the most important are leukocyte function antigen-1 (LFA-1), which is made up of two chains, CD18 and CD11. Upregulation and activation (involving steric change) in this molecule facilitate "tight" binding of neutrophils to activated vascular endothelial through the receptor for LFA-1 known as intercellular adhesion molecule-1 (ICAM-1). Through this mechanism neutrophils in the circulation come to a complete standstill, bound to the endothelium, and are then able to egress from the circulation into the tissues.

The best defined defect of this system is leukocyte adhesion deficiency type 1 (LAD-1). Mutations in the gene for CD18 result in absence or lack of functional protein, in turn resulting in a syndrome of excessive susceptibility to pyogenic infection associated with poor pus formation at sites of infection (due to failure of cells to egress from the circulation). This is also known as Job's syndrome. There is also a defect in lymphocyte-mediated cytotoxicity (which also involves LFA-1). This is usually less clinically significant, though a recent series of reports describe severe polyoma virus infections in patients treated with anti–LFA-1 for multiple sclerosis or Crohn's disease (42), suggesting a role for this molecule in cell-mediated immune mechanisms for control of this viral infection. Affected children with full-blown deficiency present with delayed separation of the umbilical cord (since separation of the cord is dependent on migration of neutrophils). There is an excess susceptibility to bacterial and fungal infections and a high mortality in early life in the full-blown form. In partial forms there is no problem with umbilical cord separation and a lower susceptibility to infection. However, inflammatory skin and gastrointestinal lesions can occur in these partial cases, which is not primarily infective and may be responsive to corticosteroid treatment (43).

Children with complete and some with partial forms of the disorder require bone marrow transplantation. Other forms of LAD have been described but are extremely rare, and detailed description is beyond the scope of this book. They involve either general abnormalities of β-integrin expression (which affect platelet as well as neutrophil function—LAD-3) or defects of selectins (LAD-2). LAD type 2 is associated with multisystem defects including brain development, and the defect lies in fucosylation of selectins as well as other molecules important in brain development (44).

Defects of Phagocytosis

Poor ability to phagocytose bacteria is a feature of neutrophils in newborn infants and may form part of genetic syndromes such as RAC-2 deficiency (45). They may also be seen as part of ill-defined syndromes of susceptibility to bacterial and fungal infections. Phagocytosis can be measured by incubating neutrophils with fluorescent-labeled bacteria in the presence of serum. After washing and quenching of remaining extracellular fluorescence (with trypan blue), the internalized fluorescence can be measured in a flow cytometer (Fig. 1.9). Susceptibility to bacterial infections, particularly *S. aureus* and fungal species, is the main clinical feature.

Defects of Microbial Killing: Chronic Granulomatous Disease

Defective killing of phagocytosed organisms can lead to serious deep-seated infections. The best characterized of these disorders is chronic granulomatous

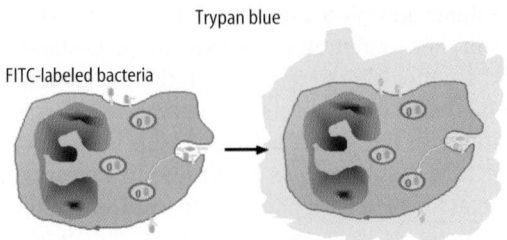

FIGURE 1.9. Methodology of phagocytosis assay. FITC, fluorescein isothiocyanate. For method see text (page 21).

disease (CGD), in which there is a defect in the reduced nicotinamide adenine dinucleotide phosphate (NADPH) oxidase system. There are four glycopeptide (gp) photo oxidase (phox) components to this enzyme system; gp91 phox is the major component and is coded on the X chromosome. Defects in this gene account for around two thirds of CGD cases. The remaining third is made up of gene defects in the other phox components (gp67, gp47, gp22), and are inherited as autosomal recessive traits.

Deep-seated bacterial and fungal infections can occur and include suppurative lymphadenitis, liver abscesses, pneumonia, osteomyelitis, and perianal abscesses. The predominating causative organisms are catalase positive (catalase being an enzyme that helps the organism inactivate hydrogen peroxide produced in the phagolysosome). Examples include *S. aureus*, *Serratia marcescens*, *Burkholderia cepacia*, and *Aspergillus* spp. (46). Infection with the last of these is particularly difficult to treat in these patients.

Noninfective granulomatous complications also occur in CGD. These affect the gastrointestinal (GI) tract, genitourinary (GU) tract (causing urinary obstruction), lungs, and skin. A noninfective colitis is the commonest of these and can mimic Crohn's disease. Corticosteroid treatment is very effective against these granulomatous complications but does increase the risk of infections.

Diagnosis of CGD can be made by using a simple nitroblue tetrazolium (NBT) slide test. Normal neutrophils when activated with phorbol myristate acetate and incubated with NBT take up the dye and reduce it to a brown/black deposit, which can be seen by light microscopy. Neutrophils from CGD patients cannot reduce the NBT and so no deposits are seen, while in the mother of boys with the X-linked form of the disease approximately 50% of the cells (depending on lyonization) show this deposit (Fig. 1.10).

Other microbicidal defects have also been described. Myeloperoxidase (MPO) deficiency is the commonest of these, affecting 1 in 2000 individuals and resulting in a mild excess of infections. Much rarer defects include deficiencies of glucose-6-phosphate dehydrogenase (G-6-PD) (mostly the G-6-PD deficiency affecting red cells is partial and does not affect neutrophil function), glutathione synthetase, glutathione reductase, pyruvate kinase, and transcobalamin 2.

Treatment of Neutrophil Function Disorders

Prophylactic treatment for neutrophil function disorders includes attention to mouth and skin hygiene, antifungal prophylaxis, and judicious use of antibiotic prophylaxis. In CGD, cotrimoxazole is used because it exhibits good cell penetration, and itraconazole because it has good activity against *Aspergillus* species. Corticosteroid treatment is very effective against noninfective granulomatous complications but does increase the risk of infections. Granulocyte colony-stimulating factor treatment and any other cytokines such as interferon-γ may be used as adjunctive treatment for episodes of severe infection such as deep abscesses. White cell infusions have also been used to treat infection or prophylactically at the time of bone marrow transplantation. Sources of white cells include single-donor volunteers recruited through the blood transfusion services, volunteer family members, or close family friends. Priming with G-CSF and dexamethasone produces a yield of neutrophils 10-fold higher and, in order to get a significant dose of white cells, is the only realistic approach in patients weighing more than 30 kg. Currently in the U.K., guidelines produced by the National Blood Service limit the use of G-CSF to family members and friends (47). This policy differs from those in other European countries and is under review.

In the more severe neutrophil function disorders, bone marrow transplantation offers the best hope for long-term survival. In the case of CGD it is usually offered to all patients who have matched sibling donors and to other patients if they develop complications. Gene therapy trials are underway for CGD.

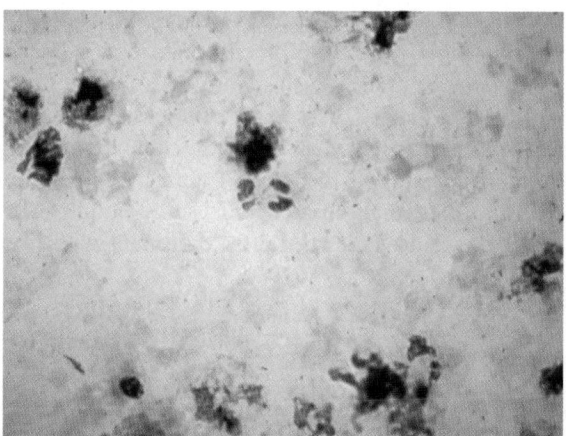

FIGURE 1.10. Nitroblue tetrazolium (NBT) reduction. Note black deposit in neutrophils in a normal individual. This is absent in chronic granulomatous disease.

Deficiencies of the Specific Adaptive Immune System

Antibody Deficiency Syndromes

Deficiency of antibody production may be a primary (genetic) or secondary. Primary deficiency may be due to an intrinsic defect in the B cells, a deficiency in T-cell help for antibody production, or a combination of both. The major primary disorders resulting in antibody deficiency are listed in Table 1.4.

Clinical Presentation

A history of recurrent bacterial infections is the hallmark of the child with antibody deficiency. Typically these infections affect the chest, sinuses, and ears (sinopulmonary infections), but other bacterial infections may include meningitis and septic arthritis/osteomyelitis (48). A variety of different bacterial pathogens may be involved, but polysaccharide-encapsulated organisms, particularly pneumococci, predominate. Most of these infections respond to oral antibiotic treatment and, as the tendency to excessive infections overlaps with the normal physiologic immunodeficiency of early childhood, the diagnosis of antibody deficiency is often delayed (49). Such delay with repeated infections in untreated individuals can lead to organ damage, particularly bronchiectasis (50).

Antibody deficiency can also present with GI symptoms, which may include chronic diarrhea and malabsorption due to *Giardia lamblia* infection, other GI infections, or celiac disease, which is more common in IgA-deficient individuals than in the general population. The role of antibody in defenses against the protozoan *G. lamblia* and the susceptibility of antibody-deficient patients to this organism are poorly understood.

Immunity to viruses is also abnormal in antibody-deficient individuals. While recovery from most virus infections is normal, as it is dependent on T-cell immunity, repeated attacks with the same virus may occur in the absence of protective antibody. In some cases, such as infections with the enterovirus group including Coxsackie and enterocytopathogenic human orphan (ECHO) viruses, there may be failure to control the infection, resulting in chronic viral infection syndromes, including chronic encephalomyelitis or dermatomyositis (48), and this can occur even after treatment with immunoglobulin replacement (51).

Specific Forms of Antibody Deficiency (Table 1.4)

X-linked agammaglobulinemia (Bruton's disease) and the other much rarer forms of B-cell developmental defects (52) are the purest forms of antibody deficiency with no associated defect of cell-mediated immunity.

Common variable immunodeficiency (CVID) is the commonest form of hypogammaglobulinemia. Onset of the disease may be at any time, but most

TABLE 1.4. Major primary antibody deficiency disorders

Diagnosis	Gene encodes	Inheritance	B cells	Immunoglobulins	Cell-mediated immunodeficiency	Clinical features
X-linked agammaglobulinemia (XLA)	Bruton's tyrosine kinase (BTK)	X-linked	Absent	Typically a panhypo-gammaglobulinemia; occasional partial deficiencies are seen	Normal	Recurrent bacterial infections, giardiasis, chronic enteroviral infections
Common variable immunodeficiency (CVID)	Mostly not known; multiple different genetic causes; gene defect identified in around 10% of cases (54)	Unknown or autosomal recessive, occasionally dominant	Usually present	Deficiency of IgG and IgA plus variable deficiency of IgM	Normal in most cases; some have a variable degree of cell-mediated immune deficiency	Recurrent bacterial infections, enteropathy, giardiasis autoimmune disease *Helicobacter* infection
Autosomal recessive hyper-IgM syndrome	AID, UNG, CD40	Autosomal recessive	Present	Absent IgG and IgA normal or raised IgM	Normal except in CD40 deficiency which behaves like X-linked hyper-IgM syndrome	Recurrent bacterial infections, persistent lymphadenopathy
X-Linked hyper-IgM syndrome	CD40 ligand	X-linked	Present	Absent IgG and IgA, normal or raised IgM	Deficient killing of intracellular organisms by macrophages	Recurrent bacterial infections, *Pneumocystis* pneumonia, tuberculosis cryptosporidiosis
Selective IgA deficiency	Unknown	Usually sporadic, may be autosomal dominant or recessive	Present	Normal IgG and IgM, absent IgA	Normal	Recurrent bacterial infections, recurrent gastrointestinal infections, celiac disease
Defective antipolysaccharide responses	Unknown	Unknown	Present	Immunoglobulin normal but deficient responses to polysaccharides	Normal	Recurrent bacterial infections, invasive pneumococcal sepsis

AID, activation induced cytidine deaminase; Ig, immunoglobulin; UNG, Uracil-N-glycosylase.

commonly it is in the second decade of life (53). Common variable immuno-deficiency includes a number of different defects, resulting in a common clinical pattern. Some of these, affecting lymphocyte function, have recently been defined (54). Some of the defects also affect T-cell function, resulting in a broader infection susceptibility to include opportunistic pathogens and a tendency to autoimmune phenomena.

The hyper-IgM syndromes result from molecular defects that affect the ability to class switch during immunoglobulin production. A number of different genetic defects have been associated with this picture (55). X-linked hyper-IgM syndrome is the best characterized and is caused by mutations in the gene for CD40 ligand. In addition to the immunoglobulin class-switching defect, there is defective cell-mediated immunity through the inability of T cells to ligate CD40 on effector cells, particularly macrophages. The much rarer CD40 deficiency is clinically similar, while the other autosomal defects result in a pure humoral immunodeficiency.

IgA deficiency is by far the commonest primary immunodeficiency defect, affecting around 1 in 500 of the population. Most individuals are asymptomatic, but some have an excess of sinopulmonary infections, and there is an increased incidence of celiac disease and other autoimmune disorders. In early childhood, IgA deficiency, often partial, is even more common due to a maturational delay in IgA production as described earlier in this chapter (page 13).

Investigation of Antibody Deficiency (Table 1.5)

Investigation should involve measurement of immunoglobulins. It is important to remember that the immunoglobulin levels will be affected by the administration of blood products. Therefore, it is a good principle to collect a serum sample before administration of blood products for assay. Immunoglobulins are measured routinely in most biochemistry laboratories, and an appropriate pediatric reference range should be used. Interpretation of results in newborn infants and particularly in premature infants is sometimes difficult and may need expert opinion. In addition to measuring total immunoglobulin levels, in children who have been appropriately immunized, measurement of antibodies against vaccine antigens such as Hib, tetanus, and diphtheria antigens is helpful. If these are low, then booster doses can be given and repeat levels taken 3 to 4 weeks later. Measurement of antibodies against polysaccharide antigens such as pneumococcal capsular polysaccharides is a useful test of humoral immunity in older children. In children younger than 2 years of age, there is naturally poor responsiveness to many of the pneumococcal polysaccharides, so that the test is not useful in distinguishing between normal and abnormal individuals. Where low pneumococcal antibody levels are found, an immunization with the polysaccharide pneumococcal vaccine, Pneumovax, followed by repeat antibody measurements will be useful. Measurement of IgG subclasses is generally not considered useful in the diagnosis of humoral immunodeficiency unless a very rare deletion in the immunoglobulin constant region genes is suspected.

TABLE 1.5. Investigation of antibody deficiency

Test	Type of test	Conditions tested for	Comments
Immunoglobulins	Nephelometry (automated) or single radial diffusion (for very low levels)	Hypogammaglobulinemia, IgA deficiency	Important to use appropriate age related normal ranges
IgG subclasses	ELISA	IgG subclass deficiencies	Poor correlation of abnormalities with infection susceptibility
Specific antibodies against protein antigens	ELISA to look at antibody to tetanus or diphtheria antigens	Defects of functional antibody production	If low levels are found, the patient should be vaccinated and then retested after 4 weeks
Polysaccharide antibody assays	Measurement of antipneumococcal antibodies to either: 1. 23 different polysaccharides in *Pneumovax* by ELISA 2. Individual pneumococcal serotypes (ELISA)	Defect of polysaccharide antibody responses	Need measurements before and after *Pneumovax* to confirm poor responses
IgE levels	Radioimmunoassay	Allergic disorders; hyper-IgE syndrome	

In addition to measuring antibodies and immunoglobulins, it is important to look at lymphocyte markers to help in the diagnosis. The enumeration of circulating B cells helps classify the type of immunoglobulin deficiency syndrome (see Table 1.5), while enumeration of T-cell numbers and T-cell function (through mitogen responsiveness) helps determine whether this is a pure humoral immunodeficiency or a combined immunodeficiency.

Complications

The most important complications result from delayed diagnosis or inadequate treatment and can lead to the development of bronchiectasis or chronic sinusitis (Fig. 1.11). Life-threatening septicemia or meningitis is rare once the diagnosis has been made and replacement immunoglobulin therapy commenced. Chronic enteroviral infections causing chronic meningoencephalitis or dermatomyositis are rare but very serious complications that are difficult to treat.

Noninfective inflammatory complications are seen mainly in CVID and include inflammatory problems such as granulomatous disease most frequently affecting the lungs, intestine, liver, and lymphoid systems (56). Autoimmune

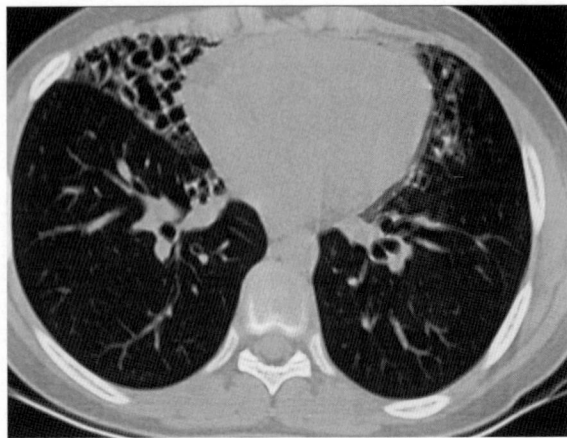

FIGURE 1.11. Chest computed tomography (CT) scan showing bronchiectasis affecting right middle and lingular lobes in an immunoglobulin-deficient child. (Reproduced with permission from Davies EG. Impaired Immunity in Children. Current Paediatrics 2006;16:16–28.)

disease is another noninfective complication found in CVID and in IgA deficiency. Most commonly it affects the hematologic system and results in cytopenias. These problems may occasionally predate the onset of infections and the diagnosis of immunodeficiency.

Treatment

In children with partial antibody deficiencies, treatment with replacement immunoglobulin is not always necessary. In pure IgA deficiency, immunoglobulin replacement therapy is not indicated, and since immunoglobulin preparations contain small amounts of IgA, there is a risk of sensitization of the individual to IgA with the potential for subsequent severe allergic reactions upon blood product administration. In children with partial antibody deficiencies, it is reasonable to use prophylactic antibiotic treatment to reduce the risk of bacterial infections. The precise regimen used varies from center to center. Daily use of cotrimoxazole covers most respiratory pathogens and has the advantage, in those with combined immunodeficiency, of covering additionally against *Pneumocystis* infection. An alternative regime that is preferred in those who are not at risk of *Pneumocystis* is to use azithromycin in a regimen of three consecutive treatment days in a 2-week period, which, because of the long half-life of this antibiotic, provides continuous prophylaxis.

For severely deficient patients, immunoglobulin replacement therapy is indicated. Immunoglobulin is derived from normal blood donors in plasma-processing plants, which are very strictly regulated. Donors are screened for the known blood-borne viruses, and the plasma processing itself incorporates at least two antiviral steps.

Immunoglobulin is normally administered by the intravenous route in a dose of 500 to 750 mg per kilogram body weight (as a 5% to 12% solution) rounded to a convenient figure and administered on a 3-week basis (3 weeks being the approximate half-life of IgG). Generally it is well tolerated, but acute side effects including fever and chills can occur and are particularly likely to occur if the treatment is administered during episodes of fever or sepsis. Rarer side effects include headaches, which may have a delayed onset of up to 48 hours, and very rarely an aseptic meningitis, the pathogenesis of which is poorly understood (57). In patients on established treatment, it is possible to switch from regular intravenous infusions to the subcutaneous route. Administration by this route utilizes more concentrated products (15% to 16% solution) administered subcutaneously by infusion pump over approximately 1 hour at a number of sites so as to get an equivalent dose to that given intravenously over a 3-week period (Fig. 1.12). Because of the restrictions of volume that can be infused, children usually need to have this done on a more frequent (usually weekly) basis. The immunoglobulin accumulates as a painless subcutaneous swelling and then dissipates as it is absorbed into the blood. The advantages of the subcutaneous route include ease of administration, which can be done by the family at home, very low incidence of acute reactions, and the fact that the immunoglobulin levels on replacement by this route remain much more constant in the blood than after bolus intravenous administration (58).

The aim of replacement immunoglobulin therapy is to maintain the IgG level in the mid-normal therapeutic range (usually 8 to 10 g/L). Most immunoglobulin-deficient children remain well on such replacement, but a few need additional prophylactic antibiotics. Those with established bronchiectasis or chronic sinus disease before immunoglobulin treatment is commenced are the ones in

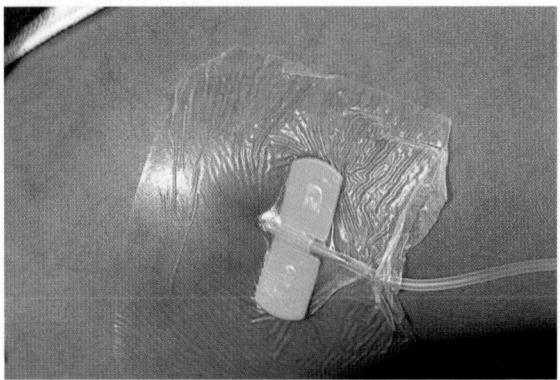

Figure 1.12. Subcutaneous administration of immunoglobulin. (Reproduced with permission from Davies EG. Impaired Immunity in Children. Current Paediatrics 2006;16:16–28.)

whom the treatment is less likely to completely prevent recurrence of the episodes of infection.

Children on immunoglobulin replacement therapy should have regular (every 3-months) monitoring of liver function tests and trough immunoglobulin levels, and an annual sample tested for hepatitis C by polymerase chain reaction (PCR) and saved for future viral evaluation.

Defects of Cell-Mediated Immunity: Combined Immunodeficiencies

Defects of cell-mediated immunity nearly always affect both T-cell immunity and antibody production. In other words, they lead to a combined immunodeficiency. This is either because the molecular defect leading to abnormal lymphocyte development affects both T cells and B cells or because the B cells fail to function and produce antibody normally in the absence of an intact T-cell system providing help. In their most complete form, these combined immunodeficiencies are labeled severe combined immunodeficiency (SCID). Affected infants are susceptible to the whole gamut of microbial pathogens. Other (less severe) combined immunodeficiencies are also recognized. Some of these disorders are associated with recognizable syndromes affecting other body systems.

Severe Combined Immunodeficiency

Infants born with SCID are at extremely high risk of life-threatening infection, both with common childhood pathogens and with opportunistic infections. They may present in a number of different ways (see below), and once stabilized and supported require treatment with a corrective therapy, usually in the form of bone marrow transplantation or, recently, gene therapy for some cases. A molecular basis for many of these disorders has now been elucidated, though there remains a sizable minority of SCID infants in whom the molecular defect remains elusive. In some cases the molecular defect does not result in an absolute deficiency of the gene product resulting in some lymphocyte development and leading to a "leaky" phenotype. Such affected infants may get added complications such as occur in Omenn's syndrome (see below). The lymphocytes that develop through the leakiness of the gene defect rarely contribute significantly to immunity but can potentially contribute to complications and to diagnostic delay.

Presentation

Infants with full-blown SCID present in the early months of life. There are three main forms of presentation:

1. Persistent or recurrent *Candida* infection of both the mucous membranes and the diaper area: Candidiasis is a relatively common problem in infancy, but its persistence and failure to respond to normal measures should arouse suspicion of a cell-mediated immune deficiency particularly if the infant has other problems such as poor weight gain, repeated infections, or chronic diarrhea.

2. Chronic diarrhea and failure to thrive: The causes of chronic diarrhea in these infants is variable. Sometimes viruses can be identified, such as rotavirus, which the infant will fail to clear and will cause chronic symptomatology. In other cases no infective agents are found, and the enteropathy is presumed to be mediated by some form of poorly understood immunodysregulatory process. In either case secondary lactose and cow's milk protein intolerance may exacerbate the problem, and appropriate nutritional management, either with elemental feeds or parenteral nutrition, will be required.

3. Interstitial pneumonitis due to *Pneumocystis jerovici*, cytomegalovirus (CMV), or respiratory viruses such as respiratory syncytial virus (RSV) or parainfluenza: This is the most severe a form of presentation of SCID, and often these infants have had a history of other less dramatic problems before they develop this complication but which failed to lead to the diagnosis being made (59). Most of these infants end up requiring respiratory support on intensive care units. and early and aggressive diagnostic strategies should be used to establish the precise microbial etiology so that optimal treatment can be given. The approach to such diagnosis is covered elsewhere in this book. It should be borne in mind that these infants often have more than one pathogen, so that the identification of, for example, RSV on a nasopharyngeal aspirate does not exclude the possibility of other pathogens such as CMV or *Pneumocystis* being involved in the pneumonitic process (Fig. 1.13).

Other less common modes of presentation of SCID include recurrent, relatively minor respiratory tract infections, which respond to oral antibiotics at least initially, and skin problems. The skin problems may take the form of maternal graft versus host disease in which maternal cells cross the placenta before or at the time of birth to the infant, who is incapable of rejecting them. Usually the rash in these cases is of a mild, reticular pattern, and severe graft versus host disease is a rare occurrence in this setting. By contrast, in Omenn's syndrome (Fig. 1.13C) the infant develops severe erythroderma, the differential diagnosis of which is Netherton's syndrome or severe atopic erythroderma. There is associated regional lymphadenopathy, hepatosplenomegaly, and often an enteropathy with severe protein loss and hypoalbuminemia.

Types

A number of different molecular types of SCID have been defined (60) (Table 1.6). In the future it is likely that there will be further genes identified to account for the cases where a molecular diagnosis cannot be made at the moment.

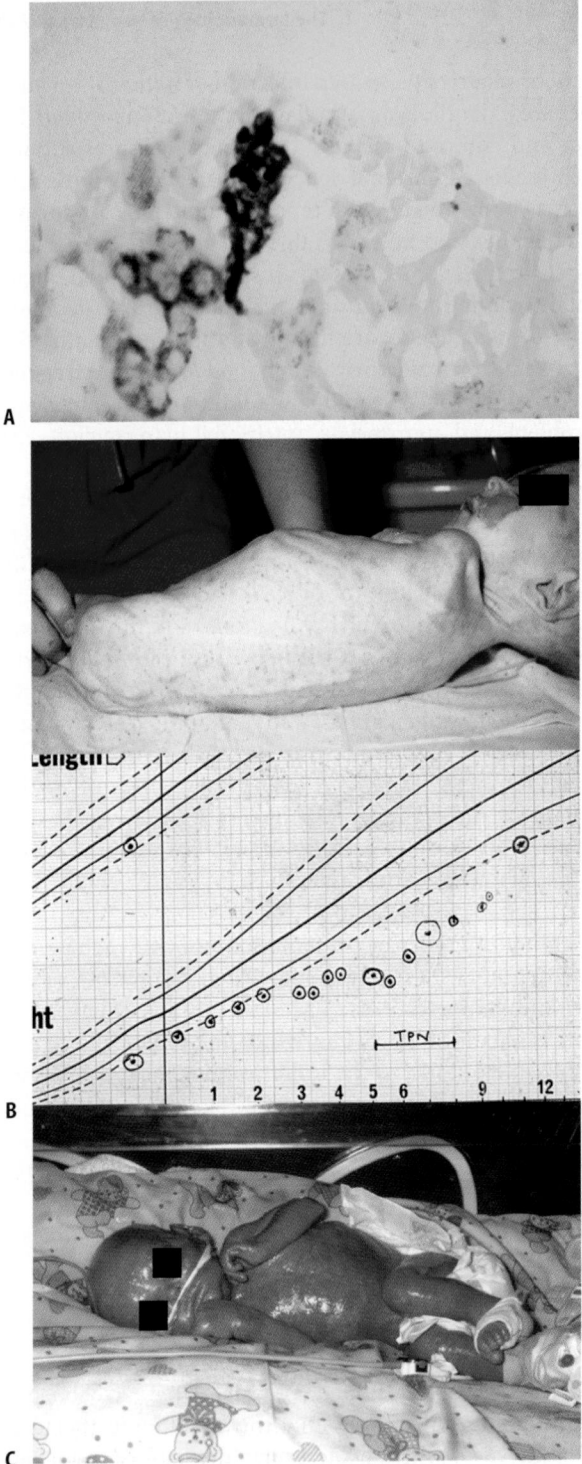

FIGURE 1.13. Severe combined immunodeficiency (SCID). (A) *Pneumocystis* pneumonia. Lung biopsy stained with Grocott–Methanamine to show organisms. (B) Severe failure to thrive. (C) Omenn's syndrome. (Reproduced with permission from Davies EG. Impaired Immunity in Children. Current Paediatrics 2006;16:16–28.)

TABLE 1.6. Main causes of severe combined immunodeficiency

Lymphocyte phenotype	Diagnosis	Gene	Inheritance
T– B+ NK–	Gamma chain (γC) deficiency or JAK 3 (Janus family kinase 3) SCID	γC codes for γ chain of several interleukin (IL) receptors. JAK3 is a kinase molecule associated with the intracytoplasmic tail of γ chain and responsible for intracellular signaling	X-linked (γ chain) or autosomal recessive (JAK3)
T– B+ NK+	Undefined SCID or IL-7 receptor α-chain deficiency	Unknown or IL-7 Rα	Autosomal recessive
T– B– NK+	T- and B-cell receptor gene rearrangement defect	Recombination activating genes (RAG) 1 and 2 or *Artemis* gene	Autosomal recessive
T– B– NK–	ADA deficiency or undefined SCID	ADA inheritance autosomal recessive	Purine metabolic enzyme defect
T+ B– NK+	Omenn's syndrome	RAG 1 or 2 or *Artemis* or undefined	Autosomal recessive

ADA, adenosine deaminase; SCID, severe combined immunodeficiency. IL-7 Rα, interleukin-7 receptor alpha chain.

T– B+ NK–

This is the commonest form of SCID. It usually results from failure of signaling through the interleukin receptors using the common γ chain (Fig. 1.13). T and NK cells have a requirement for such signaling in their development, while B cells can develop normally though they are functionally deficient, resulting in a combined humoral and cell-mediated immunodeficiency. The gene for this chain is carried on the X chromosome and accounts for around 40% of all cases. Mutations in the gene for Janus activated kinase 3 (JAK3) result in failure of signaling through the interleukin receptor, resulting in a very similar clinical and immunological picture.

T– B– NK+

This form of SCID usually results from a deficiency in the DNA recombination processes required to generate the diverse repertoire of T- and B-cell antigen receptors. NK cells do not have such a requirement in their development. Defects in genes coding for recombination activating genes, RAG 1 and 2 as well as in a gene called *Artemis* involved in this process account for most but not all cases with this phenotype. Less well defined forms of SCID with excessive radiosensitivity may also have defects involving this pathway. Omenn's syndrome is a variant of these forms of SCID, in which the particular mutations allow some enzyme activity (leakiness), which enables some DNA rearrangement to occur and a clonal expansion of T cells. These cells become switched markedly in the direction of T-helper-2 (Th2) responsiveness to produce the inflammatory changes that are seen. There is usually an eosinophilia and a raised IgE level. T cells are present often in normal numbers in the circulation, but examination of the repertoire of T-cell receptor expression shows that these are profoundly oligoclonal. B cells are usually absent from the circulation, suggesting that the leakiness does not affect the B-cell lineage.

T– B+ NK+

This autosomal recessive phenotype may be associated with a defect in the IL-7 receptor α chain or with other, as yet undefined, forms of SCID. Interleukin-7 stimulation is essential for T-cell development but not B- and NK-cell development.

Adenosine Deaminase–Deficient SCID (T– B– NK–)

Around 25% of patients with SCID have this defect. The enzyme adenosine deaminase (ADA) is involved in the purine salvage pathway. Deficiency of ADA leads to accumulation of toxic intermediaries deoxyadenosine and deoxyadenosine triphosphate. This particularly affects the lymphoid system, resulting in profound lymphopenia. Other systems are also affected, with some skeletal abnormalities such as splaying of the rib ends, mild derangement of liver function, and neurologic dysfunction, resulting in developmental delay, behavioral abnormalities, and neural deafness in many (but not all cases). These non-immunologic abnormalities are not completely correctable by bone marrow transplantation, though there may be some indirect benefit through the "detoxifying" effect of the enzyme provided in the engrafted haematopoietic cells.

Investigations

The diagnosis of SCID is suggested by one of the above clinical presentations, and often the blood count will show a lymphopenia with a lymphocyte count persistently below 2.5 (the approximate lower limit of normal for a total lymphocyte count in early infancy). Many normal infants can suffer a relative lymphopenia in the face of an acute infection, but this should return to normal when they recover, and failure to do so warrants further investigation. Confirmation of the diagnosis of SCID can be obtained by looking at the lymphocyte profile, which may show one of the patterns shown in Table 1.6. Confirmation of the absence of T-cell function can be obtained by examining responsiveness of T cells to mitogens such as phytohemagglutinin (PHA). Immunoglobulin measurements are likely to show low levels of A and M but in the early months of life maternal IgG may still be present. Since vertically acquired HIV infection may present in a similar fashion, it is important to exclude this diagnosis at an early stage. Further testing may involve detailed molecular studies to look at the particular gene defect. This may be relevant as gene therapy be comes available for a number of the genetic defects causing SCID. Precise genetic diagnosis will also facilitate genetic counseling and potential future prenatal diagnosis for the family. In the case of ADA-deficient SCID, the diagnosis can be confirmed by metabolic studies of blood and urine to look at the level of the enzyme activity in the red cells and the metabolites in the urine (Table 1.7).

TABLE 1.7. Tests of cell-mediated immunity

Test	Type of test	Conditions tested for	Comments
Lymphocyte count	Full blood count and blood film	Severe immunodeficiency disorders with lymphopenia	At least two thirds of infants with SCID have persistently low lymphocyte counts
Lymphocyte subsets	FACS analysis for range of antibodies tested (see Table 1.3)	Primary defects of lymphocyte development or secondary lymphocyte disturbance	Affected by corticosteroids and other immunosuppressive agents
Mitogenic responses	Stimulation of lymphocyte in culture with stimulants of proliferation such as phytohemagglutinin (PHA) or an anti-CD3 antibody	Defects of T lymphocyte function	Affected by steroids and other immunosuppressive treatments
Lymphocyte-proliferative response to specific antigens	Similar to mitogenic assays but using an antigen to which the child has been exposed, e.g.,*Candida* or tetanus toxoid as stimulus	Defects of lymphocyte proliferative response to antigens	Affected by steroids and other immunosuppressive treatments
Lymphocyte spectratypes	PCR test for variable regions of the T-cell receptor to look for normal variability reflecting polyclonality of T or B cells	Immunodeficiency disorders in which generation of polyclonal T and B cell receptors is impaired, e.g., *RAG* gene defects	
T-cell recombination excision cycle (TREC) analysis	PCR test for TRECs	Defects of T-cell development resulting in poor thymic output or defects of thymic function	

PCR, polymerase chain reaction; FACS, fluorescence activated cell sorting.

Treatment

Treatment of the presenting infections should be pursued vigorously, and details are covered in other parts of this book. Many SCID infants are nutritionally compromised at the time of diagnosis, and attention should be paid to this problem early in the course of their management. All blood products administered should be CMV antibody negative and irradiated to prevent the possibility of transfusion-acquired graft verses host disease. Replacement immunoglobulin therapy should be started at the earliest possible opportunity in a dose of 500 mg per kilogram body weight. If the patient is not already on therapeutic cotrimoxazole, it should be commenced in a prophylactic dose of 30 mg per kilograms per day (of the combination), and this is generally given on a daily basis to provide both antibacterial and pneumocystitis prophylaxis. Fluconazole should be commenced in a prophylactic dosage of 3 mg/kg body weight daily.

Definitive treatment involves correcting the underlying defect. For most cases this entails a bone marrow transplant. In ADA-deficient SCID, there is an alternative form of treatment for this condition using pegylated enzyme, which is injected weekly and, over a period of 2 to 3 months, usually brings about some restoration of immunity. This therapy is extremely expensive and is not completely curative in that immunity is rarely restored to normal. However, it may be a useful temporizing measure when bone marrow transplantation is not an immediate option because the child is too sick or a suitable donor is not available.

Blood should be drawn from the infant and the family as early as possible to send for tissue typing. There is a one in four chance that any full sibling will be a match, and in consanguineous families there is a possibility that other family members may match, and so an extended family search should be initiated. If a matched family donor cannot be identified, an unrelated donor search is initiated, which entails looking at volunteer adult bone marrow donor banks and at cord blood banks. Identification of an unrelated adult donor and completion of transplantation can rarely be achieved in less than 2 months, whereas a cord blood transplant may be achieved more quickly. When a matched family donor is available the transplant can proceed very quickly. An alternative approach, when an unrelated donor or cord cannot be found, is to use a parent-to-child transplant (parents share one MHC haplotype with the child, and this is called a haploidentical transplant). In this type of procedure there is T-cell depletion of the marrow with administration of a purified population of stem cells either harvested from the marrow or from peripheral blood. T-cell reconstitution after this form of graft takes a minimum of 4 months and often longer in contrast to the whole marrow transplants performed from family donors or unrelated donor. The risks of serious infection or progressive infection in children already infected with viruses such as CMV are greatly increased after such grafts, and for this reason matched family or unrelated donors are preferred. The results of bone marrow transplantation for immunodeficiency are reported regularly by the European Society for Immunodeficiencies (61).

For γ-chain–deficient x-linked SCID and ADA deficiency, an experimental program of somatic gene therapy has been reported to be successful in reconstituting immunity without the need for bone marrow transplantation. However, one potentially serious complication of this treatment is the development of lymphoproliferative disease associated with the gene inserting, and disrupting known oncogenes in the lymphoid system (62). For this reason, at the current time, gene therapy is offered only in those cases where a matched bone marrow donor cannot be found. Gene therapy has also been used in a small number of cases of ADA-deficient SCID (63).

A detailed description of the procedures involved in bone marrow transplantation for SCID is beyond the scope of this book. In general, for most forms of transplantation, chemotherapy is now used even though the infant's immune system is incapable of rejection. It has been found that the use of such conditioning therapy increases the likelihood that the new graft will take and remain in place durably. In recent years there have been advances in the use of chemotherapy for these conditions. Low-intensity conditioning, which is better tolerated by the child, has been shown to be effective in allowing complete engraftment (64). The only exception to the use of chemotherapy may be in the matched sibling donor situation, where an infusion of whole marrow without conditioning often results in a rapid engraftment with achievement of some T-cell immunity within a few weeks. This may be attempted in very sick infants and may be lifesaving. In my experience it has occasionally been used successfully for SCID infants on ventilators.

Other Well-Defined Forms of Combined Immunodeficiency

There are a number of other disorders in which there is a combination of defective T-cell function and humoral immunodeficiency, some of which are associated with syndromes. Although not as severe as SCID in terms of immunologic function, these children may present in a profoundly ill state with overwhelming infections, including those caused by opportunistic agents. Sometimes special extra tests are needed to confirm these diagnoses and these are summarized in Table 1.8.

Major Histocompatability Complex Class II Deficiency

This deficiency is inherited as an autosomal recessive trait, and affected infants suffer recurrent infections particularly with viruses. They are also prone to chronic infection with *Cryptosporidium* spp. and to *Pneumocystis jerovici* pneumonia. Failure of expression of the class II histocompatability antigens means that antigen presentation by macrophages and B cells to CD4-positive T cells, which relies on class II MHC presentation, cannot occur. The CD4 count is usually very low, as that population has failed to expand. Immunoglobulin production is deficient. These children often present later than those with SCID,

TABLE 1.8. Other tests for specific immunodeficiencies

Test	Type of test	Conditions tested for	Comments
Radiosensitivity	Lymphocyte or cultured fibroblast sensitivity to ionizing radiation	Radiation sensitivity defects, e.g., ataxia telangiectasia (AT), some forms of SCID with gene rearrangement defects	Some radio-sensitivity defects associated with SCID are still uncharacterized; α-fetoprotein measurement is a relatively sensitive screening test for AT
Chromosomal analysis	1. Specific FISH tests for 22q or 10p-deletions	DiGeorge syndrome	Not all cases of thymic aplasia have chromosomal deletions
	2. Karyotyping and chromosomal fragility	Chromosomal breakage disorders e.g. ICF (immunodeficiency centromeric instability facial abnormalities syndrome or Nijmegen breakage syndrome	
Purine/pyrimidine salvage pathway tests	Blood analysis of enzyme activity; urine analysis of metabolites	ADA and PNP deficiency	
Molecular protein analysis	FACS or Western blot analysis of specific protein in particular conditions	Known primary genetic defects, e.g., X linked agammaglobulinemia, Wiskott-Aldrich, γ-chain–deficient SCID	Allows rapid screening for suspected molecular defects
Molecular genetic analysis	Gene sequencing or other approach to detecting genetic mutations	All primary immunodeficiency disorders for which the genetic basis is known	Takes longer than protein tests. Ideally is used as a confirmatory test after protein screening

FISH, fluorescent in situ hybridization; ADA, adenosine deaminase deficiency; PNP, purine nucleoside phosphorylase; FACS, fluorescence activated cell sorting.

and by this time are often already infected with viruses such as CMV or adenovirus, which complicates their treatment. Treatment should be along the lines of SCID with supportive therapy followed by transplantation. The results of transplantation, unfortunately, are not good, and T-cell reconstitution often remains relatively poor.

Purine Nucleoside Phosphorylase Deficiency

This is another purine metabolic enzyme defect resulting in accumulation of toxic purine metabolites in lymphocytes. Presentation is usually later than in full SCID and involves recurrent infections and often autoimmune phenomena, including hemolytic anemia, due to immune dysregulation. There is generalized lymphopenia, and the diagnosis is confirmed using metabolic tests on blood and urine. Unlike ADA deficiency, there is no alternative of enzyme replacement therapy and corrective treatment is with bone marrow transplantation. The enzyme defect also affects neurologic function, and affected infants may have spastic motor problems. Anecdotally, it is believed that these neurologic problems do not usually progress if successful bone marrow transplantation has been achieved presumably because of provision of some enzyme to the brain by engrafted cells of the hematopoietic system.

X-linked Hyper–Immunoglobulin M Syndrome (CD40 Ligand Deficiency)

This x-linked defect affects the expression of CD40 ligand, a molecule expressed on the surface of T cells when they become activated as part of the immune response. Interaction of this molecule with its ligand, CD40, present on B cells facilitates class switching to allow the IgM antibody response to switch to IgG and IgA. Another important interaction with CD40 ligand is CD40 on macrophages, enabling them to become activated as part of the process of killing intracellular organisms. Affected individuals, therefore, have absence of IgA and IgG due to failure of class switching, leading to a susceptibility to pyogenic bacterial infections and also to intracellular organisms including *Pneumocystis jerovici*, cryptosporidium, and toxoplasma. The problem of chronic cryptosporidiosis can lead to a chronic enteropathy and cholangiopathy, the latter resulting in sclerosing cholangitis and cirrhosis. Management involves the use of prophylaxis against *Pneumocystis* and replacement immunoglobulin therapy. The role of bone marrow transplantation is, as yet, unclear, but it should certainly be offered to those who have a matched sibling donor and to others who are developing complications. An unexplained neutropenia also occurs in up to 50% of affected boys at some stage. This may be intermittent or persistent, and G-CSF therapy may be required (65).

X-linked Lymphoproliferative Disease (Duncan's Syndrome)

In this condition affected boys remain well until a viral infection, most commonly but not always caused by Epstein-Barr virus (EBV), produces a rapid deterioration in immune function, resulting in failure to control the virus and susceptibility to other pathogens. In the case of EBV infection, this may result in fulminating infectious mononucleosis or the development of lymphoproliferative disease or hemophagocytic lymphohistiocytosis (HLH). Some patients have a more subacute illness developing into aplastic anemia or hypogammaglobulinemia. Mutations in the gene encoding a regulatory protein SAP have been identified as the commonest cause of this disorder. SAP is associated with a surface molecule on the lymphocytes known as signaling lymphocyte activation molecule (SLAM), which is involved in regulation of lymphoprolif-eration. A second X linked gene causing this syndrome encodes a protein XIAP (X-linked inhibitor of apoptosis). The prognosis for this condition is very poor, and if the EBV infection can be controlled with measures such as monoclonal CD20 antibody, then early bone marrow transplantation should be undertaken and is potentially curative.

Syndromic Immunodeficiencies

These are genetic disorders in which immunodeficiency is only one of a number of different defects. The most important of these are summarized here.

DiGeorge Syndrome

Absent thymic development as part of DiGeorge syndrome (Fig. 1.14) may be part of the velocardiofacial syndrome most commonly associated with a 22q chromosomal microdeletion or part of other chromosomal anomalies, for example, 10p– deletion or the CHARGE syndrome (coloboma, heart anomaly, retardation, and genital and ear anomalies). Most often an associated immuno-deficiency is mild or absent. Tests may show a mild to moderate T-cell lympho-penia, which is asymptomatic or associated with a minor excess of infections or there are no abnormalities detected. Autoimmune disorders occur more frequently in this group, presumably as a result of impaired T-cell regulation. A small proportion of affected infants have complete absence of naive T cells in the circulation and behave like infants with SCID. There may be a whole spectrum of other abnormalities including hypoparathyroidism, congenital

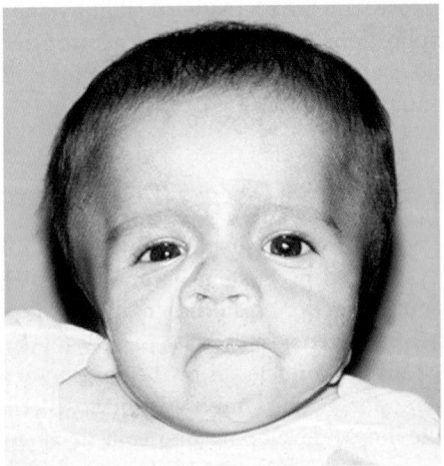

Figure 1.14. Facial characteristics in DiGeorge Syndrome. (Courtesy of Prof CBS Wood. Reproduced with permission of the family and with permission from Cant AJ, et al—see Further Reading.)

heart disease, and renal abnormalities in the 22q deletion syndrome, or the features of CHARGE syndrome if that is the diagnosis. For those with complete T-cell deficiency, a graft from a matched bone marrow donor may bring about some postthymic T-cell engraftment, which is sufficient to prevent their developing opportunistic infections. An alternative therapy that has been successfully employed by one center is to transplant cultured human thymic epithelium (derived from infants undergoing open heart surgery), which allows the body's own pre-T cells to mature (66).

Wiskott-Aldrich Syndrome

This syndrome is caused by deficiency, in all hematopoietic lineages, of a protein known as Wiskott-Aldrich associated protein (WASP) (67). This protein is involved with the functioning of the actin cytoskeleton and in a number of other cell functions. The syndrome is inherited as an x-linked condition, and affected boys suffer thrombocytopenia, with very small abnormal platelets, eczema, and recurrent infections usually affecting the sinopulmonary system. There is also an increased risk of lymphoproliferative disease. Particularly in early life, the boys are at risk of severe bleeding due to the thrombocytopenia including cerebral hemorrhages. Splenectomy may alleviate the thrombocytopenia, but increases the immune deficiency. The immune profile typically shows a low IgM level with a high IgA and poor antibody production in response to vaccines. There is usually also a generalized lymphopenia. Treatment with cotrimoxazole prophylaxis and immunoglobulin replacement therapy should be undertaken, and the patient prepared for early elective bone marrow transplantation if a donor can be identified.

Hyper–Immunoglobulin E Syndrome

This syndrome, usually inherited as an autosomal dominant condition, is also known as Job's syndrome. The gene responsible is not known. A rarer recessively inherited form has also been described (68). Affected individuals are prone to S. aureus and fungal infections of the skin and deeper organs. Pneumonias often lead to pneumatocele formation. Most patients have a chronic eczematoid or pustular dermatitis, and there are also nonimmunologic features such as bone fragility, joint hypermobility, and delayed loss of primary dentition. Diagnosis is confirmed by the finding of a very high IgE level (>5000 IU/L) in association with typical clinical features. The main differential diagnosis is severe atopic disease with secondary infections. A scoring system has been suggested to aid the diagnostic process (69). Some affected individuals also have a deficient pneumococcal antibody response, which increases the risk of repeated pneumonias and the development of bronchiectasis. Management is with prophylactic antistaphylococcal and antifungal drugs. Immunoglobulin replacement should be used in those with defective antibody responses.

Chromosome Breakage Disorders

Several of the chromosomal breakage disorders are associated with immune deficiency. The most classic of these is ataxia telangiectasia, in which, in addition to a progressive cerebellar degeneration and the appearance of skin telangiectases, affected children have deficiency of the immune system. This is variable, but usually involves a lymphopenia with a particular deficiency of CD4/CD45 RA positive cells (the naive thymic emigrant T cells). There are also immunoglobulin disturbances with absence of IgA and defective antibody responses to polysaccharide antigens. There is a high incidence of malignant disease, which may be partly due to the DNA repair disorder and partly due to the lack of immune surveillance. Despite low CD4 cell counts these patients very rarely develop opportunistic infections such as *Pneumocystis* pneumonia. They do get recurrent bacterial infections of the chest and ears, which can usually be controlled, in milder cases, by use of prophylactic antibiotics and in more severe cases by the use of regular immunoglobulin infusions (70).

Nijmegen breakage syndrome is another chromosomal repair defect with an immune deficiency affecting both T cells and immunoglobulins associated with developmental delay and microcephaly (71).

Radiographic investigations should be kept to a minimum in patients with these disorders, especially potentially high dosage procedures such as computed tomography (CT) scans.

Immunodeficiencies Leading to Hemophagocytic Lymphohistiocytosis

Hemophagocytic lymphohistiocytosis (HLH) is a devastating condition in which uncontrolled macrophage activation and proliferation caused multisystem disease with a high mortality. Familial and sporadic cases can occur. In the former genetic defects affecting immune regulation may be recognized. X-linked lymphoproliferative disease (XLP) may present in this way (see page 39). Recent work has identified a number of other genetic causes affecting proteins involved in granule exocytosis. The resultant defect in T and NK cell cytotoxic activity seems to be crucial in the lack of ability to control macrophage activation (72). Details of these conditions are given in Table 1.9. Some of the conditions involved are associated with other clinical features such as oculocutaneous albinism and neurodevelopmental defects in Chediak-Higashi syndrome and Griscelli syndrome.

Clinical Presentation

This is a multisystem disease, which may present in a multitude of different ways. Most commonly it presents with pyrexia of unknown origin, which may be associated with lymphadenopathy, hepatosplenomegaly, and pancytopenia.

TABLE 1.9. Main genetic disorders associated with the development of hemophagocytic lymphohistiocytosis (HLH)

Disorder	Gene encodes	Cutaneous	Hematologic	Neurologic	Recurrent infections
Chediak-Higashi Syndrome	Lyst 5	Partial oculocutaneous albinism	Neutropenia with abnormal neutrophils containing giant granules	Subtle behavioral abnormalities slowly progressive; learning difficulties; increased incidence of seizures	Increased incidence of bacterial infections secondary to neutrophil defect, which occurs prior to the development of HLH
Griscelli Syndrome	1. Myo 5 (not associated with HLH)	Partial oculo-cutaneous albinism	No abnormalities	Myo 5 defects are associated with severe neurodevelopmental abnormalities	None
	2. Rab 27a (Associated with HLH)	Partial oculo-cutaneous albinism	No abnormalities	Rab 27 defects may show subtle problems as in Chediak-Higashi Syndrome	Recurrent infections minimal
X-linked lymphoprolife-rative syndrome (XLP)	SAP or XIAP	None	None (prior to onset of disease	None	Mild or no infections prior to onset of disease
HLH with defective expression of perforin	Perforin	No defects of pigmentation; some cases described as having granulomatous skin eruptions	None	None	Possible
Other familial HLH disorders	1. Munc 4.13	None	None	None	Possible
	2. Syntaxin 11	None	Predisposed to myelodysplasia/ Myeloid leukemia	Unknown	None
	3. Not yet identified	None	None	None	None

Other presentations include pulmonary involvement with a pneumonitic process or neurologic involvement with seizures. Diagnosis in the early stages may be difficult. There is usually pancytopenia, and bone marrow examination may show increased numbers of activated macrophages with hemophagocytosis. It should be noted that a degree of hemophagocytosis may be found in the marrow in a number of a different inflammatory disorders and is not in itself diagnostic of HLH. Biopsies of other tissues such as liver show infiltrations of lymphocytes and macrophages, and again hemophagocytosis may or may not be seen. Very markedly raised levels of ferritin and of triglycerides in the blood are helpful diagnostic indicators though not very specific. There may also be a hypofibrinogenemia or, in more advanced cases, a frank picture of disseminated intravascular coagulopathy. The condition may be complicated by secondary opportunistic infection, making the diagnosis of the underlying disorder more difficult.

Treatment

Affected patients may require the full panoply of supportive therapy including ventilatory support for pulmonary involvement and blood product support. Immunosuppression is required to bring the macrophage activation process under control. A generally agreed protocol for treating this involves the use of dexamethasone and etoposide followed by the introduction of cyclosporin A. If there is central nervous system involvement, intrathecal methotrexate is also advised. When the triggering viral infection can be identified, it should also be treated if possible. One of the most common triggering agents is EBV, but in many cases no virus can be identified. The viral load driving the process may be reduced with the use of the anti-CD20 monoclonal antibody rituximab. This temporarily destroys the B cells acting as the main site of replication of the virus. Other viral causes may be treated as appropriate, for example, using ganciclovir for CMV. In cases of familial HLH, even if the process can be fully controlled with therapy, it is likely to recur, and a corrective bone marrow transplant is indicated. Tissue typing, therefore, should be done early so that a bone marrow donor can be identified. Transplantation should be performed promptly once the patient is in remission because early relapse may occur. The outcome of transplantation for this condition has been recently reviewed (73) and shows a moderately good success rate for unrelated donor transplants.

Hemophagocytic lymphohistiocytosis may also occur as a nonfamilial virus-driven illness. In general, it tends to occur in older individuals who do not have any of the stigmata of the known genetic disorders (see Table 1.9) or any of the known gene defects identified. As a group, these patients have a better prognosis if they survive the initial illness. In such cases bone marrow transplant is not indicated immediately after remission has been achieved.

TABLE **1.10.** Causes of secondary immunodeficiency

Associated with disease state	Iatrogenic
Malnutrition	Immunosuppressive drugs
Infections	Cytotoxic chemotherapy
Metabolic disorders	Combined, e.g., Bone Marrow
Gastrointestinal disease	Transplantation
Stress (trauma, burns, etc.)	Other drug effects, e.g., anticonvulsants
Malignancy	Splenectomy

Secondary Immunodeficiency

The immune system may be suppressed by a variety of different factors including disease states, trauma, and treatments administered (Table 1.10). The last includes treatment in the intensive care setting as summarized in Figure 1.15.

Immunosuppression from Underlying Disease

The mechanisms by which disease processes suppress immunity are not well understood. The effect of stress such as occurs after trauma, including surgery,

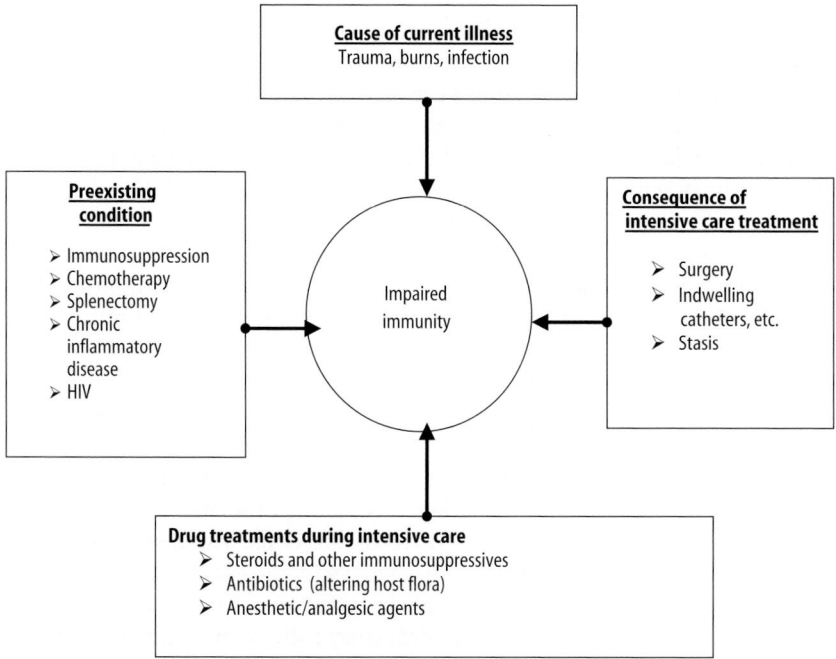

FIGURE **1.15.** Factors leading to impaired immunity in children undergoing intensive care treatment.

TABLE 1.11. Mechanisms by which infections can cause secondary immunodeficiency

Microbial agent	Mechanisms
Bacteria	Biofilm formation
	Adhesins and other virulence factors
Malaria	Phagocytosis of infected red blood cells inhibits Mø and DC function ↓ specific CD8, ↓ IFN-γ, ↓ IL-12, ↑IL-10 contribute to prolonged liver cycle
Measles	Receptors include CD46 & SLAM. ↓ T-cell Nos, ↓ T-cell activation, ↓ mitogen responses, ↓ IL-2 production
	Changes persist for several weeks
	See ref. 76
CMV	Virally encoded proteins include: an IL-10 homologue and proteins which bind to RANTES and β_2-microglobulin, ↓HLA-1 expression
EBV	Infects B cells in tonsillar tissue, latent cells become "invisible" to the immune system
	Virally encoded LMP1 & LMP2 are homologues of CD40 and B-cell receptor

CMV, cytomegalovirus; DC, dendritic cells; EBV, Epstein-Barr virus; HLA-1, human leukocyte antigen class 1; IFN, interferon; IL, interleukin; LMP, latent membrane proteins; Mø, macrophage; SLAM, signaling lymphocyte activation molecule.

can lead to suppression of lymphocyte numbers and lymphocyte proliferative responses. There may also be impairment of neutrophil function, particularly chemotaxis. These effects are almost certainly mediated by cytokines and other soluble factors. In full-blown form, these responses can lead to the systemic inflammatory response syndrome (SIRS). The immunosuppression that follows extensive burn injuries has a similar basis and is often more marked than after other injuries. Heat shock proteins and local nitric oxide production (74) seem to be involved, and recent work suggests the generation of T regulatory cells, which limit immune responsiveness (75). After burns, soluble immunosuppressive factors including lipid/protein complexes have been found in the circulation.

Infection itself can also lead to immunosuppression through the nonspecific effects of stress discussed above. Transient lymphopenia is common during the acute phase of a systemic viral or bacterial infection. More specifically, some microbes can subvert the immune response to enhance their own survival. Human immunodeficiency virus (HIV) is the most dramatic example of this. Infection with HIV is covered elsewhere in the book. Another well-studied example is the immunosuppression associated with measles infection (76). The basis of this and other examples are shown in Table 1.11.

Other causes of secondary immunodeficiency include malnutrition, particularly protein calorie malnutrition and specific trace element deficiencies such as zinc deficiency, which can lead to a T-cell functional deficiency by poorly understood mechanisms. Malignancy and metabolic disorders, both inborn (e.g., glycogen storage disease) and acquired (e.g., uremia), can affect both T-cell and neutrophil function.

Excessive plasma protein loss as is found in nephrotic syndrome (particularly when there is a nonselective proteinuria), protein losing enteropathy (especially intestinal lymphangiectasia), or chylous leaks can lead to a profoundly low immunoglobulin levels. Typically the IgG is more depressed than the IgA and IgM levels. The albumin level will always be low in this situation. Specific antibody levels to vaccine antigens are usually maintained in these circumstances, and most patients do not suffer an excess of bacterial infections, though some reports suggest this situation predisposes to giardiasis. Those with lymphangiectasia are additionally profoundly lymphopenic, typically with CD4 cells more depressed than CD8 cells. They may show cutaneous anergy, but opportunistic infections are rare.

Iatrogenic Immunosuppression

Corticosteroids, other immunosuppressive drugs, and antiproliferative (chemotherapeutic) agents all suppress immune responses. Figure 1.16 illustrates the stages of T-cell response and sites of action of some of the main classes of drugs.

Corticosteroids, which are the most used immunosuppressive agents, have a broad range of suppressive effect on T cells as well as neutrophils and inflammatory processes (77). Chemotherapy and radiotherapy also affect predominantly T cells but can also cause neutropenia. Consequently these agents can predispose to both fungal and pyogenic bacterial infections as well as the classic T-cell pathogens—viruses (Fig. 1.17), *Pneumocystis*, and intracellular bacteria such as mycobacteria and *Salmonella* spp. Purely immunosuppressive agents, on the other hand, lead predominantly to problems with T-cell pathogens. Suppression of antibody responses occurs only with high doses, and primary responses suppress more readily than secondary. Recent advances have led to the production of new "biologic" immunosuppressive agents that bring their own characteristic patterns of impaired immunity, as summarized in Table 1.12.

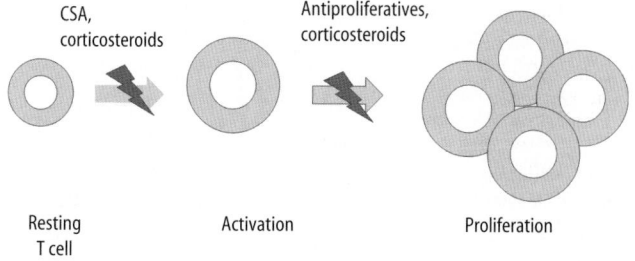

FIGURE **1.16.** Main sites of action of immunosuppressive drugs. CSA, cyclosporin A.

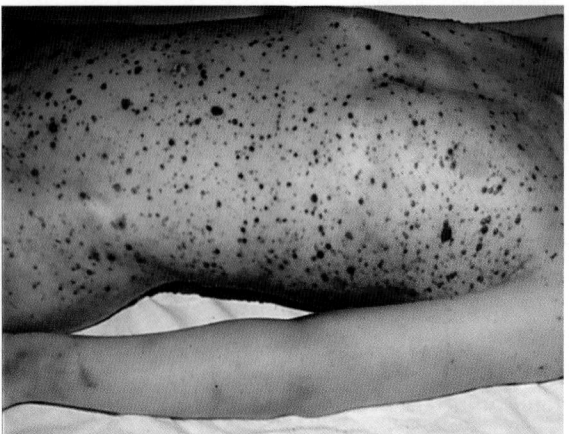

FIGURE **1.17.** Hemorrhagic chickenpox in a child on steroids and azathioprine.

Antibody deficiencies can also occur as a secondary phenomenon due to the effect of antiepileptic drugs such as phenytoin (78).

Hyposplenism

Poor splenic function is associated with reduced clearance of intravascular particles, a small reduction in IgM and alternative pathway complement function, reduced polysaccharide antibody responses and responses to intravenously administered antigens, and a reduced proportion of naive CD4 positive (CD4$^+$, CD45RA$^+$) T cells in the circulation. Patients are susceptible to sudden overwhelming sepsis particularly with pneumococcus and other capsulated organisms. Investigation for hyposplenism should be part of the workup in children with unexplained sepsis. The degree of susceptibility to infection following splenectomy for clinical reasons varies markedly with the reason for the removal (Fig. 1.18) (79).

TABLE **1.12.** Types of infection following immunosuppression with most commonly used biologic agents

- Antilymphocyte (or thymocyte) globulin, ALG (or ATG)
  - T-cell pathogens, EBV-LPD
- Anti–TNF-α
  - TB reactivation, invasive fungal disease
- Anti-CD25 (IL-2 receptor)
  - T-cell pathogens (less than ALG)
- Anti–LFA-1
  - JC virus
- Anti-CD20 (B cells)
  - Invasive bacterial sepsis, enteroviral infections

EBV-LPD, Epstein Barr virus driven lymphoproliferative disease; TNF, tumor necrosis factor.

Thalassaemia, Wiskott-Aldrich

⇓

Lymphoproliferative disease

⇓

Spherocytosis, ITP

⇓

Trauma

FIGURE 1.18. Risk of sepsis following splenectomy. ITP, idiopathic thrombocytopenic purpura. Highest risk at the top.

Management of the Child with Secondary Immunodeficiency

Recognition that a child is at risk of infection is an important first step. Attention to routine procedures for minimizing nosocomial infection should be part of normal clinical care. In the most immunosuppressed children, for example those who have received bone marrow transplantation (BMT), care in a side room with barrier nursing and ideally with a filtered air supply has been shown to improve the outcome. Prophylactic antimicrobials are helpful but have their own problems in inducing resistant flora. Nevertheless, antifungals in patients with neutropenia, penicillin in hyposplenic patients, and cotrimoxazole in those with persistent CD4 lymphopenia are inarguable. Additionally, aciclovir is of benefit in preventing *Herpes simplex* infection and possibly also CMV reactivation in very high risk situations such as post-BMT. When appropriate, immunization may be helpful. Good examples include pneumococcal and meningococcal vaccination in splenectomized individuals (80) and varicella vaccine in patients prior to solid organ transplantation. Medic alert bracelets should be considered for splenectomized individuals, and careful advice given for malaria avoidance for those patients who travel to at-risk areas.

The use of immunoglobulin infusions as prophylaxis, whilst established in those with primary immunodeficiencies, is of uncertain value in secondary immunodeficiency. It is particularly controversial in those with protein-losing states and very low IgG levels. The increment achievable by immunoglobulin infusions in such patients is very poor, though some have suggested that subcutaneous immunoglobulin may be more effective (81). The use of immunoglobulin infusions for prophylaxis or treatment in patients undergoing intensive care treatment for a variety of illnesses, though showing a marginal benefit in meta-analyses (82,83), has not become widely recommended.

Immunologic Approach to the Child in the Pediatric Intensive Care Unit

General Considerations

An illness requiring admission to the pediatric intensive care unit may be the presenting feature of an immunodeficiency in childhood. Alternatively, an admission may be necessary in a child previously diagnosed with a primary immunodeficiency or one who is immunocompromised as a result of other treatments such as chemotherapy. This section addresses the practical approach to dealing with the diagnosis and management issues from the immunologic point of view. Septicemia complicates deficiencies of the antibody/complement/neutrophil axis but is an unusual presenting feature of a combined immunodeficiency. In a child not previously suspected of having an immunodeficiency, tests may be difficult to interpret in the face of sepsis, partly from the effects of the sepsis itself such as neutropenia or from treatment with blood products that contain complement factors and immunoglobulins. In a child not known to be previously neutropenic, a finding of a low neutrophil count is most likely to be secondary to the sepsis process. Complement measurements are extremely difficult to interpret in the acute situation, and exclusion of a complement defect (for example, in a child with meningococcal sepsis) cannot really be achieved until the convalescent period. Immunoglobulin levels, on the other hand, are not affected by the sepsis processes, and so a sample taken before blood product administration is useful. Table 1.13 lists the available immunologic interventions for cases of immunodeficiency in the intensive care unit and cites limitations of these interventions.

Pneumonia

In the case of bacterial pneumonias with or without empyema, any underlying immunodeficiency is most likely to be in the antibody/complement/neutrophil system. Occasionally such clinical presentations may occur in one of the combined immunodeficiencies. Fungal pneumonias are associated with neutrophil problems or T-cell defects. Interstitial pneumonia is one of the commonest presenting features of combined immunodeficiency or HIV/AIDS. Noninfective pulmonary disease may also be indicative of underlying immunodeficiency including lymphoproliferative disease, which complicates X-linked lymphoproliferative syndrome or other combined immunodeficiencies. Hemophagocytic lymphohistiocytosis (HLH) can also lead to pulmonary involvement requiring intensive care treatment. Diagnosis of immunodeficiency complicating bacterial pneumonia and empyemas follows the same principles as for overwhelming sepsis. When combined immunodeficiency is suspected, it is important to look at lymphocyte numbers and function as well as an HIV test as early as possible, as this may have a major bearing on the management of the patient. While many children with serious infection are secondarily lymphopenic, it is normally possible, by looking at T- and B-cell numbers, to distinguish cases of severe combined immunodeficiency on an early blood sample. More subtle defects of the immune system leading to interstitial pneumonia include CD40 ligand deficiency, Wiskott-Aldrich syndrome, and MHC class II antigen deficiency. Diagnosis of these conditions requires more specialized tests. If possible, any lymphocyte tests should be sent to the laboratory before corticosteroid treatment is introduced into therapeutic regimes so as to make interpretation of the results easier.

Sepsis

Septicemia and deep-seated bacterial or fungal infections may be indicative of an underlying immunodeficiency state (84). In such circumstances the manifestation of the illness may be atypical (for example, patients with complement abnormalities may have become less shocked and ill during meningococcal sepsis). Unusual organisms may be found. Investigation may be initially misleading, with lymphopenia common as a result of the sepsis and sometimes also neutropenia, especially in neonates. Staphylococcal, gram-negative bacillary and fungal sepsis are more likely to be indicative of innate immune defects, especially neutrophil problems, while capsulate bacteria such as *Streptococcus pneumoniae* predominate in antibody deficient patients. The use of immunoglobulin for sepsis in the absence of any indication of preexisting immunodeficiency is not generally recommended, but if antibody deficiency is present, early use of immunoglobulin and watching for reactions (more common in febrile, septic patients) should be undertaken.

Meningitis

An underlying immunodeficiency should be suspected in a number of situations:

1. The infection is caused by an unusual organism, including those unusual serogroups of meningococcus which are more likely to cause infection in complement deficient individuals (see page 16).
2. The infection occurs at an unusual age for a particular organism, for example, group B streptococcal infection occurring after 3 months of age or salmonella meningitis occurring in children beyond the age of 6 months (unless the patient has sickle cell anemia).
3. There is a previous history of other invasive bacterial disease.
4. There is a history of recurrent meningitis. If caused by meningococcus, complement factor deficiencies must be excluded. As described above (see page 50), excluding complement deficiency may only be possible after a period of convalescence. Defects in the integuments surrounding the central nervous system also predispose to recurrent meningitis.

Immunoglobulin deficiency predisposes to meningitis, with any of the polysaccharide capsulated organisms, and can be excluded on a sample collected during the acute illness provided that blood products have not already been given.

Gastrointestinal Infections

Severe enteropathy is a common presenting feature of combined immunodeficiencies. It may be associated with infections such as viral gastroenteritis,

TABLE **1.13.** Possible immunologic interventions in the intensive care unit

Infection/underlying immunologic defect	Intervention	Comments
Neutropenic sepsis	G-CSF	Shortens period of neutropenia where this is secondary to chemotherapy; may induce some neutrophil production in primary neutropenias
Neutropenic sepsis	Neutrophil infusions	Most useful where there is local infection such as in the soft tissues (see page 23)
Sepsis in the presence of neutrophil defects, e.g., chronic granulomatous disease	Interferon-γ	Has been shown to be of benefit in CGD with deep-seated bacterial or fungal infections
Sepsis in the presence of neutrophil defects, e.g., chronic granulomatous disease	G-CSF	Enhances neutrophil function and prolongs neutrophil survival
Sepsis in complement deficient patients	Fresh frozen plasma	Provides all the complement factors but may exacerbate inflammation if given during the acute phase of the illness
Sepsis in complement deficient patients	MBL concentrates	Not yet available but theoretically helpful in MBL-deficient patients
Immunoglobulin deficiency with bacterial infection	Intravenous immunoglobulin infusion	Administration during acute bacterial sepsis may lead to reactions or clinical deterioration due to complement fixation
Viral infection in immunoglobulin deficient patients	IVIG	Evidence of benefit in severe enteroviral infections in both immunocompetent and immunodeficient patients and some evidence for usefulness in acute CMV infections in immunocompromised hosts
Central nervous system enteroviral infection in immunodeficient patients	Intrathecal immunoglobulin	Anecdotal reports of benefit in immunoglobulin-deficient patients with chronic enteroviral encephalitis
EBV infection in immunodeficient patients	Anti-CD20 monoclonal (rituximab)	Eliminates B cells, which are the main site of EBV replication
Cell mediated immunodeficiency with viral infections	Adoptive immunotherapy with specific cytotoxic T lymphocytes: EBV-specific CTLs CMV-specific CTLs	Little experience; can exacerbate disease by causing tissue destruction as part of cytotoxic viral killing; under trial for use prophylactically in high risk situations such as bone marrow transplantation

TABLE 1.13. *Continued*

Infection/underlying immunologic defect	Intervention	Comments
Cell-mediated immune defects with opportunistic infections	Interferon-γ	May help in killing intracellular organisms such as mycobacteria, salmonella, and fungal infections
Lymphoproliferative disease	Anti-CD20 monoclonal antibody (rituximab)	Eliminates proliferating B cells driven by Epstein-Barr virus
Lymphoproliferative disease	EBV cytotoxic T lymphocytes	May cause tissue destruction; see above

CTL, cytotoxic T lymphocyte; G-CSF, granulocyte colony-stimulating factor; IVIG, intravenous immunoglobulin; MBL, mannan-binding lectin.

cryptosporidiosis, giardiasis, or bacterial disease, but often it is an apparently noninfective immunoregulatory disorder. Diagnostic tests are particularly difficult in this group of patients because, in the presence of severe enteropathy, protein loss may lead to secondary hypogammaglobulinemia and, in the more severe cases, secondary lymphopenia.

Conclusion

Consideration of the immunologic status of children and newborn infants is of crucial importance in optimizing management in the intensive care setting. Immunity to infection may be compromised as a result of immaturity or genetic disorder or variability. It may also become compromised as result of the underlying disease itself or its treatment, including intensive care management. Awareness of these issues aids in prompt diagnosis of congenital immunodeficiencies and allows early interventions to protect the child as much as possible.

References

1. Hoffman JA, Kafatos FC, Janeway JR, Ezekowitz RA. Phylogenetic perspectives in innate immunity. Science 1999;284:1313–1318.
2. Turner MW. The role of mannose-binding lectin in health and disease. Mol Immunol 2003;40:423–429.
3. Rosenzweig SD, Holland SM. Defects in the interferon gamma and interleukin-12 pathways. Immunol Rev 2005;203:38–47.
4. Ku CL, Yang K, Bustamante J, et al. Inherited disorders of human Toll-like receptor signaling: immunological implications. Immunol Rev 2005;203:10–20.

5. Whiteside TL, Herberman RB. Role of human natural killer cells in health and disease. Clin Diagn Lab Immunol 1994;1:125–133.
6. Le Deist F, Poinsignon C, Moshous D, Fischer A, de Villartay JP. Artemis sheds new light on V(D)J recombination. Immunol Rev 2004;200:142–155.
7. Goronzy JJ, Weyand CM. T cell development and receptor diversity during aging. Curr Opin Immunol 2005;17:468–475.
8. Wang L, Kamath A, Das H, Li L, Bukowski JF. Antibacterial effect of human V gamma 2V delta 2 T cells in vivo. J Clin Invest 2001;108:1349–1357.
9. Kaufmann SH. Gamma/delta and other unconventional T lymphocytes: what do they see and what do they do? Proc Natl Acad Sci U S A 1996;93:2272–2279.
10. Kohler PF, Farr RS. Elevation of cord over maternal IgG immunoglobulin: evidence for an active placental IgG transport. Nature 1966;210:1070–1071.
11. Thorarinsdottir HK, Ludviksson BR, Vikingsdottir T, et al. Childhood levels of immunoglobulins and mannan-binding lectin in relation to infections and allergy. Scand J Immunol 2005;61:466–474.
12. Buckley RH, Dees SC, O'Fallon WM. Serum immunoglobulins. I. Levels in normal children and in uncomplicated childhood allergy. Pediatrics 1968;41:600–611.
13. Buffolano W, Lappalainen M, Hedman L, et al. Delayed maturation of IgG avidity in congenital toxoplasmosis. Eur J Clin Microbiol Infect Dis 2004;23:825–830.
14. Michie C, Harvey D. Can expression of CD45RO, a T-cell surface molecule, be used to detect congenital infection? Lancet 1994;343:1259–1260.
15. Lambert PH, Liu M, Siegrist CA. Can successful vaccines teach us how to induce efficient protective immune responses? Nat Med 2005;11:S54–62.
16. Ota MO, Vekemans J, Schlegel-Haueter SE, et al. Hepatitis B immunisation induces higher antibody and memory Th2 responses in new-borns than in adults. Vaccine 2004;22:511–519.
17. Weller S, Braun MC, Tan BK, et al. Human blood IgM "memory" B cells are circulating splenic marginal zone B cells harboring a prediversified immunoglobulin repertoire. Blood 2004;104:3647–3654.
18. Borrow R, Goldblatt D, Andrews N, et al. Antibody persistence and immunological memory at age 4 years after meningococcal group C conjugate vaccination in children in the United kingdom. J Infect Dis 2002;186:1353–1357.
19. Finn A, Heath P. Conjugate vaccines. Arch Dis Child 2005;90:667–669.
20. Goldblatt D, Turner MW, Levinsky RJ. Branhamella catarrhalis: antigenic determinants and the development of the IgG subclass response in childhood. J Infect Dis 1990;162:1128–1135.
21. Tiller TL Jr, Buckley RH. Transient hypogammaglobulinemia of infancy: review of the literature, clinical and immunologic features of 11 new cases, and long-term follow-up. J Pediatr 1978;92:347–353.
22. Roberton DM, Colgan T, Ferrante A, Jones C, Mermelstein N, Sennhauser F. IgG subclass concentrations in absolute, partial and transient IgA deficiency in childhood. Pediatr Infect Dis J 1990;9:S41–45.
23. Affentranger P, Morell A, Spath P, Seger R. Registry of primary immunodeficiencies in Switzerland. Immunodeficiency 1993;4:193–195.
24. Stray-Pedersen A, Abrahamsen TG, Froland SS. Primary immunodeficiency diseases in Norway. J Clin Immunol 2000;20:477–485.
25. Figuero J, Densen P. Infectious diseases associated with complement deficiencies. Clin Microb Rev 1991;4:359–395.

26. Tedesco F, Nurnberger W, Perissutti S. Inherited deficiencies of the terminal complement components. Int Rev Immunol 1993;10:51–64.

27. Fijen CAP, Kuijper EJ, Bulte MT, et al. Assessment of complement deficiency in patients with meningococcal disease in the Netherlands. Clin Infect Dis 1999;28:98–105.

28. Klein NJ. Mannose-binding lectin: do we need it? Mol Immunol 2005;42:919–924.

29. Fidler KJ, Wilson P, Davies JC, Turner MW, Peters MJ, Klein NJ. Increased incidence and severity of the systemic inflammatory response syndrome in patients deficient in mannose-binding lectin. Intensive Care Med 2004;30:1438–1445.

30. Klein NJ, Kilpatrick DC. Is there a role for mannan/mannose-binding lectin (MBL) in defence against infection following chemotherapy for cancer? Clin Exp Immunol 2004;138:202–204.

31. Hibberd ML, Sumiya M, Summerfield JA, Booy R, Levin M. Association of variants of the gene for mannose-binding lectin with susceptibility to meningococcal disease. Meningococcal Research Group. Lancet 1999;353:1049–1053.

32. Picard C, Casanova JL. Inherited disorders of cytokines. Curr Opin Pediatr 2004;16:648–658.

33. Hawn TR, Dunstan SJ, Thwaites GE, et al. A polymorphism in Toll-interleukin 1 receptor domain containing adaptor protein is associated with susceptibility to meningeal tuberculosis. J Infect Dis 2006;194:1127–1134.

34. Picard C, Puel A, Bonnet M, et al. Pyogenic bacterial infections in humans with IRAK-4 deficiency. Science 2003;299:2076–2079.

35. Badolato R, Fontana S, Notarangelo LD, Savoldi G. Congenital neutropenia: advances in diagnosis and treatment. Curr Opin Allergy Clin Immunol 2004;4: 513–521.

36. Dale DC, Person RE, Bolyard AA, et al. Mutations in the gene encoding neutrophil elastase in congenital and cyclic neutropenia. Blood 2000;96:2317–2322.

37. Klein C, Grudzian M, Appaswamy G, et al. HAX 1 deficiency causes autosomal recessive severe congenital neutropenia (Kostmann disease). Nat Genet 2007;39: 86–92.

38. Haurie C, Dale DC, Mackey MC. Occurrence of periodic oscillations in the differential blood counts of congenital, idiopathic, and cyclical neutropenic patients before and during treatment with G-CSF. Exp Hematol 1999;27:401–409.

39. Lalezari P, Khorshidi M, Petrosova M. Autoimmune neutropenia of infancy. J Pediatr 1986;109:764–769.

40. Anderson DC, Smith CW. Leukocyte adhesion deficiencies. In: Scriver CR, Beaudet AL, Sly WS, Valle D, eds. The Metabolic and Molecular Basis of Inherited Disease, 8th ed. New York: McGraw Hill, 2001:4829–4856.

41. Inwald D, Davies EG, Klein N. Demystified . . . adhesion molecule deficiencies. Mol Pathol 2001;54:1–7.

42. Langer-Gould A, Atlas SW, Green AJ, Bollen AW, Pelletier D. Progressive multifocal leukoencephalopathy in a patient treated with natalizumab. N Engl J Med 2005;353:375–381.

43. Bedlow AJ, Davies EG, Moss AL, Rebuck N, Finn A, Marsden RA. Pyoderma gangrenosum in a child with congenital partial deficiency of leucocyte adherence glycoproteins. Br J Dermatol 1998;139:1064–1067.

44. Etzioni A, Gershoni-Baruch R, Pollack S, Shehadeh N. Leukocyte adhesion deficiency type II: long-term follow-up. J Allergy Clin Immunol 1998;102:323–324.

45. Ambruso DR, Knall C, Abell AN, et al. Human neutrophil immunodeficiency syndrome is associated with an inhibitory Rac2 mutation. Proc Natl Acad Sci U S A 2000;97:4654–4659.
46. Winkelstein JA, Marino MC, Johnston RB Jr, et al. Chronic granulomatous disease. Report on a national registry of 368 patients. Medicine (Baltimore) 2000;79:155–169.
47. Elebute M, Massey E, Benjamin S, Stanworth S, Navarrete C, Lucas G. Clinical Guidelines for the use of granulocyte transfusions. Report of the Granulocyte Working Group of the National Blood Service. http://www.blood.co.uk/HOSPITALS/guidelines/pdf/clinical_guidelines.pdf.
48. Winkelstein JA, Marino MC, Lederman HM, et al. X-linked agammaglobulinemia: report on a United States registry of 201 patients. Medicine (Baltimore) 2006;85: 193–202.
49. Chapel HM. Consensus on diagnosis and management of primary antibody deficiencies. BMJ 1994;308:581–585.
50. Quartier P, Debre M, De Blic J, et al. Early and prolonged intravenous immunoglobulin replacement therapy in childhood agammaglobulinemia: a retrospective survey of 31 patients. J Pediatr 1999;134:589–596.
51. Cunningham CK, Bonville CA, Ochs HD, et al. Enteroviral meningoencephalitis as a complication of X-linked hyper IgM syndrome. J Pediatr 1999;134:584–588.
52. Conley ME, Broides A, Hernandez-Trujillo V, et al. Genetic analysis of patients with defects in early B-cell development. Immunol Rev 2005;203:216–234.
53. Cunningham-Rundles C, Bodian C. Common variable immunodeficiency: clinical and immunological features of 248 patients. Clin Immunol 1999;92:34–48.
54. Grimbacher B, Schaffer AA, Peter HH. The genetics of hypogammaglobulinemia. Curr Allergy Asthma Rep 2004;4:349–358.
55. Erdos M, Durandy A, Marodi L. Genetically acquired class-switch recombination defects: the multi-faced hyper-IgM syndrome. Immunol Lett 2005;97:1–6.
56. Mechanic LJ, Dikman S, Cunningham-Rundles C. Granulomatous disease in common variable immunodeficiency. Ann Intern Med 1997;127:613–617.
57. Stiehm ER. Human intravenous immunoglobulin in primary and secondary antibody deficiencies. Pediatr Infect Dis J 1997;16:696–707.
58. Gardulf A, Nicolay U, Asensio O, et al. Rapid subcutaneous IgG replacement therapy is effective and safe in children and adults with primary immunodeficiencies—a prospective, multi-national study. Clin Immunol 2006;26:177–185.
59. Soldatou A, Davies EG. Respiratory virus infections in the immunocompromised host. Paediatr Respir Rev 2003;4:193–204.
60. Fischer A, Le Deist F, Hacein-Bey-Abina S, et al. Severe combined immunodeficiency. A model disease for molecular immunology and therapy. Immunol Rev 2005;203:98–109.
61. Antoine C, Muller S, Cant A, et al. Long term survival and haematopoietic stem cell transplantation for immunodeficiencies: a survey of the European experience 1968–1999. Lancet 2003;361:553–560.
62. Thrasher AJ, Gaspar HB, Baum C, et al. Gene therapy: X-SCID transgene leukaemogenicity. Nature 2006;443:E5–6.
63. Aiuti A, Slavin S, Aker M, et al. Correction of ADA-SCID by stem cell gene therapy combined with nonmyeloablative conditioning. Science 2002;296:2410–2413.
64. Rao K, Amrolia PJ, Jones A, et al. Improved survival after unrelated donor bone marrow transplantation in children with primary immunodeficiency using a reduced-intensity conditioning regimen. Blood 2005;105:879–885.

65. Levy J, Espanol-Boren T, Thomas C, et al. Clinical spectrum of X-linked hyper-IgM syndrome. Pediatrics 1997;131:47–54.

66. Markert ML, Sarzotti M, Ozaki DA, et al. Thymus transplantation in complete DiGeorge syndrome: immunologic and safety evaluations in 12 patients. Blood 2003;102:1121–1130.

67. Thrasher AJ, Kinnon C. The Wiskott-Aldrich syndrome. Clin Exp Immunol 2000;120:2–9.

68. Grimbacher B, Holland SM, Puck JM. Hyper-IgE syndromes. Immunol Rev 2005;203:244–250.

69. Grimbacher B, Schaffer AA, Holland SM, et al. Genetic linkage of hyper-IgE syndrome to chromosome 4. Am J Hum Genet 1999;65:735–744.

70. Nowak-Wegrzyn A, Crawford TO, Winkelstein JA, Carson KA, Lederman HM. Immunodeficiency and infections in ataxia-telangiectasia. J Pediatr 2004;144:505–511.

71. The International Nijmegen Breakage Syndrome Study Group. Nijmegen breakage syndrome. Arch Dis Child 2000;82:400–406.

72. Ueda I, Ishii E, Morimoto A, Ohga S, Sako M, Imashuku S. Correlation between phenotypic heterogeneity and gene mutational characteristics in familial hemophagocytic lymphohistiocytosis (FHL). Pediatr Blood Cancer 2006;46:482–488.

73. Horne A, Janka G, Maarten Egeler R, et al. Histiocyte Society. Haematopoietic stem cell transplantation in haemophagocytic lymphohistiocytosis. Br J Haematol 2005;129:622–630.

74. Valenti LM, Mathieu J, Chancerelle Y, et al. High levels of endogenous nitric oxide produced after burn injury in rats arrest activated T lymphocytes in the first G1 phase of the cell cycle and then induce their apoptosis. Exp Cell Res 2005; 306:150–167.

75. Ni Choileain N, MacConmara M, Zang Y, Murphy TJ, Mannick JA, Lederer JA. Enhanced regulatory T cell activity is an element of the host response to injury. J Immunol 2006;176:225–236.

76. Marie JC, Kehren J, Trescol-Biemont MC, et al. Mechanism of measles virus-induced suppression of inflammatory immune responses. Immunity 2001;14:69–79.

77. Boumpas DT, Chrousos GP, Wilder RL, Cupps TR, Balow JE. Glucocorticoid therapy for immune-mediated diseases: basic and clinical correlates. Ann Intern Med 1993;119:1198–1208.

78. Callenbach PM, Jol-Van Der Zijde CM, Geerts AT, et al. Dutch Study of Epilepsy in Childhood. Immunoglobulins in children with epilepsy: the Dutch Study of Epilepsy in Childhood. Clin Exp Immunol 2003;132:144–151.

79. Hansen K, Singer DB. Asplenic-hyposplenic overwhelming sepsis: postsplenectomy sepsis revisited. Pediatr Dev Pathol 2001;4:105–121.

80. Working Party British Society Haematology. Management of splenectomised patients. BMJ 1996;312:430.

81. Stiehm ER, Casillas AM, Finkelstein JZ, et al. Slow subcutaneous human intravenous immunoglobulin in the treatment of antibody immunodeficiency: use of an old method with a new product. J Allergy Clin Immunol 1998;101:848–849.

82. Ohlsson A, Lacy JB. Intravenous immunoglobulin for preventing infection in preterm and/or low-birth-weight infants. Cochrane Database Syst Rev 2004;(1): CD000361.

83. Alejandria MM, Lansang MA, Dans LF, Mantaring JB. Intravenous immunoglobulin for treating sepsis and septic shock. Cochrane Database Syst Rev 2002;(1): CD001090.

84. Orange JS. Congenital immunodeficiencies and sepsis. Pediatr Crit Care Med 2005;6: S99–S107.

Further Reading

Cant AJ, Cale C, Gennery A, Davies EG. Immunodeficiency. In: McIntosh N, Campbell AG, eds. Forfar and Arneil's Textbook of Paediatrics, 6th ed. Edinburgh: Churchill Livingstone, 2003:1255–1295.

Steihm ER, Ochs HD, Winkelstein JA, eds. Immunologic Disorders in Infants and Children. Philadelphia: Elsevier Saunders, 2004.

2
Infections in the Critically Ill Neonate

Cheryl Jones

Epidemiology and Pathogenesis

Incidence

Approximately 1 in 200 to 1 in 1000 live-born infants in the developed world develop an episode of severe sepsis during their stay in the neonatal nursery (1–3). The incidence of neonatal sepsis is much higher in the developing world, where access to antenatal care, neonatal intensive care, hygiene, and appropriate antibiotics is limited (4,5). The risk of neonatal sepsis increases as birth weight and gestational age decrease (3,6). Therefore, the reported incidence rates for neonatal sepsis vary with the proportion of low birth weight infants in the population studied. Infants with very low birth weight (VLBW; <1500 g) represent just over 1% of all live births in the United States, yet approximately 20% of them develop an episode of severe sepsis during their time in the neonatal intensive care unit (NICU) (2). In contrast, the risk of sepsis in term infants is only 0.1% (3). Rates of neonatal sepsis do not vary with sex, but do vary with multiple births; preterm twins have higher attack rates for sepsis than preterm singletons (7).

Definitions of Early- Versus Late-Onset Sepsis and Focal Infections

Infections that arise in the first few days of life have a different set of causative organisms and a different pathogenesis to infections that arise beyond this period, so they are often considered separately. Early-onset neonatal sepsis (EONS) is usually defined as onset of infection in the first 48 to 72 hours of life, and late-onset neonatal sepsis (LONS) as onset of infection after 3 days (8,9). Some authorities extend the cut-off point between the two categories to 7 days of life (8). Late-onset neonatal sepsis may be further divided into late-onset neonatal sepsis (LLONS; >3 months of life) and very late onset neonatal sepsis (VLONS: >6 months of life) (8). The incidence of EONS is approximately 10-fold lower than LONS, but the mortality rate is higher (15% to 30% versus 10% to 20%, respectively) (2,3,10,11).

Microorganisms that Cause Neonatal Sepsis

As our ability to promote survival of extremely preterm and extremely low birth weight infants has improved, the incidence of neonatal sepsis has increased and the causative organisms have expanded from predominantly virulent bacteria to include fungal pathogens and viruses (1–3).

The National Institute of Child Health and Human Development (NICHD) in the United States has reported surveillance data of the pathogens associated with sepsis in the VLBW infant for the last decade through its Neonatal Research Network (2,11). Table 2.1 summarizes the distribution of organisms that caused EONS and LONS from this group compared to data from a survey of neonatal sepsis in all infants admitted to a NICU in United Kingdom from 1996 to 2000 (2,3,11). The type of causative organisms is similar to those reported elsewhere, including Australia (12), although as shown in Table 2.1, regional differences exist between the relative contribution made by gram-positive and gram-negative organisms to each category of neonatal sepsis. In the United States, the incidence of EONS due to group B streptococci has significantly decreased since the early 1990s, possibly due to the increased use of intrapartum antibiotics for suspected maternal sepsis, resulting in predominance of EONS due to gram-negative organisms in the latter part of the decade (13).

Gram-positive organisms are the predominant cause of LONS in most parts of the world, comprising approximately 70% of the total infections in this group, followed by gram-negative organisms (20%) (3,11). Fungi are increasingly recognized as important neonatal pathogens. They contribute to approximately 2% and 10% of cases of EONS and LONS, respectively, and occur predominantly in VLBW infants (3,11).

Pathogenesis

Early-onset neonatal sepsis is usually caused by organisms acquired from the mother's genital tract. The newborn may become infected by transplacental passage of organisms due to maternal bacteremia or viremia, or by ingesting or inhaling infected amniotic fluid, which then translocates across the respiratory epithelium into the bloodstream. Late-onset neonatal sepsis, in contrast, is caused by organisms that have colonized the infant from either the mother's genital tract or the environment, which then invade through a breach in the mucoepithelium (e.g., caused by an intravascular catheter, necrotizing enterocolitis, or gut ischemia). Early-onset neonatal sepsis affects both sexes equally, whereas males have a higher attack rate for LONS (2,3,6).

Low birth weight is the single most important independent risk factor for neonatal sepsis, followed by preterm delivery (9). Some features of the immune system are relatively immature at birth, which make the newborn, especially preterm infants, more susceptible to infection (14,15). These features are

TABLE 2.1. Distribution of pathogens that cause neonatal sepsis

Type of sepsis	EONS	LONS	EONS	LONS
Country	United States	United States	United Kingdom	United Kingdom
Year	2002–2003		1996–2000	1996–2000
Study population	VLBW infants in registry	VLBW infants in registry who survived >72 hours	All infants admitted to NICU at district hospital	All infants admitted to NICU at district hospital
Reference	2	11	3	3
No. infants in study population	5999	6215	1612	1612
No. infections reported	102	1313	24	100
Organism	Distribution of isolates (%)[a]		Infants with each isolate (%)[b]	
Gram-negative organisms	**53**	**18**	**13**	**19**
E. coli	41	5	0	9
Hemophilus influenzae	2		NS	NS
Citrobacter species	3		NS	NS
Enterobacter species	4	3	4	0
Acinetobacter anitratus	1		NS	NS
Pseucodomonas aeruginosa	1	3	0	1
Klebsiella species	1	4	0	1
Serratia species	0	2		
Other coliform	0	1	4	2
Gram-positive organisms	**45**	**70**	**95**	**89**
Group B Streptococcus	12	2	50	1
Streptococcus viridans	2	NS	4	3
Streptococcus milleri (intermedius)	NS	NS	4	1
Group A Streptococcus	1	NS	NS	NS
Group D Streptococcus	2	NS	0	1
Streptococcus pneumoniae	1	NS	4	0
Listeria monocytogenes	2	NS	NS	NS
CoNS[c]	15	48	46	83
Staphylococcus aureus	3	8	8	9
Bacillus species	4	NS	NS	NS
Enterococcus species	NS	3	NS	NS
Other gram-positive cocci	4	9	4	8
Fungi	**2**	**12**	**0**	**5**
Candida albicans	2	6	0	5
Candida parapsilosis	0	4	0	5
Other fungi	0	2	0	0

[a]Reported fraction of percentage rounded up to nearest whole digit.
[b]Infants may have more than one infection.
[c]Contaminants excluded.
EONS, early-onset sepsis; LONS, late-onset sepsis; CoNS, coagulase negative staphylococci; NS, not specified; VLBW, very low birth weight; NICU, neonatal intensive care.

TABLE **2.2.** Comparison of immature host defenses in the preterm and sick term infant

Mucoepithelial barriers	Preterm	Term
Immature skin with high insensible water loss	+ +	−
Parenteral nutrition promotes bacterial proliferation	+	+
Colonization of endotracheal and NG tubes, intravascular catheters	+	+
Biofilms on plastic catheters facilitate adhesion of pathogens	+	+
Decreased gastric acid production reduced intestinal absorption	+	−/+
Complement		
Lower levels until third trimester	+	−
Neutrophils		
Decreased bone marrow reserve	+ +	−
Immature neutrophil oxidative burst	+ +	+
Decreased gelatinase and specific granules	+ +	+
Decreased adherence and signalling	+ +	+/−
Monocytes		
Diminished number and function	+ +	−
Decreased adherence	+ +	+
Decreased opsonization and phagocytosis in response to IFN-γ	+ +	+
Diminished G-CSF production	+ +	+/−
Decreased IL-6 and IL-12 responses to lipopolysaccharide	+	+
Decreased TNF-α/ IFN-γ in response to TLR activation	+	+
Dendritic cells		
Decreased production of type 1 interferons	+	+
Decreased IL-12/ IL-23 production	+	+
NK cells		
Deficient NK cytotoxicity	+	+
Reduced IFN-γ production	+	+
T-cells, B-cells		
Decreased T-cell function and greater signalling requirements	+	+
Th2 polarization of CD4+ T-cell responses	+	+
Decreased numbers of lymphocytes in gastrointestinal tract	+	−
Decreased production of antibodies by B cells	+ +	−

G-CSF, granulocyte colony-stimulating factor IFN, interferon; IL, interleukin NG, nasogastric; NK, natural killer; TNF, tumor necrosis factor; TLR, toll like receptor.

summarised in Table 2.2. Factors that breach the normal mucoepithelial defenses, however, are more important risk factors in mature infants than immune incompetence. Critically ill infants on the NICU have the same risk factors as any child or adult admitted to an intensive care unit. These include the presence of endotracheal tubes and suctioning, prolonged ventilation, parenteral nutrition, intravascular catheters, urinary catheters, colonization with multiresistant organisms, and the widespread use of broad-spectrum antibiotics.

Clinical Manifestations and Evaluation of a Septic Neonate

Diagnosis of neonatal sepsis requires a high index of suspicion because the signs of infection are often subtle in the early stages (9). Signs may include apnea, lethargy, poor color, reduced feed tolerance, vomiting, abdominal distention, hypotension, temperature instability (both hypothermia and hyperthermia), cyanosis, or respiratory distress. While virulent bacterial infections have a greater propensity to cause shock-like syndromes, some viral and fungal pathogens can also cause acute cardiorespiratory collapse (e.g., enterovirus, herpes simplex virus, and *Candida albicans*). Infants with infections acquired in utero (congenital infections) may present clinically with jaundice, petechiae, hepatosplenomegaly, respiratory distress, disseminated intravascular coagulation, skin rashes that may be maculopapular or pustular, skin scarring (cicatrization) microcephaly, intrauterine growth retardation, eye changes (chorioretinitis or microphthalmia, cataracts), limb atrophy, and cardiac murmurs.

The presentation of neonatal sepsis varies with the age of onset. Early-onset neonatal sepsis usually presents as a fulminant multisystem disease with pneumonia, whereas LONS usually presents as slowly progressive focal infection, most commonly meningitis. The microbiologic cause of focal infections in the neonatal period, such as meningitis, pneumonia, osteomyelitis, septic arthritis, endocarditis, skin rashes, and congenital infections, are listed in Table 2.3.

Evaluation of a newborn with suspected sepsis should include a careful evaluation of maternal risk factors for neonatal sepsis, such as the results of maternal antenatal group B screen, history of maternal fever, rash or other illness during pregnancy (16,17), and a review of possible postnatal exposure to infected family members or staff. A history of vomiting or reduced feed tolerance, diarrhea, seizures, temperature instability, or cough in the infant should be sought from the nursing staff and clinical observation (9). Infants should be examined for skin lesions, abscesses, rashes, or skin changes at the site of vascular catheters. In addition, careful examination for the presence of conjunctivitis, reduced limb movements or pain on movement, signs of respiratory distress, tender distended abdomen, reduced bowel sounds, jaundice, organomegaly, fullness of the anterior fontanelle, or focal neurological signs. Infants with meningitis rarely have nuchal rigidity.

Laboratory Diagnosis of Neonatal Infections

Infants with suspected sepsis should be promptly investigated and commenced on empiric antimicrobial therapy, as there can be rapid progression to clinical demise.

Rapid Diagnosis

Elevated total white cell count is an unreliable marker of neonatal sepsis; however, the neutrophil count is abnormal in two thirds of septic neonates, and can be either raised above age norms or very low in the severely ill infant (18). Examination of the blood film may reveal immature neutrophils (band forms or bands), also called a left shift, best viewed as an increased ratio of immature to mature neutrophils, with signs of toxic changes (granulations). The platelet

TABLE 2.3. Microbiological causes of focal infections in the neonatal period

Meningitis
Group B streptococci
Escherichia coli
Listeria monocytogenes
Streptococcus
Pneumoniae
Enterococci
Other streptococci
Proteus species
Neisseria meningitidis
Staphylococus aureus
Klebsiella species
Haemophilus influenzae
Pseudomonas species
Enterobacter species
Citrobacter species
Serratia species
Salmonella species
Other gram-negative
  bacilli
Anaerobes
Mycobacterium
  tuberculosis
Campylobacter species
Coagulase-negative
  staphylococci

Osteomyelitis/septic
  arthritis
Staphylococcus aureus
Group B *streptococci*
Gram negative bacilli
Eschericia coli
Pseudomonas species
Serratia species
Enterobacter sp.
Proteus species
Klebsiella species
Salmonella species
Haemophilus influenzae
Group A streptococci
Coagulase negative
  staphylococci
Neisseria gonorrheae
Treponema pallidum
Anaerobes
Fungi

Pneumonia
Congenital/ intrauterine
Toxoplasmosis
Rubella
CMV
HSV
Enteroviruses
Adenovirus
Treponema pallidum
Listeria monocytogene
Mycobacterium tuberculosis

Early onset (first week of life)
Group B streptococci
Haemophilus influenzae
Streptococcus viridans
Eschericia coli
Listeria monocytogenes
Staphylococcus aureus
Pseudomonas species
Streptococcus pneumoniae
Late onset
RSV
Influenza
Adenovirus
Streptococcus pneumoniae
Staphylococcus aureus
Other gram-positive bacilli
Gram-negative bacilli
Chlamydia trachomatis
Mycoplasma
Pneumocystis jirovecii (formerly
  carinii)

Skin and subcutaneous tissue
Staphylococcus aureus
Group B streptococci
Candida species
Pseudomonas aeruginosa, aeromonas
Coagulase-negative staphylococci
Group A streptococci
Gram-negative bacilli
Neisseria gonorrheae
Treponema pallidum
Anaerobes
Listeria monocytogenes
Haemophilus influenzae
Aspergillus and other filamentous
  fungi

Congenital infections
CMV
Rubella
Herpes simplex virus
Treponema pallidum
Toxoplasmosis
Enterovirus
Varicella zoster virus
Human immunodeficiency
Listeria monocytogenes
Mycobacterium tuberculosis

Eye infections
Common
Neisseria gonorrheae
Chlamydia trachomatis
Staphylococcus aureus
Pseudomonas aeruginosa
Rare
Group B streptococci
Group A streptococci
Streptococcus pneumoniae
Haemophilus influenzae
Meningococci
Herpes simplex virus
Echoviruses
Adenoviruses
Candida species
Mycoplasma hominis

Endocarditis
Staphylococcus aureus
Gram-negative bacilli
Klebsiella species
Enterobacter species
Eschericia coli
Pseudomonas species
Other gram-negative bacilli
Candida species
Group B streptococci and other
  streptococci
Coagulase-negative
  staphylococci

count may be low in severe bacterial sepsis, fungal infections, and in some congenital infections.

The nonspecific clinical and hematologic signs of sepsis in the newborn period have prompted the evaluation of a number of other laboratory tests for their ability to predict neonatal sepsis, including C-reactive protein (CRP), interleukin-6, interleukin-8, and procalcitonin. Of those currently available, elevated serum CRP has the best reported sensitivity (48% to 90%), specificity (13% to 93%) and negative predictive values (49% to 98%) for neonatal sepsis (reviewed in ref. 10). The sensitivity of CRP testing is unaffected by the patient's gestational age, but appears to be organism dependent (less sensitive for gram-positive organisms, especially coagulase negative staphylococci, than for gram-negative organisms). The CRP level is elevated within 12 to 24 hours after the onset of sepsis, and remains high for 2 to 7 days after successful treatment. Serial measurements may assist in the response of bony infection, and persistently elevated CRP may indicate persistent or focal infection (19).

Microbiologic Diagnosis

Despite the increasing availability of a number of adjunctive diagnostic tests, blood culture remains the gold standard for diagnosis of neonatal sepsis. Surface swabs, tracheal aspirates, and urine (LONS only) should be sent to the laboratory for culture. Many experts recommend performing cerebrospinal fluid (CSF) examination on all septic neonates, although some question its usefulness in infants with EONS (8). Neither culture of gastric aspirates nor the performance of antigen tests for group B streptococci on urine or CSF is routinely done, due to problems with high false-negative rates or high false-positive rates, respectively (20). Molecular diagnosis (e.g., by polymerase chain reaction, PCR) has proved valuable for the diagnosis of a number of viral infections in the newborn period, for example, meningitis caused by enterovirus or herpes simplex virus, or perinatal transmission of human immunodeficiency virus or hepatitis C virus. Diagnosis of neonatal candidemia by PCR for *Candida* is currently being developed, and appears promising but is not routinely available. Infants with respiratory symptoms should also have nasopharyngeal isolates sent to the lab for immunofluorescence and viral culture and PCR.

Microbiology of Neonatal Sepsis

Bacterial Causes of Neonatal Sepsis

Lancefield Group B β-Hemolytic Streptococcus

Group B β-hemolytic streptococcus (GBS) (*Streptococcus agalactiae*) was a major cause of neonatal sepsis up until the last decade, when efforts to prevent perinatal transmission of GBS by chemoprophylaxis have resulted in a decline in incidence (21). However, GBS still remains an important cause of infection in both preterm and term infants, with an overall incidence of approximately 0.5 to 0.75 cases per 1000 live births in the United States and the United Kingdom, respectively (21–23). Maternal GBS infection also remains a common cause of stillbirths (21).

Group B β-hemolytic streptococcus remains a major cause of neonatal meningitis, septicemia, and pneumonia. It can also cause focal infections such as osteomyelitis, septic arthritis, and cellulitis. The modes of presentation vary slightly between early- and late-onset GBS disease. While both groups can present with the full spectrum of GBS disease, a greater proportion of late-onset GBS disease presents with meningitis. The outcome of GBS disease also varies with age at onset; the overall mortality rate for early-onset GBS disease is approximately 4.7% compared to 2.8% for late-onset disease (21). Preterm infants, however, especially those of less than 33 weeks' gestation, have a higher mortality rate of up to 30% (21). The risk of long-term sequelae is higher in survivors of late-onset disease compared to early-onset disease, probably related to a greater percentage manifesting as meningitis (21).

Risk factors for early-onset GBS disease include gestational age (infants <34 weeks' gestation are at significantly greater risk of GBS septicemia), low levels of type-specific antibodies against GBS in both infants with disease and their mothers, prolonged rupture of membranes (>80 hours before delivery), maternal fever during labor (>38°C), maternal colonization or urinary tract infection with GBS during pregnancy or at delivery, and birth of a previous infant with invasive GBS disease (21). Rates of maternal vaginal GBS carriage range from approximately 7% to just over 20% in the developed world. Factors associated with increased maternal GBS carriage include diabetes, age <20 years, and racial origin; rates are higher in the developing world and in African-American women in the U.S. (21). Risk factors for late-onset GBS disease are less well described than for early-onset disease. Preterm gestation, maternal race, young maternal age, and maternal GBS colonization are also independent risk factors for late-onset GBS disease (21). Transmission of GBS in breast milk, between patients, and from colonized personnel in the NICU has also been reported (9).

Optimal treatment of invasive GBS disease remains high-dose parenteral penicillin G. Duration of therapy depends on the site of infection, with prolonged courses required for central nervous system (CNS) infection or bone disease. Relapse of GBS sepsis after discontinuation of antibiotic therapy or recurrence during therapy can occur usually because penicillin has failed to eradicate GBS colonization (24). The risk of GBS disease is also high in a twin whose other twin has proven GBS disease; therefore, empiric antibiotic therapy is usually recommended in this setting. Resistance of GBS to β-lactams has not yet become a problem. Clinical isolates from Japan, however, have shown intermediate sensitivity to penicillin (25). Group B β-hemolytic streptococcus resistance to clindamycin or erythromycin, particularly with type V GBS strains, is moderately high (30% to 40%) (21). This has important implications regarding chemoprophylaxis in penicillin-allergic women.

Intrapartum antibiotics given to maternal carriers of GBS disease have been clearly shown to prevent early-onset GBS disease (21). However, controversies remain regarding use of laboratory screening-based prevention strategies versus screening based on maternal risk factors for GBS sepsis. Determination of maternal GBS carriage at 35 to 37 weeks' gestation by combined vaginal and rectal swab, however, is now the preferred method of assigning chemoprophylaxis in many centers (26). Maternal disinfectants and the use of microbicides against GBS disease to prevent vaginal transmission to the newborn have not proven efficacious in clinical trials (21). Prevention of late-onset GBS disease does not appear to be influenced by intrapartum antibiotic prophylaxis. Further interventions have yet to be identified to prevent this condition.

Group B β-hemolytic streptococcus capsular polysaccharide conjugate vaccines are being developed, although vaccination of pregnant women remains a barrier to licensure (26). The serotype distribution of invasive GBS disease in neonates varies around the world, which is an important consideration in the formulation of multivalent GBS vaccines in the future. In Europe and North America, GBS serotypes III, Ia, and V are the dominant serotypes of invasive disease. Parts of Asia including Japan, however, have a different serotype distribution, with a high proportion of serotypes VIII and VI, which are uncommon elsewhere (25). Extracellular virulence factors of GBS include lipoteichoic acid, thick polysaccharide capsule, the enzyme C5a-ase, capsular sialic acid, cyclic adenosine monophosphate (cAMP) factor, and the carbohydrate exotoxin CM101 (27). Research into the potential roles of these factors in virulence may provide further additional targets for vaccine and antimicrobial therapy in the future.

Streptococci Other than Group B

Groups A, C, D, and G β-hemolytic streptococci and the α-hemolytic *streptococci* (*Streptococcus viridans* and *S. pneumoniae*) may cause disease in the newborn period less frequently than GBS, but can nevertheless result in significant morbidity and mortality (9).

Group A streptococci (*S. pyogenes*) was an important cause of puerperal sepsis early in the last century (1,9). It is now an infrequent cause of neonatal sepsis, but recent reports of increased virulence of the organism in older children and adults may see a reemergence of this organism as a neonatal pathogen (28). Neonatal infection may be acquired intrapartum or by postpartum exposure to a caregiver with group A streptococcal pharyngitis or asymptomatic carriage. A recent review of 24 cases of invasive neonatal group A streptococcal disease found that the majority were associated with the M1 serotype and concurrent maternal infection. Neonates presented with respiratory distress, pneumonia, or toxic shock syndrome (29).

Group C and G streptococci are known causes of puerperal sepsis, and are rare causes of neonatal sepsis or meningitis (9,30). Group D streptococci (*S. bovis* and *S. mitis*) are colonic flora that have also been occasionally reported to cause neonatal sepsis (9). They are usually sensitive to penicillins and cepha-losporins in contrast to the enterococci.

Viridans streptococci are being increasingly recognized as important newborn pathogens, both in Europe and in the United States (31). These organ-isms are mouth flora and are usually α-hemolytic on blood agar, although nonhemolytic forms are reported. Most neonates with viridans streptococcal disease are born to mothers with maternal obstetric risk factors for neonatal sepsis, and present with early-onset sepsis or meningitis, although some infants show no signs of disease (31).

S. pneumoniae is an uncommon but highly virulent cause of neonatal sepsis or meningitis. Historically, neonatal pneumococcal sepsis was reported to mostly occur in the preterm infant and present with early-onset pneumonia, sepsis, and or leukopenia, and have a mortality rate of up to 50% (1,9). A recent review of 29 cases of pneumococcal disease in the newborn, however, observed that infants now presented much later (2 to 3 weeks of age), and were more likely to be full term (32). The clinical features at presentation remained similar (pneumonia, meningitis, otitis media), but the overall mortality rate was lower (10%) (30).

Staphylococcus Aureus

S. aureus was a major cause of neonatal sepsis in the middle of the last century (1,9). Although its incidence has decreased, it too remains a highly virulent neonatal pathogen. *S. aureus* is a common cause of nosocomial infection in the neonatal nursery and is particularly associated with infections caused by intra-vascular catheters (33). Congenital *S. aureus* infections have been described and are usually associated with amniotic fluid sampling prior to delivery in preterm infants (9). Postnatally acquired *S. aureus* infections usually involve the skin, and may be complicated by deep tissue abscesses, bacteremia, a sepsis-like syndrome, endocarditis, bone and joint infection (osteomyelitis and septic arthritis), pneumonia, or meningitis in up to 20% of cases (33). *S. aureus* bac-teremia can be associated with endocarditis even in the absence of a heart murmur. For this reason, some experts recommend echocardiography, espe-cially in preterm infants with persistent *S. aureus* bacteremia and in those with a central venous catheter (9).

S. aureus can also cause toxin-mediated disease in the newborn period such as staphylococcal scalded skin syndrome, which is associated with exfoliative toxins A or B. These toxins mediate disease by binding to desmoglein-1, a skin glycoprotein that plays an important role in maintaining epithelial cell-to-cell adhesion (34). It is speculated that the toxins cause conformational change of this protein, resulting in disruption of intercellular adhesion. Toxins produced by *S. aureus* can also cause toxic shock syndrome (TSS). This is usually medi-ated by the toxin TSST-1, which can be produced by both methicillin-sensitive *S. aureus* (MSSA) and methicillin-resistant *S. aureus* (MRSA). Recently, a syn-drome described as neonatal toxic shock syndrome–like exanthematous disease

(NTED) has been described in a series of Japanese neonates associated with TSST-1 production by MRSA, and is associated with a macular papula exanthematous rash and thrombocytopenia in the first weeks of life (35). The mortality of MRSA sepsis in the neonate is higher (approximately 25%) compared with MSSA infections (approximately 10%), although early-onset MSSA infections also carry a high mortality (up to 40%) (36).

Most *S. aureus* strains now are penicillin-resistant but many retain sensitivity to extended-spectrum penicillins such as oxacillin, flucloxacillin, and naprocillin. Methicillin resistance has been increasingly reported in neonatal nurseries around the world (33). Eradication of MRSA outbreaks may be brought about by strict infection control measures such use of intranasal mupirocin and handwashing with an antimicrobial detergent. Treatment of infection caused by MRSA is with vancomycin. Vancomycin-resistant *S. aureus* is an emerging problem in older children and adults and can be treated with linezolid. Community-acquired methicillin resistant *S. aureus* (CA-MRSA) is being increasingly recognized and have been reported to cause severe necrotizing infections and toxic shock–like syndromes in older infants and children (35). These strains contain genes for Panton-Valentine leukocidin and staphylococcal enterotoxin K and often retain sensitivity to clindamycin (indicated by erythromycin sensitivity on antimicrobial susceptibility testing) (37). An outbreak of CA-MRSA skin and soft tissue infections in the NICU has been reported (38).

There is currently no licensed vaccine against *S. aureus*, although a polysaccharide capsule vaccine has been shown to halve the incidence of invasive *S. aureus* disease in adult hemodialysis patients (39). Safety and efficacy of this vaccine has yet to be tested in pediatric patients.

Coagulase-Negative Staphylococci

Coagulase negative staphylococci (CoNS) is the major cause of nosocomial sepsis in the NICU (40), and is the cause of over two thirds of all late-onset infections in the newborn (3,6,11). The CoNS species that cause neonatal disease include *S. epidermitis, S. haemolyticus, S. lugdenaecus, S. capitus, S. hominis, S. aunerei,* and *S. saprophyticus. S. epidermidis* is the commonest cause of CoNS infections, resulting in up to 80% of colonization and 90% of bloodstream infections (33). The incidence rate is approximately 3.5 episodes per 1000 live births. There is a slight male predominance of infections, and it is significantly associated with very low birth weight (<1500 g) prematurity (<30 weeks' gestation), and the use of parenteral alimentation (33).

Aside from bacteremia, which is usually associated with intravascular catheters, CoNS also causes meningitis and rarely deep-seated infections such as endocarditis and osteomyelitis. It is also the commonest cause of ventricular-peritoneal shunt infections, and can be a cause of urinary tract infections associated with indwelling catheters or urinary tract instrumentation, and conjunctivitis. Coagulase negative staphylococci have also been associated with necrotizing enterocolitis, but the significance of this is controversial (33). A recent review of invasive staphylococcal disease in infants noted that while there were few differentiating features between infants with CoNS and *S. aureus* neonatal infections at the time of presentation, CoNS has less of a tendency to disseminated disease and pyogenic complications and has lower morbidity in survivors than *S. aureus* (33).

Coagulase negative staphylococci are generally resistant to penicillins, extended-spectrum penicillins, and gentamicin. Empiric therapy usually requires vancomycin, although vancomycin resistance has been increasingly recognized (33). As neonates frequently do not display clinical signs of sepsis and CoNS is a common skin contaminant in blood culture collection, interpretation of clinically significant CoNS bacteremia often requires more than one positive blood culture or other laboratory evidence of infections such as elevated CRP levels. However, in the preterm infant with clinical signs of sepsis, directed antibiotic therapy should be commenced on receipt of the single blood culture. Persistent CoNS bacteremia despite vancomycin therapy should prompt investigation for heteroresistance to vancomycin and the use of other antimicrobials such as linezolid (41,42). Therapy of CoNS bacteremia associated with intravascular lines has been successfully eradicated without central line removal (41).

Mortality from CoNS infections is reportedly lower than late-onset infections due to *S. aureus* (2% versus approximately 30%, respectively), although in a recent review, there was no difference in attributable mortality (33). Given the relatively benign morbidity of CoNS infections, attempts to reduce the incidence of CoNS colonization using prophylactic antibiotics are generally not practiced.

Enterococci

Enterococci (*Enterococcus faecalis and E. faecium*) are an increasingly recognized cause of nosocomial neonatal sepsis and often occur concurrently with infections with other organisms (11,43). *E. faecalis* causes the majority of enterococcal infections, and usually presents as sepsis in association with an intravascular catheter or necrotizing enterocolitis. It may manifest as an early-onset infection with diarrhea or respiratory distress, or as a late-onset infection associated with apnea and circulatory collapse. Enterococci are also an uncommon but important cause of catheter-associated endocarditis and have been reported in association with subcutaneous abscesses and epidural abscess (9).

Enterococci are uniformly resistant to penicillin and cephalosporins. Empiric treatment of invasive enterococcal infections is usually with ampicillin or vancomycin in combination with an aminoglycoside such as gentamicin for bactericidal synergy. However, as enterococci may be resistant to ampicillin and now also to vancomycin, therapy should be reviewed when antimicrobial susceptibility results become available. Infections with vancomycin-resistant enterococci (VRE) are becoming increasingly important in adult intensive care units and chronic care institutions. However, the majority of enterococcal infections in the NICU continue to be caused by vancomycin-sensitive organisms (43), although VRE-related endocarditis has been reported in a preterm infant and successfully treated with linezolid (42). Outbreaks of VRE colonization in the neonatal nursery have also been reported and successfully controlled with strict attention to infection control measure, including cohorting of infected infants, restricting the use of vancomycin, and attention to environmental contamination including that of incubators (44).

Listeria Monocytogenes

L. monocytogenes is a gram-positive rod that is ubiquitous in the environment. On rare occasions, it may be vertically transmitted after symptomatic maternal infection (flu-like illness, general malaise, gastrointestinal upset, amnionitis, or brown-stained liquor) or asymptomatic maternal genital carriage in approximately one third of women with infected offspring (45). Ingestion of contaminated food such as unpasteurized milk or cheeses, processed or undercooked meats, and unwashed raw vegetables has been implicated as the source of maternal infection (45).

Early-onset *Listeria* infection is associated with prematurity and may present as pneumonia or as a sepsis-like syndrome, and is rarely associated with a pale, nodular rash called granuloma infantiseptica due to the presence of granulomas on histologic examination of a skin biopsy. It accounts for less than 5% of early-onset neonatal infections (45). Late-onset *Listeria* infection may be acquired after colonization during delivery or from postnatal environmental colonization. *Listeria* has rarely been associated with outbreaks in the NICU (9).

Treatment of neonatal listeriosis is with ampicillin and gentamicin for 2 weeks, and for a minimum of 3 weeks for meningitis. Delayed sterilization of the CSF in late-onset meningitis may require the addition of trimethoprim-sulfamethoxazole or rifampicin.

Escherichia Coli and Other Enteric Gram Negative Infections

Enteric gram-negative organisms (*E. coli, Klebsiella* sp., *Citrobacter, Serratia,* and *Enterobacter*) are the second most common cause of neonatal sepsis and meningitis in the NICU and are associated with a high mortality (3,6,13). The NICHD has reported a change in the causes of neonatal early-onset sepsis over the period early 1991 to 2000, from predominantly gram-positive organisms to predominantly gram-negative organisms (53%), most commonly *E. coli* (41%) (13). A recent review has confirmed that this change has been sustained, but the difference is not increasing (2). Intrapartum maternal antibiotic prophylaxis with ampicillin or penicillin to prevent GBS may partly account for this change; however, rates of late-onset gram-negative infections are also increasing according to some reports (3,13).

Neonates are colonized by gram-negative organisms from the maternal gastrointestinal tract at the time of delivery. Early-onset gram-negative sepsis results from invasion of these organisms into the neonatal bloodstream and across the blood–brain barrier. Postpartum, neonates are colonized with gram negatives from the hands of caregivers and the environment in the NICU. Late-onset gram-negative sepsis can occur from translocation of their gastrointestinal flora into the bloodstream after a gastrointestinal insult. *E. coli* virulence factors that increase invasiveness or translocation across the blood–brain barrier include determinants of the K1 capsule, OmpA and Ibe proteins that increase binding, and cytotoxic necrotizing factor-1 that augments transcystosis (46). These factors may play a more important role in the pathogenesis of sepsis in preterm infants than in term infants, in whom host factors that cause reduced resistance are more important (10). Metabolic abnormalities such as galactosemia and mucoepithelial defects are also associated with an increased risk of neonatal gram-negative sepsis.

E. coli resistance to ampicillin in invasive isolates from neonates is increasing and has also been attributed to maternal antibiotic prophylaxis (2), although the same trend has been observed in isolates acquired by women from the community (47). Overall, the mortality and morbidity of gram-negative infections is higher than with gram-positive infections (2).

Infections due to other gram-negative enteric organisms such as *Enterobacter*, *Klebsiella*, *Serratia*, and *Citrobacter* species are a less common cause of neonatal sepsis than *E. coli*, accounting for approximately 5% of bloodstream infections, and almost 9% of LONS in the U.S. (2,13). These organisms are increasingly associated with extended antibiotic resistance patterns to aminoglycosides, third-generation cephalosporins, and carbapenems and can result in life-threatening nosocomial outbreaks in the NICU. *Enterobacter sakazakii* and the *Citrobacter* species (*C. freundii*, *C. diversus*, and *C. koseri*) have a propensity to infect the CNS of neonates and can result in ventriculitis, brain abscesses, or cysts (9). *E. sakazakii* has been associated with nosocomial infections due to contaminated powdered formula in preterm infants (48). *Citrobacter* spp. are uncommon causes of neonatal infections, but are especially associated with cerebral abscesses and necrosis and poor neurologic outcome (49). They may be acquired intrapartum and present as early-onset sepsis, or be associated with NICU outbreaks in previously well babies. *Salmonella* species are an uncommon cause of sepsis in the NICU, but infants with *salmonella* bacteremia have a higher incidence of complicated infections such as meningitis or osteomyelitis than do other age groups (9).

Treatment of invasive gram-negative infections is usually with combination ampicillin and an aminoglycoside for bactericidal synergy. If gram-negative meningitis is suspected or proven, empiric therapy is with a third-generation cephalosporin plus an aminoglycoside. Therapy should be adjusted when the causative organism and antibiotic susceptibility spectrum is known. The presence of inducible β-lactamases in many gram-negative species may warrant a change from extended spectrum cephalosporins to carbapenems. The duration of therapy is usually 14 days for uncomplicated bacteremia and a minimum of 21 days for gram-negative meningitis. Intraventricular antibiotics have been used as adjunctive therapy for the treatment of gram-negative meningitis complicated by ventriculitis and cerebral abscesses, as it can be difficult to sterilize the cerebrospinal fluid in this setting. However, the efficacy of this intervention is not supported by data from current clinical trials (50). Intravenous immunoglobulin has been given both as prophylaxis and adjunctive therapy for neonatal sepsis, but a meta-analysis did not prove its efficacy for this indication, largely due to a lack of sufficiently powered clinical trials (51).

Pseudomonas Aeruginosa and Other Nonenteric Gram-Negative Bacteria

Infections due to *P. aeruginosa* usually present as late-onset neonatal sepsis and are predominantly nosocomially acquired (52). There are rare reports of *P. aeruginosa* sepsis presenting with pneumonia in the first 72 hours of life (52,53). Clinical presentations of *P. aeruginosa* in the newborn period include conjunctivitis that can rapidly develop into endophthalmitis (54), necrotic skin infections, bacteremia, meningitis, pneumonia and lung abscesses, diarrhea, and necrotizing enterocolitis (52). Bloodstream infections in the newborn period have been associated with necrotic lesions of the lips, nose, and mouth called noma. The source of the organism is often the hands of health care workers, especially those with long or artificial nails, or equipment in the NICU associated with aqueous solutions such as ventilator humidifiers, suction catheters, multiuse drug vials, and sinks (55). Treatment of *P. aeruginosa* infections is usually with an extended-spectrum penicillin or cephalosporin such as Timentin or ceftazadime, respectively, combined with an aminoglycoside. The mortality of *P. aeruginosa* sepsis is high, with rates up to 75% reported in infants with LONS (52).

Other nonenteric gram-negative rods such as *Stenotrophomonas maltophila*, *Acinetobacter* sp., and *Burkholderia cepacia* are being increasingly recognized as nosocomial pathogens in the pediatric setting including in the NICU (56). Prolonged broad-spectrum antibiotic therapy is a risk factor for infection with these organisms, and they often have extensive antibiotic resistance.

Haemophilus Influenzae and Neisseria Meningitidis

Nontypable *H. influenzae* is a well-recognized, but uncommon cause of maternal and EONS especially in preterm infants (9). It may present as fulminant sepsis or pneumonia, as soft tissue or joint infections, or as otitis media or externa and has a high mortality rate. *H. influenzae* type b (Hib) sepsis is rare in the newborn period, likely due to transfer of passive immunity from the mother. Hib disease is now also rare in later infancy and childhood since the introduction of the Hib vaccine in the early 1990s (57). *Neisseria meningitidis* is also an uncommon cause of infection in the first month of life, but continues to be a common cause of meningitis and sepsis in early infancy and childhood, with a peak attack rate of 3 to 5 months of age, largely due to serogroup B. A *meningococcal* serogroup C conjugate vaccine has been introduced into the routine childhood immunization schedule in the U.K., and has significantly reduced the incidence of *meningococcal* serogroup C disease in infancy (58).

Anaerobic Bacteria

Anaerobic infections (*Bacteroides fragilis*, *Clostridial* species, *Fusobacterium*, *Peptostreptococcus*, *Peptococcus*, *Veillonella*, and *Actinomyces*) are an occasional cause of bacterial sepsis in the NICU (9). They most commonly occur in preterm infants and may present as a fulminant early-onset sepsis after maternal chorioamnionitis, or later as skin or subcutaneous infections such as infected cephalhematomas, scalp infections following the use of scalp electrodes during labor, omphalitis, or necrotizing fasciitis, and occasionally as meningitis and shunt infections (59). Anaerobic infections also occur in the setting of compromised intestinal mucosa in the preterm infant, such as occurs with necrotizing enterocolitis. Mortality rates from anaerobic infections in the newborn period are high. One review of over 170 neonates with anaerobic infections reported a death rate of 26% (60). *Clostridia* and *Bacteroides* accounted for the majority of infections in this series.

If an anaerobe is suspected as a cause of neonatal sepsis, it is important to ensure specimens for culture are collected appropriately, and empiric antibiotic therapy is adjusted to include anaerobic cover. Blood cultures are sent to the laboratory in both aerobic and anaerobic blood culture bottles and pus or other specimens are sent anaerobically. Standard empiric antibiotic regimens for sepsis do not adequately cover many significant anaerobes (e.g., intravenous penicillin is the treatment of choice for *Clostridia* and most other anaerobes, but it has no efficacy against β-lactamase producing *Bacteroides*). Therefore, clindamycin, metronidazole, or a penicillin or carbapenem with a β-lactamase inhibitor (e.g., Timentin, or imipenem-cilastin) should be included in any empiric regimen for suspected anaerobic sepsis until culture results are known.

Tuberculosis

An infant can become infected with *Mycobacterium tuberculosis* in two ways: after vertical transmission from a mother with active tuberculosis (TB), or after postnatal exposure to a parent or other family member, visitor, staff member, or other infant on the NICU with TB. Congenital tuberculosis is a rare complication of maternal TB and usually occurs only in offspring of women with a TB pleural effusion, TB meningitis, or disseminated TB. Fetal infection can occur transplacentally via the umbilical vein or by inhalation or ingestion of infected amniotic fluid. A series of 29 infants with congenital TB reported the following signs and their respective frequencies at diagnosis: hepatosplenomegaly (76%), respiratory distress (72%), fever (48%), lymphadenopathy (38%), abdominal distention (24%), lethargy/irritability (21%), ear discharge (17%), and papular skin lesions (14%) (61). The chest radiograph was abnormal in the majority of cases, and none had a positive Mantoux test.

Cantwell and colleagues (61) proposed the following diagnostic criteria for congenital tuberculosis: the presence of a primary hepatic complex or caseating hepatic granulomas in first week of life, documented TB infection of the placenta or maternal genital tract, or, if these were lacking, confirmed TB in an infant in the first week of life or in an older infant where extrauterine infection can be excluded (i.e., child removed at birth from mother). Infants with suspected congenital TB should be investigated by CSF examination with mycobacterial stain and culture of CSF, blood, and early-morning gastric aspirate (62). Chest radiograph, liver function tests, placental histopathologic examination and culture, and abdominal ultrasound should also be performed, and the infant should be commenced on three- or four-drug empiric antituberculous therapy pending investigations in consultation with an infectious diseases physician. The duration of therapy and number of antituberculous agents required depends on the results of investigations, the sensitivity of the maternal isolate, and the results of follow-up chest radiograph and Mantoux evaluations at 3, 6, and 12 months of age. Some experts also suggest separating the infant from the mother to reduce the risk of postnatal exposure until the mother has been stabilized on active anti-TB therapy (62). Infants of mothers with TB can breast-feed (or be fed expressed breast milk if separated) if there is no evidence of maternal TB mastitis. Nosocomial transmission from infants with congenital tuberculosis is rare, although it has been proposed after use of contaminated respiratory equipment (63).

Postnatal exposure of infants in the NICU to open TB has been reported, and carries a low but not insignificant risk of infection in the infant (63). The risk of disseminated TB infection is much higher after exposure during infancy than in later childhood or adulthood. Outbreaks should be evaluated by the infection control service. Exposed infants should be commenced on prophylactic antituberculous therapy, which is usually isoniazid plus or minus rifampicin. Some offer prophylactic neonatal bacille Calmette-Guérin (BCG) vaccination as an alternative to drug therapy (62). The duration of prophylaxis should be discussed with an infectious diseases physician, but is usually a minimum of 6 months. Many experts recommend 9 months of prophylaxis after neonatal exposure irrespective of follow-up Mantoux results, due to a high false-negative rate of Mantoux testing in infants with latent TB infection, and a high rate of later dissemination in this age group (62). Infants should be followed up with Mantoux testing and chest radiograph at 3, 6, and 12 months postexposure.

Syphilis

Maternal syphilis in pregnancy can result in stillbirth, hydrops fetalis, preterm delivery, and an embryopathy. The clinical manifestations of congenital syphilis in the newborn include a characteristic pustular rash of the hands and feet, hepatosplenomegaly, petechiae, generalized edema, and pseudoparalysis of the limbs. Abnormal findings on investigation include radiologic evidence of long bone osteitis, haemolytic anemia, thrombocytopenia, and occasionally CSF abnormalities (positive CSF Venereal Disease Research Laboratory [VDRL], elevated CSF white cell count and protein). Up to two thirds of infants may be asymptomatic in the newborn period (9). Untreated, congenital syphilis progresses over infancy and later childhood to involve the CNS, teeth, eyes, skin, bones, and joints. Antenatal screening for maternal syphilis and appropriate treatment with parenteral penicillin for mothers with positive tests significantly reduces the risk of vertical transmission. Treatment of syphilis in pregnant women with antibiotics other than parenteral penicillin has not been shown to be effective at reducing infection in the fetus (64). The risk of vertical transmission is greatest in pregnant women with active syphilis (indicated by a positive maternal non-treponemal test—VDRL or rapid plasma reagent [RPR]), and in those in whom penicillin therapy was not completed up to 3 weeks before delivery.

Serologic testing for treponemal immunoglobulin M (IgM) in the newborn should be performed on the infant's peripheral blood. Cord blood should not be used due to a high rate of maternal contamination. Detection of treponemal pallidum particle agglutination (TPPA) IgG or fluorescent treponemal antibody absorption (FTA-ABS) IgG in the newborn reflects passive maternal transfer of antibody (64). If the risk of vertical transmission is low, that is, the mother received adequate antenatal penicillin therapy, the maternal RPR/VDRL is not elevated, the infant is clinically normal at birth, and can be reliably followed up after birth, many clinicians would not perform further investigations and would await the results of serology to evaluate the need for further investigation and penicillin therapy for the infant. However, if any of these conditions are not fulfilled, or if the infant has positive treponemal IgM serology, the infant should have a CSF examination, long bone and chest x-ray, full blood count, liver function tests, and histopathologic assessment of the placenta, and should be treated with a full 10-day course of intravenous penicillin 50,000 U/kg every 6 hours (64). Infants with positive CSF VDRL results or neurologic abnormalities on examination should have a repeat CSF examination (cell count, protein, VDRL) in 6 months, and be retreated with a full course of penicillin if any parameter is abnormal.

Chlamydia Trachomatis

Chlamydia trachomatis infection can present in the newborn as either conjunctivitis or pneumonitis (65). Infants acquire the infection from their mother's genital tract. The onset of *C. trachomatis* conjunctivitis can be at any time between a few days of age to several weeks of life. It rarely results in long-term scarring. *C. trachomatis* pneumonitis typically occurs at between 2 and 19 weeks of age and is associated with a "staccato" cough, a hyperinflated chest, and interstitial sounds on auscultation. It is sometimes associated with a pearly white appearance of the tympanic membrane. Diagnosis of *C. trachomatis* in the infant is by culture of the organism from conjunctival swab or nasopharyngeal aspirates, detection of *C. trachomatis* antigen using direct fluorescence tests, or detection of *C. trachomatis* DNA by PCR or other nuclear amplification tests. Infection in the infant should prompt investigation of the mother for *C. trachomatis* and other sexually transmitted infections. Infected infants should be treated with oral erythromycin for 21 days. Topical antibiotics provide no additive benefit in the treatment of *C. trachomatis* conjunctivitis.

Fungal Infections in the Neonate

Fungi are now a major cause of sepsis in the critically ill neonate. Rates of fungal sepsis in the NICU have increased over the last two decades from approximately 0.4 cases to 2 cases per 1000 live births (2,66). Increased survival rates of VLBW infants have contributed to the increase, as these infants contribute to over 50% of identified cases of fungal sepsis in the NICU. Two decades ago, *Candida albicans* was the predominant cause of fungal sepsis, but in recent years the rates of non-*albicans Candida* species (*C. parapsilosis, C. tropicalis, C. krusei,* and *C. glabrata,* and rarely *C. lusitaniae* and *C. guilliermondii*) have significantly increased to collectively contribute to over 50% of cases of neonatal fungal sepsis in a number of large recent reviews (66).

Risk Factors for Neonatal Fungal Colonization and Sepsis

Risk factors for neonatal fungal colonization and sepsis include preterm delivery, the use of broad-spectrum antibiotics (especially third-generation cephalosporins), VLBW (<1500 g), prolonged mechanical ventilation, the use of parenteral nutrition and central or peripheral venous catheters, steroid therapy, and duration of stay in the NICU. The use of H-2 receptor antagonists is particularly associated with colonization with *C. parapsilosis,* and the use of azole antifungal prophylaxis in the NICU has been associated with an increase in the incidence of *C. glabrata* sepsis (10,67).

Pathogenesis of Neonatal Fungal Infections

Fungal colonization precedes invasive fungal disease in the majority of cases of neonatal fungal sepsis. The rates of fungal colonization in the NICU at the end of the first weeks of life range from approximately 10% in term infants to up to over 60% in VLBW infants (66). Fungi may be acquired from the mother's birth canal during delivery, or postpartum from the hands of a caregiver in the NICU. Invasive *Candida* species only rarely colonize environmental sources. *C. albicans* has the greatest capacity of the *Candida* species to attach and invade the vascular endothelium. *Candida parapsilosis* is able to form biofilms that promote growth on intravascular catheters, and this reduces fungal exposure to antifungal agents and to the host's immune defenses (e.g., cytokines) (67).

Clinical Manifestations of Neonatal Fungal Disease

Fungal infections in the newborn period may manifest as local disease of the skin and mucosa, as isolated fungemia with or without the features of shock, as endocarditis, and as disseminated infection of end organs including the kidneys, CNS, eyes, lungs, liver, bone, and joints (66,68). *Candida* may also uncommonly present as a congenital infection after fungal chorioamnionitis.

Mucocutaneous candidiasis may present in the second week of life as white-gray plaques on the mucosa, or vesicular or pustular lesions of the skin. Occasionally, it develops into a diffuse erythematous rash that eventually desquamates. In the full-term infant, it is usually not associated with systemic infection unless the infant has an underlying immunodeficiency. In preterm infants, however, especially those who received steroid therapy postnatally, there is a high risk of dissemination, and a positive fungal culture at any sterile site should prompt investigations for fungal sepsis (culture of blood, urine, and CSF) and the commencement of empiric parenteral antifungal therapy (66).

The clinical presentation of fungal sepsis in the newborn period is nonspecific. A review that compared neonatal sepsis caused by *Candida* species with that caused by CoNS noted that both presented with a slow deterioration that contrasts with the circulatory collapse associated with infection caused by gram-negative or virulent gram-positive organisms (67). However, infants with *Candida* sepsis were noted to be more unwell in appearance than infants with CoNS sepsis and to have a strong association with the risk factors for fungal sepsis outlined above, in particular prior cephalosporin use. The majority of infants with fungal sepsis develop thrombocytopenia ($<100,000/mm^3$). Fungal sepsis may present at any time from the first week of life to after many months of hospitalization in an NICU. Rates of fungemia resulting in disseminated end-organ fungal infection in the NICU range from 7% to just over 50% (66,67).

Fungal infection of the urinary tract may manifest as an uncomplicated urinary tract infection in up to two thirds of infants with fungal sepsis or as a renal abscess that can result in urinary tract obstruction, hydronephrosis, and renal failure (10,66). Renal abscess may take some time to appear on ultrasound after the onset of candiduria; therefore, imaging should be repeated when fungal urine cultures are persistent. Dissemination of fungi to the liver and lung occurs less frequently than to the urinary tract in most series (10). Pulmonary candidiasis can occur in isolation but cannot be distinguished on clinical grounds alone.

Fungi can also disseminate to the CNS and cause meningitis, ventriculitis, or cerebral abscesses. Rates of fungal CNS dissemination vary in reported series from <5% (64) to over 30% in series of VLBW infants (10). Diagnosis of CNS fungal infections requires CSF examination and CNS imaging. The CSF glucose is low in the majority of cases of fungal meningitis and the CSF protein level is often elevated, but the CSF white cell count is not always raised, especially in VLBW infants.

Fungal endophthalmitis is recognized in up to 50% of preterm infants with fungal sepsis (10), although much lower incidences have been reported (0 to 6%) with the advent of more rapid identification of fungemia with current blood culture systems (65,66). Fungal lesions in the retina appear as fluffy white lesions on ophthalmoscopic examination, although the appearance may be less distinct in the very preterm infant.

Fungal endocarditis is recognized in up to 15% of cases of neonatal fungal sepsis and carries a higher mortality than fungemia alone (10,66). Fungal endocarditis is usually associated with the presence of a central intravascular catheter, and confirmation of the diagnosis should prompt removal of the catheter and investigation for disseminated infection.

Fungal septic arthritis and osteomyelitis have occasionally been reported in the newborn and usually are a result of candidemia (66). The radiographic appearances of *Candida* osteomyelitis are of punched-out metaphyseal lesions that are often surrounded by a sclerotic margin.

Infants infected in utero with *Candida* may present at birth with a skin rash characterized by diffuse vesicular and pustular lesions on an erythematous base. Congenital candidiasis usually occurs as an isolated skin infection in term infants, but may be associated with systemic infection in preterm infants or term infants with cellular immunodeficiencies (10). Confirmation of congenital candidiasis is by histologic evidence of fungal infection in the placenta.

Fungal infections due to *Aspergillus* and other filamentous fungi are less common than *Candida* infections in the neonate (69). Infection is usually the result of environmental contamination. Neonatal infections most commonly involve the skin and present as a necrotic lesions at the site of trauma or intravascular catheters and have been associated with direct inoculation by contaminated equipment including skin tape (10,70). Dissemination in preterm infants can occur despite antifungal therapy, and is associated with a high mortality (70,71). Filamentous fungi may also present as isolated lung abscesses (70). Diagnosis requires histologic examination and culture of the infected tissue.

Other uncommon neonatal fungal infections include infection with nosocomially acquired dermatophytes that have been transferred from the hands of caregivers (usually those with infected animals) to infect the keratinized skin of neonates and cause ringworm, and *Malassezia furfur*, the cause of pityriasis versicolor. The latter has been reported to contaminate lipid parental nutrition solutions and cause fungemia (70,72).

Outcome of Neonatal Fungal Sepsis

Mortality from invasive fungal infections in the newborn period has improved over the last two decades (2,66), possibly as a result of improved blood culture systems that allow early recognition of fungemia and institution of empiric antifungal therapy (10). Estimating the attributable mortality caused by fungal infections in the NICU is difficult as these infections occur most commonly in the sickest and most premature infants. Therefore, most surveys of fungal infection in the NICU report death rates due to all causes, and do not distinguish those directly attributable to fungal diseases. All-cause mortality from preterm infants with fungal infections is approximately 30%, that is, threefold higher than those without fungal infection (2). In general, *C. albicans* carries a higher mortality rate than other *Candida* species, possibly because it tends to infect younger infants (66). Reports of morbidity in survivors of fungal sepsis in the newborn period also vary. Some studies report high rates of adverse neurodevelopmental outcome (10), chronic lung disease, and ophthalmologic abnormalities while others do not (66). The gestational ages and variations in diagnostic and prescribing practices may partly account for these differences.

Therapy for Neonatal Fungal Infection

Empiric therapy for fungal sepsis should be with parenteral amphotericin B or one of its less nephrotoxic lipid preparations. Definitive treatment of fungal infections is based on the site of infection and type of fungus identified. Central venous catheters should be promptly removed if feasible, to ensure faster resolution of infection and to limit the risk of blood-borne dissemination and endocarditis. Prophylactic oral antifungal agents have been used in preterm infants to reduce the risk of systemic fungal disease; however, a recent meta-analysis concluded that there are still insufficient data to support their use (73).

Viral Infections in the Critically Ill Neonate

Viral infections are another significant cause of mortality and morbidity in infants in the neonatal nursery. They may be acquired from the mother in utero (congenital infections), intrapartum, or postnatally either through the breast milk or by contact with an infected caregiver. Viral infections in the sick neonate can also be acquired nosocomially from infected staff, parents and visitors or other infants in the NICU, or occasionally from infected equipment.

Respiratory Syncytial Virus, Influenza, and Other Respiratory Viruses

Respiratory syncytial virus (RSV) is the major cause of bronchiolitis. Infection is by direct contact with respiratory secretions to the upper respiratory tract mucosa and is always postnatally acquired. Nosocomial outbreaks in the NICU have been reported and are often related to fomite spread on stethoscopes, gowns, or the hands of nursery staff (74). Respiratory syncytial virus infections carry a high mortality rate in the preterm, in those with underlying cyanotic cardiac conditions or chronic lung disease (especially bronchopulmonary dysplasia), or in those with cellular immunodeficiency states (75).

Respiratory syncytial virus has an incubation period of 2 to 7 days followed by the onset of upper respiratory tract symptoms with profuse clear rhinorrhea, followed by cough, and in some infants low-grade fever, wheezing, respiratory distress that can reduce oral intake, and nonspecific changes on chest radiograph. Signs of RSV infection in infants younger than 4 weeks are often nonspecific, and include apnea, lethargy, and poor feeding, with little lower respiratory tract involvement (75).

Infants in the NICU with suspected RSV or other respiratory virus infection should be isolated and investigated by immunofluorescence and viral culture of nasopharyngeal secretions. Treatment of RSV infection is largely supportive. Ribavirin is currently the only antiviral agent available that has in vitro efficacy against RSV, but randomized controlled trials have shown mixed results with respect to reduction of duration of ventilation, intensive care stay, or hospitalization (76). As it requires continuous aerosolization and has potential toxicity to health care providers, its use is generally not recommended. Respiratory syncytial virus–immunoglobulin preparations prepared either from pooled donors (RSV–intravenous immunoglobulin [IVIG]), or as a monoclonal preparation (palivizumab) have no role in established RSV infection, but have been shown to reduce the incidence and likelihood of RSV infection in at risk infants (i.e., in preterm infants with chronic lung disease) when administered as a monthly dose just prior to and during the RSV season (76). The high cost of these agents limits their routine use in most countries to those infants most at risk.

Intrauterine exposure to influenza virus has not been shown to cause a consistent syndrome of congenital defects, above the general increase in rates of deformities associated with maternal febrile illnesses during pregnancy (74).

Postnatal influenza infection is not uncommon. Infants may present with nonspecific signs of sepsis, lethargy, reduced oral intake, and apnea. Occasionally, infants develop sepsis-like syndromes, high fevers, nasal congestion, and lower respiratory tract signs. Nosocomial outbreaks in the NICU setting have been reported, and are generally mild (74). The only agent with efficacy against influenza licensed for use in children younger than 1 year of age is amantadine, and it is available only as an oral preparation (77). It is effective only against influenza type A. Its use in neonatal outbreaks has been reported, although there are limited data about its efficacy in the neonatal period (77). The recently developed neuraminidase inhibitors (oseltamavir and zanamivir) which are effective against both influenza A and influenza B are not licensed for use in patients younger than 1 year of age. Oseltamavir, which is administered orally, has been used in younger infants (77). Its use must be instituted within 36 hours of onset of symptoms to be effective.

Enterovirus (Coxsackie Viruses, Enteroviruses, Echoviruses, Poliovirus)

Enteroviral infections are a common cause of fever and aseptic meningitis in the sick newborn (78). Enterovirus infections are seasonal and show a summer to autumn predominance. They are acquired by the fecal-oral route or by respiratory inhalation. Intrauterine enterovirus infections are associated with spontaneous abortions, preterm delivery, and stillbirths, but there is no specific syndrome associated with congenital enterovirus infection. Maternal infection just prior to delivery can result in a shock-like presentation in the infant during the first week of life. Infections are often also acquired from infected family members after discharge home. Enterovirus disease may present with a wide range of clinical features in the newborn period including nonspecific febrile illness, sepsis-like syndrome, gastroenteritis, hepatitis, myocarditis, and CNS infections that range from aseptic meningitis to meningoencephalitis and transverse myelitis (78). The latter have been associated with outbreaks of enterovirus type 11. Pleconoril, an antiviral agent with demonstrated in vitro efficacy against enteroviruses, and clinical efficacy suggested by small case series (79) has not been released onto the market. Intravenous immunoglobulin has been used in the treatment of critically ill neonates with enterovirus disease, but evidence of its efficacy in this setting is limited (51).

Cytomegalovirus

Cytomegalovirus is the commonest cause of congenital infections in the developed world (80). Infants born to mothers who have primary CMV infection during pregnancy and possibly in the 2 years prior to conception carry the greatest risk of intrauterine infection and sequelae. Congenital infection is symptomatic in the newborn period in approximately 10% of cases, and may manifest as jaundice, hepatosplenomegaly, petechiae, microcephaly, chorioretinitis, intrauterine growth retardation, and inguinal hernia. Laboratory abnormalities present in the first weeks of life include conjugated hyperbilirubinemia, thrombocytopenia, elevated hepatic transaminases, and there may abnormalities on CNS imaging (computed tomography [CT] or magnetic resonance imaging [MRI]), including intracerebral calcification (which is often periventricular in distribution) and abnormal neuronal migration. Long-term neurologic sequelae include mental retardation, motor abnormalities, sensorineural hearing loss (bilateral or unilateral), visual abnormalities, and seizures (81). A poor neurologic prognosis is strongly associated with microcephaly after adjustment for reduced weight and height, and with abnormalities on CT scan, but not with isolated hematologic, hepatic, or hearing abnormalities in the newborn period (82). Infants with asymptomatic congenital CMV infection have a good prognosis; however, 10% to 15% may develop late-onset hearing abnormalities in the first years of life (83). Late-onset visual disturbances have been reported in this group, but are rare (84).

Cytomegalovirus infection acquired at the time of delivery in healthy term infants from maternal secretions, from the breast milk, or from infected family members is generally asymptomatic. Preterm infants, however, may develop severe disease, particularly pneumonitis, colitis, or hepatitis (85). Long-term neurologic sequelae and hearing loss attributed to CMV has not been consistently shown in preterm or term infants with postnatally acquired CMV infection (86).

Ganciclovir, valganciclovir, cidofovir, and foscarnet are the main antiviral agents with efficacy against CMV, but aside from ganciclovir, use in the newborn period is limited to case reports only. Indications for ganciclovir therapy for congenital CMV infection include life- or sight-threatening CMV disease. Prolonged courses of intravenous ganciclovir (up to 6 weeks) to reduce long-term CNS sequelae associated with congenital CMV infection in infants with signs of symptomatic CNS disease in the newborn period have been evaluated in a randomized controlled trial (87). Treated infants had less chance of having progressive hearing loss at 6 months compared to control infants. However, there was a large loss to follow-up, making it difficult to interpret the significance of the reported effect beyond 6 months. The use of antiviral agents to prevent the long-term sequelae of congenital CMV infection therefore still requires further study.

Herpes Simplex Virus

Neonatal herpes simplex virus (HSV) infection is a rare but highly fatal disease that can be caused by both HSV type 1 and HSV type 2. It may manifest as disease localized to the skin, eye, or mouth (SEM), as isolated encephalitis, or as a widespread disseminated infection with or without CNS involvement that presents as a shock-like illness or pneumonitis in the first week of life. Neonatal HSV infection is usually acquired intrapartum from an infected birth canal (85% of cases) or postnatally from direct contact with an infected caregiver. Herpes simplex virus can also be transmitted transplacentally (5% of cases), resulting in a congenital syndrome characterized by a triad of skin vesicles or scarring, microcephaly, and eye involvement (chorioretinitis with or without keratoconjunctivitis). Attack rates of neonatal HSV disease are highest after primary maternal genital HSV disease during pregnancy (30% to 60%), especially in the absence of maternal type–specific seroconversion well before delivery (88). Asymptomatic recurrent genital HSV disease in pregnant women is associated with the shedding of virus in the genital tract in only 1% of cases, 3% of whom transmit the virus to their newborn (89).

Treatment of neonatal HSV disease is with intravenous acyclovir, 20 mg/kg/dose given every 8 hours by infusion (90). Therapy is for 21 days for disseminated or CNS disease (or where a lumbar puncture was not performed) and for 14 days for SEM disease. Untreated HSV disease carries a high rate of neurologic dissemination and a high mortality. With the institution of early, appropriate parenteral antiviral therapy, SEM disease is rarely fatal, and carries and excellent neurologic prognosis (91), although infants with frequent recurrences of SEM HSV-2 disease may be at long-term risk for learning defects (92). Neonatal HSV encephalitis still has a mortality rate of 15% with treatment, and carries a high rate of long-term CNS sequelae (especially after HSV-2 encephalitis) in survivors (92). Disseminated HSV infection is often fatal, even with the institution of antiviral therapy (91). The nonspecific features of neonatal HSV infection means that there are often delays between the onset of symptoms and diagnosis and institution of therapy. Recurrent skin HSV lesions are common sequelae of neonatal HSV disease. Oral acyclovir prophylaxis in survivors of neonatal disease (with HSV encephalitis or frequent HSV-2 skin infections) has been evaluated in phase II randomized trials and shown to suppress the frequency of skin recurrences but was associated with a high rate of neutropenia (93). However, its effect on preventing occult CNS recurrences and long-term learning defects remains unproven. Therefore, routine suppressive antiviral prophylaxis following neonatal HSV disease cannot be routinely recommended. However, some experts would recommend long-term prophylaxis with acyclovir for the preterm infant with HSV disease, due to the high risk of early recurrence after cessation of acute antiviral therapy.

Rubella

Rubella infection during pregnancy, especially during the first trimester, carries a high risk of congenital rubella syndrome in babies born to nonimmune women (94). Congenital rubella syndrome is characterized in the newborn period by the appearance of eye defects (cataracts, retinopathy, and congenital glaucoma), sensorineural hearing loss, and cardiac abnormalities (most commonly patent ductus arteriosus) (95). Infants may also have purpuric lesions, bony abnormalities, hepatosplenomegaly, and thrombocytopenia (95). Long-term sequelae include neurologic defects (mental retardation, myelomeningocele) and diabetes mellitus (96). Diagnosis is by detection of rubella IgM in the newborn infant. Rubella virus is shed by congenitally infected infants for many years, but is only cultured in reference laboratories. There is no effective therapy. Postnatal rubella infection is a mild disease characterized by a fine, generalized maculopapular rash, occipital lymphadenopathy, and mild fever. It is not a significant problem in infants in the NICU.

Varicella Zoster Virus

Primary varicella zoster virus (VZV) infection is the cause of chickenpox, and recurrent VZV causes herpes zoster, otherwise known as shingles. Neonatal VZV infection after maternal chickenpox can result in a highly lethal, disseminated disease in infants born to mothers who developed chickenpox 5 days before to 2 days after the onset of labor (97). These infants should be given VZV immunoglobulin (VZIG) within 96 hours of the onset of maternal disease where possible, and monitored closely for the development of chickenpox, which can still be severe despite VZIG administration (98). Chickenpox in these infants should be treated with high-dose intravenous acyclovir. Preterm infants (<28 weeks) or extremely low birth weight (ELBW) infants (<1000 g) also carry a higher risk of disseminated infection irrespective of maternal VZV seropositivity, due to low levels of passively transferred maternal antibody (99). Term infants born to VZV-seronegative mothers may also be at risk of severe disease (100). These infants should also be given VZIG within 48 hours of exposure, and be treated with intravenous acyclovir. Beyond this window of high-risk exposure, VZV infection in the term infant born to a VZV IgG-seropositive mother with a prior history of chickenpox usually follows the same course as for older children and infants, that is, a vesicular eruption that is only rarely complicated by pneumonitis, or bacterial superinfection with S. aureus or group A streptococci. These infants do not require VZIG, and do not need to be treated with IV acyclovir unless they develop severe or complicated VZV infection. All infants born to mothers with perinatal VZV infection who cannot be discharged home should be placed in respiratory isolation until the end of the incubation period.

Postnatal exposure to VZV of infants in the NICU can result from contact with a mother, visiting family member, or a member of the staff with chickenpox or with herpes zoster on an exposed area (e.g., the face). Postnatal exposure of VZV also carries a risk of severe disease in preterm or ELBW infants, and in hospitalized infants ≥28 weeks or ≥1000 g born to VZV nonimmune mothers. These infants would be given VZIG, and monitored closely for the onset of chickenpox, which should be treated with IV acyclovir. All exposed infants (and mothers) who cannot be discharged from the NICU should be placed in isolation from 8 days after the earliest exposure to 21 days postexposure or 28 days if they received VZIG.

If women develop primary chickenpox during the first two trimesters of pregnancy, there is approximately a 2% risk of an embryopathy in the offspring (101). Congenital VZV infection is characterized by limb atrophy, skin cicatrization (scarring), eye abnormalities (microphthalmia, chorioretinitis), and CNS abnormalities (101). Postnatally, the diagnosis is made in the infant on clinical features, as VZV IgM rarely remains positive in the infant, and VZV cannot be cultured or detected by molecular techniques from the infant's secretions or CSF. There is no treatment for congenital VZV infection, and the condition carries a poor neurologic prognosis. These infants do not need to be placed in isolation.

Hepatitis B Virus and Hepatitis C Virus

Neither hepatitis B virus (HBV) nor hepatitis C virus (HCV) cause clinical disease in the newborn period, but both are blood-borne viruses than can be vertically transmitted from infected mothers to cause asymptomatic chronic infection in the newborn.

Perinatal transmission of HBV results in chronic HBV infection in over 90% of infants. This rate is significantly reduced by early administration of hepatitis B immunoglobulin (Hep B Ig) to infants of HBV carrier mothers (102). Rare cases of fulminant neonatal HBV infection have been reported (103). Exposed infants should receive Hep B Ig as soon as possible after delivery, ideally within 12 hours of birth, and should commence immunization with the hepatitis B vaccine (composed of recombinant HBV surface antigen) at the same time, but a different site. The course of HBV immunization should be completed as per the routine schedule. These infants should be tested after 9 months to determine if they have developed chronic HBV infection despite immunoprophylaxis.

The risk of vertical transmission of HCV is approximately 6%, and occurs almost exclusively in offspring of HCV-seropositive women who had positive HCV RNA tests (indicating viremia) around the time of delivery (104). Maternal HIV co-infection increases the risk of perinatal transmission threefold. There is no identified HCV embryopathy. Hepatitis C virus is detected in breast milk, but is not a recognized source of perinatal infection, and in healthy, HCV-seropositive women, breast-feeding is not contraindicated (105). Infants born to HCV-infected mothers should be tested for HCV infection by HCV RNA testing after 6 weeks of age (sensitivity is <25% prior to this time) or by HCV antibody tests at or beyond 18 months of age (106). Persistent maternal antibody makes interpretation of HCV antibodies tests difficult prior to this time.

Hepatitis C virus–infected infants should be referred to a pediatric infectious disease specialist for ongoing management.

Human Immunodeficiency Virus

Intrauterine or perinatal HIV transmission usually results in asymptomatic infection in the newborn period, although an HIV embryopathy with microcephaly and intrauterine growth retardation (IUGR) has been described (107). Older infants with HIV infection may present with severe pneumonitis caused by *Pneumocystis jiroveci* (formerly *P. carinii*), persistent lymphadenopathy, failure to thrive, mucosal candidiasis, recurrent otitis media, and persistent diarrhea. Vertical transmission of HIV has been reduced from approximately 25% to <5% due to perinatal interventions such as the administration of maternal antiretroviral agents in pregnancy and before the onset of labor, elective cesarean delivery, and reduced invasive fetal monitoring (scalp electrodes, forceps) if the women elect to have a vaginal delivery (108).

The HIV antibody tests cannot be used to detect vertical HIV transmission due to the presence of passively transferred maternal antibody. Infants born to HIV-infected women should be tested for HIV infection by molecular testing for HIV DNA PCR on peripheral blood mononuclear cells (ethylenediamine-tetraacetic acid [EDTA] specimen) at 48 hours, 2 to 6 weeks, and 2 to 3 months of age (109). Nearly all HIV-infected infants will have positive HIV molecular tests by 2 months of age. HIV-exposed infants should also receive antiretroviral prophylaxis until 6 weeks of age when the diagnosis of HIV infection can be confidently excluded. *Pneumocystis carinii* pneumonia (PCP) prophylaxis of HIV-exposed infants with trimethoprim-sulfamethoxazole is no longer routinely recommended where the likelihood of vertical transmission is low, that is, where perinatal interventions to prevent vertical infection have been used (109). Regimens for testing and antiretroviral prophylaxis should be tailored to the individual mother–infant pair in consultation with a pediatric infectious diseases physician. Factors such as the maternal HIV viral load, resistance patterns, and history of antiretroviral use need to be taken into account. The Children's HIV Association of the United Kingdom and Ireland (CHIVA) has made recommendations for testing and neonatal antiretroviral doses (109). Perinatal testing should always be performed after informed consent from the parent or guardian. HIV is present in breast milk of infected mothers; therefore, breast-feeding by HIV-infected women is contraindicated in the developed world (110).

Rotavirus

Disease from rotavirus is uncommon in the neonatal period. Epidemics of diarrheal disease due to rotavirus have been reported in the NICU (110,111). Most outbreaks result from transmission by hands of caregivers from a symptomatic infant. Persistent endemic asymptomatic shedding of rotavirus has also been reported in some nurseries and is associated with frequent stooling and a higher percentage of bloody, mucoid, or watery stools (112). Infection is by the fecal-oral route.

Parvovirus

Human parvovirus B19 infection is usually asymptomatic, but can result in epidemics of erythema infectiosum otherwise known as fifth disease, characterized by facial maculopapular rash and circumoral pallor ("slapped cheek"); a transient, lacy, truncal rash; polyarthralgia; myalgia; low-grade fever; and mild malaise (74). Up to 50% of women of child-bearing age are susceptible. During epidemics, 15% to 30% of seronegative women become infected, of whom half transmit the virus to their fetus. Fetal infection is usually benign, but rarely can result in severe anemia, hydrops fetalis, and, in some cases, fetal death (74). There are isolated reports of associated congenital abnormalities, but there is no proven parvovirus embryopathy (74). The newborn infant does not appear to be at any greater risk of disease from parvovirus infection.

Protozoal Infections in the Critically Ill Neonate

Toxoplasma Gondii

Toxoplasma gondii is an important cause of congenital infection, especially in Europe, where it is common to ingest undercooked meat (113). Maternal toxoplasmosis infection in the first two trimesters of pregnancy carries the highest risk of sequelae in infants, although the risk of fetal infection is lower at these times than in the third trimester (9). France and some other countries with high rates of congenital toxoplasmosis perform routine antenatal screening for maternal infection, and treat infected mothers with antiparasitic agents to reduce the risk of severe disease in the infant (114).

Infants with congenital toxoplasmosis are often asymptomatic at birth, although there are reports of fulminant disease where it was acquired around the time of delivery (115). Signs that may be present at birth include a maculopapular rash, jaundice, hepatosplenomegaly, generalized lymphadenopathy, microcephaly, and chorioretinitis (116). Late-onset neurologic sequelae occur in up to 90% of infants with congenital toxoplasmosis and includes visual loss, hearing loss, seizures, mental retardation, and hydrocephalus (116). Abnormal findings on investigation in the newborn period include intracerebral calcifications, which are usually scattered throughout the brain, and seen on CT scan, skull x-ray, or head ultrasound. Cerebrospinal fluid examination may be abnormal in the newborn period (xanthochromia, mononuclear pleocytosis, high CSF protein), even in infants who are otherwise clinically normal.

Infants who present with clinical stigmata of congenital toxoplasmosis or whose mothers have positive antenatal toxoplasmosis serology should be evaluated by performance of toxoplasmosis IgM and IgA on the infant's blood, ophthalmologic and audiologic examination, CNS imaging, CSF examination, full blood count, and liver function tests. Placental examination for toxoplasmosis (histopathology, nucleic acid tests for *Toxoplasma*) should be performed where possible. Infants with positive toxoplasmosis serology should be treated with combination antiparasitic agents (usually pyrimethamine and a sulphur-containing drug such as sulfamethoxazole in combination with folinic acid supplementation) in consultation with an infectious diseases physician (116). Therapy is usually given for 12 months to reduce the risk of long-term sequelae. Clinical trials to evaluate shorter courses of therapy are underway in the United States (116).

Pneumocystis Jiroveci

Pneumocystis jiroveci (formerly *P. carinii*) pneumonia (PCP) infection almost exclusively occurs in individuals with cellular immunodeficiency states such as congenital immunodeficiencies or HIV infection. It usually causes a pneumonitis characterized by respiratory distress, hypoxia, and dry cough with diffuse changes on chest x-ray. Rare cases have been reported of infants during the first month of life (117), but it more commonly occurs in immunocompromised children after 3 months of age. The diagnosis is made by demonstration of an organism in lower respiratory secretions (e.g., bronchoalveolar lavage specimens). Treatment is with high-dose intravenous trimethoprim-sulfamethoxazole or IV pentamidine.

Malaria

Malaria is spread to humans by transmission of one of four *Plasmodium* species (*P. falciparum*, *P. vivax*, *P. ovale*, or *P. malariae*) through the bite of an anopheline mosquito. It continues to be a major health problem in the developing world, and impacts where it is a significant cause of fetal and infant mortality (118). Malaria infection of nonimmune pregnant women carries a high risk of fetal and perinatal loss, and is associated with the delivery of low birth weight infants (118). Rarely, it can result in congenital malaria, which manifests after the first week of life as fever, anemia, splenomegaly, and jaundice (119). Many antimalarial agents are not approved for use in infancy, and drug resistance is increasing. Therefore, treatment of malaria in infancy should be performed in consultation with an infectious diseases physician.

Treatment and Prevention

Infants who appear toxic or have clinical or laboratory indicators of sepsis should be promptly commenced on empiric antibiotic therapy. Other common indications for commencing antibiotic therapy in the newborn period are as follows: the asymptomatic newborn who has two or more risk factors for sepsis (Table 2.4), one risk factor for sepsis plus respiratory distress or in the very preterm (<32 weeks' gestation) with a risk factor, the term infant with respiratory distress from birth, or the infant with persistent neutropenia (e.g., $<1 \times 10^9$/L

TABLE **2.4.** Risk factors for neonatal sepsis (8)

Spontaneous onset of preterm onset of labor <37 weeks
Prolonged rupture of membranes >18 hours
Maternal carriage of group B streptococcus
Maternal fever >37.5°C
Mother has previous baby with group B streptococcal infection

for more than 3 days) (8). The infant born with meconium aspiration or severe perinatal asphyxia should be assessed individually, as these syndromes are only occasionally associated with sepsis (8).

The empiric antibiotic regimen should be guided by the local antibiotic guidelines and the likely causative organisms of the clinical syndrome (early- or late-onset sepsis, or a focal infection). Local guidelines take into account prevailing colonizing organisms on the unit, and local antibiotic resistance patterns. Therapy should be revised when results of microbiologic cultures and supportive laboratory tests are known. If no organisms are isolated after 48 to 72 hours, it is usually advisable to stop empiric antibiotics to avoid colonization with resistant organisms. For most organisms, directed antibiotic therapy should be continued for 7 to 10 days. There are exceptions: *Listeria monocytogenes*, which requires 14 days of antibiotics; GBS or gram-negative meningitis, which requires 21 days; and endocarditis, which often requires 4 to 6 weeks of parenteral antibiotics depending on the organism isolated.

Supportive therapy also plays an important role in the treatment of the septic neonate. Respiratory support, fluid resuscitation, and correction of metabolic disturbances, particularly hypoglycemia and metabolic acidosis, are essential adjuncts to antimicrobial therapy. Other practices, including the use of exchange transfusions or colony-stimulating factors, have not been clearly shown to be efficacious in well-designed, adequately powered clinical studies (8). There are conflicting opinions about the efficacy of IVIG for the treatment of the septic neonate; however, a recent meta-analysis concluded that IVIG had no proven benefit in this setting (51). For suspected line sepsis, intravenous catheters should always be removed if a fungus is isolated from the blood culture. For proven CoNS line-associated sepsis, many infections can be successfully treated without removal of the line (40). For *S. aureus* or gram-negative line infections, the likelihood of successfully treating infections without line removal is lower, and it is often necessary to remove the infected catheter, especially if the infection is persistent or fulminant.

Antenatal interventions to reduce infections in the newborn period include strategies prior to conception (e.g., vaccination of nonimmune women against VZV and rubella prior to pregnancy), strategies during pregnancy (e.g., washing vegetables before eating them, eating cooked meat, antiretroviral therapy for HIV, antenatal screening for transmissible infections, such as HIV, hepatitis B, hepatitis C, syphilis, rubella); and peripartum strategies (e.g., maternal antibiotics for GBS carriage or maternal indicators of sepsis).

Postnatal strategies to prevent infection in the neonatal nursery include the use of prophylactic topical antifungal agents (e.g., nystatin) to prevent fungal colonization in the VLBW infants (73), strict attention to hand washing by staff and family on the neonatal nursery, and avoidance of understaffing and over-crowding of neonatal units (120). The use of gowns and masks except for surgical procedures, however, has not been shown to reduce the incidence of nosocomial infections (120).

References

1. Bizzarro MJ, Raskind C, Baltimore RS, Gallagher PG. Seventy-five years of neonatal sepsis at Yale: 1928–2003. Pediatrics 2005;116:595–602.
2. Stoll BJ, Hansen NI, Higgins RD, et al. Very low birth weight preterm infants with early onset neonatal sepsis: the predominance of gram-negative infections continues in the National Institute of Child Health and Human Development Neonatal Research Network, 2002–2003. Pediatr Infect Dis J 2005;24:635–639.
3. Haque KN, Khan MA, Kerry S, Stephenson J, Woods G. Pattern of culture-proven neonatal sepsis in a district general hospital in the United Kingdom. Infect Control Hosp Epidemiol 2004;25:759–764.
4. Vergnano S, Sharland M, Kazembe P, et al. Neonatal sepsis: an international perspective. Dis Child Fetal Neonatal Ed 2005;90:F220–224.
5. Zaidi AK, Huskins WC, Thaver D, et al. Hospital-acquired neonatal infections in developing countries. Lancet 2005;365:1175–1188.
6. Isaacs D, Barfield C, Clothier T, et al. Late onset infections of infants in neonatal units. J Paediatr Child Health 1996;32:158–161.
7. Pass MA, Khare S, Dillon HC Jr. Twin pregnancies: incidence of group B streptococcal colonization and disease. J Pediatr 1980;97:635–637.
8. Isaacs D, Moxon R. Pathogenesis and epidemiology. In: Isaacs D, Moxon R, eds. Neonatal Infections. London: WB Saunders, 1999:1–23.
9. Klein J. Bacterial sepsis and meningitis. In: Remington JS, Klein JO, eds. Infectious Diseases of the Fetus and Newborn, 5th ed. Philadelphia: WB Saunders, 2001: 943–998.
10. Kaufman D, Fairchild KD. Clinical microbiology of bacterial and fungal sepsis in very-low-birth-weight infants. Clin Microbiol Rev 2004;17:638–680.
11. Stoll BJ, Hansen N, Fanaroff AA, et al. Late-onset sepsis in very low birth weight neonates: the experience of the NICHD Neonatal Research Network. Pediatrics 2002;110:285–289.
12. May M, Daley AJ, Donath S, Isaacs D; Australasian Study Group for Neonatal Infections. Early onset neonatal meningitis in Australia and New Zealand, 1992–2002. Arch Dis Child Fetal Neonatal Ed 2005;90:F324–327.
13. Stoll BJ, Hansen N, Fanaroff AA, et al. Changes in pathogens causing early-onset sepsis in very-low-birth-weight infants. N Engl J Med 2002;347:240–247.
14. Satwani P, Morris E, van de Ven C, Cairo MS. Dysregulation of expression of immunoregulatory and cytokine genes and its association with the immaturity in neonatal phagocytic and cellular immunity. Biol Neonate 2005;88:214–227.
15. Goldblatt D. Immunisation and the maturation of infant immune responses. Dev Biol Stand 1998;95:125–132.

16. Boyer KN, Gadzala CA, Burd LI, et al. Selective intrapartum chemoprophylaxis of group B streptococcal early onset disease. I. Epidemiologic rationale. J Infect Dis 1983;148:795–801.

17. Boyer KM, Gotoff SP. Prevention of early-onset neonatal group B streptococcal disease with selective intrapartum chemoprophylaxis. N Engl J Med 1986;314: 1665–1669.

18. Rozycki HJ, Stahl GE, Baumgart S. Impaired sensitivity of a single early leukocyte count in screening for neonatal sepsis. Pediatr Infect Dis J 1987;6:267–270.

19. Warris AB, Semmekrot A, Voss A. Candidal and bacterial bloodstream infections in premature neonates; a case-control study. Med Mycol 2001;39:75–79.

20. Ingram DI, Pengergrass EL, Promberger PI et al. Group B streptococcal disease: its diagnosis with use of antigen detection, Gram's stain and the presence of apnea, hypotension. Am J Dis Child 1980;134:754–758.

21. Gibbs RS, Schrag S, Schuchat A. Perinatal infections due to group B streptococci. Obstet Gynaecol 2004;104:1062–1076.

22. Luck S, Torny M, d'Agapeyeff K, Pitt A, et al. Estimated early-onset group B streptococcal neonatal disease. Lancet 2003;361:1953–1954.

23. Weisner AM, Johnson AP, Lamagni TL, et al. Characterization of group B streptococci recovered from infants with invasive disease in England and Wales. Clin Infect Dis 2004;38:203–208.

24. Moylett EH, Fernandez M, Rench MA, et al. A 5-year review of recurrent group B streptococcal disease: lessons from twin infants. Clin Infect Dis 2000;30:282–287.

25. Matsubara K, Nishiyama Y, Katayama K, et al. Change of antimicrobial susceptibility of group B streptococci over 15 years in Japan. J Antimicrob Chemother 2001;48:579–582.

26. Daley AM, Garland SM. Prevention of neonatal group B streptococcal disease: progress, challenges and dilemmas. J Paediatr Child health 2004:40:664–668.

27. Liu GY, Nizet V. Extracellular virulence factors of group B streptococci. Front BioSci 2004;9:794–802.

28. Factor SH, Levine OS, Harrison LH, et al. Risk factors for pediatric invasive group A streptococcal disease. Emerg Infect Dis 2005;11:1062–1066.

29. Miyairi I, Berlingieri D, Protic J, Belko J. Neonatal invasive group A streptococcal disease: case report and review of the literature. Pediatr Infect Dis J 2004; 23:161–165.

30. Faix RG, Soskolne EI, Schumacher RE. Group C streptococcal infection in a term newborn infant. J Perinatol 1997;17:79–82.

31. Haffar AA, Fuselier PA, Baker CJ. Species distribution of non-group D alpha-hemolytic streptococci in maternal genital and neonatal blood cultures. J Clin Microbiol 1983;18:101–103.

32. Hoffman JA, Mason EO, Schutze GE, et al. Streptococcus pneumoniae infections in the neonate. Pediatrics 2003;112:1095–1102.

33. Healy CM, Palazzi DL, Edwards MS, Campbell JR, Baker CJ. Features of invasive staphylococcal disease in neonates. Pediatrics 2004;114:953–961.

34. Ladhani S. Understanding the mechanism of action of the exfoliative toxins of Staphylococcus aureus. FEMS Immunol Med Microbiol 2003;39:181–189.

35. Takahashi N. Neonatal toxic shock syndrome-like exanthematous disease (NTED). Pediatr Int 2003;45:233–237.

36. Isaacs D, Fraser S, Hogg G, Li HY. Staphylococcus aureus infections in Australasian neonatal nurseries. Arch Dis Child Fetal Neonatal Ed 2004;89:F331–335.

37. Ochoa TJ, Mohr J, Wanger A, Murphy JR, Heresi GP. Community-associated methicillin-resistant Staphylococcus aureus in pediatric patients. Emerg Infect Dis 2005;11:966–968.
38. Bratu S, Eramo A, Kopec R, et al. Community-associated methicillin-resistant Staphylococcus aureus in hospital nursery and maternity units. Emerg Infect Dis 2005;11:808–813.
39. Shinefield H, Black S, Fattom A, et al. Use of a Staphylococcus aureus conjugate vaccine in patients receiving hemodialysis. N Engl J Med 2002;346:491–496.
40. Hudome SM, Fisher MC. Nosocomial infections in the neonatal intensive care unit. Curr Opin Infect Dis 2001;14(3):303–307.
41. Chapman RL, Faix RG. Persistent bacteremia and outcome in late onset infection among infants in a neonatal intensive care unit. Pediatr Infect Dis J 2003;22(1): 17–21.
42. Deville JG, Adler S, Azimi PH, et al. Linezolid versus vancomycin in the treatment of known or suspected resistant gram-positive infections in neonates. Pediatr Infect Dis J 2003;22(9 suppl):S158–163.
43. Toledano H, Schlesinger Y, Raveh D, et al. Prospective surveillance of vancomycin-resistant enterococci in a neonatal intensive care unit. Eur J Clin Microbiol Infect Dis 2000;19:282–287.
44. Singh N, Leger MM, Campbell J, Short B, Campos JM. Control of vancomycin-resistant enterococci in the neonatal intensive care unit. Infect Control Hosp Epidemiol 2005;26:646–649.
45. Gellin BG, Bromme CV, Bibb WF, et al. The epidemiology of listeriosis in the United States- 1986. Am J Epidemiol 1991;133:392–401.
46. Xie Y, Kim KJ, Kim KS. Current concepts on Escherichia coli K1 translocation of the blood-brain barrier. FEMS Immunol Med Microbiol 2004;42:271–279.
47. Gupta K, Scholes D, Stamm WE. Increasing prevalence of antimicrobial resistance among uropathogens causing uncomplicated cystitis in women. JAMA 1999; 281:736–738.
48. Noriega FR, Kotloff KL, Martin MA, Schwalbe RS. Nosocomial bacteremia caused by Enterobacter sakazakiki and Leuconostoc mesenteroides resulting from extrinsic contamination of infant formula. Pediatr Infect Dis J 1990;9:447–449.
49. Doran TI. The role of Citrobacter in clinical disease of children: review. Clin Infect Dis 1999;28:384–394.
50. Shah S, Ohlosson A, Shah V. Intraventricular antibiotics for bacterial meningitis in neonates. Cochrane Database Syst Rev 2004;18:CD004496.
51. Ohlsson A, Lacy JB. Intravenous immunoglobulin for suspected or subsequently proven infection in neonates. Cochrane Database Syst Rev 2004;1:CD001239.
52. Foca MD. Pseudomonas aeruginosa infections in the neonatal intensive care unit. Semin Perinatol 2002;26:332–339.
53. Insoft RM, Sola A. Perinatally acquired Pseudomonas infection: a newly recognized maternal risk factor. Am J Perinatol 1995;12:25–26.
54. Shah SS, Gallagher PG. Complications of conjunctivitis caused by Pseudomonas aeruginosa in a newborn intensive care unit. Pediatr Infect Dis J 1998;17:97–102.
55. Foca M, Jakob K, Whittier S, et al. Endemic Pseudomonas aeruginosa infection in a neonatal intensive care unit. N Engl J Med 2000;343:695–700.
56. Ladhani S, Gransden W. Septicaemia due to glucose non-fermenting, gram-negative bacilli other than Pseudomonas aeruginosa in children. Acta Paediatr 2002;91: 303–306.

57. Heath PT, McVernon J. The UK Hib vaccine experience. Arch Dis Child 2002;86:396–399.
58. Soriano-Gabarro M, Stuart JM, Rosenstein NE. Vaccines for the prevention of meningococcal disease in children. Semin Pediatr Infect Dis 2002;13:182–189.
59. Brook I. Cutaneous and subcutaneous infections in newborns due to anaerobic bacteria. J Perinat Med 2002;30:197–208.
60. Noel GJ, Laufer DA, Edelson PJ. Anaerobic bacteremia in a neonatal intensive care unit: an eighteen-year experience. Pediatr Infect Dis J 1988;7:858–862.
61. Cantwell MF, Shehab ZM, Costello et al. Brief report: congenital tuberculosis. N Engl J Med 1994;330:1051–1054.
62. American Academy of Pediatrics. Tuberculosis. In: Pickering LD, ed. Red Book: 2003 Report of the Committee on Infectious Diseases, 26th ed. Elk Grove Village, IL: American Academy of Pediatrics, 2003:642–660.
63. Crockett M, King SM, Kitai I, et al. Nosocomial transmission of congenital tuberculosis in a neonatal intensive care unit. Clin Infect Dis 2004;39:1719–1723.
64. American Academy of Pediatrics. Syphilis. In: Pickering LD, ed. Red Book: 2003 Report of the Committee on Infectious Diseases, 26th ed. Elk Grove Village, IL: American Academy of Pediatrics, 2003:595–607.
65. American Academy of Pediatrics. Chlamydia trachomatis. In: Pickering LD, ed. Red Book: 2003 Report of the Committee on Infectious Diseases, 26th ed. Elk Grove Village, IL: American Academy of Pediatrics, 2003:238–239.
66. Makhoul IR, Kassis I, Smokin T, Tamir A, Sujov P. Review of 49 neonates with acquired fungal sepsis: further characterization. Pediatrics 2001;107:61–66.
67. Benjamin DK Jr, Ross K, McKinner RE Jr, Benjamin DK, Auten R, Fisher RG. When to suspect fungal infection in neonates: a clinical comparison of Candida albicans and Candida parapsilosis fungemia with coagulase-negative staphylococcal bacteraemia. Pediatrics 2000;106:712–718.
68. Chen JY. Neonatal candidosis associated with meningitis and endophthalmitis. Acta Paediatr Jpn 1994;36:261–265.
69. Woodruff CA, Hebert AA. Neonatal primary cutaneous aspergillosis: case report and review of the literature. Pediatr Dermatol 2002;19(5):439–444.
70. Miller MJ. Fungal infections. In: Remington JS, Klein JO, eds. Infectious Diseases of the Fetus and Newborn, 5th ed. Philadelphia: WB Saunders, 2001:813–853.
71. Herron MD, Vanderhooft SL, Byington C, King JD. Aspergillosis in a 24-week newborn: a case report. J Perinatol 2003;23:256–259.
72. Stuart SM, Lane AT. Candida and Malassezia as nursery pathogens. Semin Dermatol 1992;11:19–23.
73. Austin NC, Darlow B. Prophylactic oral antifungal agents to prevent systemic Candida infection in preterm infants. Cochrane Database Syst Rev 2004;1: CD003478.
74. Arvin A, Maldonado YA. Other viral infections of the fetus and newborn. In: Remington JS, Klein JO, eds. Infectious Diseases of the Fetus and Newborn, 5th ed. Philadelphia: WB Saunders, 2001:855–866.
75. Carbonell-Estrany X, Figueras-Aloy J, Law BJ, et al. Identifying risk factors for severe respiratory syncytial virus among infants born after 33 through 35 completed weeks of gestation: different methodologies yield consistent findings. Pediatr Infect Dis J 2004;23:S193–201.
76. Jafri HS. Treatment of respiratory syncytial virus: antiviral therapies. Pediatr Infect Dis J 2003;22:S89–92.

77. Uyeki TM. Influenza diagnosis and treatment in children: a review of studies on clinically useful tests and antiviral treatment for influenza. Pediatr Infect Dis J 2003;22(2):164–177.
78. Rittichier KR, Bryan PA, Bassett KE, et al. Diagnosis and outcomes of enterovirus infections in young infants. Pediatr Infect Dis J 2005;24:546–550.
79. Bauer S, Gottesman G, Sirota L, et al. Severe Coxsackie virus B infection in preterm newborns treated with pleconaril. Eur J Pediatr 2002;161:491–493.
80. Stagno SS. Cytomeglovirus. In: Remington JS, Klein JO, eds. Infectious Diseases of the Fetus and Newborn, 5th ed. Philadelphia: WB Saunders, 2001:389–424.
81. Boppana SB, Pass RF, Britt WJ, Stagno S, Alford CA. Symptomatic congenital cytomegalovirus infection: neonatal morbidity and mortality. Pediatr Infect Dis J 1992;11:93–99.
82. Noyola DE, Demmler GJ, Nelson CT, et al. Early predictors of neurodevelopmental outcome in symptomatic congenital cytomegalovirus infection. J Pediatr 2001;138:325–331.
83. Williamson WD, Demmler GJ, Percy AK, Catlin FI. Progressive hearing loss in infants with asymptomatic congenital cytomegalovirus infection. Pediatrics 1992;90:862–866.
84. Boppana S, Amos C, Britt W, Stagno S, Alford C, Pass R. Late onset and reactivation of chorioretinitis in children with congenital cytomegalovirus infection. Pediatr Infect Dis J 1994;13:1139–1142.
85. Cheong JL, Cowan FM, Modi N. Gastrointestinal manifestations of postnatal cytomegalovirus infection in infants admitted to a neonatal intensive care unit over a five year period. Arch Dis Child Fetal Neonatal Ed 2004;89:F367–369.
86. Kumar ML, Nankervis GA, Jacobs IB, et al. Congenital and postnatally acquired cytomegalovirus infections: long-term follow-up. J Pediatr 1984;104:674–679.
87. Kimberlin DW, Lin CY, Sanchez PJ, et al. Effect of ganciclovir therapy on hearing in symptomatic congenital cytomegalovirus disease involving the central nervous system: a randomized, controlled trial. J Pediatr 2003;143:16–25.
88. Brown ZA, Wald A, Morrow RA, Selke S, Zeh J, Corey L. Effect of serologic status and cesarean delivery on transmission rates of herpes simplex virus from mother to infant. JAMA 2003;289:203–209.
89. Brown ZA, Benedetti J, Ashley R, et al. Neonatal herpes simplex virus infection in relation to asymptomatic maternal infection at the time of labor. N Engl J Med 1991;324:1247–1252.
90. Kimberlin DW, Lin CY, Jacobs RF et al. Safety and efficacy of high-dose intravenous acyclovir in the management of neonatal herpes simplex virus infections. Pediatrics 2001;108:230–238.
91. Whitley R, Arvin A, Prober C, et al. Predictors of morbidity and mortality in neonates with herpes simplex virus infections. N Engl J Med 1991;324:450–454.
92. Corey L, Whitley RJ, Stone EF, Mohan K. Difference between herpes simplex virus type 1 and type 2 neonatal encephalitis in neurological outcome. Lancet 1988;1:1–4.
93. Kimberlin D, Powell D, Gruber W, et al. Administration of oral acyclovir suppressive therapy after neonatal herpes simplex virus disease limited to the skin, eyes and mouth: results of a phase I/II trial. Pediatr Infect Dis J 1996;15:247–254.
94. Enders G, Nickerl-Pacher U, Miller E et al. Outcome of confirmed periconceptional maternal rubella. Lancet 1988;1:144–157.

95. Peckham C. Clinical and laboratory study of children exposed in utero to maternal rubella. Arch Dis Child 1972;47:571–577.
96. Menser MA, Forrest JM. Rubella—high incidence of defects in children considered normal at birth. Med J Aust 1974;1:123–126.
97. Enders G, Miller E, Cradock-Watson J, Bolley I, Ridehalgh M. Consequences of varicella and herpes zoster in pregnancy; prospective study of 1739 cases. Lancet 1994;343:1548–1551.
98. Reynolds L, Struik S, Nadel S. Neonatal varicella: varicella zoster immunoglobulin (VZIG) does not prevent disease. Arch Dis Child Fetal Neonatal Ed 1999;81: F69–F70.
99. Conway SP, Dear PRF, Smith I. Immunoglobulin profile of the preterm baby. Arch Dis Child 1985;60:208–212.
100. Heuchan AM, Isaacs D. The management of varicella-zoster virus exposure and infection in pregnancy and the newborn period. Australasian Subgroup in Paediatric Infectious Diseases of the Australasian Society for Infectious Diseases. Med J Aust 2001;174:288–292.
101. Pastuszak AL, Levy M, Schick B, et al. Outcome after maternal varicella infection in the first 20 weeks of pregnancy. N Engl J Med 1994;330:901–905.
102. Zanetti AR, Dentico P, Del Vecchio Blanco C, et al. Multicenter trial on the efficacy of HBIG and vaccine in preventing perinatal hepatitis B. Final report. J Med Virol 1986;18:327–334.
103. Vanclaire J, Cornu C, Sokal EM. Fulminant hepatitis B in an infant born to a hepatitis Be antibody positive, DNA negative carrier. Arch Dis Child 1991;6:983–985.
104. Conte D, Fraquelli M, Prati D, et al. Prevalence and clinical course of chronic hepatitis C virus (HCV) infection and rate of HCV vertical transmission in a cohort of 15,250 pregnant women. Hepatology 2000;31:751–755.
105. American Academy of Pediatrics. Hepatitis C. In: Pickering LD, ed. Red Book: 2003 Report of the Committee on Infectious Diseases, 26th ed. Elk Grove Village, IL: American Academy of Pediatrics, 2003:336–340.
106. Hardikar W, Elliott E, Jones CA. Perinatal hepatitis C—the silent infection. Should we be testing for it and how? Med J Aust 2006;184:54–55.
107. American Academy of Pediatrics. Human Immunodeficiency Virus Infection. In: Pickering LD, ed. Red Book: 2003 Report of the Committee on Infectious Diseases, 26th ed. Elk Grove Village, IL: American Academy of Pediatrics, 2003:360–382.
108. Wilfert CM, Stringer JS. Prevention of pediatric human immunodeficiency virus. Semin Pediatr Infect Dis 2004;15:190–198.
109. Children's HIV Association of the United Kingdom and Ireland (CHIVA) Web site. http://www.bhiva.org/chiva/.
110. Jones CA. Maternal transmission of infections in breast milk. J Paediatr Child Health 2001;37:576–582.
111. Rotbart HA, Nelson WL, Glode MP, et al. Neonatal rotavirus-associated necrotizing enterocolitis: case control study and prospective surveillance during an outbreak. J Pediatr 1988;112:87–93.
112. Sharma R, Hudak ML, Premachandra BR, et al. Clinical manifestations of rotavirus infection in the neonatal intensive care unit. Pediatr Infect Dis J 2002;21: 1099–1105.
113. Cook AJ, Gilbert RE, Buffolano W, et al. Sources of toxoplasma infection in pregnant women: European multicentre case-control study. European Research Network on Congenital Toxoplasmosis. BMJ 2000;321:142–147.

114. Peyron F, Wallon M, Liou C, Garner P. Treatments for toxoplasmosis in pregnancy. Cochrane Database Syst Rev 2000;2:CD001684.
115. Armstrong L, Isaacs D, Evans N. Severe neonatal toxoplasmosis after third trimester maternal infection. Pediatr Infect Dis J 2004;23:968–969.
116. American Academy of Pediatrics. Toxoplasma gondii infections. In: Pickering LD, ed. Red Book: 2003 Report of the Committee on Infectious Diseases, 26th ed. Elk Grove Village, IL: American Academy of Pediatrics, 2003:631–636.
117. Kattan M, Platzker A, Mellins RB, et al. Respiratory diseases in the first year of life in children born to HIV-1–infected women. Pediatr Pulmonol 2001;31:267–276.
118. Shulman CE, Dorman EK. Importance and prevention of malaria in pregnancy. Trans R Soc Trop Med Hyg 2003;97:30–35.
119. Ahmed A, Cerilli LA, Sanchez PJ. Congenital malaria in a preterm neonate: case report and review of the literature. Am J Perinatol 1998;15:19–22.
120. Kilbride HW, Wirstchafter DD, Powers RJ, Sheehan MB. Implementation of evidence based potentially better practices to decreased nosocomial infections. Pediatr 2003;111:e519–533.

3
Fungal Infection in Critically Ill Children

Alok Sharma

Systemic fungal infection is a significant cause of morbidity and mortality in critically ill children. This is particularly so for children who remain for long periods in intensive care. The most common species causing infection are *Candida* and *Aspergillus*, although a wide variety of opportunistic fungi are now emerging as significant pathogens.

Treatment of fungal infections must often begin empirically, since obtaining the diagnosis can be difficult and often is delayed. Not only are fungal infections difficult to distinguish from bacterial or other infections, but the clinical manifestations of many fungal infections are shared among a variety of bacterial and fungal pathogens as well.

Fungal pathogens, especially in critically ill children, are difficult to treat and result in prolonged hospital stay, cost of care and morbidity.

Incidence

Bacteria account for most nosocomial infections. During the past 20 years, however, increases in the severity of illness of hospitalized patients, the use of invasive medical devices, and the administration of more potent broad-spectrum antibiotics have resulted in an increase in the incidence of infections due to fungi. Most notable is the sharp rise in the rate of bloodstream infections with *Candida* species and the increasing importance of uncommon fungal pathogens such as non-*albicans* species of *Candida*, *Fusarium* species, *Trichosporon* species, and dematiaceous fungi (1–3).

Systemic aspergillosis is the second most common invasive fungal infection. In certain patient groups, such as those with hematologic malignancies, the condition has been reported as occurring in up to 30% of patients in postmortem series (4).

Candida

A population-based surveillance study conducted in 1992–1993 by the Centers for Disease Control (CDC), reported that *C. albicans* as the most common species, followed in order by *C. parapsilosis*, *C. tropicalis*, and *C. glabrata* (3).

The overall increase in candidemia in recent years is complicated by the emergence of non-*albicans Candida* (NAC) species as both colonizers and pathogens causing nosocomial fungal bloodstream infection (BSI). Wingard (5), in a comprehensive review of all published reports from 1952 to 1992, found that 12 reports showed proportionally higher (>50%) isolation of NAC species. The NAC species isolated were *C. glabrata*, *C. krusei*, *C. tropicalis*, and *C. parapsilosis*. Other species, such as *C. guilliermondii*, *C. lusitaniae*, *C. dubliniensis*, *C. kefyr*, *C. lipolytica*, and *C. pelliculosa*, were occasionally isolated (3,5).

Candida albicans has been the species most often associated with neonatal infections, but there are reports of an increasing number of infections attributable to *C. parapsilosis* associated with common source outbreaks (6).

Epidemiology

Among 168 total children with candidemia, the median age was 3.5 years (interquartile range, 0.6 to 14.3). There were 189 episodes of candidemia. *Candida* species included *C. albicans* (41%), *C. parapsilosis* (24%), *C. glabrata* (13%), and *C. tropicalis* (9%).

The most common underlying diagnoses were oncologic (24%), gastrointestinal (15%), and cardiac (10%) diseases; 53% of patients were admitted to an intensive care unit (ICU), 27% to a general pediatric or surgical ward, and 20% to the oncology ward. Organ involvement was most commonly identified in the lung (58%), followed by the liver (23%), kidney (16%), brain (12%), spleen (8%), eye (8%), and heart (8%). Independent risk factors for disseminated candidiasis were persistently positive blood cultures for *Candida* (>3 days) with a central venous catheter in place, and immunosuppression (7).

Overall, the patients in neonatal and surgical ICUs appear to be at greatest risk, including children on cytotoxic chemotherapy or corticosteroid therapy, and those who are HIV infected.

T-cell defects, such as those found in chronic mucocutaneous candidiasis, make patients more susceptible to chronic *Candida* infections. Chemotherapy associated with neutropenia as well as other neutrophil disorders places patients at risk of disseminated infection.

Breaches in continuity of natural barriers to infection such as those created by central venous catheters and urinary catheters lead to *Candida* infections. Prolonged use of broad-spectrum antibiotics inhibits the normal flora and predisposes to superinfection (8).

Clinical Presentation

Critically ill children are predisposed to infection with *Candida* in various different manifestations. *Candida* infection can affect different organ systems varying from benign superficial infections to deep invasive infections.

Skin

Cutaneous infection with *Candida* is benign and usually involves wet, moist areas of skin. It is common in children on chemotherapy, steroids, and congenital or acquired immunodeficiency.

Intertrigo occurs in flexural areas. Paronychia and onychomycosis are associated with immersion of the hands in water and with diabetes mellitus. Characteristic skin lesions occur in patients with disseminated candidiasis and candidemia. Biopsy specimens of these lesions may demonstrate yeast cells, hyphae, or pseudohyphae, and cultures are positive for Candida species (8). Congenital cutaneous candidiasis is rare and presents as skin erythema with macules, papules, or pustules at birth (9).

Gastrointestinal Illness

The most common presentation is thrush. The lesions usually appear as pearly white plaques on the mucosa of the oropharynx, which when removed leave spots of punctuate bleeding. Atrophic glossitis, esophagitis, and chronic hyperplastic candidiasis are other presentations (8).

Urinary Tract

Candida infection of the urinary tract occurs in the immunocompromised host especially in diabetics, patients with indwelling catheters, and those on prolonged antibiotic therapy. It is usually asymptomatic, but children may have dysuria. Fungal balls may occur in the renal tract leading to outflow obstruction (8).

Respiratory Tract

Candida pneumonitis is rare. Primary illness results from aspiration of heavily colonized oral secretions, while the secondary form occurs because of disseminated candidemia and manifests as fungal balls in the lungs (8).

Candida *in the Neonate*

Prematures and low-birth-weight infants are at risk for *Candida* infection, as are infants who are on broad-spectrum antibiotics and those ventilated for prolonged periods. They often have compromised skin integrity, gastrointestinal disease, chronic malnutrition, and central venous or arterial catheters. The symptoms of invasive candidiasis are often nonspecific and can mimic bacterial sepsis. Sepsis in the presence of an intravascular catheter, or not responding to appropriate antibiotics, should raise the possibility of *Candida* sepsis. The most common sites of occurrence of *Candida* species are the bloodstream and urinary tract (8,10,11).

Systemic Infection

Candidemia represents bloodstream invasion of the organism, from a mucosal surface such as the gastrointestinal or urinary tract, or from an intravascular device.

The presence of satellite lesions and cotton-like chorioretinal lesions may be evidence of candidemia. *Candida* can affect the heart and cause endocarditis. Disseminated candidiasis indicates organ involvement and may occur with or without fungemia. It is common in neutropenic patients. The liver and spleen are commonly involved (7,8).

Diagnosis

The diagnosis of *Candida* as a cause of systemic and disseminated infection requires a high index of suspicion because *Candida* may be difficult to demonstrate microbiologically. The differentiation between colonization and infection is also difficult; however, the importance of *Candida* colonization as a risk factor for systemic infection is widely recognized (12).

For superficial skin infections, potassium hydroxide–prepared scrapings reveals pseudohyphae. Blood cultures have a low sensitivity in diagnosing *Candida* sepsis and disseminated candidiasis. Only 50% of patients with disseminated candidiasis have positive cultures (13). Positive blood cultures in the presence of immunosuppression and a central line are a risk factor for candidiasis (7). In predisposed neonates, a single positive blood culture should prompt thorough investigation of all end organs (11).

The significance of *Candida* in urine is unclear. In a prospective study evaluating the outcome of funguria, 65% of patients had *Candida* species in the urine but only 1.3% had documented candidemia (14).

Candiduria may indicate systemic involvement, upper renal tract involvement, or cystitis. It is not a dependable indicator of systemic or upper renal tract disease, especially in catheterized children, because of bladder colonization. However, candiduria in a premature neonate or immunocompromised setting should prompt further investigation for systemic disease. A critically ill child with candiduria should have renal imaging to look for evidence of fungal balls in the kidney (8).

The presence of *Candida* in endotracheal secretions needs to be interpreted in a clinical context, as it may indicate that the patient is colonized, and the presence of *Candida* in secretions does not differentiate colonization from invasive disease.

Isolation of *Candida* species from multiple sterile sites (e.g., gastrointestinal [GI] tract, urine, respiratory) should arouse suspicions for the possibility of disseminated candidiasis. Definitive diagnosis of organ involvement can be made by biopsy (8).

Aspergillosis

Aspergillus species are ubiquitous soil inhabitants. They are saprophytic molds, which are common on decaying material throughout the world. *Aspergillus* may grow as a harmless saprophyte in cerumen of the ear, and the paranasal sinuses may be colonized by various species (15).

Systemic aspergillosis is the second most common invasive fungal infection.

Aspergillus fumigatus is the most common species implicated in invasive aspergillosis. Other common infecting species are *A. flavus* and *A. niger* (16).

Epidemiology

Systemic aspergillosis is the second most common invasive fungal infection. In a retrospective study carried out in 2000, there were 666 cases of invasive aspergillosis among 152,231 immunocompromised children, yielding an annual incidence of 0.4% among hospitalized immunocompromised children. Children with underlying cancer accounted for the 74% of the cases. The highest incidence of invasive aspergillosis was seen in children who underwent allogeneic bone marrow transplantation and those with acute myelogenous leukemia. The overall in-hospital mortality of immunocompromised children with invasive aspergillosis was 18%. Children with malignancy and invasive aspergillosis were at increased risk for death compared with children with malignancy and without aspergillosis (17).

Risk factors for developing invasive aspergillosis include neutropenia, stem-cell transplant recipients, and solid organ transplant patients. Underlying immune dysfunction is also associated with invasive aspergillosis, particularly in patients with chronic granulomatous disease. Patients with HIV/AIDS with a low CD4 cell count are also at risk, as well as patients on high-dose systemic corticosteroids (18).

Clinical Presentation

The lungs are the most commonly involved site, followed by the nasopharynx, skin, and subcutaneous tissues. Other organs are commonly involved following systemic dissemination. Virtually any organ can be affected in invasive disease in the immunocompromised.

Infection may manifest as either relatively noninvasive disease (e.g., an aspergilloma in a pulmonary cavity, or allergic bronchopulmonary aspergillosis in patients with bronchiectasis) or invasive disease in the immunocompromised.

Invasive aspergillosis presents as a necrotizing bronchopneumonia with invasion of the pulmonary vessels. Widespread fungal embolization may then occur to the heart, gastrointestinal tract, skin, kidneys, and liver. Central nervous system (CNS) involvement in invasive aspergillosis has a poor outcome, and mortality is as high as 90% (15).

Aspergillomas occur when the fungus grows as a distinct mass of hyphae and tissue debris in a preexisting pulmonary cavity caused by a concomitant pulmonary disease due to, for example, tuberculosis or histoplasmosis. There is no tissue invasion, but in the immunocompromised, hyphae may proliferate throughout the lung and invade the bloodstream, causing dissemination (15).

Aspergillus rhinosinusitis is a potentially lethal complication of chemotherapy-induced neutropenia in patients with acute leukemia. *Aspergillus flavus* is the most common species identified as the cause. The infection is difficult to diagnose early but should be suspected when a neutropenic patient develops persistent fever without a known source, or symptoms and signs of rhinitis or sinusitis. Cavernous sinus thrombosis and CNS involvement are known complications. Anterior rhinoscopy and computed tomography (CT) scan are important for diagnosis and evaluating the extent of the disease. Confirming the presence of *Aspergillus* is done by histopathology of biopsied material (19).

Diagnosis

Although diagnosis of aspergillosis can be difficult, its early detection and treatment are important factors in improving the clinical outcome and survival rate of patients. A definitive diagnosis of invasive aspergillosis includes a positive culture for *Aspergillus* species from a sterile site and histopathologic demonstration of hyphal elements in host tissue, combined with evidence of tissue damage either microscopically or unequivocally by imaging studies.

Antifungal therapy, however, may need to be started even in the absence of definitive diagnosis because of the difficulties in diagnosis and the high risk of mortality.

The isolation of *Aspergillus* in the sputum must be interpreted cautiously and in the context of clinical presentation. Repeatedly positive sputum cultures may reflect colonization. Further, *Aspergillus* species are frequent lab contaminants (20). In a study performed to determine the significance of *Aspergillus* species in respiratory secretions, it was revealed that prolonged duration of hospitalization between initial isolation (greater than 2 weeks) and multiple isolates (greater than three) are significantly associated with the presence of disease (20).

The isolation of *A. fumigatus* or *A. flavus* from respiratory secretions does not usually represent laboratory contamination and must be interpreted in light of a known predisposition to invasive disease. In patients who are predisposed, such as granulocytopenic patients with acute leukemia, even a single isolation carries a high likelihood of invasive aspergillosis. Even in the absence of evidence of tissue invasion, antifungal therapy may be warranted in such cases (20,21).

Bronchoalveolar lavage (BAL) is a valuable tool in the investigation of *Aspergillus* pneumonia. In an investigation performed by Stover et al. (22), BAL had a diagnostic yield in 83% in all patients with invasive pulmonary aspergillosis confirmed by open lung biopsy, transbronchial biopsy, or necropsy. Although BAL fluid that is positive for *Aspergillus* species is indicative of invasive aspergillosis in a child with hematologic malignancy who is neutropenic and has new pulmonary infiltrates on chest radiographs, absence of hyphal elements or negative cultures does not exclude the diagnosis (22,23). A single positive sputum culture for *Aspergillus* should be viewed critically. A positive culture of *Aspergillus* on a BAL specimen should not be underestimated as just contamination in immunocompromised patients. It may be taken as presumptive evidence of invasive aspergillosis, and in view of the high mortality rate associated with this disease, serve as an indication for starting treatment. Further, the isolation of an *Aspergillus* species from sputum or BAL is highly predictive of invasive disease in neutropenic patients (20,21,24).

Lung biopsy remains the gold standard for diagnosis, but it must be remembered that the nature of underlying illness or the clinical condition of the child may limit this option.

Radiography is an important adjunct in diagnosing invasive aspergillosis. Thoracic CT scan is the most sensitive radiologic method of detecting early changes of invasive aspergillosis. Computed tomography should be performed early in neutropenic patients with antibiotic-resistant fever and further clinical signs of invasive aspergillosis (25).

Typical chest CT findings of invasive pulmonary aspergillosis are multiple inflammatory nodules, often with one large dominant mass. This may not be apparent on routine chest radiography. A characteristic early finding on CT scan is the "halo" sign, which consists of haziness surrounding a soft tissue nodule. With cavitation of this nodule, an air crescent sign may subsequently develop. The halo sign is characteristic of angioinvasive infection and is highly suggestive in patients with prolonged neutropenia (26,27). The halo sign, however, is not pathognomonic of invasive aspergillosis, and a study comparing the radiologic findings in invasive aspergillosis with those of candidiasis in immunocompromised patients concluded that pulmonary aspergillosis and candidiasis manifest with similar high-resolution CT findings. Centrilobular nodules and consolidation are more common in aspergillosis. While the halo sign is not pathognomonic for aspergillosis, its presence in predisposed individuals may help in early diagnosis (26,28).

Because of the difficulty of trying to cultivate *Aspergillus* species, there is ongoing research trying to develop serologic methods for the diagnosis of invasive aspergillosis. Two diagnostic assays rely on cell detection of antigens that are present in the cell wall of *Aspergillus* species: galactomannan (GM), a component of cell walls that is secreted from growing hyphae, and 1,3-β-glucan, a fungal cell wall constituent. The presence of these fungal markers may help in the diagnosis of aspergillosis as adjuncts. Comprehensive data on GM detection in children with hematologic malignancies who are at a high risk of invasive aspergillosis is still lacking (18,29).

Polymerase chain reaction (PCR) has been used in the diagnosis of aspergillosis. It has been demonstrated that PCR performed on BAL fluid has a negative predictive value that approaches 100%. Different issues are still unresolved in the use of PCR, like the best source of material (e.g., whole blood, serum, or plasma), the amplification protocol, and primer selection (18,29).

Other Fungal Infections

A variety of other fungal infections can affect critically ill children. An overview of opportunistic infections in HIV-infected children and *Pneumocystis jirovecii* is presented in Chapter 2. A brief overview of other important fungal pathogens is presented here.

Endemic Mycosis

Histoplasmosis, caused by the fungus *Histoplasma capsulatum*, a thermal dimorphic fungus, is prevalent in North, Central, and South America. The severity of illness depends on the size of the inoculum. The spectrum of this illness ranges from asymptomatic infection to severe disseminated disease. Initial symptoms consist of a flu-like illness, which may evolve into fever and cough with radiologic features of pneumonitis. These symptoms are usually self-limiting. Disseminated infection is common in HIV-infected children and infants who have cell-mediated immune defects. There is diffuse involvement of the lungs with infiltrates, and hepatosplenomegaly.

Travel to, or residence in or near, a known endemic area is a critical feature of the history. Specific laboratory tests used to diagnose histoplasmosis include culture, histopathology of specimens, serologic testing, and antigen assay.

Treatment is required for severe and disseminated infections. Amphotericin B remains the initial treatment of choice for severe infections. Following stabilization of the patient's condition, treatment may be continued with oral itraconazole (30,31).

Blastomycosis is a dimorphic fungus endemic mainly in North America. It is less common than histoplasmosis and tends to cause mainly pulmonary involvement. The clinical presentation is that of community-acquired pneumonia, which fails to respond to standard antibiotics. Diagnosis is by microscopy of respiratory secretions, or BAL specimens, because of the characteristic appearance of the fungus. Amphotericin B is the agent of choice for therapy (30).

Coccidioidomycosis

Coccidioides immitis, which exists in some isolated areas of South America, is far more common in certain areas of the western United States and adjacent areas of Mexico.

The portal of entry is the lung, and although extrapulmonary spread does occur, it is unclear how frequently dissemination occurs. In the endemic area, acute coccidioidomycosis frequently presents as an episode of community-acquired pneumonia.

The most feared complication of coccidioidomycosis is the development of meningitis. While the majority of infections are either self-limited or mild, occasional patients present with fulminant pulmonary disease, leading to acute respiratory failure, requiring ventilatory support. The majority of these patients are immunocompromised and many are HIV-infected. History of travel to an endemic area is very important and should arouse suspicion.

Diagnosis is by culture of clinical specimens, serology and skin testing, but is difficult.

For severe and life-threatening illnesses, amphotericin B is the drug of choice. For meningitis, fluconazole is the drug of choice because of its excellent CNS penetration (30,32).

Cryptococcosis

Cryptococcus neoformans is a yeast-like fungus that may infect children with T-cell immune defects such as those seen in HIV infection and acute lymphoblastic leukemia. The portal of entry is by inhalation, and it may cause a localized pneumonitis or it may hematogenously disseminate to any organ of the body. The CNS is the most common site of infection, and presentation is with a chronic meningitis.

Diagnosis is by demonstration of cryptococcal antigen in serum or cerebrospinal fluid (CSF). Demonstrating budding organisms in India ink wet preparations of CSF also establishes the diagnosis.

Cryptococcal meningitis is treated with high-dose amphotericin B, with or without flucytosine, followed by a prolonged phase of maintenance therapy with fluconazole after 2 weeks of initial therapy. Relapses are common, especially in HIV-infected children (33).

Other Opportunistic Fungi

In addition to Zygomycetes, previously uncommon hyaline filamentous fungi (such as *Fusarium* species, *Acremonium* species, *Paecilomyces* species, *Pseudallescheria boydii*, and *Scedosporium prolificans*), dematiaceous filamentous fungi, and yeast-like pathogens (such as *Trichosporon* species, *Blastoschizomyces capitatus*, *Malassezia* species, *Rhodotorula rubra*, and others) are increasingly encountered as causing life-threatening invasive infections.

As airborne pathogens, the emerging opportunistic molds may cause disease that is virtually indistinguishable from that of *Aspergillus* infection.

Apart from infection of the skin and subcutaneous tissues, these fungi may affect primarily the sinobronchial tree and have a propensity for dissemination, in particular to the CNS.

Yeast-like pathogens mostly follow a similar pattern of fungemia and disseminated infection as seen in *Candida* infections (2).

Malassezia furfur is another fungus that causes tinea versicolor and folliculitis. It may also cause septicemia in patients receiving lipid solutions, due to its propensity for lipid-rich fluids (34).

Prophylaxis and Treatment of Fungal Infections in Critically Ill Children

The availability of new antifungal agents and their improved tolerability has widened options for the use of antifungal therapy for difficult-to-treat opportunistic mycoses. The treatment, however, is largely empirical and based on a high index of clinical suspicion because of the difficulty in diagnosis.

Four classes of antifungal agents have been identified:

- Polyenes: amphotericin B, liposomal amphotericin; these agents destabilize the fungal cell membrane.
- Nucleoside analogues: for example, 5-fluorocytosine, which interferes with fungal DNA and RNA synthesis and is used as an adjunct to amphotericin B.
- Azoles: triazoles (e.g., fluconazole, itraconazole) and the newer azoles (voriconazole, posaconazole, and ravuconazole). These agents interfere with sterol synthesis and fungal cell wall integrity.
- Echinocandins: for example, caspofungin; these agents inhibit glucan synthesis, leading to increased cell wall permeability and lysis.

Basic Principles

Management of fungal infection may be prophylactic, empirical, or definitive (35).

Prophylaxis

Outcomes for invasive fungal infections historically have been suboptimal and associated with a high mortality rate; hence, prophylaxis of patients at risk for fungal infections is an important therapeutic option. This involves the use of antifungal agents to prevent a fungal infection from occurring (35).

Several drugs are available for prophylaxis against fungal infection. The ease of use of oral antifungal agents makes them an attractive option for prophylaxis, and their introduction has led to routine outpatient therapy for prophylaxis and treatment of fungal infection. The intravenous route is preferred in patients with severely impaired swallowing, patients who are vomiting, and when high steady-state concentrations of the drug are required. The drug's side effects such as fever, hypotension, rigors, and nephrotoxicity may be treatment limiting.

Fluconazole

Oral fluconazole is useful for treating mucocutaneous, oropharyngeal, urinary, and systemic *Candida* infections, as well as cryptococcal infections. However, it is ineffective against *Aspergillus* species and *C. krusei*, and has variable activity against *C. glabrata*. Excessive use of fluconazole can lead to the development of fungal resistance, which is a risk during empirical treatment and prophylaxis. The emergence of fluconazole-resistant strains and the narrow spectrum limit its use in the prophylactic setting (36).

Itraconazole

Itraconazole has a wide spectrum of antifungal activity and is the only available azole agent that is active against *Aspergillus*. The most significant problem with the itraconazole oral solution remains compliance, and gastrointestinal side effects frequently necessitate withdrawal (37).

Unlike fluconazole, itraconazole binds strongly to protein, which may explain why itraconazole accumulates in high concentration in tissues and is highly effective against superficial fungal infections, particularly in keratinized tissue. If the problems of bioavailability of oral administration of the capsules were overcome, this property of tissue accumulation could be an advantage in prophylaxis of deep fungal infection in neutropenic patients.

The itraconazole oral solution is effective against fluconazole-resistant *Candida* infection, and this property, combined with the activity of itraconazole against *Aspergillus* species, may make the new itraconazole oral solution the best prophylactic antifungal agent available (38).

Amphotericin

The bioavailability of oral amphotericin is less than 5%, limiting its use for systemic fungal infections, but there is evidence to show that it may suppress *Candida* in the gut, thus reducing the risk of candidemia (39).

Newer Agents

Voriconazole has been shown to be effective for treatment of both *Aspergillus* and *Candida* infections. Thus, voriconazole is an attractive prospective agent for prophylaxis in patients at risk for these pathogens (40). Further randomized trials are needed to assess the effectiveness of voriconazole versus other antifungals in the prophylaxis of invasive fungal infection.

Posaconazole is an extended spectrum triazole with demonstrated activity against the same range of pathogens as voriconazole, with the additional advantage of activity against Zygomycetes.

Empirical Treatment

Empirical treatment involves waiting for a predefined time period (72 to 120 hours) of persistent fever, despite broad-spectrum antibiotics, to serve as a trigger for initiating antifungal therapy for a suspected infection (35).

Febrile Neutropenia

Invasive fungal disease is a cause of major morbidity and mortality in patients with neutropenia, and recent or ongoing prolonged exposure to broad-spectrum antibiotics. An early study by Pizzo et al. (41), showed the benefit of empiric addition of an antifungal agent in patients who had persistent fever with neutropenia lasting longer than 7 days.

The major concern with empirical antifungal therapy is that, like prophylaxis, it exposes a large proportion of the at-risk patient population to unnecessary antifungal therapy when infection may not be present. However, studies of patients with febrile neutropenia demonstrate that the addition of amphotericin B to broad-spectrum antibiotics at 96 hours significantly decreased the incidence of invasive fungal infections (42).

Traditionally the agent of choice has been amphotericin B, but given the drug-related toxicities and the availability of alternatives with presumed equivalent efficacy and less toxicity, agents such as voriconazole and lipid formulations of amphotericin B have been increasingly used. A major limitation of newer agents is the increased cost of therapy (43).

A liposomal preparation of amphotericin is a good first-line treatment in febrile neutropenia (44).

Voriconazole, a second-generation triazole, can be used for empirical antifungal therapy in patients with febrile neutropenia instead of liposomal amphotericin B. Its use may reduce the frequency of proven breakthrough fungal infections, preserve renal function, and reduce the frequency of acute infusion-related toxic effects (45). In institutions where infections with drug-resistant *Candida* species such as *C. krusei* or *C. glabrata* and mold infections such as those due to *Aspergillus* species are uncommon, empiric fluconazole therapy could be a reasonable alternative (46).

Treatment of Candidiasis

Treating *Candida* in a critical care setting needs careful thought. For superficial *Candida* infections (e.g., thrush or vaginitis), topical antifungals such as nystatin or clotrimazole are usually sufficient.

Candida esophagitis and vaginitis can be effectively treated with oral fluconazole. Invasive candidiasis (uncomplicated fungemia, catheter-related fungemia, and disseminated candidiasis) requires systemic antifungal treatment. Amphotericin B has traditionally been the drug of choice, but intravenous fluconazole should be seriously considered (47).

In critical care settings, itraconazole may also be a useful drug for empirical treatment of candidemia. A randomized control trial comparing the efficacy and side effects of oral fluconazole and oral itraconazole in pediatric intensive care settings showed itraconazole to be as effective in the treatment of nosocomial candidiasis and devoid of serious side effects (48,49).

Treatment of Aspergillosis

The availability of newer antifungal agents has been an important development in the treatment of invasive aspergillosis. Amphotericin B has traditionally been the mainstay of treatment. However, in patients with invasive aspergillosis, initial therapy with voriconazole led to better responses and improved survival, and resulted in fewer severe side effects than the standard approach of initial therapy with amphotericin B (50). Voriconazole appears to have comparable safety and efficacy in children with invasive mold infections compared with adults (51).

Echinocandins such as caspofungin have been used in combination with amphotericin B or a mold-active azole, such as voriconazole, as salvage therapy in invasive aspergillosis. Empiric therapy with caspofungin compared with liposomal amphotericin B in neutropenic patients with persisting fever showed an overall response rate of approximately 34%, with less toxicity for caspofungin (52).

Further randomized trials are required to definitively assess the benefit of combination antifungal therapy.

The use of interferon-γ as an adjunct against invasive aspergillosis is based on the augmentation of immune-related mechanisms against *Aspergillus*, but actual evidence is only in the form of anecdotal reports (18).

Emerging Fungal Pathogens

Uncommon fungal pathogens are becoming more common along with the emergence of non-*albicans Candida* species and *Aspergillus*. Mold infections continue to occur predominantly among highly immunosuppressed patients, such as those who have acute leukemia and those undergoing hematopoietic stem cell or solid organ transplantation. *Aspergillus* species remain the most common molds to cause invasive infection, but other environmental molds, such as *Scedosporium*, *Fusarium*, and various Zygomycetes, including *Rhizopus* and *Mucor*, appear to be increasing in some medical centers.

The treatment of mold infections has changed markedly in recent years. Previously, amphotericin B and itraconazole were the only available agents, but many non-*Aspergillus* molds are resistant to these agents. Voriconazole is also effective for the treatment of infections with *Scedosporium, Fusarium,* and other molds. However, the Zygomycetes are resistant to voriconazole and must be treated with amphotericin B (2,51).

References

1. Jarvis WR. Epidemiology of nosocomial fungal infections, with emphasis on Candida species. Clin Infect Dis 1995;20:1526–1530.
2. Groll AH, Walsh TJ. Uncommon opportunistic fungi: new nosocomial threats. Clin Microbiol Infect 2001;7(suppl 2):8–24.
3. Pfaller MA, Diekema DJ. Role of sentinel surveillance of candidemia: trends in species distribution and antifungal susceptibility. J Clin Microbiol 2002;40: 3551–3557.
4. Bodey G, Bueltmann B, Duguid W, et al. Fungal infections in cancer patients and international autopsy survey. Eur J Clin Microbiol 1992;11:99–109.
5. Wingard JR. Importance of Candida species other than *C. albicans* as pathogens in oncology patients. Clin Infect Dis 1995;20:115–125.
6. Welbel SF, McNeil MM, Kuykendall RJ. *Candida parapsilosis* bloodstream infections is neonatal intensive care unit patients: epidemiologic and laboratory confirmation of a common source outbreak. Pediatr Infect Dis J 1996;15:998–1002.
7. Zaoutis TE, Greves HM, Lautenbach E, Bilker WB, Coffin SE. Risk factors for disseminated candidiasis in children with candidemia. Pediatr Infect Dis J 2004;23:635–641.
8. Flynn PM, Gaur A. Infectious diseases. In: Rudolph DC, Rudolph A, Hostetter MK, George L, Siegel JN, eds. Rudolph's Paediatrics, 21st ed. New York: McGraw-Hill, pp. 1087–1090.
9. Darmstadt GL, Dinulos JG, Miller Z. Congenital cutaneous candidiasis: clinical presentation, pathogenesis, and management guidelines. Pediatrics 2000;105(2): 438–444.
10. Clerihew L, Lamagni TL, Brocklehurst P, McGuire W. Invasive fungal infection in very low birthweight infants: national prospective surveillance study. Arch Dis Child Fetal Neonatal Ed 2006;91(3):F188–F192.
11. Benjamin DK, Ross K, McKinney RE, et al. When to suspect fungal infection in neonates: a clinical comparison of *Candida albicans* and *Candida parapsilosis* fungemia with coagulase-negative staphylococcal bacteremia. Pediatrics 2000; 106(4):712–718.
12. Wenzel PR. Nosocomial candidemia; risk factors and attributable mortality. Clin Infect Dis 1995;20:1531–1534.
13. Berenguer J, Buck M, Witebsky F, et al. Lysis-centrifugation blood cultures in the detection of tissue-proven invasive candidiasis. Disseminated versus single-organ infection. Diagn Microbiol Infect Dis 1993;7:103–109.
14. Kauffman CA, Vazquez JA, Sobel JD, et al. Prospective multicenter surveillance study of funguria in hospitalized patients. Clin Infect Dis 2000;30:14–18.
15. Lehman D. Infectious diseases. In: Rudolph DC, Rudolph A, Hostetter MK, George L, Siegel JN, eds. Rudolph's Paediatrics, 21st ed. New York: McGraw-Hill, pp. 1084–1085.
16. Chakrabarti A, Shivaprakash MR. Microbiology of systemic fungal infections. J Postgrad Med 2005;51:16–20.

17. Zaoutis TE, Heydon K, Chu JH, Walsh TJ, Steinbach WJ. Epidemiology, outcomes, and costs of invasive aspergillosis in immunocompromised. *Pediatrics* 2006;117(4):711–716.
18. Segal BH, Walsh TJ. Current approaches to diagnosis and treatment of invasive aspergillosis. Am J Respir Crit Care Med 2006;173(7):707–717.
19. Talbot GH, Huang A, Provencher M. Invasive aspergillus rhinosinusitis in patients with acute leukemia. Rev Infect Dis 1991;13(2):219–232.
20. Nalesnik MA, et al. Significance of Aspergillus species isolated from respiratory secretions in the diagnosis of invasive pulmonary aspergillosis. J Clin Microbiol 1980;11(4):370–376.
21. Yu VL, Muder RR, Poorsatter A. Significance of isolation of Aspergillus from the respiratory tract in diagnosis of invasive pulmonary aspergillosis. Results from a three-year prospective study. Am J Med 1986;81:249–254.
22. Stover DE, Muhammad BZ, Steven IH, et al. Bronchoalveolar lavage in diagnosis of diffuse pulmonary infiltrates in the immunosuppressed host. Ann Intern Med 1984;101:1–7.
23. Walsh TJ, Gonzalez C, Lyman CA, Chanock SJ, Pizzo PA. Invasive fungal infections in children: recent advances in diagnosis and treatment. Adv Pediatr Infect Dis 1996;11:187–290.
24. Hohenadel IA, Kiworr M, Genitsariotis R, et al. Role of bronchoalveolar lavage in immunocompromised patients with pneumonia treated with a broad spectrum antibiotic and antifungal regimen. Thorax 2001;56:115–120.
25. Caillot D, Casanovas O, Bernard A, et al. Improved management of invasive pulmonary aspergillosis in neutropenic patients using early thoracic computed tomography scan and surgery. *J Clin Oncol* 1997;15:139–147.
26. Kuhlman JE, Fishman EK, Siegelman SS. Invasive pulmonary aspergillosis in acute leukemia: characteristic findings on CT, the CT halo sign, and the role of CT in early diagnosis. Radiology 1985;157(3):611–614.
27. Kuhlman JE, Fishman EK, Burch PA, et al. Invasive pulmonary aspergillosis in acute leukemia: the contribution of CT to early diagnosis and aggressive management. Chest 1987;92:95–99.
28. Althoff SC, Muller NL, Marchiori E. Pulmonary invasive aspergillosis and candidiasis in immunocompromised patients: a comparative study of the high-resolution CT findings. J Thorac Imaging 2006;21(3):184–189.
29. Abuhammour W, Hasan RA. Treatment of invasive Aspergillosis in children with hematologic malignancies. Indian J Pediatr 2004;71(9):837–843.
30. Sarosi GA. Fungal infections and their treatment in the intensive care unit. Curr Opin Intern Med 2006;5(6):553–558.
31. Kleiman MB. Infectious diseases. In: Rudolph DC, Rudolph A, Hostetter MK, George L, Siegel JN, eds. Rudolph's Paediatrics, 21st ed. New York: McGraw-Hill, pp. 1093–1095.
32. Schleiss MR. Infectious diseases. In: Rudolph DC, Rudolph A, Hostetter MK, George L, Siegel JN, eds. Rudolph's Paediatrics, 21st ed. New York: McGraw-Hill, 19••:1090–1093.
33. Lehmann D. Infectious diseases. In: Rudolph DC, Rudolph A, Hostetter MK, George L, Siegel JN, eds. Rudolph's Paediatrics, 21st ed. New York: McGraw-Hill, pp. 1092–1093.
34. Powell DA. Infectious diseases. In: Rudolph DC, Rudolph A, Hostetter MK, George L, Siegel JN, eds. Rudolph's Paediatrics, 21st ed. New York: McGraw-Hill, pp. 1095.

35. Leather HL, Wingard JR. New strategies of antifungal therapy in hematopoietic stem cell transplant recipients and patients with hematological malignancies. Blood Rev 2006;20:267–287.
36. Slavin MA, Osborne B, Adams R, et al. Efficacy and safety of fluconazole prophylaxis for fungal infections after marrow transplantation—a prospective randomized double-blind study. J Infect Dis 1995;20(171):1545–1552.
37. Foot A, Veys P, Gibson B. Itraconazole oral solution as antifungal prophylaxis in children undergoing stem cell transplantation or intensive chemotherapy for haematological disorders. Bone Marrow Transplant 1999;24(10):1089–1093.
38. Prentice AG, Donnelly P. Oral antifungals as prophylaxis in haematological malignancy. Blood Rev 2001;15(1):1–8.
39. Ben-Ari J, Smara Z, Nahum E. Oral amphotericin B for the prevention of Candida bloodstream infection in critically ill children. Pediatr Crit Care Med 2006;7:115–118.
40. Herbrecht R, Denning DW, Patterson TF, et al. Voriconazole versus amphotericin B for primary therapy of invasive aspergillosis. N Engl J Med 2002;357:408–415.
41. Pizzo PA, Robichaud KJ, Gill FA, Witebsky FG. Empiric antibiotic and antifungal therapy for cancer patients with prolonged fever and granulocytopenia. Am J Med 1982;72(1):101–111.
42. EORTC. Empiric antifungal therapy in febrile granulocytopenic patients. EORTC International Antimicrobial Therapy Cooperative Group. Am J Med 1989;86: 668–672.
43. Wingard JR. Empirical antifungal therapy in treating febrile neutropenic patients. Clin Infect Dis 2004;39(auppl 1):S38–43.
44. McKinsey DS. Making best use of the newer antifungal drugs. Infect Med 2003;20(8):392–399.
45. Walsh TJ, Pappas P, Winston DJ, et al. Voriconazole compared with liposomal amphotericin B for empirical antifungal therapy in patients with neutropenia and persistent fever. N Engl J Med 2002;346:225–234.
46. Gaur AH, Flynn PM, Shenep JL. Optimum management of pediatric patients with fever and neutropenia. Indian J Pediatr 2004;71(9):825–835.
47. Flynn PM. Infectious diseases. In: Rudolph DC, Rudolph A, Hostetter MK, George L, Siegel JN, eds. Rudolph's Paediatrics, 21st ed. New York: McGraw-Hill, pp. 1079–1084.
48. Hiranandani M, Singhi SC, Kaur I, Chakrabarti A. Disseminated nosocomial candidiasis in a paediatric intensive care unit. Indian Pediatr 1995;32(11):1160–1166.
49. Mondal RK, Singhi SC, Chakrabarti AMJ. Randomized comparison between fluconazole and itraconazole for the treatment of candidemia in a pediatric intensive care unit: a preliminary study. Pediatr Crit Care Med 2004;5(6):561–565.
50. Herbrecht R, Denning DW, Patterson TF, et al. Voriconazole versus amphotericin B for primary therapy of invasive aspergillosis. N Engl J Med 2002;347:408–415.
51. Walsh TJ, Lutsar I, Driscoll T, et al. Voriconazole in the treatment of aspergillosis, scedosporiosis and other invasive fungal infections in children. Pediatr Infect Dis J 2002;21:240–248.
52. Aoun M. Clinical efficacy of caspofungin in the treatment of invasive aspergillosis. Med Mycol 2006;44(suppl):363–366.

4
Toxin-Mediated Diseases and Toxic Shock Syndrome

Andrew C. Steer and Nigel Curtis

Toxic shock syndrome (TSS) is an acute febrile illness caused by gram-positive bacteria that rapidly progresses to shock with multiorgan failure. The capillary leak that underlies the disease results from intense T-cell proliferation and cytokine release that is part of an inflammatory response initiated by bacterial protein exotoxins acting as superantigens. This is analogous to, but distinct from, the inflammatory cascade initiated by lipopolysaccharide (LPS) from gram-negative bacteria that leads to septic shock. Toxic shock syndrome is caused by *Staphylococcus aureus* and *Streptococcus pyogenes* (the Lancefield group A β-hemolytic streptococcus [GAS]), and has also been described in association with other non–group A streptococci. Staphylococcal TSS became well known in the late 1970s when it was described in menstruating women using tampons (1,2). Nonmenstrual cases affecting males and females were widely described in the 1980s (3). Reports of streptococcal TSS began to emerge in the mid-1980s (4). Both streptococcal TSS and staphylococcal TSS can affect the paediatric population; in fact, the first description of staphylococcal TSS was in children (5).

Since the late 1980s, gram-positive infections have assumed increasing importance as a cause of morbidity and mortality, particularly with the resurgence of severe GAS infections, including streptococcal TSS, as well as acute rheumatic fever (6,7). In contrast to severe gram-negative infections and septic shock, gram-positive–induced TSS often affects young, previously healthy individuals, including children.

Although staphylococcal TSS and streptococcal TSS share a similar pathogenesis and are both characterized by early-onset shock and multiorgan failure, there are differences in the epidemiology, clinical features, and molecular microbiology of these two diseases. One of the most striking differences is that the mortality of streptococcal TSS is far higher (30% to 50%) than staphylococcal TSS (3%).

Epidemiology

Invasive Group A Streptococcal Disease and Streptococcal Toxic Shock Syndrome

Invasive infections due to GAS are defined as isolation of GAS from a normally sterile site and include bacteremia, focal infections with or without bacteremia, and streptococcal TSS (8). Focal infections include bone and joint infections, necrotizing fasciitis (NF), pneumonia, empyema, and meningitis.

Streptococcal TSS was first described in a 37-year-old woman with GAS primary peritonitis who developed toxic shock–like features in Prague in 1984 (9). Following this case, there were further reports in adults (4,10) and subsequently in children (11–13).

Reviews of historical literature suggest that some of the severe cases of GAS infection described in the earlier part of the 20th century may have been consistent with streptococcal TSS (14,15). Invasive GAS disease became less common in the industrialized world during the middle part of the 20th century. The reduction in prevalence has not been adequately explained but is presumed to have resulted from both changes in virulence of circulating GAS strains (14) as well as improvements in living conditions; the introduction of antibiotics is believed to have had only a modest impact. Since the mid-1980s there have been increasing reports of invasive GAS disease and streptococcal TSS occurring in both adults and children (4,8–11,16–36). This has been associated with a resurgence in poststreptococcal sequelae, particularly acute rheumatic fever (6,37).

There have been a number of large prospective and retrospective population-based surveys of invasive GAS disease and streptococcal TSS in the last two decades. These are summarized in Table 4.1 and indicate that the incidence of invasive GAS disease in the developed world is approximately 3.0 per 100,000.

Streptococcal TSS can affect any age group, with children, young adults, and the elderly (over the age of 65) most at risk. Approximately 20% of all cases of invasive GAS infections occur in children. The epidemiology of streptococcal TSS and invasive GAS disease is different in children and adults (29,38). The number of cases of streptococcal TSS as a proportion of invasive GAS disease is lower in children than in adults by a factor of two (28). In the elderly, underlying chronic illness appears to be a risk factor, and in young children varicella infection and immunosuppression are risk factors.

Nearly all reports of the resurgence of invasive GAS infections and streptococcal TSS have been in developed countries, mostly the United States and in Europe. It is unclear whether the same resurgence in invasive GAS infections has also occurred in developing countries. Recent research into the etiology of bacteremia in neonates and young infants in the developing world has identified GAS as an important pathogen. In a study in four developing countries of unwell infants aged 90 days and under, there were 167 (6.8%) blood culture isolates from 2452 blood cultures (39). Of these 167 isolates, 34 (20%) were *S. aureus*, 33 (20%) were *Streptococcus pneumoniae*, 29 (17%) were GAS, and 19

TABLE 4.1. Population-based surveys of invasive group A streptococcal (IGAS) disease and streptococcal toxic shock syndrome

Location	Year	No. of IGAS cases	No (%) of childhood IGAS cases	Case fatality ratio IGAS	Incidence IGAS (per 100,000)	No. (%) of TSS cases	No of childhood TSS cases	Case fatality ratio TSS	Incidence TSS (per 100,000)
Ontario (18)	1992–1993	323	79 (24%)	NA	1.5	42 (13%)	4	81%	0.2
Arizona (17)	1985–1990	128	18 (14%)	20%	4.3	6 (5%)	NA	33%	0.2
Atlanta (24)	1994–1995	183	41 (22%)	14%	5.2	25 (14%)	3	48%	0.7
Five states USA (26)	1995–1999	2002	226 (11%)	13%	3.3	120 (6%)	6	45%	0.2
Sweden (32)	1996–1997	255	NA	11%	2.3	19 (7%)	NA	47%	0.3
Ontario (28)	1992–1996	243	243 (100%)	10%	1.9	16 (7%)	16	56%	0.13

NA, information not available.

(11%) were *Escherichia coli*. In a study in infants in Kenya, the incidence of GAS bacteremia in children under 1 year of age was 96 per 100,000 (40). In this landmark study, community-acquired bacteremia caused at least 25% of deaths in children (33% in infants), and over 70% died within 48 hours of admission (41). Studies in indigenous populations have also shown a high incidence of invasive GAS disease—82 per 100,000 in Australian Aboriginals in Queensland and 46 per 100,000 in Native Americans in Arizona (17,27).

Morbidity and mortality from invasive GAS disease is significant. Epidemiologic surveys in the United States suggest that there are about 9600 cases of invasive GAS disease each year, resulting in 1200 deaths; this rate is three to four times that of meningococcal disease (26). Although some reports suggest that the mortality rate of streptococcal TSS is lower in children (29,42), most studies suggest that adult and child case fatality rates are similar, at approximately 50% (24,28,43).

Molecular Epidemiology of Streptococcal Toxic Shock Syndrome

Most GAS isolates have the necessary genes to produce at least one streptococcal superantigen toxin (44). Eleven GAS superantigen toxins have been identified: streptococcal pyrogenic exotoxins (SPEs) A, C, and G to M; the streptococcal superantigen (SSA); and the streptococcal mitogenic exotoxin Z (SMEZ), which has 34 known allelic variants.

Staphylococcal Toxic Shock Syndrome

The epidemiology of staphylococcal TSS has best been described in the United States. It is a good example of a rapid public health response to an emerging disease epidemic.

Following the initial reports of disease (1,2,5), passive surveillance across the United States between 1980 and 1981 revealed 1407 cases of staphylococcal TSS, with 92% of these associated with menstruation, and of these cases 99% occurred

TABLE 4.2. Staphylococcal toxic shock syndrome in the United States 1979–1996

Period	No. of cases	Menstrual cases (%)	Case fatality rate
1979–1980	1392	1264 (91%)	6%
1981–1986	2835	2021 (71%)	3.5%
1987–1996	1069	636 (59%)	3.5%[a]

[a]The case fatality rate for menstrual cases was 1.8%, while for nonmenstrual cases it was 6%.
Adapted from Hajjeh et al. (50).

in women using tampons (45). Over one third of these cases occurred in women between 15 and 19 years of age. Incidence rates as high as 12.3 per 100,000 were found in women of menstruating age (1,46).

The increasing awareness of the association between tampon use and staphylococcal TSS (47), together with public health recommendations including the voluntary removal from the market of one particularly high-risk brand of hyperabsorbable tampon, led to a fall in the incidence of staphylococcal TSS over the following years (Table 4.2). The incidence rate in women of menstruating age fell to 1 per 100,000 in 1986 (48) and was 0.8 per 100,000 in the Minneapolis–St. Paul area in 2000 (49). More recently the incidence of staphylococcal TSS in women of menstruating age appears to be increasing with a reported incidence of 3.4 per 100,000 in the Minneapolis–St. Paul area in 2003 (49).

The increasing proportion of nonmenstrual cases of staphylococcal TSS has been noteworthy (50). In the United States the proportion increased from 29% in the period 1981 to 1986 to 41% in the period 1987 to 1996. Among this group there has been an increase in the number of cases following surgical procedures. Also of note is the higher case fatality rate for nonmenstrual staphylococcal TSS. This may reflect the fact that nonmenstrual patients tend to be older than otherwise healthy young women who are at risk of menstrual TSS, and therefore possibly have more comorbid conditions (3).

Molecular Epidemiology of Staphylococcal Toxic Shock Syndrome

Menstrual staphylococcal TSS is almost always associated with the superantigen toxic shock syndrome toxin-1 (TSST-1), whereas nonmenstrual cases are associated with an ever-growing number of other staphylococcal superantigen toxins including TSST-1 and staphylococcal enterotoxins (SEs) A through to R (49,51–54). Toxic shock syndrome toxin-1 was expressed by approximately 20% of *S. aureus* isolates in one study (55), but the proportion of *S. aureus* isolates that produce each superantigen toxin varies widely, and many isolates produce more than one superantigen toxin (55).

Non–Group A Streptococcal Toxic Shock Syndrome

Group C and G streptococci have also been associated with TSS (56–61). There are also case reports of TSS and NF associated with group B streptococci (62,63).

The clinical manifestations of non-GAS TSS are very similar to group A streptococcal TSS (56,60,61). Over 50% of cases are associated with soft tissue infection, particularly NF, and the mortality rate is approximately 30% to 40%. The underlying pathophysiology is believed to be similar: superantigens or laboratory evidence of superantigen production has been found in group C and G streptococcal isolates (60).

Pathogenesis

Knowledge of the pathophysiology and role of superantigens is important in understanding the clinical features and management of TSS.

Streptococcal and staphylococcal TSS are mediated by exotoxins produced by *S. pyogenes* and *S. aureus*, respectively, that act as superantigens. It has been proposed that these protein toxins play a role in the pathogenesis of a number of other diseases, including Kawasaki disease, that share common clinical features, which include the presence of an erythematous rash that desquamates, and oropharyngeal mucosal changes (64–68). It has also been proposed that superantigens are involved in the pathogenesis of autoimmune disease, atopic dermatitis, and psoriasis (69–71).

The Mechanism of Action of Superantigens

Superantigens are a family of immunomodulatory proteins that stimulate T cells by directly binding class II molecules on antigen-presenting cells (for example, B cells and macrophages) to the T-cell receptor (Fig. 4.1) (52,53,55,64,72,73). This unique mechanism differs from conventional antigen stimulation in a number of key ways:

1. Lack of antigen processing: Conventional antigens are ingested by antigen-presenting cells and broken down into peptide fragments for presentation on the antigen-presenting cell surface in the groove of the major histocompatability complex (MHC) class II molecules. Superantigens do not undergo antigen processing but interact directly with the class II molecule.

2. Lack of MHC restriction: Conventional antigen fragments are presented on the antigen-presenting cell surface in conjunction with an MHC class II molecule. T-cell recognition of this MHC-antigen complex is therefore MHC restricted. While superantigen stimulation requires MHC class II expression (MHC dependent), it is not restricted.

3. T-cell receptor Vβ specificity and intense immune activation: T-cell recognition of conventional antigen is highly specific, involving all domains of both chains of the T-cell receptor. Only a small proportion of T cells (perhaps 1 in 10^6) have a receptor that recognizes a given MHC-antigen complex and thus can be stimulated. In contrast, superantigen binding to T cells is restricted only by one portion of the variable region of the β chain of the T-cell receptor, the Vβ region. Each T cell belongs to one of only 24 different Vβ families, based

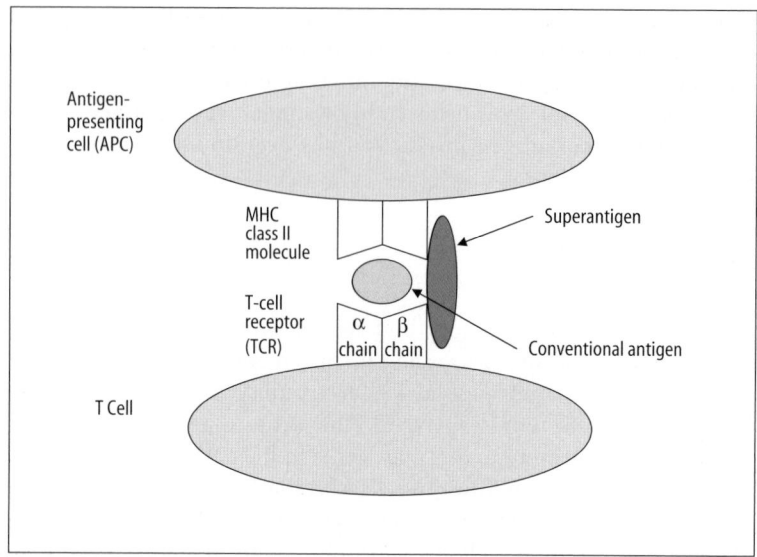

FIGURE 4.1. Composite diagram contrasting T-cell stimulation by a conventional antigen and a superantigen.

on the sequence of their Vβ domain. Each superantigen has a specificity for one or a limited set of Vβ families and can stimulate all T cells bearing those Vβ regions, irrespective of the antigen specificity of the T-cell receptor. By this mechanism superantigens are able to stimulate a large proportion (up to one in five) of all T cells. Thus, superantigen toxins are extremely potent with activity even at picomolar concentrations.

Superantigen stimulation of T cells leads to the release of cytokines both from T cells and from other cells of the immune system. These cytokines include tumor necrosis factor-α, interleukin-1, interleukin-2, and interferon-γ (Fig. 4.2). The intense cytokine release brought about by superantigens, especially the release of TNF-α, is believed to be particularly important in the pathogenesis of the capillary leak underlying toxic shock and the clinical features of TSS (74). The cascade of cytokine release and immune activation is similar to LPS-induced septic shock in gram-negative bacteremia, but there are clear differences in the pattern, cell requirements, and kinetics of cytokine release. While the mechanisms of superantigen and LPS-induced shock are distinct, another important pathologic mechanism may be the ability of superantigens to enhance endotoxic shock.

Evidence of the Role of Superantigens in Toxic Shock Syndrome

Immunologic studies of patients have provided good evidence that superantigens play a key role in the pathogenesis of TSS. The hallmark of a superantigen-mediated disease is a skewed pattern of Vβ expression in the population of T cells from patients with the disease. This is caused by the preferential stimulation and proliferation of T cells belonging to Vβ families specific to the superantigen. The specific pattern ("Vβ repertoire") should reflect the in vitro Vβ specificity (or "signature") of the causative superantigen. Staphylococcal TSS was the first disease in which an altered T-cell Vβ repertoire was detected in patients. A disproportionately high number of T cells bearing Vβ2 were found in patients with staphylococcal TSS (75). This correlated with the in vitro Vβ specificity of TSST, which stimulates T cells bearing Vβ2. Similar studies have been undertaken in streptococcal TSS (72).

Two further lines of evidence indirectly support the role of superantigen toxins in the pathogenesis of TSS: first, epidemiologic studies of the superantigen toxin-producing capability of bacterial isolates; and second, serologic studies correlating absence of neutralizing antibody to superantigen toxins with susceptibility as discussed below.

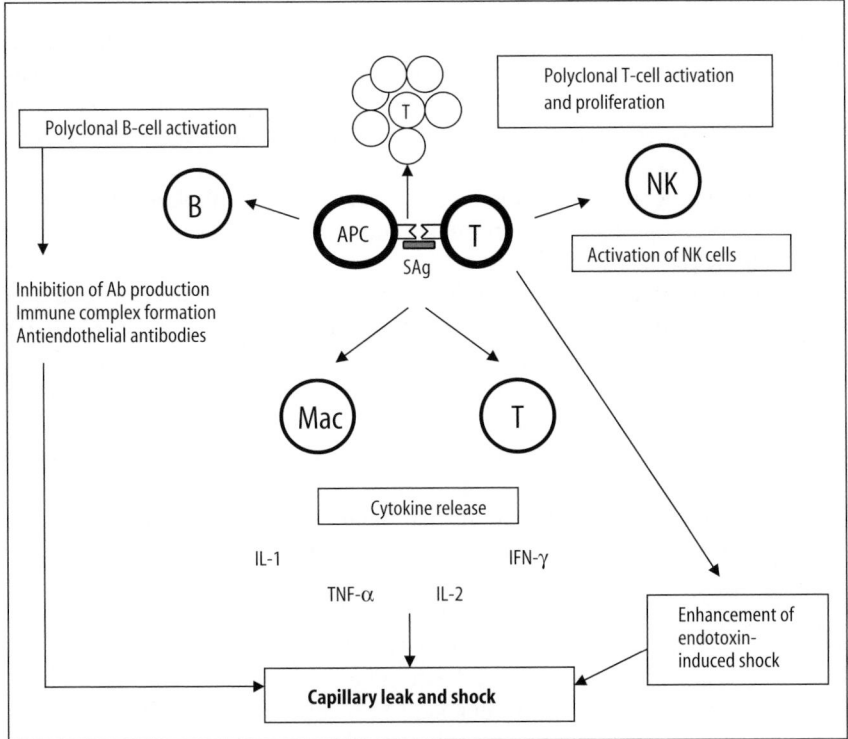

FIGURE 4.2. Immunologic consequences of superantigen activity. APC, antigen-presenting cell; IFN, interferon; IL, interleukin; Mac, macrophage; NK, natural killer; SAg, superantigen; TNF, tumor necrosis factor.

Host Factors in Superantigen-Mediated Disease

It is believed that the outcome following exposure to staphylococcal and streptococcal superantigen toxins depends on a number of factors including previous exposure, dose, route, local microenvironmental and other cofactors, as well as possible genetic factors. Lack of neutralizing antibody to a particular superantigen appears to be a prerequisite to the development of streptococcal TSS (76,77) and staphylococcal TSS (53,78). Many individuals develop protective antibodies following asymptomatic exposure to superantigen toxins with acquisition of carriage of *S. aureus* and GAS (79). This is believed to explain why only a small proportion of individuals exposed to virulent strains develop TSS, despite the finding that 20% of *S. aureus* isolates express TSST-1 (55,78,79).

Clinical Features

Both streptococcal TSS and staphylococcal TSS are characterized by fever and rash, with rapid progression to shock and multiorgan failure. The typical "sunburn"-type rash in TSS is widespread, erythematous, macular, and blanching. Characteristically, there is subsequent desquamation about 2 weeks after the initial illness. Shock is caused by the capillary leak and vasodilation resulting from massive cytokine release induced by bacterial superantigen toxins, and, untreated, leads to disseminated intravascular coagulation (DIC), myocardial suppression, hypotension, renal failure, and adult respiratory distress syndrome (ARDS).

Although diagnostic criteria for both streptococcal and staphylococcal TSS have been published (45,80), these were designed primarily as research criteria with high specificity to identify established cases. Consequently the criteria have poor sensitivity to diagnose the syndrome early in their course. Before the onset of capillary leak sufficient to cause shock with resulting end-organ dysfunction, patients may present with only fever and rash, sometimes with additional characteristic features such as conjunctivitis or mucositis. The absence of sufficient features to fulfill the formal diagnostic criteria should not deter early provisional diagnostic and empiric treatment of TSS.

It is not possible to reliably distinguish streptococcal from staphylococcal TSS from the clinical features alone, particularly early in the disease. However, there are some general differences between the two syndromes. Patients with staphylococcal TSS are more likely to have the macular erythematous rash that desquamates than are patients with streptococcal TSS. Patients with streptococcal TSS are much more likely to have positive blood cultures with rates of between 60% and 80% (17,18,26). In a landmark study of 130 patients with staphylococcal TSS, *S. aureus* was cultured from the blood in only 3% of patients (3).

In addition, streptococcal TSS is usually associated with severe focal infection such as NF or pneumonia, while in staphylococcal TSS the focus of infection

TABLE 4.3. Unique clinical features of streptococcal and staphylococcal toxic shock syndrome (TSS)

	Streptococcal TSS	Staphylococcal TSS
Mortality rate	30–60%	<3%
Positive blood cultures	60–80%	Low
Typical rash	Less common	Very common
Associations	Soft tissue infection	Tampon use
	Varicella infection	Surgical procedures
	NSAID	NSAID
		Burns
		Influenza infection

NSAID, nonsteroidal antiinflammatory drug.

may be a trivial cutaneous or subcutaneous infection. The case mortality rate of streptococcal TSS is on the order of 10 times greater than staphylococcal TSS.

There are a number of associations for both streptococcal and staphylococcal TSS; these are listed in Table 4.3 and described in more detail below.

Streptococcal Toxic Shock Syndrome

The case definition for streptococcal toxic shock was published in 1992 (Table 4.4) (80). As mentioned above, appropriate treatment should usually be started in suspected cases even if the patients do not meet the formal diagnostic criteria.

Typically patients present with fever. Approximately 50% of patients have hypotension at presentation, and nearly all develop hypotension over the following 4 hours (81). Subacute presentations in which patients deteriorate over

TABLE 4.4. Diagnostic criteria for streptococcal toxic shock syndrome (80)

1. Isolation of GAS
    A. From a sterile site (definite case)
    B. From a nonsterile site (probable case)
2. Clinical signs of severity
    A. Hypotension
        AND
    B. Two or more of the following clinical and laboratory abnormalities:
        a. Fever (>38.5°C)
        b. Rash (diffuse macular erythema with subsequent desquamation)
        c. Renal impairment
        d. Coagulopathy (platelets <100 or DIC)
        e. Liver abnormalities
        f. ARDS
        g. Extensive tissue necrosis (including necrotizing fasciitis)

ARDS, adult respiratory distress syndrome; DIC: disseminated intravascular coagulation; GAS, group A β-hemolytic streptococcus.

days are rare. Around 20% of patients with streptococcal TSS have a flu-like prodromal illness with fever, myalgia, vomiting, and diarrhea (81).

Soft tissue infection is the most common focus of infection associated with streptococcal TSS, occurring in approximately 60% of patients (18). Around 75% of these soft tissue infections progress to NF (82). The next most common associated clinical infection is pneumonia with empyema (83). Streptococcal TSS presents with bacteremia alone without a clear focus in approximately 15% of patients (18). Other clinical infections described include septic arthritis, pharyngitis, peritonitis, meningitis, tracheitis, endophthalmitis, and perihepatitis (20,82,84),

There have been increasing reports of streptococcal TSS in neonates since the mid-1980s (85,86). Maternal carriage is an important factor in early-onset neonatal invasive GAS disease, with 75% of patients having documented maternal carriage.

Streptococcal Toxic Shock Syndrome and Necrotizing Fasciitis

Group A β-hemolytic streptococcus can cause a variety of soft tissue infections ranging from pyoderma, erysipelas, and cellulitis to full-blown NF (87). In the clinical setting it is extremely important to differentiate between cellulitis and NF because of the implications for treatment and outcome.

Necrotizing fasciitis is a rapidly spreading infection of muscle fascia, subcutaneous fat, and epidermis that leads to necrosis of muscle fascia (88). It has been classified into types I and II (89). Type I refers to NF caused by polymicrobial infections, while type II refers to NF caused by GAS infection.

The case mortality rate of GAS-associated NF is 30% to 50% (88,90–92). The mortality rate increases with increasing age and in patients with underlying chronic illness. About 30% to 50% of patients with GAS-associated NF develop streptococcal TSS; these patients have a higher mortality rate than those patients who do not develop streptococcal TSS (88,90,93).

Necrotizing fasciitis may follow local blunt or penetrating trauma to the skin. It occurs most commonly in the upper limb, followed by the lower limb. In adults, the most common precipitating factor is intravenous drug use (92). In children, the most common precipitating factor is varicella infection (90).

The recognition of infection beyond the dermis is critical, as aggressive surgical debridement may reduce mortality significantly (94). Severe pain and tenderness that is disproportionate to the physical findings is the clinical hallmark that differentiates NF from more superficial infection and should alert physicians (88,95). Initially there may only be subtle skin signs that accompany the tenderness. Tense edema and the development of bluish bullae appear as the disease progresses and are useful signs in differentiating NF from cellulitis (82,91). Skin necrosis is a late sign and is associated with poor outcome.

If the diagnosis of NF is not clear, there are a number of investigations available to the clinician. There are some reports of the usefulness of magnetic resonance imaging (MRI) (96–98). The use of frozen section biopsy specimens of suspected areas of tissue may enable early recognition of NF and rapid and wide surgical debridement (99). However, if MRI is not available or if the pathology staff is unable to interpret frozen section specimens, or whenever there is a strong suspicion of NF, then surgery should not be delayed (100). Recently, a scoring system that uses hematologic and biochemical results at admission has been developed to aid the clinician in the early recognition of NF (101).

The evolution of the NF is rapid with progression to limb and life-threatening disease within 24 hours. In children, 90% of deaths occur in the first 48 hours after presentation (28).

Streptococcal Toxic Shock Syndrome and Varicella Infection

Varicella infection is the predisposing factor in about 15% to 50% of all invasive GAS disease in children (28,102). The overall incidence of invasive GAS disease in the paediatric population in Ontario between 1992 and 1996 was 1.9 per 100,000. In children with varicella the attack rate was 5.2 per 100,000 in the 2-week period following varicella infection compared with 0.09 per 100,000 in those without varicella infection; this represents a relative risk of 58 (28).

Varicella infection is a particularly important risk factor for GAS NF (93,103–106). In a series of 77 patients with NF in Canada, there were five children less than 10 years of age with NF, of which four cases followed varicella infection (90). The mechanism by which varicella predisposes to NF is not clear (105). It may be that varicella lesions act as a portal of entry to the dermal and fascial layers, or that varicella infection itself causes immunosuppression, particularly a decrease in humoral immunity (28). The latter explanation is supported by the fact that patients tend not to have secondarily infected pox lesions overlying the area of NF (93), and because streptococcal TSS and invasive GAS disease without NF also follows varicella infection (107–109). The median duration of presence of varicella lesions before developing symptoms of NF is 3 to 4 days (93,104). Once symptoms develop, it is rapidly progressive with evolution within 24 hours. Again, a high index of suspicion is critical for differentiating NF from cellulitis.

It is hoped that the availability of varicella vaccination will reduce the number of cases of invasive GAS disease and streptococcal TSS (28). At one Chicago pediatric center, rates of hospitalization for varicella-associated invasive GAS disease fell from 27% of total cases of invasive GAS disease to 2%, following implementation of the varicella vaccine in the intervening years; rates of hospitalization for invasive GAS remained static at around 1.5 per 1000 over this period (110).

Streptococcal Toxic Shock Syndrome and Nonsteroidal Antiinflammatory Drugs

A number of case reports as well as a case-control study have noted an association between the use of nonsteroidal antiinflammatory drugs (NSAIDs) and NF and streptococcal TSS (106,111–113). It may simply be that by masking fever and reducing pain, NSAIDs lead to delayed presentation. The proposed pathologic mechanism by which NSAIDs may increase the risk of TSS is inhibition of the normal feedback loop of prostaglandin on the production of TNF-α by macrophages (114). By inhibiting cyclooxygenase, NSAIDs prevent the conversion of arachidonic acid to prostaglandin E_2 (PGE_2), and this leads to unregulated production of TNF, as PGE_2 is normally a feedback inhibitor of TNF (114). This excess of cytokines may predispose to TSS (Fig. 4.3). In addition,

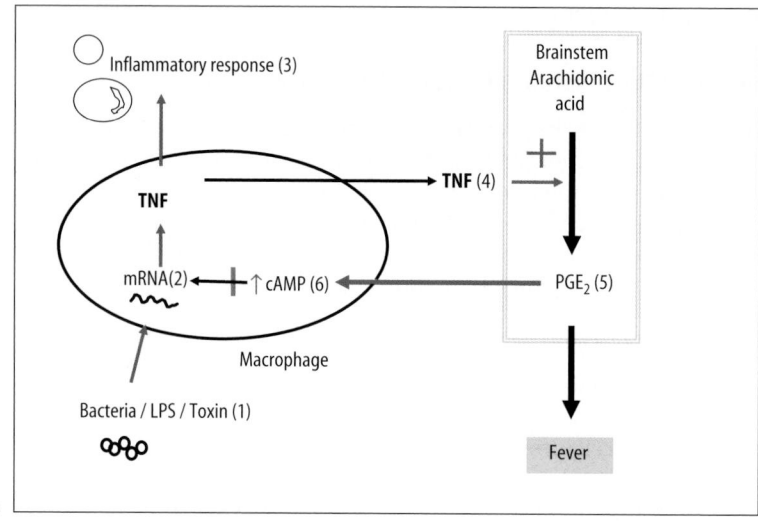

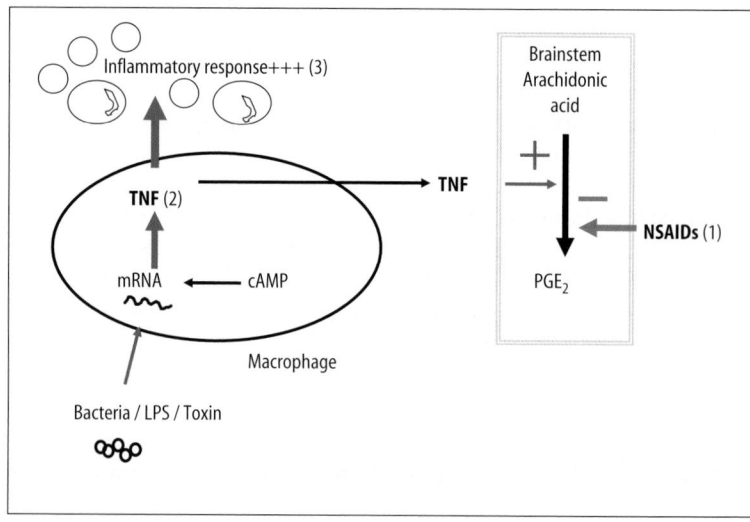

FIGURE 4.3. (A,B) The proposed mechanism by which nonsteroidal antiinflammatory drugs (NSAIDs) cause increased cytokine production that may explain their association with the development of necrotizing fasciitis (NF). cAMP, cyclic adenosine monophosphate; LPS, lipopolysaccharide; mRNA, messenger RNA.

NSAIDs have a profoundly suppressive effect on neutrophil function. There-fore, some authors recommend avoiding NSAIDs in patients without a known source for their fever (106,114–116), though this is controversial (117–119).

Staphylococcal Toxic Shock Syndrome

In the original description of staphylococcal TSS, seven children presented with fever, headache, confusion, conjunctival injection, vomiting and diarrhea, per-sistent hypotension, subcutaneous edema, and a diffuse erythematous macular rash that subsequently desquamated (5). These patients developed DIC, hepatic impairment, and renal impairment that in many cases preceded their hypoten-sion. All patients had evidence of staphylococcal infection, but *S. aureus* was not isolated from blood cultures.

These cases, along with subsequent reports of numerous cases of menstrual staphylococcal TSS, led to a case definition for staphylococcal TSS being estab-lished in 1981 (Table 4.5) (45). In these criteria, definite cases are defined as those with fever, the typical erythematous rash that subsequently desquamates, hypotension, and multiorgan dysfunction that involves at least three organs. Probable cases are defined as those that lack one of these features. However, as with streptococcal TSS, appropriate treatment should be instigated in patients with clinical features suggesting staphylococcal TSS even if the formal case definition is not met.

The rash in staphylococcal TSS is prominent—more so than in streptococcal TSS. The rash is typically diffuse, macular, and erythematous, and desquamates 1 to 2 weeks after the onset of the illness, particularly on the palms, soles, fingers, and toes. Mucosal hyperemia may be present as nonpurulent conjunc-tivitis, reddened or swollen lips, and vaginal mucosal hyperemia.

TABLE 4.5. Diagnostic criteria for staphylococcal toxic shock syndrome (45)

1. Fever (>38.9°C)
2. Hypotension
3. Rash (diffuse macular rash with subsequent desquamation)
4. Involvement of three of the following organ systems:
   a. Liver (elevated transaminases)
   b. Blood (platelets <100)
   c. Renal (raised creatinine/urea or pyuria in absence of UTI)
   d. Mucous membranes (vaginal, conjunctival, or oropharyngeal hyperaemia)
   e. Gastrointestinal (vomiting and profuse diarrhoea)
   f. Muscular (severe myalgia or raised CPK)
   g. Central nervous system (disorientation or alteration in consciousness without focal neurologic signs)
5. Exclusion of the following illnesses by negative serology
   a. Measles
   b. Leptospirosis
   c. Rocky Mountain spotted fever
6. Negative blood or cerebrospinal fluid cultures for organisms other than *S. aureus*

UTI, urinary tract infection; CPK, creatinine phosphokinase.

More recently it has been suggested that the definition of staphylococcal TSS be revised to include laboratory findings such as the production of TSST-1 by a staphylococcal isolate, isolation of *S. aureus* from a sterile site, absence of antibody to superantigen toxin at the time of the acute illness, development of antibody to the toxin in recovery from the illness (120), and expansion of TSST-1 reactive Vβ2 T cells in peripheral blood mononuclear cells (121).

Menstrual Staphylococcal Toxic Shock Syndrome

Despite the dramatic reduction in cases of menstrual staphylococcal TSS since the early 1980s, 60% of adult cases are still menstrual-related (50).

Recurrent menstrual staphylococcal TSS tends to occur in women who do not develop an adequate antibody response to TSST (78) and who have persistent vaginal carriage of *S. aureus*. In the initial studies of menstrual staphylococcal TSS, up to 30% of patients had recurrent episodes (1). Women who were not treated with an antistaphylococcal antibiotic and who continued to use tampons appeared to be at highest risk (122). Patients who have a first episode of menstrual staphylococcal TSS and have an inadequate antibody response to staphylococcal toxin should be advised not to use tampons (123,124).

Nonmenstrual Staphylococcal Toxic Shock Syndrome

Nonmenstrual staphylococcal TSS can occur in any age group and affects both sexes. It has been associated with a number of different staphylococcal infections as well as surgical procedures, childbirth, burns, and influenza infection (Table 4.6) (3). Other documented sites of infection include visceral abscesses, endocarditis, osteomyelitis, pyomyositis, mastitis, and peritonitis (125). The broad range of possible sites of infection means that the clinician must think widely when assessing a patient with staphylococcal TSS.

In children with staphylococcal TSS, the skin is most commonly the site of infection (50). In a series of eight pediatric cases, the sites of infection were cervical lymphadenitis, a surgical wound, bacteremia, and pleural fluid, and in four cases the site was not established (126). In this small series there appeared to be a higher rate of ARDS compared with adult patients.

Recurrent nonmenstrual staphylococcal TSS is less common than recurrent menstrual staphylococcal TSS but has been described (123). The case fatality

TABLE **4.6.** Sites of infections related to nonmenstrual staphylococcal toxic shock syndrome

Site of infection	Percentage of cases
Cutaneous and subcutaneous lesions	30%
Childbirth or abortion	28%
Surgical wound	18%
Vaginal infections (excluding during menstruation or related to childbirth)	5%
Other or unknown	19%

Adapted from Reingold et al. (3).

rate of nonmenstrual staphylococcal TSS is generally higher than menstrual staphylococcal TSS and varies in reports from 6% to 9% (3,50).

Staphylococcal Toxic Shock Syndrome and Surgical Procedures

Nonmenstrual staphylococcal TSS has been associated with a variety of surgical procedures including spinal surgery, genitourinary surgery, hernia surgery, and orthopedic surgery (3,127). Of particular note is an association with ear, nose, and throat surgery (127) and especially nasal packing (128,129). This is presumed to occur in patients who are nasopharyngeal carriers of superantigen toxin-producing strains of *S. aureus* with microbial entry facilitated by mucosal injury. The median interval between surgery and onset of TSS is 2 days (3).

Staphylococcal Toxic Shock Syndrome and Burns

Staphylococcal TSS was first described in children with burns in 1985; four of the seven children described died (130). An informal postal survey of burns units in the United Kingdom suggested that 2.5% of burns admissions develop staphylococcal TSS (131). Children with burns are at a particularly high risk of staphylococcal TSS because of the loss of skin integrity and high rates of *S. aureus* colonization acquired in hospital. The illness usually occurs in the first few days following the burn (132). Although most children with burns who develop TSS have extensive skin involvement (more than 5% of total body surface area), there have been reports of children with burns as small as a 2% scald (133).

Staphylococcal Toxic Shock Syndrome and Influenza Infection

There is an association between influenza infection and the development of staphylococcal TSS, with a particularly high risk in pediatric patients in whom the mortality rate is high (134).

Differential Diagnosis

The differential diagnosis of TSS includes other causes of capillary leak and shock such as gram-negative septic shock and meningococcal septicemia, as well as other diseases associated with shock such as myocarditis. The possible diagnostic difficulty in distinguishing NF and other soft tissue infection is discussed above. Other diseases characterized by fever and erythematous rash often also need to be considered. One important disease that can mimic TSS is Kawasaki disease. In fact, the clinical and laboratory features of these two diseases are so similar that when children with staphylococcal TSS were first identified in 1978 it was thought that they had a form of Kawasaki disease (James Todd, personal communication). The similarities between these diseases have led to the hypothesis that Kawasaki disease is itself a superantigen-mediated disease. The most obvious distinguishing feature is the presence of shock. However, shock can occur in Kawasaki disease, either as a result of severe myocardial involvement or, more rarely, after myocardial infarction. The clinician must be cautious, however, as Kawasaki disease may coexist with TSS or patients may have clinical features suggestive of Kawasaki disease but may develop toxic shock (135–137).

Management

Supportive Care

One of the defining features of TSS is the profound hypotension caused by toxin-mediated capillary leak. This requires volume expansion by aggressive fluid replacement. Inotropes are often required early. Renal support may also be required early; it is important to recognize that renal failure may precede hypotension (138). Patients frequently require endotracheal intubation and ventilation, particularly when ARDS develops.

Surgical Intervention

Removal of any source of infection is critical in the early management of TSS. Surgical intervention is particularly important in streptococcal TSS when there is GAS infection of soft tissue. The mainstay of treatment in NF is debridement. Wide debridement of nonviable tissue when the source of infection is NF is critical and substantially improves the outcome (82,139). In one retrospective survey of adult patients with NF, patients who had early debridement had a lower mortality rate (4%) than those with late debridement (38%) (140). In another series of patients with GAS NF, almost all patients who did not have surgical excision of necrotic tissue died (90). Most patients require repeated surgery before wound coverage is possible. Hyperbaric oxygen therapy has been proposed in the management of NF but its benefit is unproven (141). Establishing a diagnosis of NF is not always straightforward and is discussed above (see Clinical Features).

Surgical intervention is required less often in staphylococcal TSS. However, the removal of any in situ tampons and vaginal irrigation in menstrual staphylococcal TSS is extremely important. Establishing the presence of any tampons is therefore a crucial part of the examination of all postmenarche women with TSS.

Antibiotic Therapy

Penicillin is the first-line antibiotic of choice for streptococcal TSS and floxacillin the first choice for staphylococccal TSS. Floxacillin is also an effective anti-streptococcal antibiotic and should therefore be used when the etiology is uncertain, which is the case in most instances initially, and in a significant proportion of patients in whom neither *S. aureus* nor *S. pyogenes* is isolated. There is some evidence that clindamycin has advantages over β-lactam antibiotics (142). However, it is recommended that clindamycin should be added to the above standard treatment regimes rather than replace them. There is no antagonism between the penicillins and clindamycin when they are used in combination for the treatment of streptococcal TSS (143).

The advantages of clindamycin in severe gram-positive infections have been shown in laboratory experiments. These include avoidance of the Eagle effect (see below) (142), direct effects on toxin production (144), an ability to potentiate phagocytosis (145), a longer postantibiotic effect (146), and superior tissue penetration. There is less evidence, however, to support any clinical correlates of these effects.

The Eagle was first described in 1952 (147). Eagle showed that in a mouse model of streptococcal myositis, penicillin is less effective if the inoculum of streptococci is high, or if treatment is delayed. When numbers of streptococci reach a high level, they reach a steady state; at this point the growth phase of these organisms is stationary and penicillin becomes less effective because of decreased cell division and decreased concentration of penicillin binding proteins. Clindamycin is not affected by the Eagle effect, remaining 100% effective in the same mouse model (142).

In streptococcal TSS, clindamycin has direct effects on superantigen toxin synthesis (148,149). Similarly in staphylococcal TSS, clindamycin has been shown to suppress TSST-1 production (150). It has been shown that underlying this effect is the ability of clindamycin to inhibit toxin gene transcription (151).

Clindamycin has been shown to potentiate opsonization, phagocytosis, and complement fixation of both GAS and staphylococci in vitro (145). In the case of GAS, clindamycin appears to denude the organism of its hairlike structures of M-protein, an important virulence factor (145).

There has been only one clinical study of clindamycin in invasive GAS infections (152). This retrospective review of 56 children with invasive GAS infections over a 15-year period showed improved outcomes in patients with deep-seated infections treated initially with a combination of a penicillin and clindamycin when compared with those treated with a penicillin alone. In this study, surgical debridement was also associated with improved outcome. There have been no clinical trials of clindamycin in staphylococcal TSS.

In general, the use of vancomycin in TSS is avoided because of the risk of inducing multiple organism resistance to vancomycin. However, in staphylococcal TSS, vancomycin may need to replace floxacillin as first-line therapy if the infection is hospital acquired or in other situations where the proportion of methicillin resistant *S. aureus* strains is high.

Immunoglobulin Therapy

Intravenous immunoglobulin (IVIG) is widely used in a number of sepsis syndromes (153). However, there is conflicting evidence about the effect of IVIG in lowering mortality in sepsis (153,154).

Studies suggest that streptococcal TSS may be a subgroup of sepsis where IVIG has a clear role. The role of IVIG in staphylococcal TSS has been less closely studied. Given that the pathogenesis of staphylococcal TSS is similar to that of streptococcal TSS, and that superantigens of *S. aureus* and *S. pyogenes* share a common three-dimensional structure and mode of action, it seems likely that IVIG will also be beneficial in this syndrome.

Rationale for the Use of Intravenous Immunoglobulin in Toxic Shock Syndrome

Humoral immunity is important in protecting against the development of invasive streptococcal and staphylococcal disease (155). From this observation came the idea that passive immunization with IVIG could improve the outcome of TSS (156). Neutralizing antibodies to streptococcal superantigen toxins are present in IVIG (157), and plasma from patients with streptococcal TSS who have been treated with IVIG has been shown to inhibit superantigen-induced T-cell proliferation and production of cytokines in vitro (158,159).

Evidence for the Use of Intravenous Immunoglobulin in Toxic Shock Syndrome

There have been a number of case reports in adults and children describing the successful use of IVIG in TSS (160–164). However, there is only one randomized controlled trial of IVIG in TSS (165). Unfortunately, this trial was ceased prematurely because of slow patient enrollment; it enrolled 21 patients when it aimed for a total of 120. This study found a trend toward improved survival at 28 days in patients with streptococcal TSS but did not find a significant difference in mortality at 28 days. This study was unable to answer definitively whether IVIG is beneficial in streptococcal TSS (166). An earlier observational historically controlled cohort study showed a significant difference in mortality at 30 days (167). Table 4.7 summaries the results of these two studies. There have been no published comparative trials of IVIG in staphylococcal TSS. It is unlikely that another randomized controlled trial of IVIG will take place in either staphylococcal or streptococcal TSS.

Dosing of Intravenous Immunoglobulin in Toxic Shock Syndrome

There is no clear regime for dosing IVIG in TSS. The two dosing regimes used in the above two studies are presented in Table 4.8. There have, however, been randomized controlled studies of IVIG dose in Kawasaki diseases (168). In

TABLE 4.7. Summary of results of two major trials of intravenous immunoglobulin (IVIG) in streptococcal toxic shock syndrome (165,167)

Study	End point	IVIG group	Placebo/control group
Darenberg et al., 2003 (165)	Mortality at 28 days	1/10 (10%)	4/11 (36%)
Kaul et al., 1999 (167)	Mortality of 30 days	7/21 (33%)	21/32 (66%)

TABLE **4.8.** Summary of management of toxic shock syndrome

1. Supportive care
    Aggressive fluid replacement
2. Surgical intervention
    Identification and removal of any focus of infection
    Wide debridement in necrotizing fasciitis
3. Antibiotic therapy
    Empiric intravenous cover against *S. aureus* and GAS (e.g., floxacillin)
    Consider cover against methicillin-resistant *Staphylococcus aureus* (MRSA) where applicable
    Clindamycin
4. Intravenous immunoglobulin therapy (see Table 4.9)
5. Secondary prophylaxis (see Table 4.10)

Kawasaki disease a higher dose (2 g/kg single dose) is more effective than multiple smaller doses and it is has been postulated that is attributable to a higher achieved serum immunoglobulin G (IgG) level. A high dose may be required for staphylococcal TSS after observations that staphylococcal superantigens are not inhibited as efficiently as streptococcal superantigens by IVIG in vitro (165). It should also be kept in mind that there appears to be variation in the neutralizing activity of different brands and lots of IVIG preparations (169) (Table 4.9).

Secondary Prophylaxis

There has been increasing recognition of the potential risk of secondary attacks in close contacts of patients with invasive GAS disease, analogous to meningococcal disease.

Outbreaks of streptococcal TSS and invasive streptococcal disease within family clusters, schools, and communities do occur (25,30,36,170–172). These outbreaks have shown that virulent clones of GAS can spread quickly within families and communities, and that there are public health implications for prevention of secondary invasive cases.

Larger population-based studies have come to conflicting conclusions as to whether secondary prophylaxis is indicated (18,173). The attack rate in a study in Ontario for household contacts of patients with invasive GAS disease was 294 per 100,000 compared with the incidence of sporadic disease in the same population of 2.4 per 100,000 (18). The attack rate in a study in the United States

TABLE **4.9.** Two suggested dosing regimes for intravenous immunoglobulin in toxic shock syndrome (165,167)

Regimen	Day 1	Day 2	Day 3	Reference
1	2 g/kg	—	Repeat 2 g/kg if patient remains unstable	165
2	1 g/kg	0.5 g/kg	0.5 g/kg	167

TABLE 4.10. Regimen for secondary prophylaxis following streptococcal toxic shock syndrome

Recommended regimen (174,185)	Alternative regimen (18)	Regimen for β-lactam sensitive patients (18)
Penicillin V 250 mg (<10 years) 500 mg (≥10 years) b.i.d. for 10 days, PLUS Rifampicin 10 mg/kg (max 600 mg) b.i.d. for 4 days	Cephalexin 250 mg q.i.d. for 10 days	Erythromycin 250 mg q.i.d. for 10 days

for household contacts of patients with invasive GAS disease was 66 per 100,000 compared with the incidence of sporadic disease in the same population of 3.5 per 100,000 (173). In the Canadian study this represented an increased risk of over 120–fold and led authorities to recommend secondary chemoprophylaxis. In contrast, the increased risk was around 19–fold and subsequently the Centers for Disease Control and Prevention recommended against chemoprophylaxis.

The advantages of treatment are potentially preventing disease in contacts and transmission of virulent strains. The disadvantages of treatment include the unnecessary use of antibiotics in most contacts and the risk of serious side effects including anaphylaxis. In addition, there is not enough data to be certain whether prophylaxis actually prevent secondary cases.(174). Options for secondary prophylaxis following streptococcal TSS are presented in Table 4.10.

The Future

The changing epidemiology of both staphylococcal and streptococcal TSS will present further challenges in the future. The recognition of the large burden of disease from invasive bacterial infection in developing countries presents its own challenges. The problem of methicillin-resistant *S. aureus*, both hospital- and community-acquired, is likely to become an increasing clinical problem.

The cornerstone of further reducing morbidity and mortality from TSS is research into superantigen toxin pathophysiology and vaccine development. A deeper appreciation of the immunologic mechanisms by which superantigen toxins cause disease may lead to the development of new agents that more specifically target the immune response. Other bacterial virulence factors that interact with superantigens may also be important in disease pathogenesis (175). These may be additional targets for future therapy. Vaccine development for GAS is well underway (176). The most advanced vaccine candidates are those based on the M protein. These include polyvalent vaccines based on type-specific N-terminal regions of the M protein (177, 178) as well as vaccines based on the conserved C repeat region (179,180). In addition, a number of non-M proteins are the subject of research as possible epitopes for a GAS vaccine, and these include GAS carbohydrate, C5a peptidase, and SPE B (176). A number of strategies have also been proposed for vaccines to protect against *S. aureus* infection, with most research focused on capsular polysaccharides (181,182). Finally, vaccination with nontoxic superantigen toxins from both *S. aureus* and GAS have been shown to induce protective antibodies in animal models of toxic shock syndrome (183,184).

References

1. Davis JP, Chesney PJ, Wand PJ, LaVenture M. Toxic-shock syndrome: epidemiologic features, recurrence, risk factors, and prevention. N Engl J Med 1980;303: 1429–1435.
2. Shands KN, Schmid GP, Dan BB, et al. Toxic-shock syndrome in menstruating women: association with tampon use and Staphylococcus aureus and clinical features in 52 cases. N Engl J Med 1980;303:1436–1442.
3. Reingold AL, Hargrett NT, Dan BB, et al. Nonmenstrual toxic shock syndrome: a review of 130 cases. Ann Intern Med 1982;96:871–874.
4. Cone LA, Woodard DR, Schlievert PM, Tomory GS. Clinical and bacteriologic observations of a toxic shock-like syndrome due to Streptococcus pyogenes. N Engl J Med 1987;317:146–149.
5. Todd J, Fishaut M, Kapral F, Welch T. Toxic-shock syndrome associated with phage-group-I Staphylococci. Lancet 1978;2:1116–1118.
6. Veasy LG, Wiedmeier SE, Orsmond GS, et al. Resurgence of acute rheumatic fever in the intermountain area of the United States. N Engl J Med 1987;316:421–427.
7. Stevens DL. The flesh-eating bacterium: what's next? J Infect Dis 1999;179(suppl 2):S366–374.
8. Duff BA, Denny FW, Kiska DL, Lohr JA. Invasive group A streptococcal disease in children. Clin Pediatr (Phila) 1999;38:417–423.
9. Hribalova V. Streptococcus pyogenes and the toxic shock syndrome. Ann Intern Med 1988;108:772.
10. Bartter T, Dascal A, Carroll K, Curley FJ. "Toxic strep syndrome." A manifestation of group A streptococcal infection. Arch Intern Med 1988;148:1421–1424.
11. Wheeler MC, Roe MH, Kaplan EL, Schlievert PM, Todd JK. Outbreak of group A streptococcus septicemia in children. Clinical, epidemiologic, and microbiological correlates. JAMA 1991;266:533–537.
12. Wong VK, Wright HT Jr. Group A beta-hemolytic streptococci as a cause of bacteremia in children. Am J Dis Child 1988;142:831–833.
13. Christie CD, Havens PL, Shapiro ED. Bacteremia with group A streptococci in childhood. Am J Dis Child 1988;142:559–561.
14. Stevens DL. Streptococcal toxic shock syndrome. Clin Microbiol Infect 2002;8: 133–136.
15. Katz AR, Morens DM. Severe streptococcal infections in historical perspective. Clin Infect Dis 1992;14:298–307.
16. Chiobotaru P, Yagupsky P, Fraser D, Dagan R. Changing epidemiology of invasive Streptococcus pyogenes infections in southern Israel: differences between two ethnic population groups. Pediatr Infect Dis J 1997;16:195–199.

17. Hoge CW, Schwartz B, Talkington DF, Breiman RF, MacNeill EM, Englender SJ. The changing epidemiology of invasive group A streptococcal infections and the emergence of streptococcal toxic shock-like syndrome. A retrospective population-based study. JAMA 1993;269:384–389.
18. Davies HD, McGeer A, Schwartz B, et al. Invasive group A streptococcal infections in Ontario, Canada. Ontario Group A Streptococcal Study Group. N Engl J Med 1996;335:547–554.
19. Holm SE. Invasive group A streptococcal infections. N Engl J Med 1996;335:590–591.
20. Barnham MR, Weightman NC, Anderson AW, Tanna A. Streptococcal toxic shock syndrome: a description of 14 cases from North Yorkshire, UK. Clin Microbiol Infect 2002;8:174–181.
21. Eriksson BK, Norgren M, McGregor K, Spratt BG, Normark BH. Group A strepto-coccal infections in Sweden: a comparative study of invasive and noninvasive infections and analysis of dominant T28 emm28 isolates. Clin Infect Dis 2003;37:1189–1193.
22. Johnson DR, Stevens DL, Kaplan EL. Epidemiologic analysis of group A streptococ-cal serotypes associated with severe systemic infections, rheumatic fever, or uncomplicated pharyngitis. J Infect Dis 1992;166:374–382.
23. Kiska DL, Thiede B, Caracciolo J, et al. Invasive group A streptococcal infections in North Carolina: epidemiology, clinical features, and genetic and serotype analy-sis of causative organisms. J Infect Dis 1997;176:992–1000.
24. Zurawski CA, Bardsley M, Beall B, et al. Invasive group A streptococcal disease in metropolitan Atlanta: a population-based assessment. Clin Infect Dis 1998;27:150–157.
25. Cockerill FR 3rd. An outbreak of invasive group A streptococcal disease associated with high carriage rates of the invasive clone among school-aged children (comment). Pediatrics 1998;101:136–140.
26. O'Brien KL, Beall B, Barrett L, et al. Epidemiology of invasive group A streptococ-cus disease in the United States, 1995–1999. Clin Infect Dis 2002;35:268–276.
27. Norton R, Smith HV, Wood N, Siegbrecht E, Ross A, Ketheesan N. Invasive group A streptococcal disease in North Queensland (1996–2001). Indian J Med Res 2004;119(suppl):148–151.
28. Laupland KB, Davies HD, Low DE, Schwartz B, Green K, McGeer A. Invasive group A streptococcal disease in children and association with varicella-zoster virus infection. Ontario Group A Streptococcal Study Group. Pediatrics 2000;105:E60.
29. Davies HD, Matlow A, Scriver SR, et al. Apparent lower rates of streptococcal toxic shock syndrome and lower mortality in children with invasive group A streptococ-cal infections compared with adults. Pediatr Infect Dis J 1994;13:49–56.
30. Stromberg A, Romanus V, Burman LG. Outbreak of group A streptococcal bacte-remia in Sweden: an epidemiologic and clinical study. J Infect Dis 1991;164:595–598.
31. Demers B, Simor AE, Vellend H, et al. Severe invasive group A streptococcal infec-tions in Ontario, Canada: 1987–1991. Clin Infect Dis 1993;16:792–800; discussion 801–802.
32. Eriksson BK, Andersson J, Holm SE, Norgren M. Epidemiological and clinical aspects of invasive group A streptococcal infections and the streptococcal toxic shock syndrome. Clin Infect Dis 1998;27:1428–1436.
33. Torres-Martinez C, Mehta D, Butt A, Levin M. Streptococcus associated toxic shock. Arch Dis Child 1992;67:126–130.

34. Hsueh PR, Wu JJ, Tsai PJ, Liu JW, Chuang YC, Luh KT. Invasive group A strepto-
    coccal disease in Taiwan is not associated with the presence of streptococcal pyro-
    genic exotoxin genes. Clin Infect Dis 1998;26:584–589.
35. Mascini EM, Jansze M, Schellekens JF, et al. Invasive group A streptococcal disease
    in the Netherlands: evidence for a protective role of anti-exotoxin A antibodies.
    J Infect Dis 2000;181:631–638.
36. Huang YC, Hsueh PR, Lin TY, Yan DC, Hsia SH. A family cluster of streptococcal
    toxic shock syndrome in children: clinical implication and epidemiological inves-
    tigation. Pediatrics 2001;107:1181–1183.
37. Westlake RM, Graham TG, Edwards KM. An outbreak of acute rheumatic fever in
    Tennessee. Pediatr Infect Dis J 1990;9:97–100.
38. Begovac J, Kuzmanovic N, Bejuk D. Comparison of clinical characteristics of
    group A streptococcal bacteremia in children and adults. Clin Infect Dis 1996;23:
    97–100.
39. Bacterial etiology of serious infections in young infants in developing countries:
    results of a multicenter study. The WHO Young Infants Study Group. Pediatr Infect
    Dis J 1999;18:S17–22.
40. Berkley JA, Lowe BS, Mwangi I, et al. Bacteremia among children admitted to a
    rural hospital in Kenya. N Engl J Med 2005;352:39–47.
41. Mulholland EK, Adegbola RA. Bacterial infections—a major cause of death among
    children in Africa. N Engl J Med 2005;352:75–77.
42. Chuang YY, Huang YC, Lin TY. Toxic shock syndrome in children—epidemiology,
    pathogenesis and management. Pediatr Drugs 2005;7:11–25.
43. Huang YC, Huang YC, Chiu CH. Characteristics of group A streptococcal bactere-
    mia with comparison between children and adults. J Microbiol Immunol Infect
    2001;34:195–200.
44. Ferretti JJ, McShan WM, Ajdic D, et al. Complete genome sequence of an M1 strain
    of Streptococcus pyogenes. Proc Natl Acad Sci U S A 2001;98:4658–4663.
45. Reingold AL, Hargrett NT, Shands KN, et al. Toxic shock syndrome surveillance
    in the United States, 1980 to 1981. Ann Intern Med 1982;96:875–880.
46. Latham RH, Kehrberg MW, Jacobson JA, Smith CB. Toxic shock syndrome in Utah:
    a case-control and surveillance study. Ann Intern Med 1982;96:906–908.
47. Berkley SF, Hightower AW, Broome CV, Reingold AL. The relationship of tampon
    characteristics to menstrual toxic shock syndrome. JAMA 1987;258:917–920.
48. Gaventa S, Reingold AL, Hightower AW, et al. Active surveillance for toxic shock
    syndrome in the United States, 1986. Rev Infect Dis 1989;11(suppl 1):S28–34.
49. Schlievert PM, Tripp TJ, Peterson ML. Reemergence of staphylococcal toxic shock
    syndrome in Minneapolis-St. Paul, Minnesota, during the 2000–2003 surveillance
    period. J Clin Microbiol 2004;42:2875–2876.
50. Hajjeh RA, Reingold A, Weil A, Shutt K, Schuchat A, Perkins BA. Toxic shock
    syndrome in the United States: surveillance update, 1979–1996. Emerg Infect Dis
    1999;5:807–810.
51. Schlievert PM. Role of superantigens in human disease. J Infect Dis 1993;167:
    997–1002.
52. Kotb M. Bacterial pyrogenic exotoxins as superantigens. Clin Microbiol Rev 1995;8:
    411–426.
53. Llewelyn M, Cohen J. Superantigens: microbial agents that corrupt immunity.
    Lancet Infect Dis 2002;2:156–162.
54. Omoe K, Imanishi K, Hu DL, et al. Biological properties of staphylococcal
    enterotoxin-like toxin type R. Infect Immun 2004;72:3664–3667.

55. Dinges MM, Orwin PM, Schlievert PM. Exotoxins of Staphylococcus aureus. Clin Microbiol Rev 2000;13:16–34, table of contents.
56. Korman TM, Boers A, Gooding TM, Curtis N, Visvanathan K. Fatal case of toxic shock-like syndrome due to group C streptococcus associated with superantigen exotoxin. J Clin Microbiol 2004;42:2866–2869.
57. Natoli S, Fimiani C, Faglieri N, et al. Toxic shock syndrome due to group C streptococci. A case report. Intensive Care Med 1996;22:985–989.
58. Wagner JG, Schlievert PM, Assimacopoulos AP, Stoehr JA, Carson PJ, Komadina K. Acute group G streptococcal myositis associated with streptococcal toxic shock syndrome: case report and review. Clin Infect Dis 1996;23:1159–1161.
59. Sharma M, Khatib R, Fakih M. Clinical characteristics of necrotizing fasciitis caused by group G Streptococcus: case report and review of the literature. Scand J Infect Dis 2002;34:468–471.
60. Hashikawa S, Iinuma Y, Furushita M, et al. Characterization of group C and G streptococcal strains that cause streptococcal toxic shock syndrome. J Clin Microbiol 2004;42:186–192.
61. Hirose Y, Yagi K, Honda H, Shibuya H, Okazaki E. Toxic shock-like syndrome caused by non-group A beta-hemolytic streptococci. Arch Intern Med 1997;157:1891–1894.
62. Crum NF, Wallace MR. Group B streptococcal necrotizing fasciitis and toxic shock-like syndrome: a case report and review of the literature. Scand J Infect Dis 2003;35:878–881.
63. Reich HL, Crawford GH, Pelle MT, James WD. Group B streptococcal toxic shock-like syndrome. Arch Dermatol 2004;140:163–166.
64. Curtis N. Kawasaki disease and toxic shock syndrome—at last the etiology is clear? Adv Exp Med Biol 2004;549:191–200.
65. Leung DY, Meissner HC, Fulton DR, Murray DL, Kotzin BL, Schlievert PM. Toxic shock syndrome toxin-secreting Staphylococcus aureus in Kawasaki syndrome. Lancet 1993;342:1385–1388.
66. Curtis N, Zheng R, Lamb JR, Levin M. Evidence for a superantigen mediated process in Kawasaki disease. Arch Dis Child 1995;72:308–311.
67. Curtis N, Chan B, Levin M. Toxic shock syndrome toxin-secreting Staphylococcus aureus in Kawasaki syndrome. Lancet 1994;343:299.
68. Abe J, Kotzin BL, Jujo K, et al. Selective expansion of T cells expressing T-cell receptor variable regions V beta 2 and V beta 8 in Kawasaki disease. Proc Natl Acad Sci U S A 1992;89:4066–4070.
69. Valdimarsson H, Baker BS, Jonsdottir I, Powles A, Fry L. Psoriasis: a T-cell-mediated autoimmune disease induced by streptococcal superantigens? Immunol Today 1995;16:145–149.
70. Michie CA, Davis T. Atopic dermatitis and staphylococcal superantigens. Lancet 1996;347:324.
71. Leung DY, Travers JB, Norris DA. The role of superantigens in skin disease. J Invest Dermatol 1995;105:37S–42S.
72. Petersson K, Forsberg G, Walse B. Interplay between superantigens and immuno-receptors. Scand J Immunol 2004;59:345–355.
73. Proft T, Sriskandan S, Yang L, Fraser JD. Superantigens and streptococcal toxic shock syndrome. Emerg Infect Dis 2003;9:1211–1218.
74. Miethke T, Wahl C, Heeg K, Echtenacher B, Krammer PH, Wagner H. T cell-mediated lethal shock triggered in mice by the superantigen staphylococcal entero-toxin B: critical role of tumor necrosis factor. J Exp Med 1992;175:91–98.

75. Choi YW, Herman A, DiGiusto D, Wade T, Marrack P, Kappler J. Residues of the variable region of the T-cell-receptor beta-chain that interact with S. aureus toxin superantigens. Nature 1990;346:471–473.
76. Basma H, Norrby-Teglund A, Guedez Y, et al. Risk factors in the pathogenesis of invasive group A streptococcal infections: role of protective humoral immunity. Infect Immun 1999;67:1871–1877.
77. Eriksson BK, Andersson J, Holm SE, Norgren M. Invasive group A streptococcal infections: T1M1 isolates expressing pyrogenic exotoxins A and B in combination with selective lack of toxin-neutralizing antibodies are associated with increased risk of streptococcal toxic shock syndrome. J Infect Dis 1999;180: 410–418.
78. Stolz SJ, Davis JP, Vergeront JM, et al. Development of serum antibody to toxic shock toxin among individuals with toxic shock syndrome in Wisconsin. J Infect Dis 1985;151:883–889.
79. Vergeront JM, Stolz SJ, Crass BA, Nelson DB, Davis JP, Bergdoll MS. Prevalence of serum antibody to staphylococcal enterotoxin F among Wisconsin residents: implications for toxic-shock syndrome. J Infect Dis 1983;148:692–698.
80. The Working Group on Severe Streptococcal Infections. Defining the group A streptococcal toxic shock syndrome. Rationale and consensus definition. JAMA 1993;269:390–391.
81. Stevens DL. Invasive group A streptococcus infections. Clin Infect Dis 1992;14: 2–11.
82. Stevens DL. Streptococcal toxic-shock syndrome: spectrum of disease, pathogenesis, and new concepts in treatment. Emerg Infect Dis 1995;1:69–78.
83. Muller MP, Low DE, Green KA, et al. Clinical and epidemiologic features of group a streptococcal pneumonia in Ontario, Canada. Arch Intern Med 2003;163:467–472.
84. Burns JA, Brown J, Ogle JW. Group A streptococcal tracheitis associated with toxic shock syndrome. Pediatr Infect Dis J 1998;17:933–935.
85. Miyairi I, Berlingieri D, Protic J, Belko J. Neonatal invasive group A streptococcal disease: case report and review of the literature. Pediatr Infect Dis J 2004;23: 161–165.
86. Mahieu LM, Holm SE, Goossens HJ, Van Acker KJ. Congenital streptococcal toxic shock syndrome with absence of antibodies against streptococcal pyrogenic exotoxins. J Pediatr 1995;127:987–989.
87. Bisno AL, Stevens DL. Streptococcal infections of skin and soft tissues. N Engl J Med 1996;334:240–245.
88. Chelsom J, Halstensen A, Haga T, Hoiby EA. Necrotising fasciitis due to group A streptococci in western Norway: incidence and clinical features. Lancet 1994;344: 1111–1115.
89. Giuliano A, Lewis F Jr, Hadley K, Blaisdell FW. Bacteriology of necrotizing fasciitis. Am J Surg 1977;134:52–57.
90. Kaul R, McGeer A, Low DE, Green K, Schwartz B. Population-based surveillance for group A streptococcal necrotizing fasciitis: clinical features, prognostic indicators, and microbiologic analysis of seventy-seven cases. Ontario Group A Streptococcal Study. Am J Med 1997;103:18–24.
91. Ward RG, Walsh MS. Necrotizing fasciitis: 10 years' experience in a district general hospital. Br J Surg 1991;78:488–489.
92. Wall DB, de Virgilio C, Black S, Klein SR. Objective criteria may assist in distinguishing necrotizing fasciitis from nonnecrotizing soft tissue infection. Am J Surg 2000;179:17–21.

93. Brogan TV, Nizet V, Waldhausen JH, Rubens CE, Clarke WR. Group A streptococcal necrotizing fasciitis complicating primary varicella: a series of fourteen patients. Pediatr Infect Dis J 1995;14:588–594.

94. Sudarsky LA, Laschinger JC, Coppa GF, Spencer FC. Improved results from a standardized approach in treating patients with necrotizing fasciitis. Ann Surg 1987;206:661–665.

95. Dahl PR, Perniciaro C, Holmkvist KA, O'Connor MI, Gibson LE. Fulminant group A streptococcal necrotizing fasciitis: clinical and pathologic findings in 7 patients. J Am Acad Dermatol 2002;47:489–492.

96. Brothers TE, Tagge DU, Stutley JE, Conway WF, Del Schutte H Jr, Byrne TK. Magnetic resonance imaging differentiates between necrotizing and non-necrotizing fasciitis of the lower extremity. J Am Coll Surg 1998;187:416–421.

97. Zittergruen M, Grose C. Magnetic resonance imaging for early diagnosis of necrotizing fasciitis. Pediatr Emerg Care 1993;9:26–28.

98. Schmid MR, Kossmann T, Duewell S. Differentiation of necrotizing fasciitis and cellulitis using MR imaging. AJR Am J Roentgenol 1998;170:615–620.

99. Stamenkovic I, Lew PD. Early recognition of potentially fatal necrotizing fasciitis. The use of frozen-section biopsy. N Engl J Med 1984;310:1689–1693.

100. Wong CH, Wang YS. The diagnosis of necrotizing fasciitis. Curr Opin Infect Dis 2005;18:101–106.

101. Wong CH, Khin LW, Heng KS, Tan KC, Low CO. The LRINEC (Laboratory Risk Indicator for Necrotizing Fasciitis) score: a tool for distinguishing necrotizing fasciitis from other soft tissue infections. Crit Care Med 2004;32:1535–1541.

102. Doctor A, Harper MB, Fleisher GR. Group A beta-hemolytic streptococcal bacteremia: historical overview, changing incidence, and recent association with varicella. Pediatrics 1995;96:428–433.

103. Falcone PA, Pricolo VE, Edstrom LE. Necrotizing fasciitis as a complication of chickenpox. Clin Pediatr (Phila) 1988;27:339–343.

104. Vugia DJ, Peterson CL, Meyers HB, Kim KS, Arrieta A, Schlievert PM, et al. Invasive group A streptococcal infections in children with varicella in Southern California. Pediatr Infect Dis J 1996;15:146–150.

105. Wilson GJ, Talkington DF, Gruber W, Edwards K, Dermody TS. Group A streptococcal necrotizing fasciitis following varicella in children: case reports and review. Clin Infect Dis 1995;20:1333–1338.

106. Zerr DM, Alexander ER, Duchin JS, Koutsky LA, Rubens CE. A case-control study of necrotizing fasciitis during primary varicella. Pediatrics 1999;103:783–790.

107. Cowan MR, Primm PA, Scott SM, Abramo TJ, Wiebe RA. Serious group A beta-hemolytic streptococcal infections complicating varicella. Ann Emerg Med 1994;23:818–822.

108. Bradley JS, Schlievert PM, Sample TG, Jr. Streptococcal toxic shock-like syndrome as a complication of varicella. Pediatr Infect Dis J 1991;10:77–79.

109. Tyrrell GJ, Lovgren M, Kress B, Grimsrud K. Varicella-associated group A streptococcal disease in Alberta, Canada 2000–2002. Clin Infect Dis 2005;40:1055–1057.

110. Patel RA, Binns HJ, Shulman ST. Reduction in pediatric hospitalizations for varicella-related invasive group A streptococcal infections in the varicella vaccine era. J Pediatr 2004;144:68–74.

111. Rimailho A, Riou B, Richard C, Auzepy P. Fulminant necrotizing fasciitis and nonsteroidal anti-inflammatory drugs. J Infect Dis 1987;155:143–146.

112. Brun-Buisson CJ, Saada M, Trunet P, Rapin M, Roujeau JC, Revuz J. Haemolytic streptococcal gangrene and non-steroidal anti-inflammatory drugs. Br Med J (Clin Res Ed) 1985;290:1786.

113. Krige JE, Spence RA, Potter PC, Terblanche J. Necrotising fasciitis after diflunisal for minor injury. Lancet 1985;2:1432–1433.

114. Stevens DL. Could nonsteroidal antiinflammatory drugs (NSAIDs) enhance the progression of bacterial infections to toxic shock syndrome? Clin Infect Dis 1995;21:977–980.

115. Curtis N. Non-steroidal anti-inflammatory drugs may predispose to invasive group A streptococcal infections. Arch Dis Child 1996;75:547.

116. Zerr DM, Rubens CE. NSAIDS and necrotizing fasciitis. Pediatr Infect Dis J 1999;18:724–725.

117. Ford LM, Waksman J. Necrotizing fasciitis during primary varicella. Pediatrics 2000;105:1372–1373; author reply 1373–1375.

118. Lesko SM, O'Brien KL, Schwartz B, Vezina R, Mitchell AA. Invasive group A streptococcal infection and nonsteroidal antiinflammatory drug use among children with primary varicella. Pediatrics 2001;107:1108–1115.

119. Forbes N, Rankin AP. Necrotizing fasciitis and non steroidal anti-inflammatory drugs: a case series and review of the literature. N Z Med J 2001;114:3–6.

120. McCormick JK, Yarwood JM, Schlievert PM. Toxic shock syndrome and bacterial superantigens: an update. Annu Rev Microbiol 2001;55:77–104.

121. Matsuda Y, Kato H, Yamada R, et al. Early and definitive diagnosis of toxic shock syndrome by detection of marked expansion of T-cell-receptor VBeta2–positive T cells. Emerg Infect Dis 2003;9:387–389.

122. Davis JP, Vergeront JM. The effect of publicity on the reporting of toxic-shock syndrome in Wisconsin. J Infect Dis 1982;145:449–457.

123. Andrews MM, Parent EM, Barry M, Parsonnet J. Recurrent nonmenstrual toxic shock syndrome: clinical manifestations, diagnosis, and treatment. Clin Infect Dis 2001;32:1470–1479.

124. Kain KC, Schuzler M, Chow AW. Clinical spectrum of nonmenstrual toxic shock syndrome (TSS): comparison with menstrual TSS by multivariate discriminant analyses. Clin Infect Dis 1993;16:100–106.

125. Parsonnet J. Nonmenstrual toxic shock syndrome: new insights into diagnosis, pathogenesis, and treatment. Curr Clin Top Infect Dis 1996;16:1–20.

126. Wiesenthal AM, Todd JK. Toxic shock syndrome in children aged 10 years or less. Pediatrics 1984;74:112–117.

127. Graham GDR, O'Brien M, Hayes JM. Postoperative toxic shock syndrome. Clin Infect Dis 1995;20:1250–1258.

128. Nahass RG, Gocke DJ. Toxic shock syndrome associated with use of a nasal tampon. Am J Med 1988;84:629–631.

129. Weber R, Keerl R, Hochapfel F, et al. Packing in endonasal surgery. Am J Otolaryngol 2001;22:306–320.

130. Frame JD, Eve MD, Hackett ME, et al. The toxic shock syndrome in burned children. Burns Incl Therm Inj 1985;11:234–241.

131. Edwards-Jones V, Dawson MM, Childs C. A survey into toxic shock syndrome (TSS) in UK burns units. Burns 2000;26:323–333.

132. Childs C, Edwards-Jones V, Heathcote DM, Dawson M, Davenport PJ. Patterns of Staphylococcus aureus colonization, toxin production, immunity and illness in burned children. Burns 1994;20:514–521.

133. Johnson D, Pathirana PD. Toxic shock syndrome following cessation of prophylactic antibiotics in a child with a 2% scald. Burns 2002;28:181–184.

134. MacDonald KL, Osterholm MT, Hedberg CW, et al. Toxic shock syndrome. A newly recognized complication of influenza and influenzalike illness. JAMA 1987;257: 1053–1058.

135. Hall M, Hoyt L, Ferrieri P, Schlievert PM, Jenson HB. Kawasaki syndrome-like illness associated with infection caused by enterotoxin B-secreting Staphylococcus aureus. Clin Infect Dis 1999;29:586–589.

136. Davies HD, Kirk V, Jadavji T, Kotzin BL. Simultaneous presentation of Kawasaki disease and toxic shock syndrome in an adolescent male. Pediatr Infect Dis J 1996;15:1136–1138.

137. Curtis N, Goodsall A, Levin M. Evidence that staphylococcal toxic shock syndrome and Kawasaki Disease share a common etiology. Pediatr Res 2000;47:18.

138. Stevens DL. The toxic shock syndromes. Infect Dis Clin North Am 1996;10: 727–746.

139. Wong CH, Chang HC, Pasupathy S, Khin LW, Tan JL, Low CO. Necrotizing fasciitis: clinical presentation, microbiology, and determinants of mortality. J Bone Joint Surg Am 2003;85–A:1454–1460.

140. Bilton BD, Zibari GB, McMillan RW, Aultman DF, Dunn G, McDonald JC. Aggressive surgical management of necrotizing fasciitis serves to decrease mortality: a retrospective study. Am Surg 1998;64:397–400; discussion 400–401.

141. Catena F, La Donna M, Ansaloni L, Agrusti S, Taffurelli M. Necrotizing fasciitis: a dramatic surgical emergency. Eur J Emerg Med 2004;11:44–48.

142. Stevens DL, Gibbons AE, Bergstrom R, Winn V. The Eagle effect revisited: efficacy of clindamycin, erythromycin, and penicillin in the treatment of streptococcal myositis. J Infect Dis 1988;158:23–28.

143. Kohn J, Evans AJ. Group A streptococci resistant to clindamycin. Br Med J 1970;2:423.

144. Mascini EM, Jansze M, Schouls LM, Verhoef J, Van Dijk H. Penicillin and clindamycin differentially inhibit the production of pyrogenic exotoxins A and B by group A streptococci. Int J Antimicrob Agents 2001;18:395–398.

145. Gemmell CG, Peterson PK, Schmeling D, et al. Potentiation of opsonization and phagocytosis of Streptococcus pyogenes following growth in the presence of clindamycin. J Clin Invest 1981;67:1249–1256.

146. Craig WA, Vogelman B. The postantibiotic effect. Ann Intern Med 1987;106: 900–902.

147. Eagle H. Experimental approach to the problem of treatment failure with penicillin. I. Group A streptococcal infection in mice. Am J Med 1952;13: 389–399.

148. Stevens DL, Bryant AE, Hackett SP. Antibiotic effects on bacterial viability, toxin production, and host response. Clin Infect Dis 1995;20(suppl 2):S154–157.

149. Sriskandan S, McKee A, Hall L, Cohen J. Comparative effects of clindamycin and ampicillin on superantigenic activity of Streptococcus pyogenes. J Antimicrob Chemother 1997;40:275–277.

150. Schlievert PM, Kelly JA. Clindamycin-induced suppression of toxic-shock syndrome—associated exotoxin production. J Infect Dis 1984;149:471.

151. Herbert S, Barry P, Novick RP. Subinhibitory clindamycin differentially inhibits transcription of exoprotein genes in Staphylococcus aureus. Infect Immun 2001;69:2996–3003.

152. Zimbelman J, Palmer A, Todd J. Improved outcome of clindamycin compared with beta-lactam antibiotic treatment for invasive Streptococcus pyogenes infection. Pediatr Infect Dis J 1999;18:1096–1100.
153. Werdan K. Intravenous immunoglobulin for prophylaxis and therapy of sepsis. Curr Opin Crit Care 2001;7:354–361.
154. Alejandria MM, Lansang MA, Dans LF, Mantaring JB. Intravenous immunoglobulin for treating sepsis and septic shock. Cochrane Database Syst Rev 2002: CD001090.
155. Darenberg J, Soderquist B, Normark BH, Norrby-Teglund A. Differences in potency of intravenous polyspecific immunoglobulin G against streptococcal and staphylococcal superantigens: implications for therapy of toxic shock syndrome. Clin Infect Dis 2004;38:836–842.
156. Stevens DL. Rationale for the use of intravenous gamma globulin in the treatment of streptococcal toxic shock syndrome. Clin Infect Dis 1998;26:639–641.
157. Norrby-Teglund A, Kaul R, Low DE, McGeer A, Andersson J, Andersson U, et al. Evidence for the presence of streptococcal-superantigen-neutralizing antibodies in normal polyspecific immunoglobulin G. Infect Immun 1996;64:5395–5398.
158. Norrby-Teglund A, Kaul R, Low DE, McGeer A, Newton DW, Andersson J, et al. Plasma from patients with severe invasive group A streptococcal infections treated with normal polyspecific IgG inhibits streptococcal superantigen-induced T cell proliferation and cytokine production. J Immunol 1996;156:3057–3064.
159. Andersson U, Chauvet JM, Skansen-Saphir U, Andersson J. Pooled human IgG modulates cytokine production in lymphocytes and monocytes. J Immunol Methods 1994;175:201–213.
160. Barry W, Hudgins L, Donta ST, Pesanti EL. Intravenous immunoglobulin therapy for toxic shock syndrome. JAMA 1992;267:3315–3316.
161. Nadal D, Lauener RP, Braegger CP, et al. T cell activation and cytokine release in streptococcal toxic shock-like syndrome. J Pediatr 1993;122:727–729.
162. Lamothe F, D'Amico P, Ghosn P, Tremblay C, Braidy J, Patenaude JV. Clinical usefulness of intravenous human immunoglobulins in invasive group A Streptococcal infections: case report and review. Clin Infect Dis 1995;21:1469–1470.
163. Perez CM, Kubak BM, Cryer HG, Salehmugodam S, Vespa P, Farmer D. Adjunctive treatment of streptococcal toxic shock syndrome using intravenous immunoglobulin: case report and review. Am J Med 1997;102:111–113.
164. Murthy BV, Nelson RA, Mannion PT. Immunoglobulin therapy in non-menstrual streptococcal toxic shock syndrome. Anaesth Intensive Care 2003;31:320–323.
165. Darenberg J, Ihendyane N, Sjolin J, et al. Intravenous immunoglobulin G therapy in streptococcal toxic shock syndrome: a European randomized, double-blind, placebo-controlled trial. Clin Infect Dis 2003;37:333–340.
166. Stevens DL. Dilemmas in the treatment of invasive Streptococcus pyogenes infections. Clin Infect Dis 2003;37:341–343.
167. Kaul R, McGeer A, Norrby-Teglund A, et al. Intravenous immunoglobulin therapy for streptococcal toxic shock syndrome—a comparative observational study. The Canadian Streptococcal Study Group. Clin Infect Dis 1999;28:800–807.
168. Newburger JW, Takahashi M, Beiser AS, et al. A single intravenous infusion of gamma globulin as compared with four infusions in the treatment of acute Kawasaki syndrome. N Engl J Med 1991;324:1633–1639.
169. Norrby-Teglund A, Basma H, Andersson J, McGeer A, Low DE, Kotb M. Varying titers of neutralizing antibodies to streptococcal superantigens in different

preparations of normal polyspecific immunoglobulin G: implications for therapeutic efficacy. Clin Infect Dis 1998;26:631–638.

170. Schwartz B, Elliott JA, Butler JC, et al. Clusters of invasive group A streptococcal infections in family, hospital, and nursing home settings. Clin Infect Dis 1992;15:277–284.

171. Gamba MA, Martinelli M, Schaad HJ, et al. Familial transmission of a serious disease—producing group A streptococcus clone: case reports and review. Clin Infect Dis 1997;24:1118–1121.

172. Auerbach SB, Schwartz B, Williams D, et al. Outbreak of invasive group A streptococcal infections in a nursing home. Lessons on prevention and control. Arch Intern Med 1992;152:1017–1022.

173. Prevention of Invasive Group ASIWP. Prevention of invasive group A streptococcal disease among household contacts of case patients and among postpartum and postsurgical patients: recommendations from the Centers for Disease Control and Prevention (erratum appears in Clin Infect Dis. 2003 Jan 15;36(2):243). Clin Infect Dis 2002;35:950–959.

174. Carapetis JR. Current issues in managing group A streptococcal infections. Adv Exp Med Biol 2004;549:185–190.

175. Curtis N. Invasive group A streptococcal infection. Curr Opin Infect Dis 1996;9: 191–192.

176. Kotloff KL, Dale JB. Progress in group A streptococcal vaccine development. Pediatr Infect Dis J 2004;23:765–766.

177. Hu MC, Walls MA, Stroop SD, Reddish MA, Beall B, Dale JB. Immunogenicity of a 26-valent group A streptococcal vaccine. Infect Immun 2002;70:2171–2177.

178. Kotloff KL, Corretti M, Palmer K, et al. Safety and immunogenicity of a recombinant multivalent group a streptococcal vaccine in healthy adults: phase 1 trial. JAMA 2004;292:709–715.

179. Batzloff M, Yan H, Davies M, Hartas J, Good M. Preclinical evaluation of a vaccine based on conserved region of M protein that prevents group A streptococcal infection. Indian J Med Res 2004;119(suppl):104–107.

180. Batzloff MR, Hayman WA, Davies MR, Zeng M, Pruksakorn S, Brandt ER. Protection against group A streptococcus by immunization with J8–diphtheria toxoid: contribution of J8–and diphtheria toxoid-specific antibodies to protection. J Infect Dis 2003;187:1598–1608.

181. Fattom AI, Horwith G, Fuller S, Propst M, Naso R. Development of StaphVAX, a polysaccharide conjugate vaccine against S. aureus infection: from the lab bench to phase III clinical trials. Vaccine 2004;22:880–887.

182. Maira-Litran T, Kropec A, Goldmann D, Pier GB. Biologic properties and vaccine potential of the staphylococcal poly-N-acetyl glucosamine surface polysaccharide. Vaccine 2004;22:872–879.

183. Hu DL, Omoe K, Sasaki S, et al. Vaccination with nontoxic mutant toxic shock syndrome toxin 1 protects against Staphylococcus aureus infection. J Infect Dis 2003;188:743–752.

184. Roggiani M, Stoehr JA, Olmsted SB, et al. Toxoids of streptococcal pyrogenic exotoxin A are protective in rabbit models of streptococcal toxic shock syndrome. Infect Immun 2000;68:5011–5017.

185. Tanz RR, Poncher JR, Corydon KE, Kabat K, Yogev R, Shulman ST. Clindamycin treatment of chronic pharyngeal carriage of group A streptococci. J Pediatr 1991;119:123–128.

5
Vaccines for the Prevention of Admission to the Pediatric Intensive Care Unit

Shelley Segal, Matthew Snape, Dominic Kelly, and Andrew J. Pollard

Infectious diseases precipitate the majority of acute medical admissions to the pediatric intensive care unit (PICU) despite the availability of a wide variety of antimicrobial agents. In previously healthy children, specific therapy is likely to have only a minimal impact on the continuing severity of the disease, since it is usually the host response to the infection that determines progression, and strategies that avoid admission are clearly preferable. Prophylactic immunization offers the potential for prevention of PICU admission for many of the major pathogens affecting children. Indeed, vaccines already exist for many of the causes of the major infectious syndromes presenting to PICU (Table 5.1).

The continuing expansion of immunization programs around the world provides the promise of a further reduction in critical illness in children over the next decade using the vaccines listed in Table 5.1. Perhaps most notable for developed countries is the increasing coverage of influenza vaccine for healthy children and the active development of vaccines for respiratory syncytial virus and serogroup B *Neisseria meningitidis*. However, two thirds of the world's deaths in children less than 5 years of age are caused by vaccine-preventable diseases such as bacterial pneumonia, rotavirus diarrhea, and measles. These figures highlight the need to continue development of vaccines against these major killers, but at the same time to invest in delivery of currently available vaccines for nations with limited resources.

Invasive Bacterial Diseases

Haemophilus Influenzae *Type b*

Haemophilus influenzae type b (Hib) is a prominent cause of invasive bacterial disease in unvaccinated populations, particularly in infants and children less than 5 years of age. Although there are six capsular types (a to f), only type b has been associated with a significant incidence of disease. Children may be admitted to the intensive care unit with septicemia, meningitis, epiglottitis, or pneumonia, and may have associated osteomyelitis or septic arthritis. The

Table 5.1. Vaccines available to prevent common causes of major infectious syndromes

Syndrome	Vaccines available	Vaccines in development
Meningitis	*Haemophilus influenzae* type b, *Streptococcus pneumoniae*, *Neisseria meningitidis*, *Salmonella* typhi, *Mycobacterium tuberculosis*	Group B streptococcus Serogroup B *Neisseria meningitidis*
Septic shock	*Neisseria meningitidis*, *Streptococcus pneumoniae*, *Haemophilus influenzae* type b influenza, adenovirus	Group A streptococcus, Group B streptococcus, Herpes simplex virus
Severe dehydration	Rotavirus, cholera	
Encephalitis	Varicella, measles, mumps, Japanese encephalitis, yellow fever, tick-borne encephalitis, polio, rabies	Cytomegalovirus, herpes simplex virus, Epstein-Barr virus (EBV)
Respiratory failure, upper airway obstruction, and croup	*Haemophilus influenzae* type b, *Streptococcus pneumoniae*, *Neisseria meningitidis*, adenovirus, pertussis, influenza, diphtheria	RSV, parainfluenza, EBV
Hepatic failure	Hepatitis A and B	Hepatitis C
Miscellaneous	Tetanus	HIV, malaria

RSV, respiratory syncytial virus.

age-specific incidence and epidemiology of invasive disease vary widely at a regional level. In the prevaccine era the United States had incidence rates of 60/100,000 to 100/100,000 children under 5 years, in comparison to the United Kingdom, where rates were 36/100,000 (1). The disease burden is highly seasonal with higher rates of infection in the winter months. In high incidence regions, the burden of disease is shifted to the earlier months of life compared to lower incidence regions. In addition, certain genetically defined groups appear more susceptible (e.g., native Alaskans and Navajo Indians) where rates exceed 100/100,000 in children under the age of 5 years. In a developed system of health care, the mortality for Hib meningitis in the prevaccine era was less than 3% (2). However, significant numbers of children develop neurologic sequelae, most commonly sensorineural deafness.

The first Hib vaccines used the bacterial polysaccharide capsule polyribosyl ribitol phosphate (PRP) as the sole vaccine antigen. Early trials in the 1970s showed that this gave significant antibody responses and protection from invasive disease in children above 2 years of age (3). However, younger children failed to develop antibodies to the vaccine and remained susceptible. This relationship of age to immune response is a feature of many similar plain polysaccharide vaccines, which generate T-cell–independent responses. Booster doses were necessary for long-term protection, as antibody responses were short lived and induced no immunologic memory.

The covalent linking of a protein carrier (diphtheria toxoid; tetanus toxoid; meningococcal outer membrane protein; or CRM197, a diphtheria toxoid) to Hib polysaccharide results in a vaccine that is able to recruit T cells to the antigen-specific immune response. Vaccines based on this principle of conjugation are immunogenic in infants and generate long-term memory. The introduction of these protein-polysaccharide conjugate vaccines into routine infant immunization schedules, from the late 1980s onwards, has been associated with a significant decrease in the incidence of invasive disease and pneumonia caused by Hib (4). An important feature of Hib protein-polysaccharide vaccines is that they induce significant herd immunity through a reduction in nasopharyngeal carriage. Herd immunity is an important component of protective efficacy, particularly when individual specific antibody levels are low either through lack of vaccination or because of the interval since infant immunization. Concerns that the reduction in Hib carriage might lead to an increase in disease caused by non–type-b strains appear unwarranted based on long-term surveillance data.

While vaccine efficacy is usually greater than 90%, Hib disease has been seen in vaccinated children. A U.K. study showed that prematurity and immunoglobulin deficiency were risk factors for children with sporadic vaccine failure (5). The U.K. has also seen a resurgence of Hib disease in vaccinated children from 1999 to 2003 (6). This was associated with the use of a less immunogenic Hib/acellular pertussis combination vaccine (7). Children presented more frequently with epiglottitis and at an older age than those with disease in the pre-vaccine era. This is a reminder that Hib disease cannot be completely excluded even in a vaccinated population.

When a child does present with invasive Hib disease, national guidelines on the prophylaxis of contacts and the immunization of unvaccinated children should be followed to prevent secondary cases.

Invasive Hib disease and Hib lower respiratory tract infection remain significant causes of mortality and morbidity in many developing countries where routine infant immunization with conjugate vaccines is unaffordable. Hib conjugate vaccines are highly efficacious in these settings and can prevent almost all admissions to intensive care with Hib disease.

Neisseria Meningitidis

Neisseria meningitidis is a gram-negative diplococcus capable of causing invasive disease in the form of meningitis or septicemia, and is one of the leading causes of septic shock in otherwise healthy children and the most common infectious cause of death in children in the U.K. A mortality rate for children with invasive meningococcal disease admitted to PICUs of 35% has been reported (8), although more recent reports place this figure between 2% and 9% (8,9).

The organism is classified according to the nature of its polysaccharide capsule into 13 different serogroups of which five—A, B, C, W135, and Y— cause the vast majority of invasive meningococcal disease. While serogroup A was responsible for epidemics in Europe during both world wars, it is now predominantly a problem in sub-Saharan Africa, where 750,790 cases of invasive meningococcal disease were reported from 1992 to 2002, with 52,880 deaths (10). Currently serogroup B and C cause the majority of disease in the developed world, with serogroup Y also being a major cause of disease in North America (11). Recent epidemics related to the Hajj and in sub-Saharan Africa have been due to serogroup W135 (12). A considerable increase in invasive meningococcal disease was seen in many countries through the 1990s, in part related to the emergence of a hyperinvasive clone (variously categorized as electrophoresis type (ET)-15 or sequence type (ST)-11 (13). Although in Europe this clone predominantly bears the serogroup C polysaccharide capsule, it is also capable of bearing the capsule of other serogroups.

Plain Polysaccharide Meningococcal Vaccines

Plain polysaccharide vaccines against either N. meningitidis serogroup A and C or A, C, W135, and Y have been available since the 1960s (14). Although immunogenic in adults in the short term, with the exception of serogroup A they do not generate an immune response in children under the age of 2 years. Also, as they do not induce immunologic memory, long-term protection is not achieved. Plain polysaccharide meningococcal ACWY vaccine, however, is currently recommended for all Hajj pilgrims and for travelers to sub-Saharan Africa (15).

Meningococcal Serogroup C Protein: Polysaccharide Conjugate Vaccine

In response to the emergence of the serogroup C hyperinvasive ST 11 clone in the 1990s, three different versions of a meningococcal C conjugate (MenC) vaccine were produced. These vaccines built on the success of the technology used in the Hib vaccine, that is, the conjugation of a plain polysaccharide capsule to a carrier protein. Unlike the plain polysaccharide vaccines, this technology had been shown to induce a T-cell response, thus providing protection to children under the age of 2 years and inducing immunologic memory. Of the new MenC vaccines, two used CRM197 (a mutant diphtheria toxoid) as the carrier protein, the third using tetanus toxoid.

These MenC vaccines were first used in the U.K. in 1999, and had a dramatic effect on the incidence of invasive serogroup C meningococcal disease (Fig. 5.1). The vaccine was also shown to reduce nasopharyngeal carriage of meningococcal serogroup C and to provide herd immunity (17).

The MenC vaccines have subsequently been introduced into the routine immunization schedule in Ireland, Spain, Belgium, the Netherlands, Canada, and Australia, where this effect has been replicated (13).

Currently MenC vaccines are routinely administered to infants as a three-dose schedule at 2, 3, and 4 months (in the U.K.) or 2, 4, and 6 months (as in

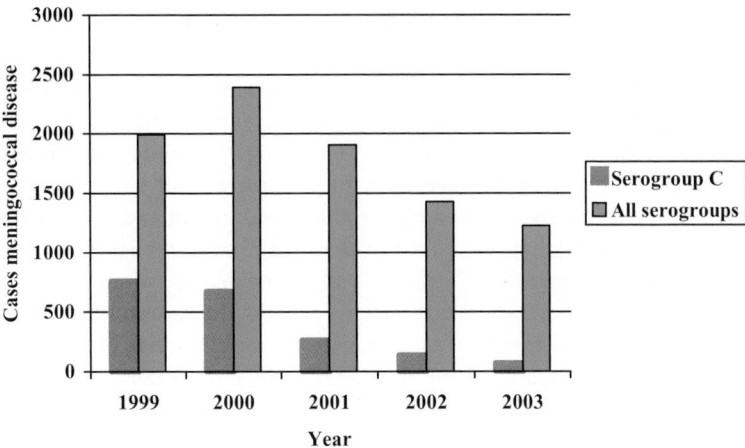

FIGURE 5.1. Cases of invasive meningococcal disease in England, Wales, and Northern Ireland. (Adapted from quarterly reports of enhanced surveillance for meningococcal disease conducted by Health Protection Agency, published in CDR weekly from 1999 to present. [One such report is ref. 16.] http://www.hpa.org.uk/cdr/.)

Spain and Ireland). Subsequent studies have shown comparable immunogenicity between a two- and three-dose infant MenC (using the tetanus conjugate) schedule, potentially allowing for a reduction in the number of doses routinely administered to this age group (18). An alternative approach of administering a single dose to toddlers at 12 to 14 months has been adapted by countries such as Australia and the Netherlands (13).

The duration of protection is as yet unknown; however, recent publications suggest a waning of immunity 18 months after the 2-, 3-, and 4-month immunization regimen used in the U.K. (19). This is potentially of clinical significance given that prior to the introduction of the MenC vaccine a second peak in incidence was seen in late adolescence. It is therefore possible that this regimen will be adapted to include a booster dose after 1 year of age. Given the uncertainty regarding duration of immune protection from MenC immunization, it should be emphasized that all household contacts of index cases with serogroup C meningococcal disease should receive appropriate chemoprophylaxis, regardless of their immunization status.

Concern that the reduction in serogroup C meningococcal disease would be offset by an increase in disease caused by other serogroups has to date proved unfounded in the U.K. (Fig. 5.1). However, there have been reports from Spain of emergence of a hyperinvasive serogroup B clone, which previously had a serogroup C capsule, which occurred following the introduction of MenC vaccines (20), highlighting the necessity of ongoing surveillance for this disease.

Further Development of Meningococcal Vaccines

Although initial trials of a protein polysaccharide conjugate vaccine protecting against serogroups A, C, W135, and Y showed disappointing immunogenicity in infants (21), development of combination conjugate meningococcal vaccines is ongoing, and one vaccine has recently been approved for use in the U.S.

Serogroup B meningococci, which are the predominant cause of disease in infants, have a capsule that is chemically identical to structures on some human tissues and is therefore a "self antigen" and very poorly immunogenic (22). Attempts to make a polysaccharide vaccine against the serogroup B organism have been unsuccessful and have raised concerns about the risk of autoimmune disease. Beneath the capsule of the meningococcus is an outer membrane that contains lipopolysaccharide and many different proteins. A number of these are currently under investigation as possible vaccine candidates either alone or as combinations of purified proteins (23). In the 1970s investigators noted that immunogenicity of these outer membrane proteins was improved when they were presented in the correct conformation and that this could be achieved by purifying vesicles made from the neisserial outer membrane. Outer membrane vesicle (OMV) vaccines have been studied in several efficacy trials and have shown reasonable protection in older children and adults but not in those most at risk, the under-4-year age group (24–28). Furthermore, protection appears to be limited mainly to the strain from which the vaccine has been made, making this a useful vaccine to consider for clonal outbreaks, but new strategies are required for endemic disease. An OMV vaccine was introduced during 2004 in New Zealand to control a prolonged clonal outbreak of serogroup B meningococcal disease; initial efficacy estimates are promising and suggest that the vaccine is safe and elicited a promising immune response against the candidate vaccine strain (29).

When a child does present with invasive meningococcal disease, national guidelines on the prophylaxis of contacts and the immunization of unvaccinated children (where an appropriate vaccine is available) should be followed to prevent secondary cases.

Without a highly efficacious vaccine against all strains that cause invasive serogroup B meningococcal infection, children will continue to be admitted to the intensive care unit with meningococcal disease.

Streptococcus Pneumoniae

S. pneumoniae is a major cause of bacterial pneumonia, sepsis, and meningitis, with children often presenting to the PICU with severe community-acquired infection. S. pneumoniae has 90 known serotypes, with a limited number of serotypes accounting for the majority of invasive disease isolates (30–32).

A 23-valent pneumococcal polysaccharide vaccine has been available since the 1970s but is poorly immunogenic in young children and has no effect on nasopharyngeal carriage. In February 2000 a heptavalent pneumococcal protein-polysaccharide conjugate vaccine (Pnc7) was licensed for use in the U.S. The first randomized controlled trial in more than 37,000 children showed that Pnc7 prevented 94% of invasive pneumococcal cases (33–37). Both this trial and a smaller study in Finland found a reduction in cases of otitis media of about 6% but with an associated increase in otitis media caused by non–vaccine-type organisms (serotype replacement) (38). It is not yet clear whether serotype replacement will be a major problem beyond mucosal infection and lead to a rise in invasive disease. The seven-valent pneumococcal vaccine does not cover all disease-causing serotypes, prompting the ongoing development of higher valency vaccines. It does, however, produce a cross-protective serogroup response extending to nonimmunized adults via herd immunity.

A high proportion of children presenting to the intensive care unit with pneumococcal septicemia have hyposplenism (detected by the presence of Howell-Jolly bodies on the blood film). Vaccination against pneumococcal disease (and the need for penicillin prophylaxis) should be considered for all children who are admitted with invasive pneumococcal disease.

The expense of the conjugate vaccine, however, is a fundamental disadvantage in developing countries, which carry the main burden of disease. Furthermore, the number of serotypes that can be covered in a vaccine may limit coverage in time and even currently in some geographic locations. For these reasons, the development of cheaper and more broadly cross-protective protein-based pneumococcal vaccines is being pursued.

The complete genome sequence of both virulent and nonvirulent isolates of *S. pneumoniae* has provided new classes of genes as potential targets for vaccine design and provides insight into the mechanisms of host–bacteria interaction (39–40). Proteins within the pneumococcal cell membrane are known to be essential in pneumococcal pathogenicity. Vaccine candidates recently considered include choline-binding proteins (Cbps), pneumolysin, Ply, LytA, PsaA, and PspA proteins (41,42). The antigenic relatedness of pneumococcal proteins to those of other commensal streptococci needs careful evaluation in order to avoid disruption of the balance of harmless commensals in the nasopharynx.

Currently pneumococcal protein-polysaccharide conjugate vaccines offer much promise in preventing the most prevalent pneumococcal serotypes causing disease worldwide. These vaccines have the potential to virtually eliminate admissions to the intensive care unit with pneumococcal disease.

Tuberculosis

One third of the world's population is infected with *Mycobacterium tuberculosis* (TB), with pediatric intensive care presentations consisting mainly of disseminated TB, often in a host with underlying immunocompromise, and TB meningitis (TBM).

Bacille Calmette-Guérin (BCG), the only vaccine currently licensed for prevention of tuberculosis, is up to 77% effective against disseminated TB and between 0% and 80% effective against infectious pulmonary TB. Its effectiveness in reducing morbidity and mortality from disseminated meningeal and miliary TB has justified its use as a neonatal vaccine. Neonatal vaccination provides protection against childhood disease but protection wanes over time. Bacille Calmette-Guérin is safe and well tolerated, with adverse reactions being rare. If development was successful, an improved TB vaccine could be employed either for naive individuals (and would need to be at least as immunogenic and safe as BCG) or a booster vaccine that would supplement BCG and lead to lasting immunity in adults (43).

Leading candidates for priming vaccines include recombinant BCG or M tuberculosis, vaccae, or microti. In an augmented BCG vaccine, deleted genes lost from the parental strain could be added, or increased expression of genes already known to induce an effective immune response might be explored. Recombinant BCG is due to enter clinical trails shortly, after studies showed better protective immunity than was found with the parent strains (44–46). Modified *M. tuberculosis* generates good protection in mouse models and is safe in severe combined immunodeficiency (SCID) mice. This animal model of T-cell immunodeficiency has become increasingly relevant because of the rising incidence of HIV and TB co-infection.

The advantage of a booster vaccine is that the well-established infant BCG program could be maintained while the booster vaccine would be added to maintain effective T-cell memory. Approaches include the use of a subunit vaccine, which may include either a recombinant protein (ESAT-6, Ag85B) or DNA vaccination. DNA vaccination involves the vector delivery of a plasmid encoding a gene product that leads to both CD4 and CD8 responses to the target protein (46). Immunization with more than one gene product may be required to ensure broad protection, and evidence suggests that efficacy is greater using the adjuvant effects of cytokines or a prime/boost vector approach (48,49). Assessing both safety and efficacy of these approaches will need to be undertaken in trials that are currently being designed. A major challenge in the development of a TB vaccine is the evaluation of efficacy against latent infection. There are potential risks of disease reactivation, and preclinical animal data may be difficult to interpret since human T-cell responses may be quite different. Better immunologic correlates of protective immunity are also required. The biggest challenge, however, remains the safe and affordable delivery to the world's poorest individuals and the impact that HIV has on the rising incidence of TB infection.

Salmonella Typhi

Salmonella enteritidis serotype typhi (salmonella typhi) is responsible for 600,000 deaths per year, mainly in resource-poor countries. Presentations to intensive care include intestinal perforation, empyema, myocarditis, respiratory distress, meningitis, coma, and shock. Three different vaccine preparations are available: heat inactivated phenol-preserved whole cell vaccine (HI), purified Vi polysaccharide vaccine (Vi), and a live attenuated oral vaccine (Ty21a). Vaccine efficacy with the HI vaccines has been highly variable in different studies (including challenge studies), with estimates ranging from 0% to 89%

(50–52). Protection with the Vi polysaccharide vaccine ranges from 55% to 72%, and up to 96% efficacy has been documented for the Ty21a vaccine (53–56).

A protein-polysaccharide conjugate vaccine (cf. Hib and MenC) is in clinical development using the Vi polysaccharide with *Pseudomonas aeruginosa* exotoxin A as the carrier protein (56). This vaccine produced an efficacy of 91% in a field trial in Vietnam, and has the potential for programmatic use since it is immunogenic in young children (56). New attenuated live oral vaccines are also in development.

Streptococcus Pyogenes

Invasive group A streptococcal (GAS) infections are particularly associated with chickenpox and include septicemia, necrotizing fasciitis, meningitis, empyema, and other focal infections (57). Development of vaccines for prevention of GAS infection has been driven both to prevent these rare serious infections and more so to prevent rheumatic fever, and also because of the economic impact of GAS upper respiratory infection. Phase 1 studies of a promising M-protein–based vaccine have recently been reported (58,59), and further evaluation is underway. Other trials have been undertaken with a live recombinant *S. gordonii* vaccine in adult volunteers showing this to be safe and well tolerated. This is a potential vector for protein-based vaccines.

Since there is an increased incidence of severe infections with group A streptococci following chickenpox, use of the varicella vaccine in the routine immunization schedule in the second year of life could have a major impact on severe infections due to this organism.

Group B Streptococcus

Severe diseases caused by group B streptococci (GBS) include meningitis, septicemia, and pneumonia, and they occur chiefly in early infancy. Passive transfer of maternal antibody provides protection against invasive disease in this age group, and the vaccine strategy that has been developed is therefore the immunization of women either before or during pregnancy (60). Early trials have shown the feasibility of protein-polysaccharide conjugate vaccines (using the GBS polysaccharide capsule and tetanus toxoid as a protein carrier) in pregnant women. A pentavalent vaccine (containing polysaccharides from the predominant serogroups) could prevent more than 90% of invasive GBS disease (60).

Respiratory Infections

Recent prospective surveillance data from the United States suggest that 1.8% of children younger than 5 years of age are hospitalized each year due to an acute respiratory illness (61). Rates of hospitalization from both respiratory syncytial virus (RSV) and influenza appear to be increasing in the pediatric age group (62), and recent events such as the emergence of severe acute respiratory distress syndrome (SARS) and Avian influenza have alerted the general public to the potential threat posed by respiratory illnesses. The burden of respiratory disease has the potential to be reduced, not only by the development of new vaccines against viruses such as RSV, but also by optimizing the use of existing vaccines against illnesses such as influenza and pertussis.

Pertussis

Unlike other organisms targeted by routine immunizations, pertussis remains a significant cause of morbidity and mortality in developed countries. A gram-negative bacillus, *Bordetella pertussis*, is highly contagious, has no known host other than humans, and can cause complications including pneumonia, seizures, and encephalopathy. In one prospective survey from the PICU of an inner London Hospital, 19.8% of admissions from respiratory failure, apnea, or acute life-threatening episodes showed evidence of infection or household contact with pertussis (63). It is estimated that it is responsible for approximately nine deaths per year in the U.K. (64) and 15 deaths per year in the U.S. (65), the majority of these being in the under 6-month age group. This disease burden persists despite immunization levels of 95% in the U.K., and is predominantly due to transmission to incompletely immunized infants from older household contacts whose postimmunization immunity has waned (63).

Pertussis Vaccines

The whole-cell pertussis vaccine, consisting of a suspension of killed *B. pertussis*, has now largely been replaced in developed countries by the acellular pertussis vaccines. These vaccines combine between two and five selected antigenic cell components with aluminium-based adjuvants. They have a significantly improved side-effect profile when compared with whole-cell pertussis vaccine. The acellular vaccines also achieve an immunogenicity that approaches or equals the whole-cell vaccine (66). Immunity from all pertussis vaccines is known to wane, necessitating the need of booster doses to maintain immunity (67). No monovalent pertussis vaccine is available, the vaccine being incorporated into combination vaccines containing other components of the primary immunization schedule.

Routine primary immunization against pertussis consists of three doses of vaccine in infancy. Countries such as the U.K. have elected to have an accelerated schedule of immunization at 2, 3, and 4 months, rather than the 2-, 4-, and 6-month schedule used in the U.S. and Australia, in an effort to provide earlier protection in the vulnerable age of early infancy (68–70). Although older children and adults are less likely to suffer the complications of pertussis, booster doses of vaccine are administered in later childhood in order to maintain the herd immunity necessary to protect infants. The number and timing of these booster doses varies according to local guidelines. The possibility of routinely immunizing adolescents and adults against pertussis in order to enhance this herd immunity has been raised; however, limitations in the understanding of pertussis immunity and transmission have meant that the effectiveness of such an intervention is uncertain (64).

In addition to immunization, pertussis infections can also be prevented by chemoprophylaxis. If the household contacts of a patient diagnosed with pertussis include an infant who has not completed the primary immunizations, current guidelines advocate the use of a prophylactic 7-day course of erythromycin estolate for all in the household (71). The same guidelines apply for immunocompromised or chronically ill household contacts.

Respiratory Syncytial Virus

By the age of 2 years, almost all children have been infected by RSV, with approximately 50% of these being infected twice (72). It is estimated that each year the virus is responsible for the hospitalization of 120,000 infants and more than 200 deaths in the U.S. alone (73). Populations particularly at risk are premature infants and those with chronic lung disease and congenital heart abnormalities. In the U.S. from 1990 to 1999, RSV was the leading cause of death in ex-premature infants (74). It is becoming apparent that RSV is also responsible for considerable morbidity and mortality in the elderly, with reports of infection rates of residents of an elderly care home of 5% to 10%, with a mortality of 5% of those infected (72). Patients receiving chemotherapy and recipients of bone marrow transplants are also at risk, with a mortality of 50% in those that develop RSV pneumonia.

Respiratory syncytial virus is a RNA virus of the Paramyxoviridae family, with two major subtypes: A and B. Infection with RSV can manifest as isolated apnea as well as bronchiolitis and pneumonia. As implied by the rates of reinfection outlined above, immunity following RSV infection is only partial and evidence of infection can be found in 46% of members of families of infected infants (72). Given that the majority of infections in older children and healthy adults manifest themselves as mild upper respiratory tract infections, it is apparent that immunity against severe disease is achieved even if immunity against infection is not.

Respiratory Syncytial Virus Vaccines

Protection against RSV is currently available only in the form of passive immunization. Two products have been used for this purpose: RSV intravenous immunoglobulin (RSV-IVIG) and monoclonal anti-RSV antibody (palivizumab). Monthly administration of RSV-IVIG to premature infants (<35 weeks) or bronchopulmonary dysplasia over the RSV season has been shown to result in a 41% reduction in RSV-related hospitalization (75). It does, however, have the disadvantage of requiring intravenous administration of a 15 mL/kg fluid load and being a human blood product. In comparison, Palivizumab administered to a similar population group via monthly intramuscular injections was shown to result in a 55% reduction in hospitalization (76). Palivizumab was also shown to benefit children under the age of 2 with congenital heart disease, with a 45% reduction in RSV hospitalization (77).

Despite these results, the considerable expense of palivizumab has restricted its use even in at risk populations. The American Academy of Pediatrics (70) recommends its use in all children in the following categories:

- Under the age of 2 years and have required medical therapy for chronic lung disease within the 6 months prior to the onset of the RSV season
- Born at 28 weeks' gestation or less and facing their first RSV season
- Born from 29 to 32 weeks' gestation and are less than 6 months old at the time of their first RSV season
- Born between 32 and 35 weeks' gestation and are less than 6 months old at the time of their first RSV season, and two or more additional risk factors for severe RSV are present
- Under the age of 2 and have hemodynamically significant congenital heart disease

In contrast, the U.K. Joint Committee on Vaccination and Immunization (JCVI) has recommended the routine use of palivizumab only in children under the age of 2 who are currently receiving home oxygen therapy (78). The committee suggested that children with congenital heart disease and other chronic illnesses, and those with chronic lung disease not receiving oxygen at home, should be considered on a case-by-case basis. It was also advised that children born at less than 32 weeks should not receive palivizumab in the absence of any other indications.

While passive immunization is of some use to a selected group of infants, a vaccine that provides active immunity against RSV disease is required to make a significant impact on the disease burden at a community level. Respiratory syncytial virus vaccine development has been hampered by the initial trials in the 1960s with a formalin inactivated RSV vaccine that resulted in hospitalization of nearly 80% of participants receiving the active vaccine versus 5% in controls (72). This effect was possibly related to alterations in the T-helper-1 (Th1)/Th2 response to wild-type infection, although the causes are remain incompletely understood.

Current RSV vaccine development focuses on both live attenuated and subunit vaccines. As yet the live vaccines studied have been either under- or overattenuated, a problem that it is hoped will be surmounted by the use of genetic engineering. Subunit vaccines incorporating RSV F and G glycoproteins, antigens capable of producing neutralizing and protective antibodies, are also in development (79).

Influenza

Immunization of elderly populations against influenza is now recommended practice in most developed countries. Greater recognition of the burden of influenza-related disease in children and their role as a reservoir of infection for the community as a whole has focused attention on the benefits of childhood influenza immunization. This interest has recently culminated in an American Academy of Pediatrics recommendation that all children between the ages of 6 and 24 months be immunized against influenza on a yearly basis (80). Admissions to the PICU with influenza include infants with viral sepsis syndrome, and children with respiratory failure (especially infants), croup, secondary bacterial pneumonia, or influenza encephalitis.

Influenza-related disease is most commonly caused by types A and B. Influenza A is further classified on the basis of two surface antigens: hemagglutinin (H1, H2, or H3) and neuraminidase (N1 or N2). Influenza A is able to undergo antigenic shift, in which a new hemagglutinin or neuroaminidase emerges, potentially resulting in the influenza pandemics seen in 1918, 1957, and 1968. In addition, both influenza A and B undergo antigenic drift, minor changes in the existing surface antigens that occurs approximately every 2 years. Both influenza A and B can result in the familiar illness of malaise, fever, cough, and myalgia, as well as the more serious complications including pneumonia, bronchiolitis, croup, and encephalitis. In the winter of 2003–2004, 24 pediatric deaths from influenza were seen in the U.K. (81) and over 152 deaths in U.S., the majority of whom were in previously healthy children (82).

Influenza Vaccines

Both inactivated and live attenuated vaccines are available against influenza. Three types of inactivated vaccines are available: split virion (containing denatured virus particles), surface antigen inactivated (containing the key neuraminidase and hemagglutinin antigens), and surface antigen inactivated virosome (containing the neuroaminidase and hemagglutinin antigens reconstituted into a virosome). These are all administered intramuscularly (83). The live attenuated vaccine is administered intranasally and is not as yet licensed in the U.K., having received a license in the U.S. in 2003 (82). Both the inactivated and live attenuated vaccines are trivalent, protecting against two influenza A strains and one influenza B strain.

Antigenic drift results in seasonal variations within these strains, and the vaccines are updated annually based on World Health Organization (WHO) surveillance data. A variable degree of cross-protection exists between antigenically drifted strains, potentially resulting in partial vaccine efficacy against strains not included in the vaccine.

All the inactivated vaccines have equivalent safety and immunogenicity. Efficacy in children varies from 31% to 91% against influenza A and 45% against influenza B (84). Efficacy of the live attenuated vaccine is between 79% and 90%

in children (82). Concerns about a possible increased risk of asthma/reactive airway disease in children aged 18 to 35 months has limited the live attenuated vaccine's license to children over 5 years of age; however, further evaluation of this risk is ongoing.

Currently, guidelines in the U.K. (83) recommend that, in a pediatric population, influenza vaccines be considered in those over the age of 6 months with any of the following conditions:

- Chronic lung disease, including asthma
- Chronic heart disease
- Diabetes
- Chronic renal disease
- Immunosuppression

Children between 6 and 35 months should receive 0.25 to 0.5 mL of the vaccine according to the manufacturer's instructions; all other age groups receive 0.5 mL. The vaccine should be administered annually between the months of September and early November, and for those under 13 years of age receiving the vaccine for the first time, two doses of the vaccine should be administered within 4 to 6 weeks of each other. Although not specifically recommended, the caregivers and siblings of a child in the at-risk groups identified above may also choose to receive the vaccine in order to reduce the risk of transmission within a family. Guidelines in the U.S. have recently extended their recommendations to include all children between 6 and 24 months, as well as older children at increased risk of disease (80). Recent difficulties with vaccine shortages, however, have highlighted the difficulties faced by manufacturers in meeting the increased demand for vaccine that this represents (85). Health care workers derive personal benefit from influenza vaccination and may also reduce the risk of spread to their patients in the PICU.

Concern regarding the possibility of recombination between avian influenza, A (H5N1), and a human influenza virus, potentially precipitating a pandemic, has led the U.S. government to manufacture 2 million doses of a monovalent H5N1 vaccine. It has been observed that this would be sufficient to immunize only a fraction of those at risk of severe disease, raising important issues of prioritizing vaccine use in a pandemic situation (86).

Diphtheria

Corynebacterium diphtheriae causes an acute infection characterized by membranous inflammation of the upper respirator tract. Admission to an intensive care unit for this disease is likely to be related to upper airway obstruction or myocardial injury with circulatory collapse.

A toxoid vaccine was developed in the early 1920s by Ramon (87) by inactivation of diphtheria toxin by heat and formalin action. This highly efficacious vaccine is now used widely (usually in combination with tetanus toxoid and pertussis vaccine), and the disease is very unusual in vaccinated populations.

However, outbreak studies have clearly demonstrated that the vaccine efficacy is not 100%, and the eradication of disease from vaccinated populations indicates that herd immunity plays a role in addition to the direct protection afforded to the individual (88,89). Unvaccinated individuals remain susceptible if exposed to the bacterium.

Treatment of diphtheria in the intensive care unit consists of passive immunization through administration of an antitoxin serum prepared from horses (90).

Adenovirus

Adenoviruses cause various severe diseases that may result in admission to the intensive care unit, including encephalitis, sepsis syndrome in infants, or respiratory failure. No vaccine has been used for childhood immunization. However, a live enteric-coated oral adenovirus vaccine (containing serotypes 4 and 7) was routinely administered to U.S. military personnel from 1971 until 1999 to prevent the substantial adenovirus morbidity that affects trainees at recruit centers, with efficacy up to 90% (91). Manufacture of the adenovirus vaccine that was previously used ceased in 1996 but remanufacture is planned.

Parainfluenza

Human parainfluenza viruses (serotypes 1 to 3), cause severe respiratory tract infections in infants and young children, some of whom require admission to the intensive care unit. Live virus vaccines developed from bovine parainfluenza virus or from attenuated human parainfluenza virus are under development (92).

Dehydration

Cholera

Vibrio cholerae causes water-borne acute diarrhea and vomiting, and leads to profound dehydration, with a mortality of up to 40% without aggressive fluid replacement. The disease is caused by two serogroups, O1 and O139. Critical illness results from hypovolemia, renal failure, electrolyte disturbances (especially hypokalemia and metabolic acidosis), thrombosis, pulmonary edema, and hypoglycemia.

A killed injectable whole-cell vaccine has an efficacy of about 50% for 6 months (93). More recently a killed oral vaccine has been used with efficacy of 60% to 100% and a live oral vaccine with efficacy of 91% against severe diarrhea in North American volunteers, but no protection in an endemic area (94–97). Both oral vaccines provide their protection against serogroup O1 but not O139. Improving water supply and sanitation are known to be highly effective in prevention of cholera.

Rotavirus

Rotavirus is a rare but important cause of admission with life-threatening illness in industrialized countries, with up to 40 deaths per year reported in the U.S. From a global perspective, rates of severe dehydration from rotavirus are enormous, with up to 1500 deaths per day reported. Intensive care unit admission is usually with hyponatremic dehydration and metabolic acidosis in a child with a history of vomiting and diarrhea.

The first rotavirus vaccine (Rotashield; Wyeth Vaccines), a simian-human reassortant rotavirus vaccine, was highly efficacious in clinical trials (up to 90% against severe disease) and given to 1 million children in the U.S. during 1998–1999 before being withdrawn from the market because of a suspected association with intussusception (98).

A bovine-human reassortant rotavirus vaccine (RotaTeq; Merck) and human rotavirus vaccine (Rotarix; GlaxoSmithKline) have recently completed clinical trials with efficacy reported as 90% or more against severe disease (98–101). Neither of these vaccines is reported to have been associated with intussusception in trials of more than 50,000 infants by each company. Rotarix received approval for use in Mexico in 2004.

Encephalitis

Encephalitis is an important cause of encephalopathy in children and associated with significant morbidity and mortality. From a global perspective, there are a large number of potential causative organisms whose prevalence varies widely depending on region and season. The use of live attenuated vaccines has made these infections rare in most industrialized countries. However, they remain among the most important causes of encephalitis in regions of the world with low vaccine uptake or limited health care infrastructure. In routinely immunized populations living in temperate climates, studies indicate the importance of (1) enteroviruses, (2) herpes viruses, (3) respiratory viruses, and (4) *Mycoplasma pneumoniae* (102,103). In many other areas of the world, flaviviruses are the most important cause of encephalitis (104).

Enteroviruses

Enteroviruses cause a wide range of illnesses including febrile exanthems, gastroenteritis, upper respiratory tract infections, and more rarely aseptic meningitis and encephalitis. Poliovirus, while not a cause of encephalitis, is the only enterovirus for which a vaccine is in widespread use. Some types of enterovirus appear to be particularly neurovirulent. Enterovirus type 71 has been associated with epidemic disease with a high frequency of brainstem encephalitis, most recently in a large outbreak in Taiwan (105). A formalin inactivated vaccine was developed following an epidemic in Eastern Europe, but there are no efficacy data for this vaccine (106). Both a formalin-inactivated vaccine and a DNA vaccine are reported to be under development by a group in Taiwan (106). Since 1997, epidemic disease type 71 enterovirus infection has been prevalent in the Asian-Pacific region and such vaccines may be of value in limiting the size of outbreaks (106).

Herpes Viruses

Of the herpes viruses, varicella zoster virus (VZV) and herpes simplex virus (HSV) are most likely to cause encephalitis. Herpes simplex virus type 1 is the commonest cause of sporadic encephalitis. There is widespread exposure to the virus in childhood, and most encephalitis is due to primary infection with HSV type 1 in immunocompetent individuals. There are currently no licensed HSV vaccines, and recent trials have been based on HSV type 2 glycoproteins to afford protection against genital herpes in adults (107). Early recognition of encephalitis and presumptive treatment of HSV with acyclovir remains the most important intervention for this infection in the absence of any preventative strategy.

For VZV, the introduction of the live attenuated Oka stain vaccine in the U.S. in 1990 has been associated with an 84% reduction in clinical varicella infection between 1990 and 2003 (108). This reduction in incidence has been associated with a reported decrease in associated pediatric invasive group A streptococcal disease and is likely to be associated with a similar decline in encephalitis (109). There are still uncertainties regarding the long-term efficacy of vaccine protection, and outbreaks have occurred in fully vaccinated populations (110). Lower efficacy may be associated with younger age at primary immunization (111). Varicella zoster virus disease may present in an atypical fashion in the partially immune vaccinated child, giving rise to diagnostic difficulties (110).

Respiratory Viruses

Respiratory viruses (e.g., influenza and parainfluenza) are associated with encephalitis in case series, although their role in pathogenesis is unclear (102,103). There are substantial public health benefits in promoting vaccination against influenza in groups at high risk of respiratory morbidity. Such concerns are more important determinants of vaccination strategies than the burden of encephalitis that may be related to these organisms. Vaccines for respiratory viruses were reviewed above.

Flaviviruses

Flaviviruses are the commonest causes of encephalitis in many areas of the world. Their distribution is governed by multiple factors including the insect vectors, host factors, and climatic variation. These viruses include Japanese encephalitis, tick-borne encephalitis, West Nile virus, and a large number of more regionally limited viruses (e.g., St. Louis encephalitis virus). Japanese encephalitis is currently confined to Asia, where it is estimated to cause over 30,000 to 50,000 cases and 10,000 deaths a year (104). However the area in which it is endemic has been increasing, with cases reported more recently in Northern Australia (112). A formalin-inactivated vaccine (Bikken vaccine) is the only commercially distributed vaccine available. It has an efficacy of around 80% in trials, and may give cross-protection against West Nile virus and Dengue virus. Although there have been previous concerns, the current inactivated vaccine is associated with a low rate of adverse affects (113). A live attenuated vaccine has been widely used in China. However, it is not licensed outside of China.

West Nile virus has extended its geographic range, with a rapid spread across the U.S. since its introduction on the east coast in 1999. Although vaccines are in development, none are licensed.

Tick-borne encephalitis (TBE) has a major public health impact in central/eastern Europe. In some areas it is the commonest cause of encephalitis, with seasonal peaks in June/July and September/October. Its range extends from central Europe across Russia to the Pacific coast and northeastern China. Several inactivated TBE vaccines are commercially available, and newer less reactogenic formulations were introduced in 2002. Although there have been no formal efficacy trials, there have been significant reductions in disease incidence in countries such as Austria, where the vaccines are used widely (114). A recent consensus has been reached on the need for routine childhood immunization in children in endemic areas (115).

Rabies Vaccines

Rabies infection causes a fatal acute encephalitis with profound central nervous system manifestations, characterized by either hydrophobic spasms or paralysis. It is a rare infection in the U.K., and the diagnosis is unlikely to have been established before admission to the intensive care unit. Globally, children are at the greatest risk of infection.

Dogs infect most human patients, but several wild mammal species are rabies reservoirs including foxes, wolves, and bats. European bat Lyssavirus (EBLV) causes an identical illness and is transmitted in the U.K. by Daubenton's bats (116).

Once symptoms have developed, no treatment has proved effective, and death is inevitable (although there is a very recent single case report of survival with uncertain neurologic deficit). However, preexposure vaccination is highly effective in preventing disease. Two rabies vaccines are licensed for use in the U.K.: human-diploid-cell vaccine and purified chick-embryo-cell vaccine (117). Prophylaxis is recommended for people at occupational risk and for travelers to areas where dog rabies is endemic, mainly in Asia and Africa. Evidence of immunity persists for 5 to 10 years in most people (117).

If exposure to rabies virus has occurred, wound care (thorough washing with soap and water) together with passive and active rabies immunization is essential and should be given as soon as possible. The risk of infection is increased in severe exposure, if bites are on the head, neck, or hands, or are multiple or deep. Postexposure treatment is thought to inactivate virus while it is still in the wound before it gains access to the nervous system. Passive immunization with human rabies immune globulin (RIG) infiltrated around the wound lowers mortality substantially. Although the protection from current rabies vaccines and RIG may be less efficient against EBLV than against classic genotype 1 rabies infection, there is currently no other treatment. This uncertainty increases the importance of preexposure vaccination and the urgency of postexposure treatment in anyone exposed to rabies-related viruses (117).

Management

For many of the causative organisms of encephalitis, treatment options are limited or nonexistent, emphasizing the importance of routine immunization programs and appropriate vaccinations for travelers, where a vaccine exists. From a public health perspective, a regional approach needs to be taken according to important local causes of encephalitis if serious life-threatening infections are to be avoided. Japanese encephalitis vaccine has been incorporated into the WHO Expanded Program of Immunizations in some countries (e.g., Thailand). For travelers, advice on which vaccines should be used will vary depending on the areas to be visited, the season, and the degree of anticipated exposure. In the PICU patient with encephalitis, the variety of infections that may present in this way is a challenge for diagnosis and treatment. The potential for alterations in geographic spread for some organisms (e.g., flaviviruses) increases the difficulties. This necessitates a detailed travel history for the patient with encephalitis, including the extent of exposure in each area visited, and in addition a thorough assessment of vaccination status.

Miscellaneous

Tetanus

In the year 2000, tetanus was responsible for 309,000 deaths globally, approximately 200,000 of which were in the neonatal period (118). In contrast, in England and Wales there were 54 notified cases of tetanus in the decade from 1992 to 2001, 11 of which were fatal (119). There was no tetanus reported in the under 5-year age group, and only one case in the 5- to 14-year age group. Similarly, in the U.S. from 1998 to 2000, there were 30 cases, only 12 of whom were under 20 years old (with one case of neonatal tetanus) (120). Given that *Clostridium tetani* spores remain ubiquitous in the environment, the relative rarity of tetanus in developed countries is testament to the effectiveness of the combination of improved hygiene and routine immunization against this frequently fatal disease. Recent outbreaks of tetanus in injecting drug users in the U.K. and elsewhere in Europe (121), however, emphasize the importance of maintaining vigilance against this disease and an effective tetanus immunization program.

Tetanus Prevention

Active immunization against tetanus uses formaldehyde inactivation of the tetanus toxin, rendering it into the innocuous tetanus toxoid (122). As with pertussis vaccines, this is not available as a monovalent vaccine, but rather in combination with other routine immunizations. A full course of tetanus immunization consists of five doses, with three of them being given in infancy, followed by two booster doses in later childhood or adolescence. The timing of both these primary and booster doses varies according to local practices, as does the recommendation for booster doses every 10 years. In developing countries it is recommended that tetanus toxoid, given in a combination vaccine with absorbed diphtheria and whole-cell pertussis, be administered at 6, 10, and 14 weeks. It is also recommended that tetanus toxoid be administered to all pregnant mothers to provide transplacental immunity to the newborn (123).

Passive immunization against tetanus, in the form of tetanus immunoglobulin, is also available for treatment of incompletely immunized patients with tetanus prone wounds (122). These are defined as follows:

- Wounds or burns requiring surgical treatment that is delayed more than 6 hours after injury or sustained more than 6 hours prior to treatment
- Puncture-type wounds
- Wounds with a significant degree of devitalized tissue or containing foreign bodies
- Wounds with contact with soil or manure
- Compound fractures
- Patients with a wound or burn who have evidence of systemic sepsis

In this context tetanus toxoid alone does not provide timely protection against the development of tetanus. It therefore frequently falls to the pediatric intensivist to decide whether a dose of tetanus immunoglobulin is required following a tetanus prone wound or burn. No immunoglobulin is required if a child has had the primary immunizations and is not overdue for any of the booster immunizations (124). If, on the other hand, the primary immunizations are not complete or the child is due for a booster immunization, both tetanus toxoid (in the age-appropriate combination) and tetanus immunoglobulin should be administered at separate sites.

Malaria

Malaria causes over one million deaths each year with a large proportion occurring in children under 5 years of age. There may be up to 500 million cases per annum worldwide. Severe malaria includes cerebral malaria, and entails complications such as severe anemia, hypoglycemia, acute renal failure, and pulmonary edema.

The acquisition of effective antimalarial immunity in endemic populations depends on repeated asymptomatic infection, which provides long-term maintenance of immunologic protection. Thus most severe disease occurs in relatively immunologically naive individuals, such as children and travelers from nonendemic areas.

Pre-Erythrocytic Vaccines

Immunization with irradiated sporozoites provides protective immunity but the logistics of scaling up production of irradiated sporozoites (or infected mosquitoes) under good manufacturing practice, and of delivering them affordably, has prevented development of this approach. Subunit vaccines must contend with several inherent disadvantages compared with those from whole-organism vaccines, including difficulties in retaining crucial antibody-binding sites, their inability to provide the broad range of major histocompatibility complex (MHC) class II binding motifs that are required to induce a T-cell response, and their inability to induce long-term antigen persistence. Pre-erythrocytic vaccines are designed to target sporozoites or schizont-infected liver cells and thus prevent the release of primary merozoites from infected hepatocytes (Fig. 5.2).

Phase 2 safety and immunogenicity trials of RTS,S/AS02A in malaria-naive and malaria-immune subjects confirmed that the vaccine is safe and immunogenic (125). A large phase 3 trial in Mozambique recently showed this vaccine provides protection in children against both infection, and a range of clinical illness caused by *Plasmodium falciparum*, with efficacy against severe disease being 58% (126). However, protective immunity conferred by this vaccine wanes over time.

Other Pre-Erythrocytic Stage Vaccine Candidates

Three phase 1 clinical trials in healthy, malaria-naive adults are underway, with the optimal *P. falciparum*/hepatitis B core particle vaccine candidate, termed ICC-1132, that uses hepatitis B core antigen as a delivery platform. To date, the vaccine appears to be safe and well tolerated (127), and a sporozoite challenge trial in Oxford is currently underway. Pf CS 282–383 long synthetic peptide vaccine incorporates a C-terminal sequence from a *P. falciparum* clone (128). The vaccine formulations are well tolerated and induce antibodies.

The availability of a number of candidates has led to several prime-boost studies in which two different candidates are administered sequentially in an effort to enhance cell-mediated immune responses. Among the best studied candidates are the thrombospondin-related adhesive protein (TRAP or SSP2) and several liver-stage antigens, including LSA-1, LSA-3, and exported antigen 1 (EXP-1); LSA-3 is a well-conserved blood-stage as well as pre-erythrocytic antigen.

Plasmid DNA or recombinant attenuated live viral vectors such as adenovirus, fowlpox, and modified vaccinia Ankara (MVA) have been employed for prime-boost vaccination in a number of studies. The most advanced of these

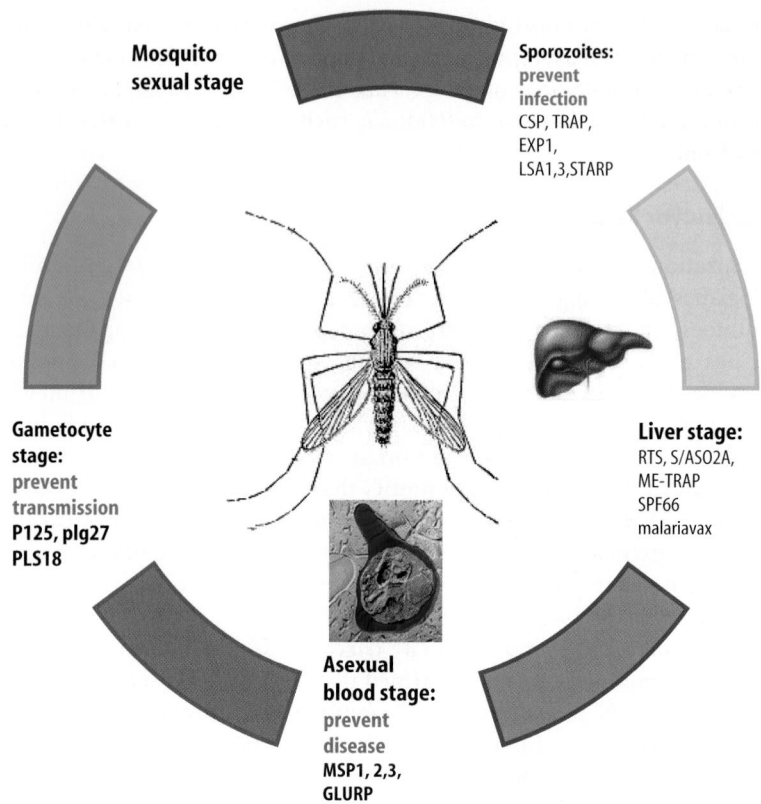

FIGURE 5.2. Malaria vaccine strategies. TRAP or SSP2, thrombospondin-related adhesive protein; LSA-1, LSA-3, liver-stage antigens 1–3; EXP-1, exported antigen 1; MSP, merozoite surface protein; GLURP, glutamine rich protein; ME-TRAP, multiple epitope-thrombospondin-related adhesion protein; SPf66, synthetic polypeptide vaccine; STARP, sporozoite threonine and asparagine-rich protein.

involves a multi-epitope string fused to TRAP sporozoite or liver-stage antigens, including CS, LSA-1, and LSA-3 (129). Several phase 1 and phase 2a sporozoite challenge studies have been conducted in healthy malaria-naive adults in the U.K., to identify prime-boost vaccination regimens that optimize the cell-mediated immune response and generate protective immune responses. On the basis of good safety profiles, a phase 2b proof of concept trial of a DNA/MVA prime-boost regimen is being conducted in Gambia. An MVA vaccine administered with RTS,S/AS02A in a prime-boost regimen is also being evaluated (130).

Asexual Stage Vaccines

A second strategy for the development of a malaria vaccine is to target immune responses against the asexual stage of the parasite. The rationale for this approach is based on the observations that maternal antibodies provide a window of protection against clinical malaria in early infancy, and that following repeated attacks of malaria individuals living in endemic areas acquire the ability to control parasite replication. The principal target of current asexual stage vaccine development is the merozoite, the stage that is initially released from the infected hepatocyte and rapidly invades and replicates in circulating red blood cells. The best studied antigens include merozoite surface protein 1 (MSP-1), MSP-2, MSP-3, GLURP, and apical membrane antigen 1 (AMA-1) (131–136). Antibodies to these molecules are reported to block invasion of merozoites. Merozoite surface protein 1, AMA-1, and MSP-3 have been produced as candidate malaria vaccines and have been shown to protect nonhuman primates from uncontrolled asexual stage parasitemia.

Vaccines that Block Transmission

Preclinical studies conducted have demonstrated that antibodies directed against several sexual stage antigens are capable of preventing the development of infectious sporozoites in the salivary glands of Anopheles mosquitoes. Sexual stage antigen targets have proven to be complex proteins with precise molecular folding requirements, and formulation of adequately immunogenic vaccines has been difficult. Animal studies have been undertaken in *P. vivax* antigen Pvs25 and its *P. falciparum* ortholog Pfs25 (137,138).

Future Developments

A number of promising vaccines are entering trials, with research being driven by the large amount of information generated through bioinformatics and gene expression studies. However, generating a sustained immune response to a number of antigens investigated thus far remains elusive.

Human Immunodeficiency Virus

Children with human immunodeficiency virus (HIV) infection may present to the PICU with AIDS-defining illnesses caused by various opportunistic infections. Over 20 years have passed since HIV was discovered and shown to be the cause of AIDS, yet we do not have a safe and effective vaccine to prevent infection or to ameliorate disease. As a result, the disease burden of HIV/AIDS is enormous and continues to grow. Highly effective antiretroviral therapies highly active antiretroviral therapy (HAART) have helped to decrease the rate of disease progression, but many developing countries lack available resources or infrastructure to deliver HAART effectively, and a safe and inexpensive AIDS vaccine is desperately needed.

Natural infection with HIV does not result in protective immunity or viral clearance by the host immune system. HIV establishes persistent, lifelong infection. The virus is difficult to neutralize with antibodies, and causes progressive destruction and impaired regeneration of $CD4^+$ T-helper cells. It evolves rapidly to escape from both cellular and humoral antiviral immune responses. In addition, HIV evades immune surveillance and resists eradication from the host via other mechanisms that include the downregulation of MHC class I molecules from the surface of infected cells by the HIV Nef protein. It also establishes a state of proviral latency in long-lived CD4$^+$ T cells that provides a persistent, yet immunologically invisible, reservoir of virus infection. Diverse evidence supports the importance of the cellular immune response in HIV containment. CD8$^+$ T lymphocytes can inhibit the replication of HIV in CD4$^+$ T lymphocytes in vitro, probably through direct cytotoxicity and the production of soluble factors including β-chemokines. The clinical status of infected individuals is associated with the level of virus-specific CD8$^+$ cytotoxic T lymphocytes (CTLs) in their peripheral blood; high levels are predictive of good clinical status. The early containment of HIV replication in acutely infected individuals coincides with the emergence of an HIV-specific CTL response.

Vaccine strategies are being pursued that focus on eliciting antiviral CD8$^+$ T-cell responses to control the level of HIV replication in vivo. However, because virus-specific CD8$^+$ T cells recognize CD4$^+$ target cells only after they are infected, it is highly unlikely that a CD8$^+$ T-cell–based vaccine could achieve sterilizing immunity by preventing the establishment of persistent HIV infection. The rationale therefore for potential efficacy of a CD8$^+$ T-cell–based AIDS vaccine is that reduction of the set-point level of viral load within an infected individual may be expected to slow his/her rate of progression to AIDS while simultaneously reducing likelihood of subsequent HIV transmission.

Current Strategies

Attenuated viruses have provided safe and effective protection against smallpox, measles, and polio. However, in the case of HIV, because of the genetic diversity of the virus within a single host, immunity is generated only against a restricted number of viruses in the population.

Recombinant envelope glycoprotein-based HIV vaccine strategies have been investigated but failed to induce antibodies that were broadly reactive against primary HIV isolates (139,140).

Genes of HIV and simian immunodeficiency virus (SIV) can be engineered into microorganisms that have proved safe and effective as live attenuated vaccines, such as vaccinia or BCG. As these engineered viruses and bacteria replicate in the inoculated individual, immunity is developed to both the vector and the HIV gene product. Since these are live, both humoral and cellular immune responses are generated (141,142). The best studied of the live vectors are the poxviruses. Although vaccinia virus might be an effective vector for HIV genes, safety issues preclude its use as an HIV vaccine. Therefore, most work using poxviruses as vectors for HIV immunization has been done with viruses that undergo an abortive replication cycle in human cells. These viruses include modified vaccinia Ankara (MVA) (143) and the avian poxviruses canarypox and fowlpox (FPV). These recombinant vectors have proved immunogenic in nonhuman primates. Early-phase human clinical trials with recombinant MVA and FPV HIV constructs are ongoing (used singly or as heterologous prime-boost vaccination), including a phase II assessment at sites in the U.K. and Kenya (144,145). Recent studies with recombinant adenovirus vectors have been particularly promising, showing that recombinant adenovirus can elicit HIV-specific T-cell immune responses (143).

Future Developments

With a growing appreciation of the importance of CTL in containing HIV replication, efforts are being made to develop immunogens that elicit high-frequency HIV-specific CTL responses. Such vaccines are not likely to confer sterile protection against HIV infection. However, nonhuman primate studies have suggested that these vaccines may elicit immune responses that contain the spread of HIV and slow the progression of disease in individuals who become infected.

Conclusion

The development of new technologies such as reverse vaccinology has revolutionized vaccine research. In the coming decade we are likely to see the widespread introduction of a number of new vaccines that will have a dramatic impact on the nature of admission to PICU. The greatest challenge will be in the dissemination of vaccine developments to the less developed, resource-poor countries, which have the highest disease burden.

References

1. Levine OS, Schwartz B, Pierce N, Kane M. Development, evaluation and implementation of Haemophilus influenzae type b vaccines for young children in developing countries: current status and priority actions. Pediatr Infect Dis J 1998;17(9 suppl): S95–113.
2. Herson VC, Todd JK. Prediction of morbidity in Haemophilus influenzae meningitis. Pediatrics 1977;59(1):35–39.
3. Peltola H, Kayhty H, Sivonen A, Makela H. Haemophilus influenzae type b capsular polysaccharide vaccine in children: a double-blind field study of 100,000 vaccinees 3 months to 5 years of age in Finland. Pediatrics 1977;60(5):730–737.
4. Heath PT. Haemophilus influenzae type b conjugate vaccines: a review of efficacy data. Pediatr Infect Dis J 1998;17(9 suppl):S117–122.
5. Heath PT, Booy R, Griffiths H, et al. Clinical and immunological risk factors associated with Haemophilus influenzae type b conjugate vaccine failure in childhood. Clin Infect Dis 2000;31(4):973–980.
6. Trotter CL, Ramsay ME, Slack MP. Rising incidence of Haemophilus influenzae type b disease in England and Wales indicates a need for a second catch-up vaccination campaign. Commun Dis Public Health 2003;6(1):55–58.

7. McVernon J, Andrews N, Slack MP, Ramsay ME. Risk of vaccine failure after Haemophilus influenzae type b (Hib) combination vaccines with acellular pertussis. Lancet 2003;361(9368):1521–1523.

8. Booy R, Habibi P, Nadel S, et al. Reduction in case fatality rate from meningococcal disease associated with improved health care delivery. Arch Dis Child 2001;85:386–390.

9. Thorburn K, Baines P, Thomson A, Hart CA. Mortality in severe meningococcal disease. Arch Dis Child 2001;85(5):382–385.

10. World Health Organization. Prevention and Control of Epidemic Meningococcal Disease in Africa. Ouagadougou, Burkina Faso: Department of Communicable Disease Surveillance and Response, 2003.

11. Pollard AJ. Global epidemiology of meningococcal disease and vaccine efficacy. Pediatr Infect Dis J 2004;23(12 suppl):S274–279.

12. Ouedraogo-Traore R, Hoiby EA, Sanou I, et al. Molecular characteristics of Neisseria meningitidis strains isolated in Burkina Faso in 2001. Scand J Infect Dis 2002;34(11):804–807.

13. Snape MD, Pollard AJ. Meningococcal polysaccharide-protein conjugate vaccines. Lancet Infect Dis 2005;5:21–30.

14. Gotschlich EC, Goldschneider I, Artenstein MS. Human immunity to the meningococcus. IV. Immunogenicity of group A and group C meningococcal polysaccharides in human volunteers. J Exp Med 1969;129(6):1367–1384.

15. Department of Health. Health advice to travellers to Hajj and Umrah. http://www.dh.gov.uk/PolicyAndGuidance/HealthAdviceForTravellers/LatestHealthUpdates%20/fs/en?CONTENT_ID=4054061&chk=LstRft.

16. Health Protection Agency. Enhanced surveillance of meningococcal disease: October to December 2004. Communicable Disease Report 2004;14:5–8.

17. Ramsay ME, Andrews NJ, Trotter CL, Kaczmarski EB, Miller E. Herd immunity from meningococcal serogroup C conjugate vaccination in England: database analysis. BMJ 2003;326(7385):365–366.

18. Borrow R, Goldblatt D, Finn A, et al. Immunogenicity of, and immunologic memory to, a reduced primary schedule of meningococcal C-tetanus toxoid conjugate vaccine in infants in the United kingdom. Infect Immun 2003;71(10):5549–5555.

19. Trotter C, Andrews N, Kaczmarski E, Miller E, Ramsay ME. Effectiveness of meningococcal serogroup C conjugate vaccine 4 years after introduction. Lancet 2004; 364:365–367.

20. Perez-Trallero E, Vicente D, Montes M, Cisterna R. Positive effect of meningococcal C vaccination on serogroup replacement in Neisseria meningitidis. Lancet 2002;360(9337):953.

21. Rennels MB, King JCJ, Ryall R, al. e. Dosage escalation, safety and immunoethnicity study of four dosages of a tetravalent meningococcal polysaccharide diphtheria toxoid conjugate vaccine in infants. Paediatr Infect Dis J 2004;23:429–435.

22. Finne J, Bitter-Suermann D, Goridis C, Finne U. An IgG monoclonal antibody to group B meningococci cross-reacts with developmentally regulated polysialic acid units of glycoproteins in neural and extraneural tissues. J Immunol 1987; 138(12):4402–4407.

23. Ruggeberg JU, Pollard AJ. Meningococcal vaccines. Paediatr Drugs 2004; 6(4):251–266.

24. de Moraes JC, Perkins BA, Camargo MC, et al. Protective efficacy of a serogroup B meningococcal vaccine in Sao Paulo, Brazil. Lancet 1992;340(8827):1074–1078.

25. Milagres LG, Ramos SR, Sacchi CT, et al. Immune response of Brazilian children to a Neisseria meningitidis serogroup B outer membrane protein vaccine: comparison with efficacy. Infect Immun 1994;62(10):4419–4424.

26. Sierra GV, Campa HC, Varcacel NM, et al. Vaccine against group B Neisseria meningitidis: protection trial and mass vaccination results in Cuba. NIPH Ann 1991;14(2):195–207; discussion 208–210.

27. Bjune G, Grønnesby JK, Høiby EA, Closs O, Nøkleby H. Results of an efficacy trial with an outer membrane vesicle vaccine against systemic serogroup B meningococcal disease in Norway. NIPH Ann 1991;14(2):125–130; discussion 130–132.

28. Noronha CP, Struchiner CJ, Halloran ME. Assessment of the direct effectiveness of BC meningococcal vaccine in Rio de Janeiro, Brazil: a case-control study. Int J Epidemiol 1995;24(5):1050–1057.

29. Wong S, Lennon D, Jackson C, et al. New Zealand epidemic strain meningococcal B outer membrane vesicle vaccine in children aged 16–24 months. Pediatr Infect Dis J 2007;26(4):345–350.

30. Dawson KG, Emerson JC, Burns JL. Fifteen years of experience with bacterial meningitis. Pediatr Infect Dis J 1999;18(9):816–822.

31. Djuretic T, Ryan MJ, Miller E, Fairley CK, Goldblatt D. Hospital admissions in children due to pneumococcal pneumonia in England. J Infect 1998;37(1): 54–58.

32. Greenwood B. The epidemiology of pneumococcal infection in children in the developing world. Philos Trans R Soc Lond B Biol Sci 1999;354(1384):777–785.

33. Black S, Shinefield H, Fireman B, et al. Efficacy, safety and immunogenicity of heptavalent pneumococcal conjugate vaccine in children. Northern California Kaiser Permanente Vaccine Study Center Group. Pediatr Infect Dis J 2000; 19(3):187–195.

34. Black S, Shinefield H. Safety and efficacy of the seven-valent pneumococcal conjugate vaccine: evidence from Northern California. Eur J Pediatr 2002;161(suppl 2): S127–131.

35. Black SB, Shinefield HR, Hansen J, Elvin L, Laufer D, Malinoski F. Postlicensure evaluation of the effectiveness of seven valent pneumococcal conjugate vaccine. Pediatr Infect Dis J 2001;20(12):1105–1107.

36. Shinefield H, Black S, Ray P, Fireman B, Schwalbe J, Lewis E. Efficacy, immunogenicity and safety of heptavalent pneumococcal conjugate vaccine in low birth weight and preterm infants. Pediatr Infect Dis J 2002;21(3):182–186.

37. Shinefield HR, Black S, Ray P, et al. Safety and immunogenicity of heptavalent pneumococcal CRM197 conjugate vaccine in infants and toddlers. Pediatr Infect Dis J 1999;18(9):757–763.

38. Eskola J, Kilpi T, Palmu A, et al. Efficacy of a pneumococcal conjugate vaccine against acute otitis media. N Engl J Med 2001;344(6):403–409.

39. Hoskins J, Alborn WE Jr, Arnold J, et al. Genome of the bacterium Streptococcus pneumoniae strain R6. J Bacteriol 2001;183(19):5709–5717.

40. Tettelin H, Saunders NJ, Heidelberg J, et al. Complete genome sequence of Neisseria meningitidis serogroup B strain MC58. Science 2000;287(5459):1809–1815.

41. Hakenbeck R, Balmelle N, Weber B, Gardes C, Keck W, de Saizieu A. Mosaic genes and mosaic chromosomes: intra- and interspecies genomic variation of Streptococcus pneumoniae. Infect Immun 2001;69(4):2477–2486.

42. Jedrzejas MJ, Lamani E, Becker RS. Characterization of selected strains of pneumococcal surface protein A. J Biol Chem 2001;276(35):33121–33128.

43. Nor NM, Musa M. Approaches towards the development of a vaccine against tuberculosis: recombinant BCG and DNA vaccine. Tuberculosis (Edinb) 2004;84(1–2):102–109.

44. Horwitz MA, Harth G, Dillon BJ, Maslesa-Galic S. Recombinant bacillus Calmette-Guerin (BCG) vaccines expressing the Mycobacterium tuberculosis 30-kDa major secretory protein induce greater protective immunity against tuberculosis than conventional BCG vaccines in a highly susceptible animal model. Proc Natl Acad Sci U S A 2000;97(25):13853–13858.

45. Pym AS, Brodin P, Majlessi L, et al. Recombinant BCG exporting ESAT-6 confers enhanced protection against tuberculosis. Nat Med 2003;9(5):533–539.

46. Smith DA, Parish T, Stoker NG, Bancroft GJ. Characterization of auxotrophic mutants of Mycobacterium tuberculosis and their potential as vaccine candidates. Infect Immun 2001;69(2):1142–1150.

47. Delogu G, Li A, Repique C, Collins F, Morris SL. DNA vaccine combinations expressing either tissue plasminogen activator signal sequence fusion proteins or ubiquitin-conjugated antigens induce sustained protective immunity in a mouse model of pulmonary tuberculosis. Infect Immun 2002;70(1):292–302.

48. McShane H, Brookes R, Gilbert SC, Hill AV. Enhanced immunogenicity of CD4(+) t-cell responses and protective efficacy of a DNA-modified vaccinia virus Ankara prime-boost vaccination regimen for murine tuberculosis. Infect Immun 2001; 69(2):681–686.

49. Palendira U, Kamath AT, Feng CG, et al. Coexpression of interleukin-12 chains by a self-splicing vector increases the protective cellular immune response of DNA and Mycobacterium bovis BCG vaccines against Mycobacterium tuberculosis. Infect Immun 2002;70(4):1949–1956.

50. Hornick RB, Greisman SE, Woodward TE, DuPont HL, Dawkins AT, Snyder MJ. Typhoid fever: pathogenesis and immunologic control. N Engl J Med 1970; 283(13):686–691.

51. Hejfec LB, Salmin LV, Lejtman MZ, et al. A controlled field trial and laboratory study of five typhoid vaccines in the USSR. Bull WHO 1966;34(3):321–339.

52. Ashcroft MT, Singh B, Nicholson CC, Ritchie JM, Sorryan E, Williams F. A seven-year field trial of two typhoid vaccines in Guyana. Lancet 1967;2(7525): 1056–1059.

53. Klugman KP, Koornhof HJ, Robbins JB, Le Cam NN. Immunogenicity, efficacy and serological correlate of protection of Salmonella typhi Vi capsular polysaccharide vaccine three years after immunization. Vaccine 1996;14(5):435–438.

54. Acharya IL, Lowe CU, Thapa R, et al. Prevention of typhoid fever in Nepal with the Vi capsular polysaccharide of Salmonella typhi. A preliminary report. N Engl J Med 1987;317(18):1101–1104.

55. Wahdan MH, Serie C, Cerisier Y, Sallam S, Germanier R. A controlled field trial of live Salmonella typhi strain Ty 21a oral vaccine against typhoid: three-year results. J Infect Dis 1982;145(3):292–295.

56. Lin FY, Ho VA, Khiem HB, et al. The efficacy of a Salmonella typhi Vi conjugate vaccine in two-to-five-year-old children. N Engl J Med 2001;344(17):1263–1269.

57. Pollard AJ, Isaacs A, Hermione Lyall EG, et al. Potentially lethal bacterial infection associated with varicella zoster virus. BMJ 1996;313(7052):283–285.

58. Kotloff KL, Corretti M, Palmer K, et al. Safety and immunogenicity of a recombinant multivalent group a streptococcal vaccine in healthy adults: phase 1 trial. JAMA 2004;292(6):709–715.

59. Kotloff KL, Dale JB. Progress in group A streptococcal vaccine development. Pediatr Infect Dis J 2004;23(8):765–766.
60. Baker CJ, Edwards MS. Group B streptococcal conjugate vaccines. Arch Dis Child 2003;88(5):375–378.
61. Griffin MR, Walker FJ, Iwane MK, Weinberg GA, Staat MA, Erdman DD. Epidemiology of respiratory infections in young children: insights from the new vaccine surveillance network. Pediatr Infect Dis J 2004;23(11 suppl):S188–192.
62. Glezen WP. The changing epidemiology of respiratory syncytial virus and influenza: impetus for new control measures. Pediatr Infect Dis J 2004;23(11 suppl): S202–206.
63. Crowcroft NS, Booy R, Harrison T, et al. Severe and unrecognised: pertussis in UK infants. Arch Dis Child 2003;88(9):802–806.
64. Crowcroft NS, Britto J. Whooping cough—a continuing problem. BMJ 2002;324(7353):1537–1538.
65. Centre for Communicable Disease Control and prevention. Pertussis—United States, 1997–2000. Morbidity and Mortality Weekly, Centre for Communicable Disease Control and Prevention 2002;51:73–76.
66. Miller E. Overview of recent clinical trials of acellular pertussis vaccines. Biologicals 1999;27(2):79–86.
67. Van Buynder PG, Owen D, Vurdien JE, Andrews NJ, Matthews RC, Miller E. Bordetella pertussis surveillance in England and Wales: 1995–7. Epidemiol Infect 1999;123(3):403–411.
68. Salisbury DM, Begg NT. Immunisation against infectious diseases 1996 (The Green Book)—Pertussis update 2004. http://www.dh.gov.uk/assetRoot/04/08/73/86/04087386.pdf.
69. Australian Technical Advisory Group on Immunisation. Australian Immunisation Handbook, 8th ed. Sydney: Department of Health and Ageing, 2003.
70. American Academy of Pediatrics. Red Book 2003, 26th ed. American Academy of Pediatrics, 2003.
71. Dodhia H, Crowcroft NS, Bramley JC, Miller E. UK guidelines for use of erythromycin chemoprophylaxis in persons exposed to pertussis. J Public Health Med 2002;24(3):200–206.
72. Collins CL, Pollard AJ. Respiratory syncytial virus infections in children and adults. J Infect 2002;45(1):10–17.
73. Welliver RC. Review of epidemiology and clinical risk factors for severe respiratory syncytial virus (RSV) infection. J Pediatr 2003;143(5 suppl):S112–117.
74. Thompson WW, Shay DK, Weintraub E, et al. Mortality associated with influenza and respiratory syncytial virus in the United States. JAMA 2003;289(2):179–186.
75. PREVENT Study Group. Reduction of respiratory syncytial virus hospitalization among premature infants and infants with bronchopulmonary dysplasia using respiratory syncytial virus immune globulin prophylaxis. The PREVENT Study Group. Pediatrics 1997;99(1):93–99.
76. IMpact-RSV Study Group. Palivizumab, a humanized respiratory syncytial virus monoclonal antibody, reduces hospitalization from respiratory syncytial virus infection in high-risk infants. The IMpact-RSV Study Group. Pediatrics 1998;102(3 pt 1):531–537.
77. Feltes TF, Cabalka AK, Meissner HC, et al. Palivizumab prophylaxis reduces hospitalization due to respiratory syncytial virus in young children with hemodynamically significant congenital heart disease. J Pediatr 2003;143(4):532–540.

78. Immunisation JCoVa. Joint Committee of Vaccination and Immunisation: minutes of meeting held on Friday November 1, 2002. http://www.advisorybodies.doh.gov.uk/jcvi/mins01nov02.htm.

79. Polack FP, Karron RA. The future of respiratory syncytial virus vaccine development. Pediatr Infect Dis J 2004;23(1 Suppl):S65–73.

80. Centre for disease control and prevention. Recommended Childhood and Adolescent Immunisation Schedule—United States, July–December 2004. Centre for Disease Control and Prevention. MMWR 2004;53:Q1–Q3.

81. Health Protection Agency. HPA National Influenza Report: Summary of Activity for 2003/04 Season, 2004.

82. Greenberg HB, Piedra PA. Immunization against viral respiratory disease: a review. Pediatr Infect Dis J 2004;23(11 suppl):S254–261.

83. Salisbury DM, Begg NT. Immunisation Against Infectious Disease (The Green Book)—Influenza update, 2004.

84. Ruben FL. Inactivated influenza virus vaccines in children. Clin Infect Dis 2004;38(5):678–688.

85. Centers for Disease Control and Prevention. Updated Interim Influenza Vaccination Recommendations—2004–05 Influenza Season. http://www.cdc.gov/flu/protect/whoshouldget.htm.

86. Quirk M. USA to manufacture two million doses of pandemic flu vaccine. Lancet Infect Dis 2004;4(11):654.

87. Ramon G. Sur le pouvoir floculant et sur les proprietes immunisantes d'une toxin diphterique rendue anatoxique (anatoxine). C R Acad Sci 1923;177:1338–1340.

88. Brennan M, Vitek C, Strebel P, et al. How many doses of diphtheria toxoid are required for protection in adults? Results of a case-control study among 40- to 49-year-old adults in the Russian Federation. J Infect Dis 2000;181(suppl 1): S193–196.

89. Fox JP, Elveback L, Scott W, Gatewood L, Ackerman E. Herd immunity: basic concept and relevance to public health immunization practices, 1971. Am J Epidemiol 1995;141(3):187–197; discussion 185–186.

90. Hrobjartsson A, Gotzsche PC, Gluud C. The controlled clinical trial turns 100 years: Fibiger's trial of serum treatment of diphtheria. BMJ 1998;317(7167):1243–1245.

91. Peckinpaugh RO, Pierce WE, Rosenbaum MJ, Edwards EA, Jackson GG. Mass enteric live adenovirus vaccination during epidemic ARD. JAMA 1968;205(1): 75–80.

92. Murphy BR, Hall SL, Kulkarni AB, et al. An update on approaches to the development of respiratory syncytial virus (RSV) and parainfluenza virus type 3 (PIV3) vaccines. Virus Res 1994;32(1):13–36.

93. Mosley WH, Aziz KM, Rahman AS, Chowdhury AK, Ahmed A. Field trials of monovalent Ogawa and Inaba cholera vaccines in rural Bangladesh—three years of observation. Bull WHO 1973;49(4):381–387.

94. Sack DA, Tacket CO, Cohen MB, et al. Validation of a volunteer model of cholera with frozen bacteria as the challenge. Infect Immun 1998;66(5):1968–1972.

95. Sanchez JL, Vasquez B, Begue RE, et al. Protective efficacy of oral whole-cell/recombinant-B-subunit cholera vaccine in Peruvian military recruits. Lancet 1994;344(8932):1273–1276.

96. Suharyono, Simanjuntak C, Witham N, et al. Safety and immunogenicity of single-dose live oral cholera vaccine CVD 103-HgR in 5–9-year-old Indonesian children. Lancet 1992;340(8821):689–694.

97. Richie EE, Punjabi NH, Sidharta YY, et al. Efficacy trial of single-dose live oral cholera vaccine CVD 103-HgR in North Jakarta, Indonesia, a cholera-endemic area. Vaccine 2000;18(22):2399–2410.

98. De Vos B, Vesikari T, Linhares AC, et al. A rotavirus vaccine for prophylaxis of infants against rotavirus gastroenteritis. Pediatr Infect Dis J 2004;23(10 suppl): S179–182.

99. Vesikari T, Karvonen A, Puustinen L, et al. Efficacy of RIX4414 live attenuated human rotavirus vaccine in Finnish infants. Pediatr Infect Dis J 2004;23(10): 937–943.

100. Clark HF, Bernstein DI, Dennehy PH, et al. Safety, efficacy, and immunogenicity of a live, quadrivalent human-bovine reassortant rotavirus vaccine in healthy infants. J Pediatr 2004;144(2):184–190.

101. Clark HF, Lawley D, Shrager D, et al. Infant immune response to human rotavirus serotype G1 vaccine candidate reassortant WI79-9: different dose response patterns to virus surface proteins VP7 and VP4. Pediatr Infect Dis J 2004;23(3): 206–211.

102. Koskiniemi M, Rautonen J, Lehtokoski-Lehtiniemi E, Vaheri A. Epidemiology of encephalitis in children: a 20–year survey. Ann Neurol 1991;29(5):492–497.

103. Kolski H, Ford-Jones EL, Richardson S, et al. Etiology of acute childhood encephalitis at the Hospital for Sick Children, Toronto, 1994–1995. Clin Infect Dis 1998;26(2):398–409.

104. Solomon T. Flavivirus encephalitis. N Engl J Med 2004;351(4):370–378.

105. Ho M, Chen ER, Hsu KH, et al. An epidemic of enterovirus 71 infection in Taiwan. Taiwan Enterovirus Epidemic Working Group. N Engl J Med 1999;341(13): 929–935.

106. McMinn PC. An overview of the evolution of enterovirus 71 and its clinical and public health significance. FEMS Microbiol Rev 2002;26(1):91–107.

107. Stanberry LR, Spruance SL, Cunningham AL, et al. Glycoprotein-D-adjuvant vaccine to prevent genital herpes. N Engl J Med 2002;347(21):1652–1661.

108. Centers for Disease Control and Prevention. Decline in annual incidence of varicella—selected states, 1990–2001. MMWR Morb Mortal Wkly Rep 2003; 52(37):884–885.

109. Patel RA, Binns HJ, Shulman ST. Reduction in pediatric hospitalizations for varicella-related invasive group A streptococcal infections in the varicella vaccine era. J Pediatr 2004;144(1):68–74.

110. Vazquez M. Varicella infections and varicella vaccine in the 21st century. Pediatr Infect Dis J 2004;23(9):871–872.

111. Vazquez M, LaRussa PS, Gershon AA, et al. Effectiveness over time of varicella vaccine. JAMA 2004;291(7):851–855.

112. Daley AJ, Dwyer DE. Emerging viral infections in Australia. J Paediatr Child Health 2002;38(1):1–3.

113. Shlim DR, Solomon T. Japanese encephalitis vaccine for travelers: exploring the limits of risk. Clin Infect Dis 2002;35(2):183–188.

114. Heinz FX, Kunz C. Tick-borne encephalitis and the impact of vaccination. Arch Virol Suppl 2004(18):201–205.

115. Kunze U, Asokliene L, Bektimirov T, et al. Tick-borne encephalitis in childhood—consensus 2004. Wien Med Wochenschr 2004;154(9–10):242–245.

116. McColl KA, Tordo N, Aguilar Setien AA. Bat lyssavirus infections. Rev Sci Tech 2000;19(1):177–196.

117. Rai Chowdhuri AN, Bhatia R, Ichhpujani RL. Immunoprophylaxis against rabies. J Commun Dis 1984;16(1):43–48.
118. Vandelaer J, Birmingham M, Gasse F, Kurian M, Shaw C, Garnier S. Tetanus in developing countries: an update on the Maternal and Neonatal Tetanus Elimination Initiative. Vaccine 2003;21(24):3442–3445.
119. Health Protection Agency. Tetanus Notifications by age group and sex, 2004. www.hpa.org.uk/infections/topics_az/tetanus/data_not_age_sex.htm.
120. Centre for Disease Control and Prevention. Tetanus Surveillance—United States, 1998–2000. Morbidity and Mortality Weekly 2003. http://www.cdc.gov/mmwr/preview/mmwrhtml/ss5203a1.htm.
121. Health Protection Agency. Ongoing outbreak of tetanus in injecting drug users. Health Protection Agency CDR Weekly 2004;14:4–6.
122. Salisbury DM, Begg NT. Immunisation against infectious diseases 1996 (The Green Book)—Tetanus chapter update, 2004. http://www.dh.gov.uk/assetRoot/04/08/73/89/04087389.pdf.
123. World Health Organization. Core Information for Development for Immunization Policy: 2002 update.
124. Health Protection Agency. Immunoglobulin Handbook: Indications and Dosage for Normal and Specific Immunoglobulin Preparations Issued by the Health Protection Agency, 2004.
125. Kester KE, McKinney DA, Tornieporth N, et al. Efficacy of recombinant circumsporozoite protein vaccine regimens against experimental Plasmodium falciparum malaria. J Infect Dis 2001;183(4):640–647.
126. Alonso PL, Sacarlal J, Aponte JJ, et al. Efficacy of the RTS,S/AS02A vaccine against Plasmodium falciparum infection and disease in young African children: randomised controlled trial. Lancet 2004;364(9443):1411–1420.
127. Birkett A, Lyons K, Schmidt A, et al. A modified hepatitis B virus core particle containing multiple epitopes of the Plasmodium falciparum circumsporozoite protein provides a highly immunogenic malaria vaccine in preclinical analyses in rodent and primate hosts. Infect Immun 2002;70(12):6860–6870.
128. Roggero MA, Weilenmann C, Bonelo A, et al. Plasmodium falciparum CS C-terminal fragment: preclinical evaluation and phase I clinical studies. Parassitologia 1999;41(1–3):421–424.
129. Schneider J, Gilbert SC, Blanchard TJ, et al. Enhanced immunogenicity for CD8+ T cell induction and complete protective efficacy of malaria DNA vaccination by boosting with modified vaccinia virus Ankara. Nat Med 1998;4(4):397–402.
130. Moorthy VS, Pinder M, Reece WH, et al. Safety and immunogenicity of DNA/modified vaccinia virus Ankara malaria vaccination in African adults. J Infect Dis 2003;188(8):1239–1244.
131. Holder AA, Guevara Patino JA, Uthaipibull C, et al. Merozoite surface protein 1, immune evasion, and vaccines against asexual blood stage malaria. Parassitologia 1999;41(1–3):409–414.
132. Garraud O, Diouf A, Nguer CM, et al. Different Plasmodium falciparum recombinant MSP1(19) antigens differ in their capacities to stimulate in vitro peripheral blood T lymphocytes in individuals from various endemic areas. Scand J Immunol 1999;49(4):431–440.
133. Pan W, Ravot E, Tolle R, et al. Vaccine candidate MSP-1 from Plasmodium falciparum: a redesigned 4917 bp polynucleotide enables synthesis and isolation of

full-length protein from Escherichia coli and mammalian cells. Nucleic Acids Res 1999;27(4):1094–1103.

134. Anders RF, Crewther PE, Edwards S, et al. Immunisation with recombinant AMA-1 protects mice against infection with Plasmodium chabaudi. Vaccine 1998; 16(2–3):240–247.

135. Hodder AN, Crewther PE, Anders RF. Specificity of the protective antibody response to apical membrane antigen 1. Infect Immun 2001;69(5):3286–3294.

136. Oeuvray C, Theisen M, Rogier C, Trape JF, Jepsen S, Druilhe P. Cytophilic immunoglobulin responses to Plasmodium falciparum glutamate-rich protein are correlated with protection against clinical malaria in Dielmo, Senegal. Infect Immun 2000;68(5):2617–2620.

137. Carter R. Transmission blocking malaria vaccines. Vaccine 2001;19(17–19):2309–2314.

138. Gozar MM, Muratova O, Keister DB, Kensil CR, Price VL, Kaslow DC. Plasmodium falciparum: immunogenicity of alum-adsorbed clinical-grade TBV25–28, a yeast-secreted malaria transmission-blocking vaccine candidate. Exp Parasitol 2001;97(2):61–69.

139. Cohen J. Public health. AIDS vaccine still alive as booster after second failure in Thailand. Science 2003;302(5649):1309–1310.

140. Cohen J. Public health. AIDS vaccine trial produces disappointment and confusion. Science 2003;299(5611):1290–1291.

141. Shen L, Chen ZW, Miller MD, et al. Recombinant virus vaccine-induced SIV-specific CD8+ cytotoxic T lymphocytes. Science 1991;252(5004):440–443.

142. Hirsch VM, Fuerst TR, Sutter G, et al. Patterns of viral replication correlate with outcome in simian immunodeficiency virus (SIV)-infected macaques: effect of prior immunization with a trivalent SIV vaccine in modified vaccinia virus Ankara. J Virol 1996;70(6):3741–3752.

143. Shiver JW, Emini EA. Recent advances in the development of HIV-1 vaccines using replication-incompetent adenovirus vectors. Annu Rev Med 2004;55:355–372.

144. Evans TG, Keefer MC, Weinhold KJ, et al. A canarypox vaccine expressing multiple human immunodeficiency virus type 1 genes given alone or with rgp120 elicits broad and durable CD8+ cytotoxic T lymphocyte responses in seronegative volunteers. J Infect Dis 1999;180(2):290–298.

145. Gupta K, Hudgens M, Corey L, et al. Safety and immunogenicity of a high-titered canarypox vaccine in combination with rgp120 in a diverse population of HIV-1–uninfected adults: AIDS Vaccine Evaluation Group Protocol 022A. J Acquir Immune Defic Syndr 2002;29(3):254–261.

6
Pathophysiology of Pediatric Sepsis

Jan A. Hazelzet

Sepsis is a major cause of morbidity and mortality among children. Sepsis-associated mortality has decreased progressively since the 1960s to around 9% among infants in the early 1990s (1). Despite this improvement over time, severe sepsis is still one of the leading causes of death in children. In 1995 there were an estimated 4400 deaths in the United States, and an estimated annual cost of nearly $2 billion (2). Worldwide, especially in developing countries, the toll of sepsis in terms of mortality and costs is probably much higher, although exact figures are lacking. For this reason much effort has been dedicated to unraveling the pathophysiology of sepsis in order to develop new therapies.

The pathophysiology of pediatric sepsis has much in common with that of sepsis in adults. However, there are differences based on, for example, etiologic microorganism, immune maturation and the absence of aging. Much of the knowledge we have is based on research in neonatal sepsis, meningococcal sepsis, or multiple organ dysfunction syndrome (MODS), in older children. In particular, meningococcal sepsis has given us much insight into the probable proinflammatory response during a "heavy hit" of toxins. But we are increasingly recognizing the importance of the individual host response and its interaction with the microbial products.

Pathogen Recognition

The innate immune system is the first line of defense against infection and is activated when a pathogen crosses the host's natural defense barriers. First, pathogens need to be recognized. It is not the intact or complete microbe that is recognized, but separate molecular parts. These structures are called *pathogen-associated molecular patterns* (PAMPs) and include endotoxins (lipopolysaccharide [LPS]), peptidoglycan, lipoteichoic acid, lipopeptides, flagellin, mannose, and viral RNA. These structures are essential for survival of the microorganism and therefore do not undergo major mutations (3). In gramnegative sepsis, particularly that due to meningococcal infection, LPS has been widely studied. By the late 1980s, the relation among the level of LPS and mortality and severity was demonstrated in meningococcal disease (4). However, recent studies show the importance of other membrane structures in the pathophysiology of sepsis, for instance in their capacity to activate the complement system (5).

Low levels of LPS can very effectively be neutralized by substances like alkaline phosphatase (6) and cholesterol (7) and removed from the circulation. The significance of physiologic low levels of these natural neutralizers in children is unclear. On the other hand, during pregnancy these levels are much higher than normal, so they indeed seem to have physiologic importance.

When the level of LPS exceeds a certain "unknown" high level, the innate immune system is activated because it is recognized by nonspecific pathogen recognition proteins or receptors. Examples are C-reactive protein (CRP), procalcitonin (PCT), mannose-binding lectin (MBL), surfactant protein A, and complement protein C3. There are also specific proteins that recognize LPS, such as lipopolysaccharide-binding protein (LBP). All of these proteins and receptors are considered to be positive acute-phase proteins, and the production of these proteins is upregulated during stress and severe infectious episodes. This suggests that the plasma levels of these proteins and receptors will increase during acute infection.

Signal Transduction

Lipopolysaccharide-binding protein in serum binds to LPS from the bacteria and transfers it to CD14. CD14 is a receptor anchored in the outer leaflet of the plasma membrane of monocytes and macrophages, although it also exists as a soluble plasma protein that attaches LPS to CD14negative cells, such as endothelial cells.

CD14 is located in the extracellular space and therefore cannot induce cellular activation without a transmembrane signal transducing co-receptor (3,8,9). Usually, a complex is formed between LPS/LBP, CD14, and a secreted protein (MD2), with Toll-like receptor-4 (TLR-4), one of the recently described family of Toll-like receptors. MD2 is associated with the extracellular domain of TLR-4 and augments TLR-4–dependent LPS responses in vitro. It is now becoming clear that apart from the TLRs, other cell-surface receptors are also involved, such as Nod1 and Nod2 and triggering receptors expressed on myeloid cells-1 (TREM-1) (9), which can be considered as pattern recognition receptors. When a PAMP binds to a pattern recognition receptor, it activates several intracellular signaling pathways, resulting in the activation of transcription factors (nuclear factor κB [NF-κB], activator protein-1 (AP-1), Fos, Jun, etc.). These transcription factors control the expression of immune response genes and the release of numerous effector molecules, such as cytokines. Cytokines as well as chemokines have an essential role in orchestrating the innate and acquired immune responses to an invading pathogen (3).

Inflammatory Response

The recognition of PAMPs leads to the activation of various immune cells such as neutrophils, macrophages, monocytes, dendritic cells, T cells, and endothelial cells, and also to the activation of the complement system, the coagulation system, and the neuroendocrine system. Although the process seems to be very similar, there are differences between the different and typical forms of sepsis (gram-positive/negative, viral, fungal, toxic shock, etc.), which might be explained by the interaction between microbial products and specific pattern recognition receptors expressed on immune cells. These specific receptors then activate specific intracellular signaling pathways and transcription factors for each group of PAMPs, resulting in expression of genes for immune response, leading to a specific response (Fig. 6.1) (3). The purpose of the activation of the innate immune system is to eliminate microbes from what is meant to be a microbe-free space, like the bloodstream or the lungs. The complement system plays an important role in this process. Complement activation occurs via either the classic lectin pathway or the alternative pathway, which converge at the level of C3 and share a sequence of terminal components (Fig. 6.2). During sepsis the alternative and lectin pathways are probably important. One of the mechanisms in the alternative pathway is CRP binding to complement proteins, which then will be activated. In a group of 50 patients with meningococcal sepsis, mortality was independently related to the levels of C3b/c and C3–CRP complexes. As confirmation that this pathway is important, levels of complement activation products correlated well with the predicted risk of mortality (PRISM) score and capillary leakage (10).

For the lectin pathway, the liver-derived serum protein, mannan-binding lectin (MBL) is the pathogen recognition protein leading to activation. Mannan-binding lectin binds microbial surface carbohydrates and mediates opsono-phagocytosis directly and by activation of the lectin complement pathway. A wide variety of clinical isolates of bacteria, fungi, viruses, and parasites are bound by MBL. Three polymorphisms in the structural gene (MBL2) and two promoter gene polymorphisms are commonly found that result in production of low serum levels of MBL (11). Clinical studies have shown that MBL insufficiency is associated with increased risk for meningococcal disease (12) and serious infections related to chemotherapy (13), and low MBL levels appear to predispose pediatric intensive care unit (ICU) patients to systemic inflammatory response syndrome (SIRS) and patients with SIRS to sepsis (14). Following activation, the complement system plays a pivotal role in opsonization and phagocytosis, and the membrane attack complex (the end product of the terminal pathway) for immunoglobulin binding. The very potent C3a and C5a are involved in many inflammatory processes (Fig. 6.3). Despite the fact that complement undoubtedly plays a role in host defense against many microbial pathogens, it appears to be most important in protection against encapsulated bacteria, especially *Neisseria meningitidis*, but also *Streptococcus pneumoniae*, *Haemophilus influenzae*, and, to a lesser extent, *Neisseria*

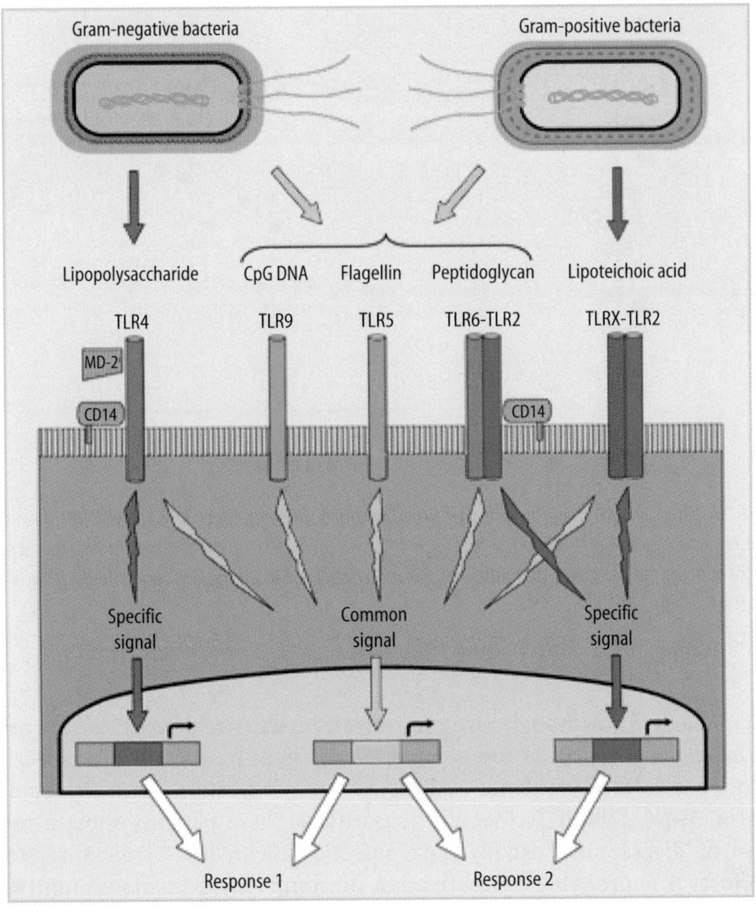

Gram-negative bacteria

Gram-positive bacteria

Lipopolysaccharide   CpG DNA   Flagellin   Peptidoglycan   Lipoteichoic acid

TLR4   TLR9   TLR5   TLR6-TLR2   TLRX-TLR2

MD-2

CD14   CD14

Specific
signal

Common
signal

Specific
signal

Response 1   Response 2

Figure 6.1. Interaction between bacterial products and pattern recognition receptors expressed on immune cells. Components of bacterial cell walls (such as lipopolysaccharide, peptidoglycan, lipoteichoic acid, flagellin, and unmethylated CpG DNA sequences) interact with specific Toll-like receptors (TLRs) expressed on immune cells. The receptors then activate intracellular signaling pathways and transcription factors, resulting in expression of the gene for immune response (3).

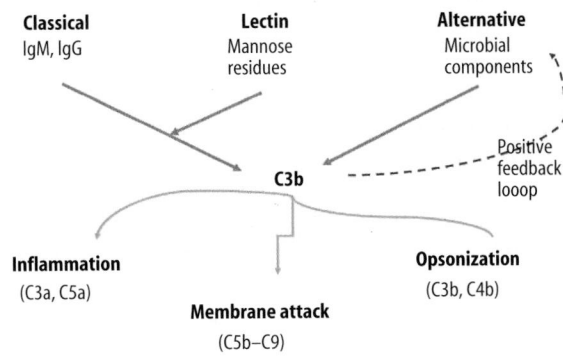

Figure 6.2. Complement system with its three activation pathways. The mannose-binding lectin pathway is antibody independent and is part of the rapid innate immune response fully engaged in the first 12 hours. Ig, immunoglobulin. (Adapted from ref. 70.)

Classical
IgM, IgG

Lectin
Mannose
residues

Alternative
Microbial
components

Positive
feedback
looop

C3b

Inflammation
(C3a, C5a)

Opsonization
(C3b, C4b)

Membrane attack
(C5b–C9)

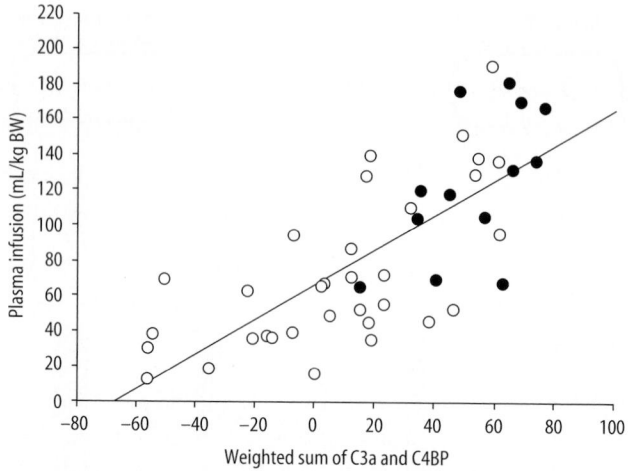

FIGURE 6.3. Total amount of plasma infused (in milliliters per kilogram of body weight [BW]) versus the weighted sum of the initial levels of C3a and C4BP ($73.1 \times (\log 10 C3a)\ 1.0 \times C4BP$) in surviving (open circles) and nonsurviving (solid circles) patients. The line represents the least-squares regression line for all data points ($r = 0.77$; $p < .001$). (From ref. 10.)

gonorrhoeae (15). Although rare (an overall prevalence of <0.03%), a number of deficiencies in parts of the complement system have been described (15), leading to increased incidence and recurrence of infections with encapsulated bacteria. Most striking is that the majority of these patients show a milder course of disease and usually have infections with less virulent microbes. Therefore, it is probably overactivation or complement-mediated injury that is more important in severity and outcome (10). Decreased levels of natural inhibitors of the complement system like C1 esterase inhibitor lend support to this idea (10,16).

Leukocytes, particularly neutrophils, are engaged in a complicated process by which they are attracted to the infectious focus, involving slowing down by margination to the vessel wall, adhesion by several specific adhesion molecules, rolling, and finally passing through the vessel wall to the focus of infection. During this process, neutrophils can lyse and deliver their granules with active substances like elastase, lactoferrin, and granzyme. These substances lead to local tissue injury. Serum levels of neutrophil granule products correlate closely with severity of disease in patients with meningococcal disease (10,17). C3a and C5a also probably play an important role in both leukocyte and platelet activation (18). C3a and C5a are chemoattractants, and are involved in leukocyte-endothelial cell interactions. Excessive production of C5a is harmful, resulting in paralysis of neutrophil function, increased apoptosis, and capillary leakage (19).

Capillary Leakage

Capillary leakage is one of the early key features in sepsis, and this is related to an increase in vascular permeability. The vascular permeability in vivo is not completely elucidated yet, but is most likely an active process and not just dependent on differences in static hydrostatic or oncotic pressures. It is a complicated interaction among aquaporin channels, intercellular junctions with actively opening or closing gaps, negatively charged endothelial membrane-binding proteins, and an active anticoagulant lining, in other words a quiescent endothelium with optimal integrity (20). During sepsis, influenced by cytokines, chemokines, interacting leukocytes and platelets, intermediate active coagulation proteins such as thrombin, as well as complement and arachidonic acid products, the endothelium becomes active and changes from anticoagulant to procoagulant, and from an antiapoptotic to proapoptotic condition (20). This will actively open intercellular junctions by cellular contraction leading to increased permeability. It is difficult to prove in vivo which of the active substances are the most potent. In a study of children with meningococcal sepsis, the amount of fluid necessary for volume resuscitation was closely correlated to the levels of complement activation products. Multiple regression analysis of the various categories of variables showed that the levels of C3a ($p < .001$) and C4BP ($p < .001$) were independently related to the total amount of plasma infused; Figure 6.3 represents the relation ($r = 0.77$; $p < .001$) between the total amount of plasma infused and the weighted sum (using the regression coefficients as the weight) of C3a and C4BP ($73 \times (\log 10 C3a)$ $1.0 \times C4BP$) (10).

Vasodysregulation

The typical adult septic cardiovascular profile is that characterized by low systemic vascular resistance (SVR) and an increased cardiac output. This low SVR necessitating vasopressor therapy is caused by an imbalance between (endothelial-derived) vasodilating and vasoconstricting agents in favor of vasodilatation. Nitric oxide (NO) probably has the biggest influence. Interestingly, both experimental and clinical studies have shown that in pediatric sepsis the cardiovascular profile is characterized by a high SVR and a decreased cardiac output (21–23). These differences are not fully understood, and in our experience the typical infant cardiovascular response exists until the age of 3 years and leads to differences in choice for inotropic and vasopressor therapy (21).

Myocardial Failure

The myocardial failure seen in adult sepsis has been extensively studied both in animals and in humans (24). Myocardial depression as manifested by decreased cardiac output is uncommon in adult patients. However, biventricular dilatation and depressed ejection fraction can be demonstrated. Depression is reversible in 7 to 10 days. Circulating myocardial depressant factors together with intramyocardial capillary leakage and edema, as well as adrenergic receptor desensitization, are possible explanations (24). In pediatric patients, at least in the younger ones, there is not a uniform hyperdynamic response, but a more hypodynamic response (21,23,25). This means a decreased cardiac output and stroke volume and an increased SVR (21,23). The myocardial dysfunction seen in meningococcal sepsis has been studied for the presence of a myocardial depressant substance (26–28). Using serum samples of patients with meningococcal sepsis in an in vitro model of myocardial contractility analysis in rat cardiac myocytes, it could be demonstrated that interleukin-6 (IL-6) was capable of causing significant myocardial depression. Interleukin-6 is a central, mainly proinflammatory cytokine, crucial in the acute-phase response. The levels of IL-6 increase dramatically in meningococcal sepsis and are directly related to severity of disease and outcome.

Coagulation Response

The response of the coagulation system during acute inflammation has received increasing research attention during recent years. One of the reasons for this increasing attention is probably the recognition that coagulation is an integral part of the host immune response. Another reason is the fact that presence of disseminated intravascular coagulation (DIC) is related to a more severe clinical picture, a higher degree of organ dysfunction, and a higher mortality. In DIC, coagulation pathways are activated, and there is dysfunction of the natural inhibitory pathways and an inhibited fibrinolytic system. The natural inhibitory pathways are of particular interest as potential therapies may be based around these systems (29,30). Coagulation may occur in the flowing blood, on the endothelial surface, at endothelial lesions, in the perivascular tissues, and in areas not directly linked to the vascular bed, and may or may not be associated with the formation of fibrin clots (29). During sepsis, tissue factor is upregulated in activated monocytes and endothelial cells as a response to endotoxin and other PAMPs, or subsequently produced cytokines activating coagulation in the flowing blood. This will lead to an increased production of thrombin. Thrombin is a short-lived intermediate, because it is neutralized by antithrombin. However, it plays a central role in coagulation and inflammation. Thrombin is a multifunctional enzyme and generates procoagulant, anticoagulant, inflammatory, and mitogenic responses (31); the presence of thrombin will lead to activation, aggregation, and lysis of leukocytes and platelets, activation of endothelial adhesion molecules, and cytokine expression (IL-6). Endothelial permeability increases by contraction of endothelial cells, and cellular proliferation is stimulated. Thrombin is a procoagulant. It leads to the formation of fibrin; activates coagulation factors V, VIII, IX, and XI; and leads to the expression of tissue factor (TF) and von Willebrand factor (vWF) as well as the aggregation of platelets. However, it is also an anticoagulant by participating in the activation of protein C (Fig. 6.4) (31). There are two other important mechanisms involving coagulation that become important during sepsis. One is the depression of natural anticoagulant systems such as antithrombin and protein C; and the other is the inhibition of the fibrinolytic pathway by the production of plasminogen activator inhibitor-1 (PAI-1) and thrombin activatable fibrinolysis inhibitor (TAFI) (Figs. 6.4 and 6.5).

Reduced levels of antithrombin and protein C (PC) may be caused by a decreased production related to impaired liver function, extravasation out of the intravascular compartment due to increased capillary leakage, age dependency (adult PC levels are not reached until the age of 5), and consumption, for example the conversion of PC to activated PC (APC).

The protein C system has been extensively studied, not only because the decreased function of this natural anticoagulant pathway may be particularly problematic in sepsis, but also because of the other properties of the protein C system (Fig. 6.5). Activated PC, and probably also PC, has specific immunomodulating properties. In vitro, APC inhibits tumor necrosis factor-α (TNF-α) elaboration from monocytes and blocks leukocyte adhesion to selectins, as well as influencing apoptosis (31). The protein C pathway is initiated when

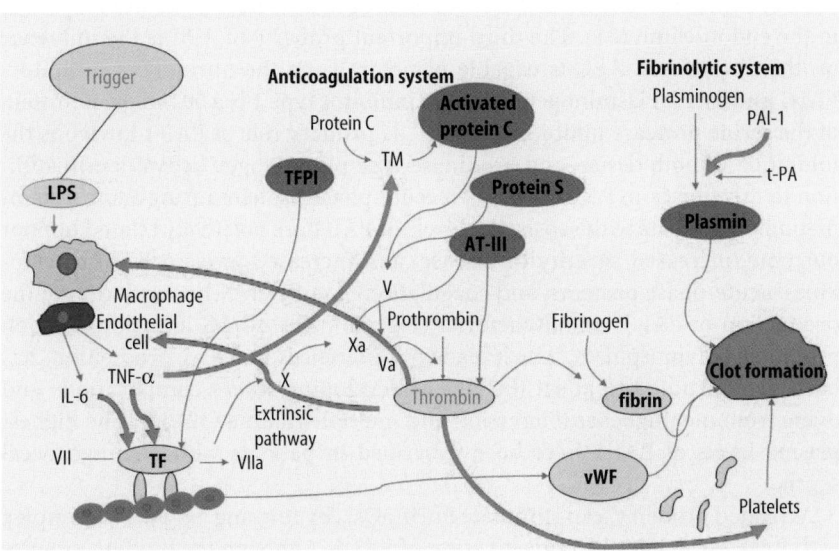

FIGURE 6.4. The coagulation, anticoagulation, and fibrinolytic system during normal circumstances (black arrows), and the effect after an infectious trigger with LPS (lipopolysaccharide). AT, anti-thrombin; IL, interleukin; PAI, plasminogen activator inhibitor; TFPI, tissue factor pathway inhibitor; TNF, tumor necrosis factor; t-PA, tissue-type plasminogen activator; vWF, von Willebrand factor.

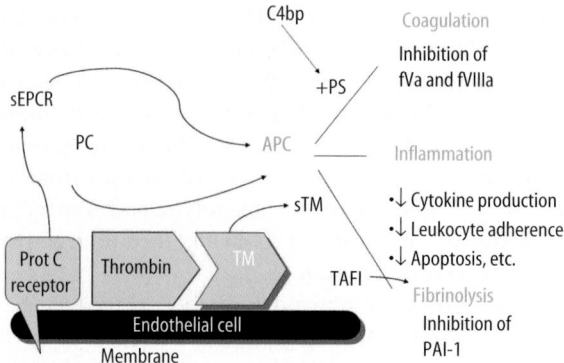

FIGURE 6.5. The protein C pathway. APC, activated protein C; PC, protein C; sEPCR, soluble endothelial protein C receptor; (s)TM, (soluble) thrombomodulin; TAFI, thrombin activatable fibrinolysis inhibitor.

thrombin binds to thrombomodulin (TM) on the surface of the endothelium. An endothelial cell protein C receptor (EPCR) augments protein C activation by the thrombin–TM complex more than 10–fold in vivo. The EPCR is shed from the endothelium by inflammatory mediators and thrombin. It can undergo translocation from the plasma membrane to the nucleus, where it redirects gene expression. During translocation it can carry APC to the nucleus, possibly accounting for the ability of APC to modulate inflammatory mediator responses in the endothelium (31). The third important property of APC is the influence on the fibrinolysis. APC is capable of neutralizing the fibrinolysis inhibitors PAI-1 and TAFI. Plasminogen activator inhibitor type 1 is a 50–kd glycoprotein of the serine protease inhibitor family. The primary role of PAI-1 in vivo is the inhibition of both tissue- and urokinase-type plasminogen activators. In addition to this function, PAI-1 acts as an acute-phase protein during acute inflammation. In patients with sepsis, the levels of PAI-1 are positively related to poor outcome, increased severity of disease, and increased levels of various cytokines, acute-phase proteins, and coagulation parameters. The regulation of the production of PAI-1 is multifactorial (Fig. 6.6). The 4G/5G insertion/deletion promoter polymorphism, which leads to differences in PAI-1 production, has been demonstrated to affect the risk of developing severe complications and dying from meningococcal infection and multiple trauma (32–34). The highest plasma levels of PAI-1 have been described in patients with meningococcal sepsis.

Activated protein C can stimulate fibrinolysis by forming a tight 1:1 complex with PAI-1, which leads to inactivation of PAI-1. Although the binding kinetics of activated protein C with PAI-1 is relatively slow, the reaction rate is increased dramatically by vitronectin. Thus, because activated protein C complexes to PAI-1, these findings are probably interrelated. High levels of thrombin lead to high levels of activated protein C, activated protein C will complex to PAI-1, and, finally, there is a depletion of protein C (32). This is a possible explanation for the extremely low levels of PC found in meningococcal disease. The purpura-picture seen in meningococcal disease is similar to that seen in congenital protein C deficiency. From a therapeutic point of view, meningococcal sepsis has been considered as a PC deficiency state and many open-label studies have been published using PC concentrate. However, since the positive effects of recombinant APC (rAPC) in baboons with sepsis (35), and some in vitro studies suggesting that the activation process in vivo of PC to APC might be disturbed during sepsis, much therapeutic effort in adult sepsis has been aimed at recom-binant human APC (rhAPC), despite the fact that APC is an anticoagulant and can lead to bleeding. These efforts have resulted in a large randomized con-trolled trial in adults with sepsis, showing a positive result on mortality (36). A pediatric study of the use of rhAPC in severe pediatric has recently been stopped at the second interim analysis because of futility. In meningococcal sepsis there has been one study suggesting a disturbed activation process on the basis of semiquantitative analysis of expression of thrombomodulin and the endothelial protein C receptor in the dermal microvasculature of children with severe

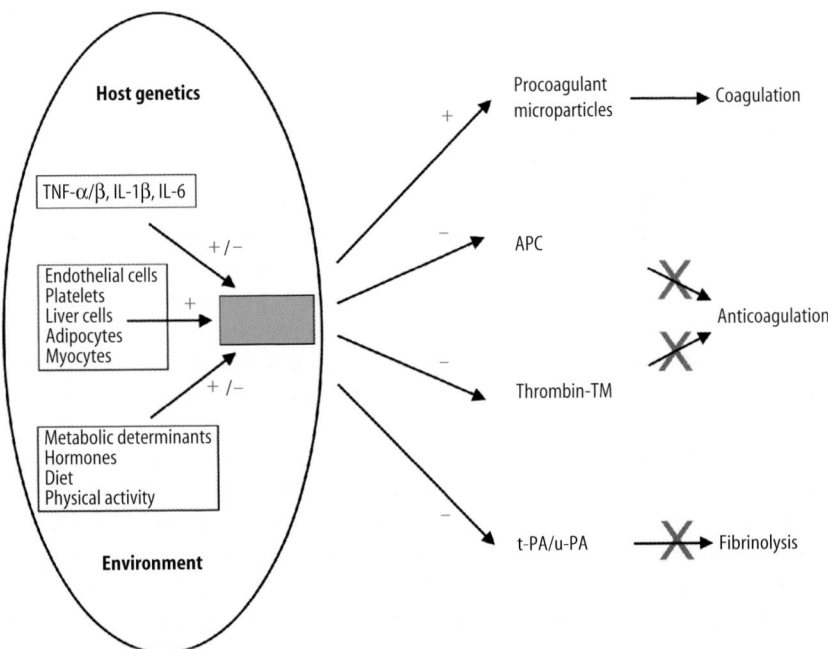

Figure 6.6. Genetic and environmental influences on the expression of plasminogen activator inhibitor type 1 (PAI-1) and the importance of PAI-1 in the coagulation and fibrinolysis pathways. APC, activated protein C; t-PA, tissue-type plasminogen activator; TM, thrombomodulin; u-PA, urokinase-type plasmino-gen activator. (From ref. 32.)

meningococcemia with purpuric or petechial lesions (37). However, a randomized, placebo-controlled dose-finding study in the same patient category of the use of protein C concentrate showed activation of PC to APC, even in the most severely ill patients, with a dose-dependent improvement in coagulation parameters (38).

Thrombin-activatable fibrinolysis inhibitor, also known as carboxypeptidase R, has been implicated as an important negative regulator of the fibrinolytic system. In addition, TAFI is able to inactivate inflammatory peptides, such as the complement factors C3a and C5a. The role of TAFI in the hemostatic and innate immune response to sepsis is still unclear. Recently a study analyzed the prevalence of the Thr325Ile dimorphism in the TAFI gene, which is associated with increased TAFIa stability and activity, in 50 patients who survived meningococcal disease, in 176 first-degree relatives of a consecutive patient series with meningococcal disease, and in 212 controls from the same geographic region. The TAFI 325 Ile/Ile genotype was slightly more common among parents of patients with meningococcal disease than in controls (11% vs. 7.1%, $p=.24$). This difference was pronounced among the subgroup of parents of nonsurviving patients (19.2%, $p=.03$). Patients whose parents were carriers of the TAFI 325 Ile/Ile genotype had a 1.6–fold higher risk (95% confidence interval [CI] 0.7–3.7) of contracting meningococcal disease and a 3.1–fold increased risk (95% CI 1.0–9.5) of dying from the infection compared with all other genotypes (39). This finding has not yet been reproduced.

Neuroendocrine System

The endocrine system is highly interrelated with the immune and neural systems. The neuroimmunoendocrine axis is subject to clear biphasic changes in the acute and chronic phases of critical illness. The distinction between acute (activated anterior pituitary function and inactivated peripheral anabolic pathways) and prolonged critical illness (reduced neuroendocrine stimulation) as different neuroendocrine paradigms has brought a new approach to the critically ill patient. It is unclear whether these phases reflect beneficial or harmful adaptations (40,41).

The acute-phase response to critical illness is well recognized, with abrupt and massive release of stress hormones, including adrenocorticotropic hormone (and cortisol), catecholamines, vasopressin, glucagon, and growth hormone. These hormones help to maintain effective circulation and thus tissue oxygenation; increase generation of energy substrate in the form of glucose, fatty acids, and amino acids from body stores, including liver and muscle; and heighten synthesis of both mitochondrial and nonmitochondrial adenosine triphosphate (ATP). Tissue oxygen consumption (VO_2) and total energy expenditure are initially increased, with intracellular metabolism boosted by up to 200%. There is a concurrent shutdown of less vital systems such as gonadal function, and anabolism is inhibited through various pathways.

One manifestation of the acute response to critical illness is the induction of insulin resistance, a metabolic state in which a normal concentration of insulin produces a subnormal biologic response. Although underlying mechanisms are not well understood, increased secretion of stress hormones, cytokines, and nitric oxide has been implicated. This enhances the acute response to critical illness by promoting the production of energy substrates through stimulation of hepatic gluconeogenesis and release of free fatty acids from fat, which, in turn, induce further resistance to insulin at the cellular level.

In the later phase, after an undefined period of critical illness of hours to days, the hormonal profile alters substantially with concentrations of vasopressin that seem inappropriately low, onset of the sick euthyroid syndrome, and reduced adrenal responsiveness to adrenocorticotropic hormone, often despite hypercortisolemia. Causation remains to be established, though cytokines and nitric oxide have been implicated at hypothalamic, pituitary, and end-organ levels.

Some of these later endocrine changes can themselves be the consequence of the acute-phase response. Thus, the secretion of growth hormone can be suppressed by cortisol, whereas gonadotropins are suppressed by both cortisol and prolactin. Cortisol also modulates thyroid-hormone metabolism, partly through inducing preferential formation of the metabolically inactive reverse triiodothyronine (rT_3), and partly by a suppressive effect on secretion of thyroid-stimulating hormone (41). This has been extensively reviewed recently (42). From the many endocrine mechanisms important during sepsis, two have received much attention because of their possibly beneficial interventions. These two are hyperglycemia/insulin resistance and relative adrenal insufficiency.

In a large, prospective, randomized, controlled study, strict blood glucose control with intensive insulin therapy strongly reduced mortality and morbidity of surgical intensive care patients (43). Most of the clinical benefits of intensive insulin therapy appear to be related to prevention of hyperglycemia, which has been demonstrated to adversely affect outcome. Part of the improvement is related to protection of the mitochondrial compartment and innate immunity, from glucose toxicity. Also, direct insulin effects may contribute to the improved outcome. The beneficial nonglycemic metabolic actions of insulin include a partial correction of the abnormal serum lipid profile and counteraction of the catabolic state evoked by critical illness. The prevention of excessive inflammation and myocardial protection illustrate other nonmetabolic direct antiinflammatory and antiapoptotic properties of insulin, although lowering of glucose levels may have played a role in these events as well (44).

Adrenal insufficiency has been recognized, and attempted treatments were initiated almost from the time sepsis was first described. In patients with severe sepsis, numerous factors predispose to glucocorticoid insufficiency, including drugs, coagulation disorders, and inflammatory mediators. These factors may compromise the hypothalamic-pituitary axis (i.e., secondary adrenal insufficiency) or the adrenal glands (i.e., primary adrenal failure), or may impair glucocorticoid access to target cells (i.e., peripheral tissue resistance). Conversely, transient functional impairment in hormone synthesis may be a common complication of severe sepsis. Glucocorticoids interact with a specific cytosolic glucocorticoid receptor, which undergoes conformational changes, sheds heat shock proteins, and translocates to the nucleus. Glucocorticoids may also interact with membrane-binding sites at the surface of the cells. This topic has been reviewed recently (45,46). Most of these studies have been performed in adults.

In children, endocrine changes during sepsis have hardly been studied. Growth hormone (GH) secretion is acutely enhanced in response to stress and illness, while, at the same time, the serum concentration of its main peripheral effector molecule, insulin-like growth factor-I (IGF-I), is low (47,48). In pediatric patients with meningococcal sepsis, nonsurvivors had extremely high GH levels (49), indicating the presence of peripheral GH resistance. In two pediatric studies, thyroid function was analyzed during sepsis. Both showed decreased levels in the more severely ill and nonsurvivors, indicating an euthyroid sick syndrome (50,51). Adrenal function during pediatric sepsis has been studied mostly in meningococcal disease (52–55), but also in sepsis of other etiology (56), studies showing relative and absolute adrenal insufficiency. The effect of corticosteroid therapy in pediatric sepsis remains to be elucidated.

Immune Status

Until recently sepsis was considered to be a merely proinflammatory clinical picture, with an extreme example being meningococcal sepsis. Outcome and severity was related directly to the levels of a number of proinflammatory cytokines and chemokines, although levels of antiinflammatory cytokines are increased (57). Some doubts about the predominant proinflammatory character did arise following a study of first-degree relatives of patients with meningococcal sepsis. A whole-blood stimulation test in the blood of these persons showed the relation between high IL-10 (antiinflammatory) and low TNF levels and a bad outcome (58). A later study in febrile patients with community-acquired infection showed that an antiinflammatory cytokine profile of a high ratio of IL-10 to TNF-α was associated with fatal outcome (59). From animal studies as well as ex vivo and pathology studies in humans, it is becoming more and more clear that after an insult like sepsis, trauma, or hypoxia, an initial predominantly proinflammatory response prevails, but following the acute insult, into the convalescent period, an antiinflammatory pattern or even an immune paralysis arises, with increased susceptibility to new infections and incapability to clear bacteria (60,61). This pattern can be described as macrophage deactivation, T-cell anergy, and the rapid apoptotic loss of lymphoid tissues.

Initial efforts to treat the septic patient have been disappointing, and therapeutic efforts to modify the immune response during sepsis syndromes will require a more thorough understanding of the innate and acquired immune responses and the increased apoptosis in the lymphoid tissue (62).

In pediatric sepsis, sporadic but similar findings have been reported: in a group of 82 patients in the early postoperative period, those with decreased monocyte human leukocyte antigen (HLA)-DR expression represented a subpopulation at greatly increased risk of later sepsis/SIRS development (63). In another study, plasma IL-10, IL-6, and an organ failure index (OFI), indicating the number of failing organ systems, were determined in 53 children on days 1 to 3 of sepsis and in control children on day 1. Children with three or more organ failures had higher plasma IL-10 levels than children with less than three organ failures (days 1 and 3; $p<.05$). Children who developed sequential pulmonary/hepatic/renal failure had higher IL-10 levels (days 1 to 3; $p<.05$). Nonsurvivors had higher IL-10 levels (day 3; $p<.05$) (64). Better recognition of the immune phase in our patients may have therapeutic consequences (62,65).

Genetic Differences and Predisposition

It is becoming more and more obvious that not every individual will have the susceptibility to infectious disease, nor will each individual, when infected, develop the same severity of disease or have the same outcome. The host response during sepsis is so complex that it would be naive to suppose a completely identical course in all individuals.

Single nucleotide polymorphisms (SNPs) are the most common type of stable genetic variation in the population. A SNP occurs in approximately 1 of 1000 base pairs, with the most frequent being a C to T substitution. There are several different ways that SNPs can lead to an aberrant gene product (66). First, sequence variation in the 5' untranslated region (UTR) could disrupt messenger RNA (mRNA) translation, and mutations in the 3' UTR could affect mRNA cleavage, stability, and export (3). Second, promoter polymorphisms that alter DNA binding of transcription factors have the potential of decreasing or increasing gene expression. Third, frameshift mutations or variation that results in early termination in transcription may lead to a defective or truncated protein. Fourth, splice site mutations that occur in intron/exon boundaries also have the potential of altering mRNA processing or protein function. Finally, nonsynonymous SNPs in exons could alter protein function or activity.

It has been estimated that 10% of all SNPs in the genome are functional, thereby having the potential of altering some biologic process (67).

In the last 5 years, there has been increasing interest in conducting disease–gene association–based studies aimed at determining the role of genetic variations in the inflammatory response to infection. The majority of these studies have been case-control studies using a candidate gene approach. A second approach has involved the identification and study of multiple SNPs or haplotypes that are in linkage disequilibrium with one another. This method increases the statistical power for detecting the association between genotype and outcome. Both study designs have generated important information in deciphering the role of genetic variation on clinical outcomes in sepsis (66). A number of recent reviews have described important polymorphisms playing a role in sepsis in general and meningococcal sepsis in particular (66,68,69). The challenge of the future will be to determine which polymorphisms or which combinations of polymorphisms will really play a role and lead to changes in policy, and to be able to determine these individually in the early phase of the disease.

References

1. Stoll BJ, Holman RC, Schuchat A. Decline in sepsis-associated neonatal and infant deaths in the United States, 1979 through 1994. Pediatrics 1998;102(2):e18.
2. Watson RS, Carcillo JA, Linde-Zwirble WT, Clermont G, Lidicker J, Angus DC. The epidemiology of severe sepsis in children in the United States. Am J Respir Crit Care Med 2003;167(5):695–701.
3. Bochud PY, Calandra T. Pathogenesis of sepsis: new concepts and implications for future treatment. BMJ 2003;326(7383):262–266.
4. Brandtzaeg P, Kierulf P, Gaustad P, Dobloug J, Mollnes TE, Sirnes K. Systemic meningococcal disease: a model infection to study acute endotoxinemia in man. Prog Clin Biol Res 1988;272:263–271.
5. Sprong T, Moller AS, Bjerre A, et al. Complement activation and complement-dependent inflammation by Neisseria meningitidis are independent of lipopolysaccharide. Infect Immun 2004;72(6):3344–3349.
6. Verweij WR, Bentala H, Huizinga-van der Vlag A, et al. Protection against an Escherichia coli-induced sepsis by alkaline phosphatase in mice. Shock 2004; 22(2):174–179.
7. Vermont CL, den Brinker M, Kakeci N, et al. Serum lipids and disease severity in children with severe meningococcal sepsis. Crit Care Med 2005;33(7):1610–1615.
8. Riedemann NC, Guo RF, Ward PA. Novel strategies for the treatment of sepsis. Nat Med 2003;9(5):517–524.
9. Cohen J. TREM-1 in sepsis. Lancet 2001;358(9284):776–778.
10. Hazelzet JA, de Groot R, van Mierlo G, et al. Complement activation in relation to capillary leakage in children with septic shock and purpura. Infect Immun 1998;66(11):5350–5356.
11. Eisen DP, Minchinton RM. Impact of mannose-binding lectin on susceptibility to infectious diseases. Clin Infect Dis 2003;37(11):1496–1505.
12. Hibberd ML, Sumiya M, Summerfield JA, Booy R, Levin M. Association of variants of the gene for mannose-binding lectin with susceptibility to meningococcal disease. Meningococcal Research Group. Lancet 1999;353(9158):1049–1053.
13. Peterslund NA, Koch C, Jensenius JC, Thiel S. Association between deficiency of mannose-binding lectin and severe infections after chemotherapy. Lancet 2001; 358(9282):637–638.
14. Fidler KJ, Wilson P, Davies JC, Turner MW, Peters MJ, Klein NJ. Increased incidence and severity of the systemic inflammatory response syndrome in patients deficient in mannose-binding lectin. Intensive Care Med 2004;30(7):1438–1445.
15. Figueroa JE, Densen P. Infectious diseases associated with complement deficiencies. Clin Microbiol Rev 1991;4(3):359–395.

16. Caliezi C, Wuillemin WA, Zeerleder S, Redondo M, Eisele B, Hack CE. C1–Esterase inhibitor: an anti-inflammatory agent and its potential use in the treatment of diseases other than hereditary angioedema. Pharmacol Rev 2000;52(1):91–112.

17. van Woensel JB, Biezeveld MH, Hack CE, Bos AP, Kuijpers TW. Elastase and granzymes during meningococcal disease in children: correlation to disease severity. Intensive Care Med 2005;31(9):1239–1247.

18. Albrecht EA, Ward PA. Complement-induced impairment of the innate immune system during sepsis. Curr Allergy Asthma Rep 2004;4(5):359–364.

19. Guo RF, Riedemann NC, Ward PA. Role of C5a-C5aR interaction in sepsis. Shock 2004;21(1):1–7.

20. Aird WC. The role of the endothelium in severe sepsis and multiple organ dysfunction syndrome. Blood 2003;101(10):3765–3777.

21. Ceneviva G, Paschall JA, Maffei F, Carcillo JA. Hemodynamic support in fluid-refractory pediatric septic shock. Pediatrics 1998;102(2):e19.

22. Hazelzet JA, Stubenitsky R, Petrov AB, et al. Cardiovascular aspects of experimental meningococcal sepsis in young and older awake piglets: age-related differences. Shock 1999;12(2):145–154.

23. Mercier JC, Beaufils F, Hartmann JF, Azema D. Hemodynamic patterns of meningococcal shock in children. Crit Care Med 1988;16(1):27–33.

24. Krishnagopalan S, Kumar A, Parrillo JE, Kumar A. Myocardial dysfunction in the patient with sepsis. Curr Opin Crit Care 2002;8(5):376–388.

25. Booker PD. Pharmacological support for children with myocardial dysfunction. Paediatr Anaesth 2002;12(1):5–25.

26. Pathan N, Hemingway CA, Alizadeh AA, et al. Role of interleukin 6 in myocardial dysfunction of meningococcal septic shock. Lancet 2004;363(9404):203–209.

27. Pathan N, Sandiford C, Harding SE, Levin M. Characterization of a myocardial depressant factor in meningococcal septicemia. Crit Care Med 2002;30(10):2191–2198.

28. Thiru Y, Pathan N, Bignall S, Habibi P, Levin M. A myocardial cytotoxic process is involved in the cardiac dysfunction of meningococcal septic shock. Crit Care Med 2000;28(8):2979–2983.

29. Dempfle CE. Coagulopathy of sepsis. Thromb Haemost 2004;91(2):213–224.

30. Faust SN, Heyderman RS, Levin M. Disseminated intravascular coagulation and purpura fulminans secondary to infection. Baillieres Best Pract Res Clin Haematol 2000;13(2):179–197.

31. Esmon CT. Crosstalk between inflammation and thrombosis. Maturitas 2004;47(4):305–314.

32. Hermans PW, Hazelzet JA. Plasminogen activator inhibitor type 1 gene polymorphism and sepsis. Clin Infect Dis 2005;41(suppl 7):S453–458.

33. Hermans PW, Hibberd ML, Booy R, et al. 4G/5G promoter polymorphism in the plasminogen-activator-inhibitor-1 gene and outcome of meningococcal disease. Meningococcal Research Group. Lancet 1999;354(9178):556–560.

34. Menges T, Hermans PW, Little SG, et al. Plasminogen-activator-inhibitor-1 4G/5G promoter polymorphism and prognosis of severely injured patients. Lancet 2001;357(9262):1096–1097.

35. Taylor FB Jr, Chang A, Esmon CT, et al. Protein C prevents the coagulopathic and lethal effects of Escherichia coli infusion in the baboon. J Clin Invest 1987;79(3):918–925.

36. Bernard GR, Vincent JL, Laterre PF, et al. Efficacy and safety of recombinant human activated protein C for severe sepsis. N Engl J Med 2001;344(10):699–709.

37. Faust SN, Levin M, Harrison OB, et al. Heyderman RS. Dysfunction of endothelial protein C activation in severe meningococcal sepsis. N Engl J Med 2001;345(6): 408–416.

38. De Kleijn ED, De Groot R, Hack CE, et al. Activation of protein C following infusion of protein C concentrate in children with severe meningococcal sepsis and purpura fulminans: a randomized, double-blinded, placebo-controlled, dose-finding study. Crit Care Med 2003;31(6):1839–1847.

39. Kremer Hovinga JA, Franco RF, Zago MA, Ten Cate H, Westendorp RG, Reitsma PH. A functional single nucleotide polymorphism in the thrombin-activatable fibrinolysis inhibitor (TAFI) gene associates with outcome of meningococcal disease. J Thromb Haemost 2004;2(1):54–57.

40. Beishuizen A, Thijs LG. The immunoneuroendocrine axis in critical illness: beneficial adaptation or neuroendocrine exhaustion? Curr Opin Crit Care 2004;10(6): 461–467.

41. Singer M, De Santis V, Vitale D, Jeffcoate W. Multiorgan failure is an adaptive, endocrine-mediated, metabolic response to overwhelming systemic inflammation. Lancet 2004;364(9433):545–548.

42. Ellger B, Debaveye Y, Van den Berghe G. Endocrine interventions in the ICU. Eur J Intern Med 2005;16(2):71–82.

43. van den Berghe G, Wouters P, Weekers F, et al. Intensive insulin therapy in the critically ill patients. N Engl J Med 2001;345(19):1359–1367.

44. Vanhorebeek I, Langouche L, Van den Berghe G. Glycemic and nonglycemic effects of insulin: how do they contribute to a better outcome of critical illness? Curr Opin Crit Care 2005;11(4):304–311.

45. Annane D, Cavaillon JM. Corticosteroids in sepsis: from bench to bedside? Shock 2003;20(3):197–207.

46. Prigent H, Maxime V, Annane D. Science review: mechanisms of impaired adrenal function in sepsis and molecular actions of glucocorticoids. Crit Care 2004; 8(4):243–252.

47. Gardelis JG, Hatzis TD, Stamogiannou LN, et al. Activity of the growth hormone/insulin-like growth factor-I axis in critically ill children. J Pediatr Endocrinol Metab 2005;18(4):363–372.

48. Onenli-Mungan N, Yildizdas D, Yapicioglu H, Topaloglu AK, Yuksel B, Ozer G. Growth hormone and insulin-like growth factor 1 levels and their relation to survival in children with bacterial sepsis and septic shock. J Paediatr Child Health 2004;40(4):221–226.

49. de Groof F, Joosten KF, Janssen JA, et al. Acute stress response in children with meningococcal sepsis: important differences in the growth hormone/insulin-like growth factor I axis between nonsurvivors and survivors. J Clin Endocrinol Metab 2002;87(7):3118–3124.

50. den Brinker M, Joosten KF, Visser TJ, et al. Euthyroid sick syndrome in meningococcal sepsis: the impact of peripheral thyroid hormone metabolism and binding proteins. J Clin Endocrinol Metab 2005;90(10):5613–5620.

51. Yildizdas D, Onenli-Mungan N, Yapicioglu H, Topaloglu AK, Sertdemir Y, Yuksel B. Thyroid hormone levels and their relationship to survival in children with bacterial sepsis and septic shock. J Pediatr Endocrinol Metab 2004;17(10):1435–1442.

52. De Kleijn ED, Joosten KF, Van Rijn B, et al. Low serum cortisol in combination with high adrenocorticotrophic hormone concentrations are associated with poor

outcome in children with severe meningococcal disease. Pediatr Infect Dis J 2002;21(4):330–336.

53. den Brinker M, Joosten KF, Liem O, et al. Adrenal insufficiency in meningococcal sepsis: bioavailable cortisol levels and impact of interleukin-6 levels and intubation with etomidate on adrenal function and mortality. J Clin Endocrinol Metab 2005;90(9):5110–5117.

54. Lichtarowicz-Krynska EJ, Cole TJ, Camacho-Hubner C, et al. Circulating aldosterone levels are unexpectedly low in children with acute meningococcal disease. J Clin Endocrinol Metab 2004;89(3):1410–1414.

55. van Woensel JB, Biezeveld MH, Alders AM, et al. Adrenocorticotropic hormone and cortisol levels in relation to inflammatory response and disease severity in children with meningococcal disease. J Infect Dis 2001;184(12):1532–1537.

56. Pizarro CF, Troster EJ, Damiani D, Carcillo JA. Absolute and relative adrenal insufficiency in children with septic shock. Crit Care Med 2005;33(4):855–859.

57. Netea MG, van der Meer JW, van Deuren M, Kullberg BJ. Proinflammatory cytokines and sepsis syndrome: not enough, or too much of a good thing? Trends Immunol 2003;24(5):254–258.

58. Westendorp RG, Langermans JA, Huizinga TW, et al. Genetic influence on cytokine production and fatal meningococcal disease. Lancet 1997;349(9046):170–173.

59. van Dissel JT, van Langevelde P, Westendorp RG, Kwappenberg K, Frolich M. Anti-inflammatory cytokine profile and mortality in febrile patients. Lancet 1998;351(9107):950–953.

60. Oberholzer A, Oberholzer C, Moldawer LL. Sepsis syndromes: understanding the role of innate and acquired immunity. Shock 2001;16(2):83–96.

61. Hotchkiss RS, Karl IE. The pathophysiology and treatment of sepsis. N Engl J Med 2003;348(2):138–150.

62. Hotchkiss RS, Tinsley KW, Karl IE. Role of apoptotic cell death in sepsis. Scand J Infect Dis 2003;35(9):585–592.

63. Allen ML, Peters MJ, Goldman A, et al. Early postoperative monocyte deactivation predicts systemic inflammation and prolonged stay in pediatric cardiac intensive care. Crit Care Med 2002;30(5):1140–1145.

64. Doughty L, Carcillo JA, Kaplan S, Janosky J. The compensatory anti-inflammatory cytokine interleukin 10 response in pediatric sepsis-induced multiple organ failure. Chest 1998;113(6):1625–1631.

65. Docke WD, Randow F, Syrbe U, et al. Monocyte deactivation in septic patients: restoration by IFN-gamma treatment. Nat Med 1997;3(6):678–681.

66. Arcaroli J, Fessler MB, Abraham E. Genetic polymorphisms and sepsis. Shock 2005;24(4):300–312.

67. Wjst M. Target SNP selection in complex disease association studies. BMC Bioinformatics 2004;5:92.

68. Dahmer MK, Randolph A, Vitali S, Quasney MW. Genetic polymorphisms in sepsis. Pediatr Crit Care Med 2005;6(3 suppl):S61–73.

69. Emonts M, Hazelzet JA, de Groot R, Hermans PW. Host genetic determinants of Neisseria meningitidis infections. Lancet Infect Dis 2003;3(9):565–577.

70. Carcillo JA. Mannose-binding lectin deficiency provides a genetic basis for the use of SIRS/sepsis definitions in critically ill patients. Intensive Care Med 2004; 30(7):1263–1265.

7
The Epidemiology of Severe Infections in Children

Mary E. Hartman, R. Scott Watson, Joseph A. Carcillo, and
Derek C. Angus

The Global Burden of Infectious Disease

Infectious diseases account for the majority of admissions to hospitals in the developing world (1,2). The Global Burden of Disease study, sponsored by the World Health Organization (WHO) and the World Bank, estimates that the majority of the nearly 11 million annual pediatric deaths in the world are due to infectious causes (2,3). Just over 1.6 million of these deaths are among neonates. The majority of cases occur in developing countries (2), and half of all infection-related deaths occur in just seven countries: India, China, Nigeria, Pakistan, Bangladesh, Ethiopia, and Zaire (3). Diarrheal and respiratory illnesses account for almost half of the deaths, while malaria, AIDS, and measles are responsible for another 17% (4).

However, these staggering statistics tell only part of the story. In the past two decades, prevention efforts have dramatically affected the incidence and prevalence of many infections in all parts of the world. The burden of infectious disease is now disproportionately carried by those who do not have reliable access to basic preventive medicine, nutrition, sanitation, and other social services. In addition, case fatality from infections, even serious infections, has rapidly dropped for those who received prompt treatment. For example, Bang and colleagues (5) have demonstrated that mortality from neonatal sepsis in rural India dropped as low as 3% with antibiotic treatment. Nhan et al. (6) have shown that rapid resuscitation of dengue shock syndrome can virtually eliminate mortality. Thus, the majority of deaths from infection occur in the world's poorest countries with the highest burden of disease and inadequate access to health care resources.

This chapter discusses the most common infectious syndromes responsible for global morbidity and mortality and their causes. Differences in incidence, prevalence, and outcome across world regions are also discussed, as well as strategies for eliminating some of the disparities.

Challenges to Epidemiologic Study

Global epidemiologic study of infections in children has been limited, in large part due to the technical difficulty of large-scale studies. Availability of qualified research work forces, challenges of standardized data collection, and high costs of medical supplies and personnel all make large-scale epidemiologic research difficult (7,8). In addition, care is not standardized within or between countries. To reduce the impact of these factors, studies are often conducted in hospital settings where care and data collection are more easily standardized (7,9). However, studies from tertiary centers face other problems of generalizability because hospital-based studies capture only a small fraction of the population of ill children. In many parts of the developing world, ill children are often cared for in rural areas, outside of hospital resources in cities (10,11). Studies in academic centers, therefore, may identify the treated incidence of many diseases, but not the true incidence.

In addition, advances in subspecialty care for children have complicated matters by generating new and disparate populations of children at risk for serious infections. For example, a very low birth weight infant in a neonatal intensive care unit (NICU) has different infectious and mortality risks than a 10-year-old neutropenic oncology patient, who, in turn, has different risks than a previously healthy 18-year-old. Medical advances have also changed the natural history of serious infections. As described above, mortality rates from many infections are already low in many countries, and quickly dropping in others. Studies that include mortality as an end point must be large enough to reliably quantify its frequency.

Incidence of Serious Infections in Children

Entire books have been devoted to each of the diseases and organisms, and it is beyond the scope of this chapter to introduce them all with a comparable level of detail. Instead, we introduce the reader to the scope and nature of serious infections in children and highlight the organisms most responsible for these diseases.

Infectious Syndromes

Sepsis

In 1992, the American College of Chest Physicians/Society of Critical Care Medicine Consensus Conference met to standardize the definitions of sepsis and severe sepsis so that they might be more clearly applied in research and clinical practice (12). The group defined "sepsis" as a systemic inflammatory response syndrome resulting from infection; "severe sepsis" as sepsis associated with organ dysfunction, hypoperfusion, or hypotension; and "septic shock" as sepsis with arterial hypotension despite adequate fluid resuscitation (12). These defini-tions now serve as criteria for inclusion in randomized controlled trials for sepsis therapies (13–19) and are increasingly employed by medical practitioners around the world. One of the significant advantages of this standard terminol-ogy is that it has allowed us to begin to understand the magnitude of sepsis. We now understand that sepsis and severe sepsis are quite common and important causes of serious morbidity and mortality in both children and adults.

For example, in the United States, the Centers for Disease Control and Pre-vention (CDC) lists sepsis as the seventh leading cause of death for children 1 to 4 years of age, and eighth for children 5 to 9 years of age (20). The largest epidemiologic study of pediatric severe sepsis in the U.S. to date is by Watson et al. (21), who identified cases of severe sepsis through discharge data from children hospitalized in seven large states in 1995. In this study, over 42,000 cases and 4400 deaths (for a hospital mortality of 10.5%) from severe sepsis were found among U.S. children that year. Almost half of the patients (48%) were less than 1 year old. Severe sepsis was more common among boys than girls, and more common in children with underlying illness. In preliminary analyses of data from 1999, Watson et al. (22) also found that rates of severe sepsis increased (up 11% over the 4-year period), while at the same time hos-pital mortality decreased. The increased incidence was due to increased numbers of very low birth weight (VLBW) babies in the U.S. and an increased rate of sepsis among those babies. Although hospital mortality from 1995 to 1999 was unchanged among previously healthy children, it decreased to 9.0% overall in 1999 because of lower mortality among children with underlying illness. The three most common pathogens for children with severe sepsis in the U.S. were staphylococcus (all types), streptococcus (all types), and fungus, though viral etiologies were not examined (21).

In a single-center study in Montreal, Canada, Proulx et al. (23) examined the incidence of sepsis and related conditions in a university pediatric intensive care unit (PICU). This group examined approximately 1000 admissions to their intensive care unit between 1991 and 1992, and identified 245 cases of sepsis (23% of all PICU admissions), 46 cases of severe sepsis (4%), and 25 cases of septic shock (2%). Among the children with sepsis, 18% developed multiple organ dysfunction syndrome, and 6% died. Al Zwaini et al. (24) studied 118 neonates admitted to the main referral hospital in Al-Anbar, Iraq, with positive blood cultures. The incidence of neonatal septicemia for babies born at that hospital was 9.2 per 1000 live births, and mortality was 28%. *Staphylococcus aureus* (39%), *Klebsiella pneumoniae* (30%), and *Escherichia coli* (21%) consti-tuted 90% of all isolates. In a single-center study of neonates in Trinidad between 1996 and 1997, Ali (25) described a population with the highest rates of neonatal sepsis in the Caribbean. They found an incidence of 10 cases of bacterial sepsis per 1000 live births, with a mortality rate of 27%. Gram-negative organisms accounted for 63% of all positive blood cultures.

When shock persists in septic shock, multiple organ system failure (MOSF) often ensues. However, the details about this sequence of events is poorly understood and its effects on mortality are still being studied. Kutko et al. (26) studied 96 cases of septic shock in 80 patients at a large academic PICU over 2 years to determine the impact of MOSF on mortality in septic shock. Over 70% of sepsis cases occurred in patients with cancer (19% of whom had undergone a bone marrow transplant), and half occurred in patients with neutropenia. Indwelling catheters were present in over 58% of cases. Multiple organ system failure was present in almost 73% of cases at some point in time during the PICU course, and mortality for this group was 18.6%. A finding common among these studies were that there were few or no deaths among children who were previously healthy, and no deaths among patients without MOSF.

Bacteremia

Bacteremia has been studied in numerous settings to identify and quantify community-acquired and nosocomial infections. Several recent single-center studies indicate that the rate of pediatric bloodstream infections (BSIs) in developed countries varies from 11 to 39 per 1000 hospital admissions (27,28), with a hospital mortality rate between 2% and 27% (27,29). The wide range in both incidence and mortality are likely due to the different populations studied. Approximately half of all BSIs occur in children <1 year old, half are community acquired, and less than 15% occur in previously healthy children (28). Intravascular catheters are the most common predisposing factor for bacteremia, occurring in up to 40% of all BSIs (28). One of the largest population-based studies looking at rates of bacteremia in the developing world was conducted by Berkley et al. (10), who studied over 19,000 children at a rural hospital in Kenya between 1998 and 2002. They found bacteremia in 6.6% of admitted patients, or 505 annual cases of community-acquired bacteremia per 100,000 children younger than 5 years old (and 1457 cases per 100,000 infants).

In developed countries, approximately two thirds of organisms isolated from bacteremic patients are gram positive, one quarter are gram-negative aerobic organisms, and 5% to 11% are fungi (27,28). Anaerobes are rarely isolated (0.4% to 1.4% of isolates) (27,28). For example, Perez et al. (29) reviewed 213 episodes of pediatric bacteremia over 7 years in a Spanish university hospital and found *Streptococcus pneumoniae* to be the most common etiologic agent overall; *Neisseria meningitidis* was found to be the most common cause of community-acquired bacteremia among previously healthy children (28). *E. coli* and group B streptococcus (*Streptococcus agalactiae*) are the two most prevalent pathogens in neonatal infections in developed countries, but their prevalence in neonatal infections in developing countries is unclear (8).

As discussed elsewhere in this chapter, *Haemophilus influenzae* type B, *S. pneumoniae*, and *N. meningitidis* are all important causes of bacteremia and sepsis in developing countries. In addition, nontyphi *Salmonella* and *S. aureus* are important causes of bacteremia and serious infection in many parts of the developing world (30–32). The WHO Young Infants Study Group investigation of bloodstream infections in infants in Africa, India, the Middle East, and the West Indies found that *Klebsiella* species, *E. Coli*, *S. aureus*, and group B streptococcus were the most common organisms isolated from blood cultures (32). In contrast, the Berkley study from Kenya (mentioned above) found that *S. pneumoniae*, non-typhi *Salmonella*, *H. influenzae*, and *E. coli* accounted for over 70% of isolated organisms from blood cultures (10). In their study of febrile, hospitalized Malawian children, Walsh et al. (30) found that non-typhi *Salmonella* accounted for two thirds of the positive blood cultures, followed by *S. pneumoniae*, which accounted for 16.4%. Galanakis et al. (33) studied 3339 neonates admitted to an NICU in a single hospital in Greece from 1989 to 1998, and found that the most common organisms isolated from blood cultures for this group of babies were gram-negative bacilli (42%), coagulase-negative staphylococci (34%), and streptococci (17%).

Diarrheal Illness

Infectious diarrhea remains a major cause of death in developing countries, and despite improved sanitation and clean water, it remains a major cause of morbidity and hospitalization in developed countries (34,35). In general, developing countries experience a prevalence of diarrheal illness nearly three times higher than that in developed countries (36) because malnutrition and insufficient access to clean water and sanitation are substantial contributors to the problem. Current estimates indicate that over 1 billion people in developing countries have poor access to safe water and 2.4 billion have inadequate sanitation (36). In the 1980s approximately 3.3 million children died from diarrhea annually. In the 1990s, the number of these deaths dropped to 2.5 million annually, but the largest proportion of this drop occurred in developed countries (35). The incidence in developing countries remained stable due to the continued unreliability of social, political, and health care services. Those most affected were children less than 1 year old, who had much higher rates than those 1 to 4 years old (8.5 vs. 3.8 deaths per 1000 children per year in developing countries) (35).

Globally, most diarrheal illness is caused by viruses. Rotavirus is a common, highly contagious virus that is responsible for up to 60% of all diarrheal illnesses in children, and is responsible for an estimated 870,000 deaths in children around the world every year (36). Rotavirus predominantly affects children less than 2 years old, and epidemics of the virus peak in the winter months in temperate climates In developed countries, rotavirus and pathogenic *E. coli* are the most common cause of diarrheal illness. *Campylobacter*, *Salmonella*, *Shigella*, and *Yersinia* species are also common causes, and *Shigella* species are the most common cause of dysentery (bloody diarrhea). *Shigella* species alone account for almost 15% of all childhood deaths from diarrhea worldwide. Enterotoxigenic *E. coli* is the bacteria most commonly associated with diarrhea, and is well known as the leading cause of traveler's diarrhea. Both rotavirus and enterotoxigenic *E. coli* cause watery diarrhea that is self-limited in most developing countries, but can progress to severe dehydration and death if appropriate therapy is not instituted.

Respiratory Illness

Acute respiratory infections, particularly pneumonia, continue to be one of the leading causes of hospitalization and death among children in developing countries (37), and pneumonia in children under 5 years of age is the leading cause of child mortality in the world (38). Recent estimates of the incidence of pneumonia in developing countries is 0.29 episodes per child-year (38). This equates to 151 million new cases annually, 11 to 20 million (7% to 13%) of which are severe enough to require hospital admission. In the developed world, large population-based studies report that the incidence of community-acquired pneumonia among children younger than 5 years of age is approximately 0.026 episodes per child-year. Thus, more than 95% of all episodes of clinical pneumonia in young children worldwide occur in developing countries.

In developing countries, a multitude of bacteria and viruses cause severe pneumonia. *S. pneumoniae* is among the most important of these, as it causes both pneumonia and invasive pneumococcal disease (39–41). Numerous studies indicate that *H. influenzae* species are also an important cause of pneumonia in children in developing countries (42), as well as influenza and measles (43,44). These are discussed below in more detail (see Epidemiology of Specific Microbes).

Community-acquired pneumonia in children in Europe and North America is often due to viral infection, with 50% or fewer being caused by bacteria (45). However, viral infection often predisposes to bacterial infection (46), and evidence is mounting that studies of pneumonia in children in developed countries have underestimated the importance of *S. pneumoniae* as an etiologic agent (47). For example, Michelow et al. (48) studied children with lower respiratory tract infections (LRIs) in Dallas, Texas. Typical respiratory bacteria accounted for 60% of the identified LRIs (of which 73% were *S. pneumoniae*), viruses accounted for 45%, and mixed bacterial/viral infections accounted for another 23%. Atypical bacteria were responsible for 25% of cases (14% had *Mycoplasma pneumoniae* and 9% had *Chlamydia pneumoniae*). The greatest inflammation and disease severity was noted among children with typical bacterial or mixed bacterial/viral infections.

Epidemiology of Specific Microbes

Bacterial Disease

Meningococcus

N. meningitidis is a highly infectious bacterium that is the leading cause of meningitis and rapidly fatal sepsis worldwide (49). Approximately one third of all deaths related to bacterial meningitis are caused by *N. meningitidis*, of which serogroups A, B, C, Y, and W135 are the most common (50). It is associated with mortality rates between 10% and 20%, and survival is often complicated by chronic morbidity such as hearing impairment, cognitive deficits, and amputation (49,51). Group A meningococcal meningitis alone remains a leading cause of mental retardation in Africa (49,51). Meningococcal disease disproportionately affects children, in whom the attack and fatality rates can be up to 20 times that of adults (49). Many parts of the world report only sporadic cases of meningococcus-related meningitis, but sub-Saharan Africa contains the "meningitis belt" where major outbreaks of *N. meningitidis* occur (49). In these countries, rates of meningitis can range from 10 to 1000 cases per 100,000 population (43,49). In Burkina Faso, rates can increase over 30 times and then return to baseline within several months (43). Case fatality for these epidemics often exceed 30%, with children younger than 1 year often having the highest fatality rate (43).

In contrast, rates of *N. meningitidis* during outbreaks in the United Kingdom from 1991 to 1999 fluctuated between 27 and 45 per 100,000 children (52). The incidence of meningococcal meningitis in Romania between 2000 and 2002 was 40 per 100,000 children per year for children younger than 1 year old, and 16 per 100,000 children per year for children 1 to 5 years old (53). The case fatality rate during this epidemic was 5.5% (53). Baseline rates of meningococcus infection in many other parts of the developed world are even lower. For example, Moura et al. (54) found rates of meningitis from different strains of meningococcus in New York City in 2000 ranged from 0.08 to 0.23 per 100,000 population, with a case fatality of 17%.

Streptococcus

Streptococcus Pneumoniae

The most common organism responsible for invasive bacterial infection in young children is *Streptococcus pneumoniae* (41). Bacteremia accounts for over 50% of invasive pneumococcal disease, followed by pneumonia and meningitis (41). In the U.S., *S. pneumoniae* is the leading cause of bacterial meningitis in young children, responsible for 25% to 40% of cases (41,55). In many other parts of the world, it is second only to *N. meningitidis* (41,55,56). Mortality in children with pneumococcal meningitis is at least twice as high as in children with meningococcal meningitis, and the survivors have among the highest incidence of sequelae of all meningitides (41). The annual incidence of invasive pneumococcal disease among children less than 2 years old in industrialized countries has been reported to be as high as 160 cases per 100,000 (55,57). However, the impact of pneumococcal disease on young children is especially profound in developing countries, where it causes an estimated 1.2 million deaths of young children annually, mostly due to pneumonia (41,55).

Group B Streptococcus

Group B *streptococcus* (GBS) is the most common cause of invasive infections in newborns, causing life-threatening perinatal infection, bacteremia without an identified focus, meningitis, or pneumonia. The global incidence of GBS disease varies from 0.41 to 5.5 per 1000 live births, with differences in incidence according to race, socioeconomic factors, and variations in medical practice (58). In the U.S., the incidence of early- and late-onset GBS infections have been steadily declining over the last two decades, with current rates estimated to be between 0.4 to 0.7 cases per 1000 live births (59). Similar rates are found in many parts of Europe. For example, Kalliola et al. (58) reviewed hospital records of Finnish infants over a 10-year period and found an incidence of 0.76 cases per 1000 live births and case fatality of 8.0%. The most common clinical diagnosis was bacteremia (77%), followed by meningitis (17%) and pneumonia (3%) (58).

Haemophilus Influenzae Type b

Haemophilus influenzae type b (Hib) is a predominant cause of bacterial meningitis (with *S. pneumoniae* and *N. meningitidis*) and the second most common cause of bacterial pneumonia in early childhood in developing countries (56,60). Globally, Hib is responsible for 300,000 to 400,000 childhood deaths each year (60). Hib meningitis has a very high rate of adverse sequelae (up to 35%) among the top three causes of meningitis in sub-Saharan Africa (56). The annual incidence of Hib meningitis varies dramatically around the globe due to the differential access to conjugate vaccine, which has approximately 98% efficacy against invasive Hib diseases, but is still used primarily in developed countries (60). For example, Hib meningitis affects 14 per 100,000 Guatemalan children, with a mortality of 14% (39), compared with only 3.5 per 100,000 children in Sweden (61).

Mycobacterium Tuberculosis

Tuberculosis (TB) is still an important global contributor to childhood morbidity and mortality (62–64). Infection with *Mycobacterium tuberculosis* causes a wide spectrum of illness, from asymptomatic carrier states to fatal, systemic disease (64). As opposed to adults, children are much more likely to experience extrapulmonary manifestations of TB, including meningitis (64). According to the WHO, 1.3 million new cases and 450,000 deaths are caused by tuberculosis annually among children younger than 15 years of age (65), which is approximately 10% of all TB cases (64).

The global epidemiology of pediatric TB varies dramatically, and is strongly associated with rates not only of adult disease but also of poverty, overcrowding, and HIV infection. Particularly hardest hit are the countries in Southeast Asia and sub-Saharan Africa, where HIV has become pandemic. In these countries, TB has become a leading cause of death in young adults and their children (62). Reported rates of TB in these countries can be as high as 1100 cases per

100,000 population, much higher than the rates in Western Europe and the U.S. (less than 10 cases per 100,000 population) (64). Migration also has a strong influence on the epidemiology of pediatric TB. In large cities of Western Europe, for example, rates of TB are increasing due to large numbers of immigrant families from endemic nations (64). This is often occurring despite declining rates of TB among native children (64,66).

Viral Diseases

Measles

Measles is a highly infectious virus that can cause pneumonia, diarrhea, encephalitis, and death (67). The WHO estimates that nearly 1.5 million people died in 1997 from measles, half of them in Africa (43). Baseline case fatality rates of 5% to 25% are common in developing countries, in contrast to the less than 1% case fatality rate during recent epidemics in the U.S. (1,68).

Factors associated with severe measles include younger age, overcrowding, poor access to care, preexisting medical conditions, and malnutrition (68). Because these factors frequently coexist, the relative contribution of each to measles morbidity is unclear (68). However, malnutrition has been implicated most markedly and repeatedly. O'Donovan analyzed measles mortality among 507 hospitalized children in Kenya and found progressively higher rates among children as the degree of wasting increased (69). Children at the 50th percentile of ideal body weight or greater experienced no measles mortality, those mildly malnourished had a 10% mortality rate, and those severely malnourished had a mortality rate of almost 50%.

Currently, measles is not endemic in the U.S. However, imported measles cases continue to occur and can result in limited indigenous transmission (67). In 2002, a record low 0.15 measles cases per million population was reported in the U.S., a 59% decrease from the incidence reported in 2000, which had been the lowest previously (67). This compares with an incidence between 2.36 and 3.37 per 100,000 population in the European Vaccine Network in 2001 to 2002 (70) and 88.7 per 100,000 population in the 1996–97 measles outbreak in Romania (71). In the U.S. and Europe in 2002, up to 70% of measles cases were in unvaccinated, vaccine-eligible individuals (67,70).

Influenza

Worldwide pandemics of human influenza virus caused extensive morbidity and mortality in the 20th century (44). The most recent international epidemiologic data on influenza is from 2004 (72). From May through October of that year, influenza A viruses circulated worldwide and were associated with mild-to moderate levels of disease activity. Influenza A viruses predominated in Africa, Asia, and Oceania (Australia, New Caledonia, and New Zealand). In South America, influenza A outbreaks occurred in Argentina, Chile, and Paraguay. During that same time, influenza B was associated with widespread outbreaks in Brazil, but less so elsewhere.

During the 2003–2004 influenza season in the U.S., over 20,000 cases of influenza virus were reported. Influenza A represented the overwhelming majority (79.1%) of cases (73). The overall hospitalization rate from the beginning to the end of influenza season for children aged 0 to 17 years was 0.8 to 12 per 10,000 children and was considerably higher (1.9 to 7.8 per 10,000) in children aged 0 to 4 years.

Complications from influenza infection include pneumonia, encephalitis, and myocarditis, and the frequency and severity of these complications varies by strain of virus (74). Epidemiologic data from Houston, Texas, from 1975 to 1985 indicates that risk of lower respiratory tract illness associated with influenza virus infection is highest (7.8 per 100) in children younger than 2 years of age (75).

Avian Influenza A Infections

Since December 2003, nine countries in Asia (Cambodia, China, Indonesia, Japan, Laos, Malaysia, South Korea, Thailand, and Vietnam) reported outbreaks of avian influenza A infection affecting poultry and other animals (72). During the first 10 months of 2004, a total of 44 laboratory-confirmed cases of avian influenza A virus infection in humans had been reported in Vietnam and Thailand. Of these 44 patients, 32 died. The cases were associated with severe respiratory illness requiring hospitalization (72). The cumulative case-fatality for confirmed avian influenza A cases since January 2004 is 73%. Currently, the disease has spread to most parts of Europe, Central Asia, and Africa, with more human cases being described almost daily. There is now a real possibility of worldwide infection of domestic fowl with H5N1 avian influenza A, and the increased risk of spread to other animal species and pandemic influenza in humans.

Poliomyelitis

Poliovirus is the cause of acute flaccid paralysis, commonly known as polio. Most infections with poliovirus are asymptomatic, and less than 1% result in paralysis. Paralysis rates are highest with poliovirus type 1, the most frequent cause of epidemics (76). Polio is predominantly a disease of the very young, with 70% to 90% of cases occurring in those younger than 3 years of age (76). The disease is seasonal, especially in temperate countries, with peaks in the hot and humid summer months. In the tropics, the seasonal peak is less pronounced. Before the advent of poliovirus vaccines, an estimated 600,000 new cases of paralytic polio occurred worldwide every year (76).

In 1988, the World Health Assembly passed a resolution calling for the global eradication of poliomyelitis by the year 2000 (76). Since that time, the number of countries with endemic poliovirus has decreased from 125 to seven (77). Through an increase in vaccine coverage and improvements in surveillance of acute flaccid paralysis, the global number of reported polio cases has decreased by 82% in the last 16 years (from 35,251 to 6339) (78). Unfortunately, important reservoir countries remain, particularly in Africa, the eastern Mediterranean, and Southeast Asia (76,77). Rates of polio in these areas can be as high as 42 cases per 100,000 children (79). Three WHO regions (Americas, Europe, and Western Pacific) appear to be free of indigenous wild poliovirus (72). However, sporadic cases associated with the polio vaccine continue to be reported, particularly in areas of low vaccine coverage (80).

Human Immunodeficiency Virus/Acquired Immunodeficiency Syndromes

Human immunodeficiency virus (HIV) infection and acquired immunodeficiency syndrome (AIDS) currently pose one of the greatest challenges to global public health (81). As a blood-borne and sexually transmitted infection, HIV has variable patterns of transmission and impact among world regions. HIV and AIDS are the leading cause of death in Africa and the fourth leading cause of death worldwide (81). According to the CDC, life expectancy in African countries most affected by HIV/AIDS has declined by 10 years, and infant mortality rates have doubled (81). In addition, HIV/AIDS can have devastating effects on families, social systems, and economies.

Considerable heterogeneity of rates of HIV and AIDS exist in HIV-infected countries throughout the world, and the differences have been attributed to risk factors associated with the spread of HIV and AIDS. These include migration, economic and political instability, drug use, and poverty (81). Sub-Saharan Africa is currently the region of the world most severely affected by HIV and AIDS (81). In 2000, an estimated 25.3 million persons in sub-Saharan Africa were infected with HIV, and the average prevalence of HIV infection among persons aged 15 to 49 years was 8.8%. In 2001, Botswana had the highest prevalence, with 36% of the adult population infected with HIV. The Caribbean is the second most affected world region, with an adult prevalence of 2.1%.

Human immunodeficiency virus has had a profound global impact on morbidity and mortality rates in children. Approximately 3.8 million children younger than 15 years old died as a result of AIDS between 1984 and 1999 (82). Millions more have been and will continue to be orphaned by AIDS (82,83). The predominant means of new HIV infection in children is via vertical transmission. In 2002, approximately 800,000 children worldwide acquired HIV, the majority vertically from their mothers (84). While multidrug regimens available to pregnant women have all but eliminated this in developed countries, these regimens are less feasible and often cost-prohibitive in most of the developing world (85).

Other

Malaria

Malaria is a parasitic infection caused by any of the four species of plasmodia that affect humans: *P. vivax*, *P. falciparum*, *P. malariae*, and *P. ovale*. *P. falciparum* is the most recently evolved and the most virulent (86). Symptoms of malaria range from an asymptomatic carrier state in partially immune persons to acute catastrophic cerebral illness and death (86). Acute, severe malaria is often associated with respiratory and neurologic symptoms, and can have mortality rates up to 20%, with frequent neurologic morbidity in survivors (86–88). Malaria can also be chronically debilitating, with prolonged anemia and cognitive and behavioral disorders (86). Its socioeconomic impact on endemic countries, because of health costs and missed schooldays and work-days is difficult to overstate.

The global burden of malaria is difficult to quantify because of the presence of asymptomatic individuals and because many febrile illnesses in endemic areas mimic malaria. Confirmatory diagnostic testing is often unavailable or unreli-able, particularly in rural areas (86). Furthermore, case detection and reporting largely underestimate current rates of malaria because of inadequate surveil-lance in many countries. Nonetheless, a recent review by the WHO concluded that roughly 1 million deaths occur from the direct effects of malaria annually in Africa, more than 75% of them in children (89). In sub-Saharan Africa, more than half of the beds in pediatric wards may be occupied by children with severe malaria (88). The impact of malaria on the pregnant woman and her fetus has only recently been appreciated (86). In particular, low birth weight and increased infant and childhood mortality can result from an infected placenta.

Preventive Strategies for Severe Infections

Vaccination

Most infectious diseases are on the decline, due in part to better nutrition, less crowded living conditions, and effective antibiotic therapies. However, it is difficult to name a medical intervention that has done as much to reduce child-hood morbidity and mortality from infection as has immunization (56,90,91). The importance of vaccination is paramount now, as prevention is a key to fighting the rising rates of multidrug resistant bacteria. Many people are famil-iar with the history of polio eradication in the Western Hemisphere, but vacci-nation against Hib, measles, rubella, diphtheria, tetanus, pertussis, polio, and influenza has lowered the burden of these diseases dramatically as well in the last half century (56,91).

Recent availability of varicella, hepatitis B, and polyvalent pneumococcal and meningococcal vaccines is changing the epidemiology of many other serious infections (91). Vaccination against one infection may reduce morbidity from others as well (92–94). For example, Stensballe et al. (95) have found that bacille Calmette-Guérin (BCG) vaccination may have a nontargeted, protective effect against lower respiratory infections of all causes. However, at current prices, many vaccines are too expensive for many areas of the world (56). In addition, political instability has lowered the quality and availability of health care in many countries. Therefore, despite the availability of a safe, effective, and inexpensive measles vaccine for over 40 years, measles remains the leading vaccine-preventable killer of children around the world (96). While Hib has been dramatically reduced in large parts of Europe, the Americas, and Australia, most children in Africa are unvaccinated against Hib and continued to be disabled or killed by this organism (56,97). Polio remains endemic only in countries where vaccination rates are at or below 50% (79).

Epidemics of these infections in developed countries are also related to drops in vaccination rates. For example, in the 1980s in the U.S., four major childhood illnesses showed increases in the case rate, and the U.S. experienced epidemics of measles, mumps, rubella, and *Bordetella pertussis* (98). Predating these epidemics was a decline in the immunization levels of 2-year-olds (98). This decline coincided with vaccine price increases, an increase in the percentage of children in poverty, and a decline in the rate of poor children receiving Aid to Families with Dependent Children (AFDC) and Medicaid (98). An estimated 100,000 excess cases of disease resulted from the low levels of immunization (98).

Prevention of Mother-to-Child Transmission of Human Immunodeficiency Virus

Until a vaccine against HIV is developed, prevention of mother-to-child transmission remains the most important means of reducing the number of pediatric HIV infections (99). Human immunodeficiency virus may be transmitted in utero across the placenta, during the birth process, or after birth, through breast-feeding (82). For many years, not enough was known about HIV transmission from mother to child for steps to be taken that would help HIV-infected women give birth to uninfected babies (82). The transmission rate of HIV from mother to child varies from <10% when mothers and newborns are treated to 40% when neither is treated and the mother is breast-feeding. However, most children who are at risk of acquiring HIV come from areas of the world in which finding safe and economically feasible alternatives to breast milk is difficult. Strategies for feeding of infants by HIV-infected mothers in those areas are urgently needed (82). Efforts designed to increase availability and affordability of antiretroviral medications could have an enormous impact of the epidemiology of HIV in children.

Sanitation and Nutrition

Conflict and economic decline have severely disrupted civil and health service infrastructures in many parts of the world. Proper sanitation and nutrition are unaffordable in many countries, and the consequences, especially for children, are enormous. Unsanitary conditions contribute to approximately 1.5 million childhood deaths each year through the ingestion of unsafe drinking water and exposure to improper waste disposal (4). In addition, civil unrest has led to large refugee populations whose camps are crowded and have scarce sanitation and poor water supply. Starvation and inadequate nutrition are ubiquitous in many of these camps, as they are often "camps" in name alone. With no water and no food sources, they are simply gatherings of people—up to tens of thousands of people—who have clumped together for protection from violence (100). These camps are an ideal environment for the spread of infectious disease. Current estimates by the United Nations indicate that there were some 6.2 million refugees globally at the end of 2003 (101). The great majority of refugees were in Central Asia, Southwest Asia, North Africa, and the Middle East, accounting for 2.7 million refugees (101). Many of the refugee deaths are among children, whose deaths are often attributable to preventable and treatable infections such as malaria, diarrhea, and pneumonia (101). Support for these populations need not be technologically complex. Many simple and inexpensive nutritional supplements, such as zinc (18,102,103) or other vitamins (104,105) can reduce morbidity and mortality from many causes of serious infection in children. Safe and proper housing, sanitation services, public works, and health care will also dramatically lower the rates of childhood morbidity and mortality from many causes in the developing world.

Conclusion

Infections are among the most important global health care challenges today. Millions of children suffer and die from serious infections each year, many of which are preventable with technology that is available today. However, resource-poor developing countries have inadequate access to both preventive and therapeutic options for many of these diseases. As a result, the epidemiology of serious infections in children is disproportionately located in the developing world. Strategies aimed at reducing the incidence, prevalence, and mortality from infection are primarily social in nature, not medical. Global improvements in the standard of living would substantially reduce the burden of infectious disease in children.

Acknowledgments. The authors wish to thank Ellen Wald, MD, and Marian Michaels, MD, for their thoughtful contributions.

References

1. Accorsi S, Fabiani M, Lukwiya M, Onek PA, Mattei PD, Declich S. The increasing burden of infectious diseases on hospital services at St Mary's Hospital Lacor, Gulu, Uganda. Am J Trop Med Hyg 2001;64(3–4):154–158.
2. Murray CJ, Lopez AD. Mortality by cause for eight regions of the world: Global Burden of Disease Study. Lancet 1997;349(9061):1269–1276.
3. Hill K, Pande R, Mahy M, et al. Trends in Child Mortality in the Developing World: 1960 to 1996. New York: UNICEF, 2005:1.
4. Black RE, Morris SS, Bryce J. Where and why are 10 million children dying every year? Lancet 2003;361(9376):2226–2234.

5. Bang AT, Bang RA, Baitule SB, Reddy MH, Deshmukh MD. Effect of home-based neonatal care and management of sepsis on neonatal mortality: field trial in rural India. Lancet 1999;354(9194):1955–1961.

6. Nhan NT, Phuong CXT, Kneen R, et al. Acute management of dengue shock syndrome: a randomized double-blind comparison of 4 intravenous fluid regimens in the first hour. Clin Infect Dis 2001;32(2):204–213.

7. Osrin D, Vergnano S, Costello A. Serious bacterial infections in newborn infants in developing countries. Curr Opin Infect Dis 2004;17(3):217–224.

8. Bacterial etiology of serious infections in young infants in developing countries: results of a multicenter study. The WHO Young Infants Study Group. Pediatr Infect Dis J 1999;18(10 suppl):S17–S22.

9. Cotton MF, Burger PJ, Bodenstein WJ. Bacteraemia in children in the south-western Cape. A hospital-based survey. S Afr Med J 1992;81(2):87–90.

10. Berkley JA, Lowe BS, Mwangi I, et al. Bacteremia among children admitted to a rural hospital in Kenya. N Engl J Med 2005;352(1):39–47.

11. Mulholland EK, Ogunlesi OO, Adegbola RA, et al. Etiology of serious infections in young Gambian infants. Pediatr Infect Dis J 1999;18(10 suppl):S35–S41.

12. Definitions for sepsis and organ failure and guidelines for the use of innovative therapies in sepsis. American College of Chest Physicians/Society of Critical Care Medicine Consensus Conference. Crit Care Med 1992;20(6):864–874.

13. Annane D, Sebille V, Charpentier C, et al. Effect of treatment with low doses of hydrocortisone and fludrocortisone on mortality in patients with septic shock. JAMA 2002;288(7):862–871.

14. Rivers E, Nguyen B, Havstad S, et al., for the Early Goal-Directed Therapy Collaborative Group. Early goal-directed therapy in the treatment of severe sepsis and septic shock. N Engl J Med 2001;345(19):1368–1377.

15. Briegel J, Forst H, Haller M, et al. Stress doses of hydrocortisone reverse hyperdynamic septic shock: a prospective, randomized, double-blind, single-center study (see comments). Crit Care Med 1999;27(4):723–732.

16. Reinhart K, Meier-Hellmann A, Beale R, et al. Open randomized phase II trial of an extracorporeal endotoxin adsorber in suspected Gram-negative sepsis. Crit Care Med 2004;32(8):1662–1668.

17. Molnar Z, Mikor A, Leiner T, Szakmany T. Fluid resuscitation with colloids of different molecular weight in septic shock. Intensive Care Med 2004;30(7): 1356–1360.

18. Bertolini G, Iapichino G, Radrizzani D, et al. Early enteral immunonutrition in patients with severe sepsis: results of an interim analysis of a randomized multi-centre clinical trial. Intensive Care Med 2003;29(5):834–840.

19. Busund R, Koukline V, Utrobin U, Nedashkovsky E. Plasmapheresis in severe sepsis and septic shock: a prospective, randomised, controlled trial. Intensive Care Med 2002;28(10):1434–1439.

20. Center for Disease Control. National Vital Statistics Report 2002;50(16):1.

21. Watson RS, Carcillo JA, Linde-Zwirble WT, Clermont G, Lidicker J, Angus DC. The epidemiology of severe sepsis in children in the United States. Am J Respir Crit Care Med 2003;167(5):695–701.

22. Watson RS, Linde-Zwirble WT, Lidicker J, et al. The increasing burden of severe sepsis in U.S. children. Crit Care Med 2001;29(suppl):(12)A8(abstr).

23. Proulx F, Fayon M, Farrell CA, Lacroix J, Gauthier M. Epidemiology of sepsis and multiple organ dysfunction syndrome in children. Chest 1996;109(4): 1033–1037.

24. Al Zwaini EJ. Neonatal septicaemia in the neonatal care unit, Al-Anbar governorate, Iraq. East Mediterr Health J 2002;8(4–5):509–514.

25. Ali Z. Neonatal bacterial septicaemia at the Mount Hope Women's Hospital, Trinidad. Ann Trop Paediatr 2004;24(1):41–44.

26. Kutko MC, Calarco MP, Flaherty MB, et al. Mortality rates in pediatric septic shock with and without multiple organ system failure. Pediatr Crit Care Med 2003;4(3):333–337.

27. Wisplinghoff H, Seifert H, Tallent SM, Bischoff T, Wenzel RP, Edmond MB. Nosocomial bloodstream infections in pediatric patients in United States hospitals: epidemiology, clinical features and susceptibilities. Pediatr Infect Dis J 2003;22(8): 686–691.

28. Gray JW. A 7-year study of bloodstream infections in an English children's hospital. Eur J Pediatr 2004;163(9):530–535.

29. Perez LA, Gimenez M, Rodrigo C, Alonso A, Prat C, Ausina V. Seven-year review of paediatric bacteraemias diagnosed in a Spanish university hospital. Acta Paediatr 2003;92(7):854–856.

30. Walsh AL, Phiri AJ, Graham SM, Molyneux EM, Molyneux ME. Bacteremia in febrile Malawian children: clinical and microbiologic features. Pediatr Infect Dis J 2000;19(4):312–318.

31. Graham SM, Molyneux EM, Walsh AL, Cheesbrough JS, Molyneux ME, Hart CA. Nontyphoidal Salmonella infections of children in tropical Africa. Pediatr Infect Dis J 2000;19(12):1189–1196.

32. Bacterial etiology of serious infections in young infants in developing countries: results of a multicenter study. The WHO Young Infants Study Group. Pediatr Infect Dis J 1999;18(10 suppl):S17–S22.

33. Galanakis E, Krallis N, Levidiotou S, Hotoura E, Andronikou S. Neonatal bacteraemia: a population-based study. Scand J Infect Dis 2002;34(8):598–601.

34. Davidson G, Barnes G, Bass D, et al. Infectious diarrhea in children: Working Group Report of the First World Congress of Pediatric Gastroenterology, Hepatology, and Nutrition. J Pediatr Gastroenterol Nutr 2002;35(suppl 2):S143–S150.

35. Kosek M, Bern C, Guerrant RL. The global burden of diarrhoeal disease, as estimated from studies published between 1992 and 2000. Bull WHO 2003;81(3):197–204.

36. Thapar N, Sanderson IR. Diarrhoea in children: an interface between developing and developed countries. Lancet 2004;363(9409):641–653.

37. Nascimento-Carvalho CM, Lopes AA, Gomes MD, et al. Community acquired pneumonia among pediatric outpatients in Salvador, Northeast Brazil, with emphasis on the role of pneumococcus. Braz J Infect Dis 2001;5(1):13–20.

38. Rudan I, Tomaskovic L, Boschi-Pinto C, Campbell H. Global estimate of the incidence of clinical pneumonia among children under five years of age. Bull WHO 2004;82(12):895–903.

39. Asturias EJ, Soto M, Menendez R, et al. Meningitis and pneumonia in Guatemalan children: the importance of Haemophilus influenzae type b and Streptococcus pneumoniae. Rev Panam Salud Publica 2003;14(6):377–384.

40. Poehling KA, Lafleur BJ, Szilagyi PG, et al. Population-based impact of pneumococcal conjugate vaccine in young children. Pediatrics 2004;114(3):755–761.

41. Ispahani P, Slack RC, Donald FE, Weston VC, Rutter N. Twenty year surveillance of invasive pneumococcal disease in Nottingham: serogroups responsible and implications for immunisation. Arch Dis Child 2004;89(8):757–762.

42. Shann F. Haemophilus influenzae pneumonia: type b or non-type b? Lancet 1999;354(9189):1488–1490.

43. World Health Organization. Communicable Disease Surveillance and Response. WHO Website, 2005.

44. Tam JS. Influenza A (H5N1) in Hong Kong: an overview. Vaccine 2002;20(suppl 2):S77–S81.

45. Drummond P, Clark J, Wheeler J, Galloway A, Freeman R, Cant A. Community acquired pneumonia—a prospective UK study. Arch Dis Child 2000;83(5): 408–412.

46. Nichol KP, Cherry JD. Bacterial-viral interrelations in respiratory infections of children. N Engl J Med 1967;277(13):667–672.

47. Shann F. Bacterial pneumonia: commoner than perceived. Lancet 2001;357(9274): 2070–2072.

48. Michelow IC, Olsen K, Lozano J, et al. Epidemiology and clinical characteristics of community-acquired pneumonia in hospitalized children. Pediatrics 2004;113(4): 701–707.

49. Tzeng YL, Stephens DS. Epidemiology and pathogenesis of Neisseria meningitidis. Microbes Infect 2000;2(6):687–700.

50. Chonghaile CN. Meningitis in Africa—tackling W135. Lancet 2002;360(9350): 2054–2055.

51. World Health Organization. Control of Epidemic Meningococcal Disease. WHO Practical Guidelines, 2nd ed. Geneva: World Health Organization, 1998:1.

52. Heyderman RS, Ben Shlomo Y, Brennan CA, Somerset M. The incidence and mortality for meningococcal disease associated with area deprivation: an ecological study of hospital episode statistics. Arch Dis Child 2004;89(11):1064–1068.

53. Luca V, Gessner BD, Luca C, et al. Incidence and etiological agents of bacterial meningitis among children <5 years of age in two districts of Romania. Eur J Clin Microbiol Infect Dis 2004;23(7):523–528.

54. Moura AS, Pablos-Mendez A, Layton M, Weiss D. Epidemiology of meningococcal disease, New York City, 1989–2000. Emerg Infect Dis 2003;9(3):355–361.

55. Hausdorff WP, Bryant J, Paradiso PR, Siber GR. Which pneumococcal serogroups cause the most invasive disease: implications for conjugate vaccine formulation and use, part I. Clin Infect Dis 2000;30(1):100–121.

56. Peltola H. Burden of meningitis and other severe bacterial infections of children in Africa: implications for prevention. Clin Infect Dis 2001;32(1):64–75.

57. Dagan R, Engelhard D, Piccard E, Englehard D. Epidemiology of invasive childhood pneumococcal infections in Israel. The Israeli Pediatric Bacteremia and Meningitis Group. JAMA 1992;268(23):3328–3332.

58. Kalliola S, Vuopio-Varkila J, Takala AK, Eskola J. Neonatal group B streptococcal disease in Finland: a ten-year nationwide study. Pediatr Infect Dis J 1999;18(9): 806–810.

59. Baltimore RS. Neonatal sepsis: epidemiology and management. Paediatr Drugs 2003;5(11):723–740.

60. Saha SK, Baqui AH, Darmstadt GL, et al. Invasive Haemophilus influenzae type B diseases in Bangladesh, with increased resistance to antibiotics. J Pediatr 2005;146(2):227–233.

61. Garpenholt O, Hugosson S, Fredlund H, Giesecke J, Olcen P. Invasive disease due to Haemophilus influenzae type b during the first six years of general vaccination of Swedish children. Acta Paediatr 2000;89(4):471–474.

62. Starke JR. Childhood tuberculosis in the 1990s. Pediatr Ann 1993;22(9):550–560.

63. Al Dossary FS, Ong LT, Correa AG, Starke JR. Treatment of childhood tuberculosis with a six month directly observed regimen of only two weeks of daily therapy. Pediatr Infect Dis J 2002;21(2):91–97.

64. Walls T, Shingadia D. Global epidemiology of paediatric tuberculosis. J Infect 2004;48(1):13–22.

65. Kochi A. The global tuberculosis situation and the new control strategy of the World Health Organization. Tubercle 1991;72(1):1–6.

66. Ussery XT, Valway SE, McKenna M, Cauthen GM, McCray E, Onorato IM. Epidemiology of tuberculosis among children in the United States: 1985 to 1994. Pediatr Infect Dis J 1996;15(8):697–704.

67. Epidemiology of measles—United States, 2001–2003. MMWR Morb Mortal Wkly Rep 2004;53(31):713–716.

68. Belamarich PR. Measles and malnutrition. Pediatr Rev 1998;19(2):70–71.

69. O'Donovan C. Measles in Kenyan children. East Afr Med J 1971;48(10):526–532.

70. Muscat M, Glismann S, Bang H. Measles in Europe in 2001–2002. Eur Surveill 2003;8(6):123–129.

71. Measles outbreak—Romania, 1997. MMWR Morb Mortal Wkly Rep 1997;46(49): 1159–1163.

72. Update: influenza activity—United States and worldwide, May–October 2004. MMWR Morb Mortal Wkly Rep 2004;53(42):993–995.

73. Update: influenza activity—United States, 2003–04 season. MMWR Morb Mortal Wkly Rep 2003;52(49):1197–1202.

74. Togashi T, Matsuzono Y, Narita M, Morishima T. Influenza-associated acute encephalopathy in Japanese children in 1994–2002. Virus Res 2004;103(1–2): 75–78.

75. Glezen WP, Taber LH, Frank AL, Gruber WC, Piedra PA. Influenza virus infections in infants. Pediatr Infect Dis J 1997;16(11):1065–1068.

76. Hull HF, Ward NA, Hull BP, Milstien JB, de Quadros C. Paralytic poliomyelitis: seasoned strategies, disappearing disease. Lancet 1994;343(8909):1331–1337.

77. Global progress toward certifying polio eradication and laboratory containment of wild polioviruses–August 2002–August 2003. MMWR Morb Mortal Wkly Rep 2003;52(47):1158–1160.

78. One thousand days until the target date for global poliomyelitis eradication. MMWR Morb Mortal Wkly Rep 1998;47(12):234.

79. Gaspar M, Morais A, Brumana L, Stella AA. Outbreak of poliomyelitis in Angola. J Infect Dis 2000;181(5):1776–1779.

80. Update: Outbreak of poliomyelitis–Dominican Republic and Haiti, 2000–2001. MMWR Morb Mortal Wkly Rep 2001;50(39):855–856.

81. The global HIV and AIDS epidemic, 2001. MMWR Morb Mortal Wkly Rep 2001;50(21):434–439.

82. Pancharoen C, Thisyakorn U. Pediatric acquired immunodeficiency syndrome in Asia: mother-to-child transmission. Clin Infect Dis 2002;34(suppl 2):S65–S69.

83. Akinsete I. HIV infection in children. Niger Pop 1993;42–44.

84. Thorne C, Newell ML. Prevention of mother-to-child transmission of HIV infection. Curr Opin Infect Dis 2004;17(3):247–252.

85. Thorne C, Newell ML. Mother-to-child transmission of HIV infection and its prevention. Curr HIV Res 2003;1(4):447–462.

86. Breman JG. The ears of the hippopotamus: manifestations, determinants, and estimates of the malaria burden. Am J Trop Med Hyg 2001;64(1–2 suppl):1–11.

87. Singhal T. Management of severe malaria. Indian J Pediatr 2004;71(1):81–88.
88. Planche T, Agbenyega T, Bedu-Addo G, et al. A prospective comparison of malaria with other severe diseases in African children: prognosis and optimization of management. Clin Infect Dis 2003;37(7):890–897.
89. Snow RW, Craig M, Deichmann U, Marsh K. Estimating mortality, morbidity and disability due to malaria among Africa's non-pregnant population. Bull WHO 1999;77(8):624–640.
90. de la HF, Higuera AB, Di Fabio JL, et al. Effectiveness of Haemophilus influenzae type b vaccination against bacterial pneumonia in Colombia. Vaccine 2004;23(1): 36–42.
91. Baker JP, Katz SL. Childhood vaccine development: an overview. Pediatr Res 2004;55(2):347–356.
92. Aaby P, Hedegaard K, Sodemann M, et al. Childhood mortality after oral polio immunisation campaign in Guinea-Bissau. Vaccine 2005;23(14):1746–1751.
93. Veirum JE, Sodemann M, Biai S, et al. Routine vaccinations associated with divergent effects on female and male mortality at the paediatric ward in Bissau, Guinea-Bissau. Vaccine 2005;23(9):1197–1204.
94. Aaby P, Bhuiya A, Nahar L, Knudsen K, de Francisco A, Strong M. The survival benefit of measles immunization may not be explained entirely by the prevention of measles disease: a community study from rural Bangladesh. Int J Epidemiol 2003;32(1):106–116.
95. Stensballe LG, Nante E, Jensen IP, et al. Acute lower respiratory tract infections and respiratory syncytial virus in infants in Guinea-Bissau: a beneficial effect of BCG vaccination for girls community based case-control study. Vaccine 2005;23(10): 1251–1257.
96. Measles deaths drop dramatically as vaccine reaches world's poorest children. J Adv Nurs 2004;48(3):312.
97. Makela PH. Conjugate vaccines—a breakthrough in vaccine development. Southeast Asian J Trop Med Public Health 2003;34(2):249–253.
98. Teitelbaum MA, Franklin PC. Vaccine-preventable illness in U.S. children 1980–1992. Stat Bull Metrop Insur Co 1994;75(4):2–9.
99. Hashimoto H, Kapiga SH, Murata Y. Mass treatment with nevirapine to prevent mother-to-child transmission of HIV/AIDS in sub-Saharan African countries. J Obstet Gynaecol Res 2002;28(6):313–319.
100. Brown H. Disease and hunger in Sudan. Lancet 2004;364(9435):654.
101. United Nations High Commission for Refugees. The State of the World's Refugees 2006; Oxford University Press, Oxford UK.
102. Thakur S, Gupta N, Kakkar P. Serum copper and zinc concentrations and their relation to superoxide dismutase in severe malnutrition. Eur J Pediatr 2004;163(12): 742–744.
103. Schapiro JM, Libby SJ, Fang FC. Inhibition of bacterial DNA replication by zinc mobilization during nitrosative stress. Proc Natl Acad Sci U S A 2003;100(14): 8496–8501.
104. Benn CS, Bale C, Sommerfelt H, Friis H, Aaby P. Hypothesis: Vitamin A supplementation and childhood mortality: amplification of the non-specific effects of vaccines? Int J Epidemiol 2003;32(5):822–828.
105. Ahmed J, Zaman MM, Ali SM. Immunological response to antioxidant vitamin supplementation in rural Bangladeshi school children with group A streptococcal infection. Asia Pac J Clin Nutr 2004;13(3):226–230.

8
Novel Challenges in Infection in the Pediatric Intensive Care Unit Setting

Laura Jones and Mike Sharland

Managing infections in immunosuppressed and immunodeficient patients in the pediatric intensive care unit (PICU) setting poses ever-increasing challenges. They are a population already susceptible to viral and fungal infections, in addition to severe bacterial sepsis. Resistant bacterial, viral, and fungal isolates are becoming increasingly common, making the management of these patients even more complex.

Bacterial Infections

Resistance

Microbes have always had the capacity to evolve in response to their environment and thus the ability to evade antibiotic therapy [1]. Multidrug-resistant organisms causing nosocomial infections are becoming increasingly prevalent, due in part to the increased empiric use of broad-spectrum antibiotics (especially vancomycin, carbapenems, and the fluoroquinolones) [2,3]. In addition, patients in the PICU have multiple predisposing factors for infections with resistant organisms, especially with staphylococcal and enterococcal species [4]. These include central vascular catheter insertion, organ dysfunction, parenteral feeding, prolonged hospital stay, poor nutrition, and poor glycemic control.

Mechanisms of resistance causing particular clinical problems include the presence of β-lactamases, alteration in the penicillin-binding proteins, and transmission of mobile genetic elements responsible for resistance (transposons) [1,5].

Staphylococci

Staphylococci remain one of the most common bacteria causing infections worldwide, but approximately 95% now produce β-lactamases, enzymes capable of hydrolyzing the β-lactam ring of penicillins, cephalosporins, and related drugs. Methicillin-resistant *Staphylococcus aureus* (MRSA) has spread rapidly and is now an increasing problem (6). In the United Kingdom between 1990 and 2001, 376 cases of staphylococcal bacteremia in children were notified to the Public Health Laboratory Service. The proportion of cases due to MRSA rose considerably during this period to between 10% and 15% (with the highest prevalence occurring in neonatal units). In adults in the U.K., around 45% of staphylococcal bacteremia is now due to MRSA. In the United States, MRSA is now a significant problem in children. A different spectrum of disease is being recognized more recently, particularly in children with Panton-Valentine leukocidin (PVL) toxin-producing strains: younger infants presenting with severe necrotizing pneumonia, and marked thrombophlebitis have been increasingly described. Methicillin-resistant *S. aureus* has also become an increasing problem elsewhere, especially in neonatal units (7,8).

Methicillin resistance is conferred by the *Mec A* gene, carried on transposons, and results in an altered penicillin-binding protein 2a, an enzyme on the bacterial inner membrane that is the target of the antibiotic (1,5). This conformational change is responsible for resistance to all the β-lactam antibiotics. Risk factors for MRSA, in common with other resistant bacteria, are previous hospital stay, ICU admission, indwelling devices, and prolonged antibiotic exposure. However, there are an increasing number of reports of community-acquired MRSA (CA-MRSA) occurring in previously healthy children with no apparent risk factors. A high index of suspicion is required for CA-MRSA infection, and empiric therapy should be guided by local epidemiologic and microbiologic advice.

Extended Spectrum β-Lactamases

Bacterial β-lactamases are responsible for resistance to the β-lactam antibiotics. Initially the extended spectrum cephalosporins were more stable against the β-lactamases, but their overuse has led to the emergence of organisms that produce extended spectrum β-lactamases (ESBLs). The gene encoding for these are located on transposons, allowing dissemination among G bacilli (1,5). There is increasing recognition that bacteria can transfer cassettes of multidrug-resistant (MDR) genes. The ESBL-producing microbes were first reported in the 1990s, but since 2003, strains of *Escherichia coli*, which produce an ESBL called CTX-M type, have become widespread and are highly resistant to multiple antibiotics including the carbapenems. The ESBLs have been isolated from both hospital patients and those in the community, and there is evidence to suggest that they are carried in fecal matter and thus may be spread by the food chain. Currently in the U.K., approximately 3% of *E. coli* isolates and 8% of *Klebsiella* isolates are known to be ESBL producers, emphasizing the need for both increased surveillance and for laboratories to have the ability to detect ESBL producers. In London, about 0.5% of isolates from children with febrile neutropenia are from ESBL-producing organisms resistant to piperacillin, ciprofloxacin, aminoglycosides, and carbapenems (9).

Vancomycin-Resistant Enterococci

Enterococci are normal inhabitants of the human gastrointestinal tract, but may become the predominant organisms in situations where broad-spectrum antibiotics such as the second- and third-generation cephalosporins have killed most of the host's gram-negative enteric bacteria. Enterococci are particularly associated with indwelling devices and are intrinsically resistant to many antimicrobials. They can also develop resistance by transfer of plasmids through transposons (5). Enterococci may be resistant to β-lactam antibiotics due to the production of β-lactamases or due to mutations in the penicillin-binding protein (1). Resistance to aminoglycosides has been detected due the presence of aminoglycoside-modifying agents. Resistance to vancomycin is mediated through transposons and alterations in the cell wall components, which result in a decreased affinity for vancomycin. Risk factors associated with vancomycin-resistant enterococci (VRE) are previous exposure to antibiotics, especially glycopeptides; parenteral feeding; and a prolonged stay in intensive care.

Penicillin-Resistant Pneumococci

Penicillin-binding proteins are involved in the synthesis of the bacterial cell wall, and they bind to β-lactam antibiotics. Pneumococcal resistance to penicillin is due to a decreased affinity for penicillin and related drugs, caused by the penicillin-binding proteins being altered (10,11). Nurseries and hospitals are potential environments for dissemination of resistant organisms such as the pneumococcus, as they are readily spread by droplets. Pneumococci resistant to macrolides are also now recognized, and is due to modification of an enzyme that methylates 23s RNA (the *erm B* gene). A second mechanism of resistance, encoded by the *mef* gene, involves an active efflux pump that removes macrolides from the bacterial cell (12). In the U.K. the prevalence of penicillin-resistant pneumococci (PRP) in blood isolates is decreasing, and is currently around 3%, having peaked at 7%. However, in North America and many European countries (especially Spain and Eastern Europe) the prevalence of PRP is between 20% and 40%. Therefore, children coming from areas of such high prevalence must be considered to be at risk of PRP bacteremia.

Management and Treatment of Resistant Infections

The prevention and control of resistant organisms involves active surveillance and thorough adherence to aseptic techniques and hand washing. Strict infection control measures remain vital, as clonal spread of resistant organisms within units has been described, particularly for MDR *Klebsiella*. No randomized trial has been conducted in children, studying the benefits of isolating patients, but the infection control department should be notified immediately about a child with an MDR organism. Wherever possible, these children should be nursed in an isolation room, with appropriate barrier nursing procedures.

The use of empirical antibiotics within an intensive therapy unit (ITU) setting was not shown to be beneficial for prevention of resistant staphylococcal infections in a recent Cochrane review of placebo-controlled trials (13).

There remains a real need for all PICUs to adopt a strict policy for antibiotic use. This might include a possible first-line regimen with as narrow a spectrum as possible, clear stop dates for all antibiotics prescribed, and the early cessation of antibiotics after negative septic screens. Modifying broad-spectrum coverage in the light of microbiologic results has been shown to reduce the incidence of resistant organisms in intensive care units, but a policy of routinely rotating the antimicrobials in use within these units has not yet been shown to be beneficial.

Methicillin-Resistant Staphylococcus Aureus

Most patients with possible serious MRSA infections are treated with glycopeptide antibiotics, pending culture results. In adults there have only been rare *S. aureus* isolates containing the *van A* gene, which have reduced sensitivity to vancomycin (6). Rifampicin is a potent antistaphylococcal drug, but resistance develops if it is used alone; it may, however, be of benefit when used in combination with other agents for the treatment of MRSA. Methicillin-resistant *S. aureus* may be treated effectively by clindamycin therapy, although staphylococci carrying the *erm* gene can mutate to convey expression of clindamycin resistance, following prolonged single-agent use. In the U.S., in areas where CA-MRSA is increasingly prevalent, clindamycin, or if a life-threatening infection is present, vancomycin, is often used as a first-line antibiotic treatment for children presenting to the emergency room with suspected staphylococcal infection.

Coagulase-negative staphylococci (CoNS) causing line infections are usually methicillin resistant (the *Mec A* gene is conferred, as described above). For these infections vancomycin would be the treatment of choice in addition to the consideration of line removal.

Linezolid, an oxazolidinone, is a bacteriostatic antibiotic with 100% oral bioavailably. It inhibits bacterial protein synthesis by binding to the 50S ribosomal subunit and thus prevents formation of essential components of messenger RNA (mRNA). There is no cross-resistance with other antibiotics due to its unique mechanism of action.

Linezolid is active against gram-positive bacteria, especially those that are resistant to other antimicrobials, such as VRE, MRSA and PRP. It is also active against some gram-negative bacteria and anaerobes. It is well tolerated in children and has been shown to be as effective as vancomycin in patients with MRSA infections (14–17). Rare reports of resistance have been associated with prolonged use (more than 4 weeks), and the presence of indwelling catheters, artificial indwelling prostheses, and endocarditis. Side effects include rash, headache, diarrhea, nausea, and vomiting, and deranged liver function tests.

Quinupristin/dalfopristin (18) is a new parenteral streptogramin that inhibits bacterial protein synthesis. It is very active against gram-positive bacteria, notably MRSA, VRE, and resistant pneumococci, and is useful for patients who are allergic to β-lactam antibiotics and vancomycin. It is not active against *Enterococcus faecalis*. This may be due to the use of streptogramin antibiotics (particularly virginiamycin) in animal feeds, which has led to the creation of reservoirs of resistant organisms within the food chain.

Extended Spectrum β-Lactamases

The main current treatment option for infections caused by ESBL gram-negative bacilli are the carbapenems, if they remain sensitive. For organisms with very widespread resistance, older antibiotics such as aztreonam or colisitin may be required, although dosing and toxicity data are limited in children.

Vancomycin-Resistant Enterococci

Alternative possible treatment options for VRE, apart from linezolid or the streptogramins, include the use of an aminoglycoside, together with high-dose penicillin, or teicoplanin. Less commonly used options include daptomycin and the ketolides.

Penicillin-Resistant Pneumococci

Possible treatment options for PRP include high-dose systemic penicillin, as PRP can still be treated satisfactorily by penicillin if the drug levels greatly exceed the minimum inhibitory concentration (MIC). Other options for PRP include the extended-spectrum cephalosporins, glycopeptides, carbapenems, and some of the fluoroquinolones—moxifloxacin and gatifloxacin(19). Most macrolide-resistant pneumococci are still currently sensitive to the ketolides, synthetic derivatives of erythromycin A.

Combination Antimicrobial Therapy

Little evidence exists about the benefit of combination therapy for gram-negative sepsis. A meta-analysis of 17 studies comparing combination therapy versus monotherapy with mortality as the outcome measure, suggested there was no added benefit (20). Possible benefits of combination therapy were highlighted, however: the possible synergistic effects, the potential for reducing antimicrobial resistance, and the increased chance that the bacteria would be susceptible to at least one of the antibacterials. The subanalysis of five studies looking at combination therapy for pseudomonas bacteremia did show an improved mortality, but these were pooled data from widely varying studies and this analysis is therefore to be interpreted with caution.

Fungal Infections

Fungal infections, notably *Candida*, are now reported to be the fourth commonest nosocomial bloodstream infection (after CoNS, *S. aureus*, and enterococci), and they are difficult both to diagnose and to treat (21). They are increasingly common in the PICU setting due to the increasing numbers of both immunodeficient and immunosuppressed patients. The widespread use of broad-spectrum antibiotics suppresses normal gut bacteria and promotes the overgrowth of *Candida*, a commensal of the gut, oropharynx, and skin. Breaks in the mucosal surface, burns, and any abdominal surgery increase the risk of fungal (especially candidal) sepsis. Fungal translocation can also occur across intact bowel wall membranes and may occur if the fungal burden is sufficient. Total parenteral nutrition (TPN) increases the risk; as gut mucosal atrophy increases, the risk of bacterial and fungal translocation also increases due to disruption of the normal gut flora.

In ITU settings, there is an increasing incidence of *Candida* species other than *Candida albicans*, notably *C. glabrata*, *C. tropicalis*, and *C. parapsilosis*. This is significant, as non-*albicans Candida* species, especially *C. glabrata*, are much more resistant to azoles (e.g., fluconazole). *Candida* sepsis related to indwelling catheters has a better outcome than *Candida* sepsis from other sources.

Aspergillus is also an increasingly common cause of pneumonia and osteomyelitis and infections involving the eyes, sinuses, nervous system, cardiovascular system, and skin. There is increasing recognition of *Aspergillus* species other than *A. fumigatus*, for example, *A. nidulans*, *A. flavus*, and *A. niger*, all of which may be more resistant to amphotericin.

Fungal infections are especially prevalent in neutropenic patients, where persistent fever despite broad-spectrum antibiotics, may be the only clinical indicator. Empirical treatment is often warranted in these patients.

Three classes of antifungals are commonly used in the PICU: polyene macrolides (amphotericin preparations), triazoles (fluconazole, and more recently voriconazole), and fluorinated pyrimadines (e.g., flucytosine). More recently the echinocandins (caspofungin, micofungin) have also been used. Side effects are class dependent: renal toxicity with polyene macrolides, myelosuppression with flucytosine, and gastrointestinal upset and deranged liver function with the azoles. Antifungal regimes vary between units, but currently, first-line empirical treatment is usually amphotericin. For febrile neutropenic patients, voriconazole and caspofungin may also be appropriate as first-line therapy.

Polyene Macrolides

Amphotericin was first introduced in 1956. It is fungicidal; binds to ergo-sterol, the principal sterol in the fungal cell membrane; and causes fungal cell death by increasing the permeability of the cell. It has a long half-life, has limited resistance but it penetrates poorly into the cerebrospinal fluid (CSF), and is not absorbed when given orally. The lipid formulations are less nephrotoxic, but more expensive than conventional amphotericin. In the U.K., it is currently the recommended first-line therapy for empirical antifungal therapy, and for disseminated candidiasis. There are case reports of high-dose amphotericin (up to 10 mg/kg) being successful in severe fungal infections, where lower doses have failed, but this is associated with very high cost and toxicity.

Fluorinated Pyrimidines

Flucytosine, converted to fluorouracil by enzymes within the fungal cell, disrupts fungal DNA synthesis and nuclear division. It has good CSF penetration and may be used in a synergistic combination with amphotericin. Resistance to flucytosine is conferred by a reduction in enzymatic activity and can develop during treatment. As it can cause bone marrow suppression, it is essential to monitor blood counts during treatment.

Triazoles

Fluconazole, by interfering with a cytochrome P-450–dependent enzyme, 14α-demethylase, impairs synthesis of ergosterol, essential for fungal cell membranes. It is well absorbed orally and has good CSF penetration; however, there are multiple drug interactions due to the inhibition of P-450. Mutations in genes encoding for 14α-demethylase confer resistance to all azoles and some *Candida* species are inherently less susceptible to azoles than to amphotericin.

Voriconazole is very potent against *Aspergillus*, *Cryptococcus*, and *Candida*. Recent studies have confirmed that it is well tolerated in children and as effective as liposomal amphotericin in neutropenic patients (22,23). Transient visual disturbances and altered liver function tests are the commonest side effects.

There is an active debate about whether voriconazole or amphotericin should be the first-line therapy for suspected fungal infection. Many adult centers have now moved to voriconazole as first-line use, although large trial data are still lacking in children.

Echinocandins

Caspofungin and micafungin inhibit 1,3,β$_2$-glucan synthesis, which is essential for the fungal cell membrane. They have a wide spectrum of activity against *Candida*, *Pneumocystis*, *Aspergillus*, and *Histoplasma*, but require parenteral administration and are poorly absorbed orally. Only fungi that have little or no glucan are resistant (e.g., mucorales and crpytococcus).

Caspofungin has been shown to be an effective empirical treatment for febrile neutropenic patients (23,24). Micafungin is fungicidal for *Candida* and fungistatic for *Aspergillus*.

Side effects of the echinocandins include deranged liver function tests. They should be avoided with concomitant use with cyclosporin A due to drug interactions.

Caspofungin is increasingly being used in combination therapy for severe fungal infection unresponsive to first-line therapy (25).

Novel Antifungals

New azoles under clinical development include Tak 187 and ER 30346. Niktlo-mycin 2, a chitin synthetase inhibitor, is currently undergoing phase 1 trials. Aureobasin a cyclic peptide is also undergoing trials, as is azoxybacillin, Ro 9156S, which inhibits regulation of genes required for the assimilation of fungal specific sulphate. Work is also progressing on specific inhibitors of known virulence factors, such as *C. albicans* phospholipases, which mediate cell penetration.

Viral Infections

Influenza

Oseltamivir is currently recommended for postexposure prophylaxis of at risk groups exposed to influenza, that is, those who have been in close household contact with influenza within the preceding 48 hours. At-risk persons are those who are immunocompromised or over 65 years of age, or older than 13 years of age with conditions such as diabetes mellitus, or those with chronic respiratory, cardiovascular, or renal disease and who are not vaccinated with the current strain. Amantadine is not recommended as postexposure prophylaxis (26).

Amantadine and rimantadine, tricyclic amines, both have activity against influenza A. Amantadine, which has good oral bioavailability, interferes with virus replication by blocking the M2 protein, an ion channel essential for uncoating the virus once it is inside the host cell. Side effects include nausea and anorexia. Neurologic effects such as agitation are also recognized but are not common. Rimantadine acts in a similar way to amantadine, but does not cross the blood–brain barrier and therefore has no neurologic side effects. Unfortunately, resistance to both these treatments has been shown to develop quickly where their use is widespread (27). Currently neither of these antivirals is recommended as treatment for, or prophylaxis of, influenza A.

Oseltamivir and zanamivir, inhibitors of viral neuramidase, are effective against both influenza A and B, by preventing detachment of virions from the cell surface (28). They have been shown to reduce the mean duration of symptoms when given within 48 hours of their onset, and are currently recommended in the U.K. for immunocompromised patients and those with chronic respiratory or renal disease (29). Oseltamivir has good oral bioavailability and has also been shown to be active against potential pandemic strains H5N1 and H9N2.

The most common side effects reported are gastrointestinal (vomiting). Zanamivir has to be administered in aerosol form (inhaled) and can cause bronchospasm.

There are limited data in children, although very early treatment in healthy children suggests that there is a reduction of duration of symptoms of around 1 day (30). There are no data on the effectiveness of these drugs in infants or the immunocompromised. However, there now are case reports of resistance to both oseltamivir and zanamivir. Kiso et al. (31) analyzed influenza A virus (H3N2) from 50 children before and during treatment with oseltamivir. They found neuraminidase mutations (conferring resistance to neuramidase inhibitors) in nine children and virus was detected even after 5 days of treatment, indicating residual infectivity. It is likely that children with the least ability to clear the virus (infants, immunocompromised) are those most likely to develop resistance.

Severe Acute Respiratory Distress Syndrome

Relatively few cases of severe acute respiratory distress syndrome (SARS), caused by the coronavirus, have been reported in children. Numerous antimicrobial therapies have been tried with no clear effect. Ribavirin, with or without concomitant steroids, has been used in an increasing number of patients. However, in the absence of clinical indicators, its effectiveness has not been proven. Vaccines are being investigated but are not yet available.

Avian Influenza

There are as yet no reported pediatric cases of avian influenza, due to H5N1, in the Western world, though there are an increasing number of cases reported in the developing world. Presenting symptoms have included fever, sore throat, and cough progressing to severe respiratory distress, secondary to viral pneumonia. In addition, encephalopathy, disseminated intravascular coagulopathy, and severe gastrointestinal dysfunction is reported. Previously healthy adults and children, and some with chronic medical conditions, have been affected.

The M2 inhibitors (amantadine and rimantadine) and the neuraminidase inhibitors (oseltamivir and zanamivir) have been licensed for the prevention and treatment of humans infected with avian influenza in some countries. Initial analysis of viruses isolated from the recently fatal cases in Vietnam indicates that the viruses are invariably resistant to the M2 inhibitors. Further testing is under way to confirm the resistance of amantadine and the effectiveness of neuraminidase inhibitors against the current H5N1 strains.

Enteroviruses

Although the majority of enteroviral infections in children are benign, they can cause sepsis, encephalitis, and meningitis, of which the latter peaks in the summer and autumn (32). Polymerase chain reaction (PCR) of the CSF is the most rapid diagnostic test. Pleconaril binds to the virus protein capsid and interferes with viral replication by affecting viral attachment and uncoating. It is well absorbed orally and has been shown to be partially effective in mild disease, with symptoms improving within 24 to 48 hours (33). However, recent studies have confirmed that it is of no benefit in enteroviral meningitis. The Collaborative Antiviral Study Group (CASG) 106 trial of pleconaril in severe neonatal disease is currently on hold.

Cytomegalovirus

Ganciclovir and foscarnet remain first-line therapy for systemic cytomegalovirus (CMV) infection (34). A recent study of combination therapy in adult transplant patients showed no added benefit when compared to single-agent therapy (35). Valganciclovir, the prodrug of ganciclovir, has been shown to be well absorbed orally in the treatment of infants with congenital CMV in the CASG 109 trial (36). A further study is planned to compare the outcome of 6 weeks of treatment versus 6 months of treatment.

Conclusion

It is becoming more widely recognized that there is an increasing risk of children presenting with critical illness to the PICU and of those within the PICU developing life-threatening nosocomial sepsis with multidrug-resistant organisms. However, if every PICU treats all children with suspected sepsis with very broad-spectrum antibiotics (such as the carbapenems and glycopeptides), inevitably this will drive antimicrobial resistance on their unit still further. There is a real and urgent need for further clinical studies defining the risk factors that are most likely to predict those children presenting with severe infections due to resistant organisms.

With a fall in the number of cases of bacteremia due to community-acquired infections such as *Haemophilus influenzae* type b (Hib) and meningococci and pneumococci due to widespread vaccination against these organisms, the management of children with severe sepsis of unknown etiology is going to become more complicated. There is an increased probability that children will present with resistant gram-positive bacteremia, and this includes MRSA and other resistant organisms.

There is a need for improved national data collection about PICU-related sepsis, microbiologic isolates, and antimicrobial resistance rates. Each PICU must have in place an annual review of its microbiology isolates and antibiotic policies, to compare with national data.

Antibiotic prescribing choices have impact directly on the microbiologic flora in each unit. As the management of MDR infections becomes ever more complex and new antimicrobials are introduced, perhaps it is sensible for all PICUs to introduce regular multidisciplinary infection rounds with pediatric infectious disease and microbiology specialists.

References

1. Gold HS, Mollering RC Jr. Antimicrobial-drug resistance. N Engl J Med 1996;335(19): 1445–1453.
2. Lieberman JM. Appropriate antibiotic use and why it is important: the challenges of bacterial resistance. Pediatr Infect Dis J 2003;22(12):1143–1151.
3. Farr BM, Salgado CD, Karchmer TB, Sherertz RJ. Can antibiotic-resistant nosocomial infections be controlled? Lancet Infect Dis 2001;1(1):8–45.
4. Urrea M, Pons M, Serra M, Latorre C, Palomeque A. Prospective incidence study of nosocomial infections in a pediatric intensive care unit. Pediatr Infect Dis J 2003;22(6):490–494.
5. Clark NM, Hershberger E, Zervosc MJ, Lynch JP 3rd. Antimicrobial resistance among gram-positive organisms in the intensive care unit. Curr Opin Crit Care 2003;9(5):403–412.
6. Khairulddin N, Bishop L, Lamagni TL, Sharland M, Duckworth G. Emergence of methicillin resistant Staphylococcal Aureus (MRSA) bacteraemia among children in England and Wales, 1990–2001. Arch Dis Child 2004;89:378–379.
7. De Man P, Verhoeven BA, Verbrugh HA, Vos MC, van den Anker JN. An antibiotic policy to prevent emergence of resistant bacilli. Lancet Infect Dis 2000;355(9208): 973–978.
8. Nambiar S, Singh N. Change in epidemiology of health care-associated infections in a neonatal intensive care unit. Pediatr Infect Dis J 2002;21(9):839–842.
9. HPA Report. Investigation into multidrug resistant ESBL producing E Coli strains causing infections in England. 2005.
10. Buckingham S, McCullers JA, Lujan-Zilbermann J, Knapp K, Orman K, English K, Pneumococcal meningitis in children: relationship of antibiotic resistance and to clinical characteristics and outcomes. Pediatr Infect Dis J 2001;20(9):837–843.
11. Garau J. Treatment of drug resistant Pneumococcal pneumonia. Lancet Infect Dis 2002;2:404–415.
12. Jacobs MR. Worldwide trends in antimicrobial resistance among common respiratory tract pathogens in children. Pediatr Infect Dis J 2003;22(8):S109–119.
13. Liberati A, D'Amico R, Pifferi, Torri V, Brazzi L. Antibiotic prophylaxis to reduce respiratory tract infections and mortality in adults receiving intensive care. Cochrane Database Syst Rev 2004;1:CD000022.
14. Wilcox M, Nathwani D, Dryden M. Linezolid compared with teicoplanin for the treatment of suspected or proven Gram-positive infections. J Antimicrob Chemother 2004;53(2):335–344.
15. Jantausuch B, Deville J, Adler S, et al. Linezolid for the treatment of children with bacteraemia or nosocomial pneumonia caused by resistant Gram positive bacterial pathogens. Pediatr Infect Dis J 2003;22:S164–171.
16. Saiman L, Goldfarb J, Kaplan S, et al. Safety and tolerability of linezolid in children. Pediatr Infect Dis J 2003;22:S193–200.
17. Jacqueline C, Navas D, Batard E, et al. In vitro and in vivo synergistic activities of linezolid combined with subinhibitory concentrations of imipenem against methicillin-resistant Staphylococcus aureus. Antimicrob Agents Chemother 2005;49(1):45–51.
18. Raad I, Hachem R, Hana H, et al. Treatment of vancomycin resistant enterococcal infections in the immunocompromised host: quinopristin-dalfopristin in combination with minocycline. Antimicrob Agents Chemother 2001;3202–3204.

19. Keating GM, Scott LJ. Moxifloxacin: a review of its use in the management of bacterial infections. Drugs 2004;64(20):2347–2377.
20. Safdar N, Handelsman J, Maki G. Does combination antimicrobial therapy reduce mortality in Gram-negative bacteraemia? A Meta analysis. Lancet Infect Dis 2004;4:519–527.
21. Denning D, Kibbler CC, Barnes R. British Society for Medical Mycology proposed standards of care for patients with invasive fungal infection. Lancet Infect Dis 2003;3:230–240.
22. Walsh TJ, Pappas P, Winston DJ, et al. Voriconazole compared with liposomal amphotericin B for empirical antifungal therapy in patients with neutropaenia and persistent fever. N Engl J Med 2002;34624(4):225–234.
23. Walsh TJ, Karlsson MO, Driscoll T, et al. Pharmacokinetics and safety of intravenous voriconazole in children after single- or multiple-dose administration. Antimicrob Agents Chemother 2004;48(6):2166–2172.
24. Walsh TJ, Teppler H, Donowitz GR, et al. Caspofungin versus liposomal amphotericin B for empirical antifungal therapy in patients with persistent fever and neutropenia. N Engl J Med 2004;351(14):1391–1402.
25. Safdar A, Rodriguez G, Rolston KV, et al. High-dose caspofungin combination antifungal therapy in patients with hematologic malignancies and hematopoietic stem cell transplantation. Bone Marrow Transplant 2007;39(3):157–164.
26. National Institute for Clinical Excellence. Guidance on the use of zanamivir, oseltamivir and amantadine for the treatment of influenza. 2005.
27. Mc Kimm-Breschkin JL. Management of influenza virus infections with neuroaminidase inhibitors: detection, incidence and implications of drug resistance. Treat Respir Med 2005;4(2):107–116.
28. Brooks MJ, Sasadeusz JJ, Tannock GA. Antiviral chemotherapeutic agents against respiratory viruses: where are we now and what's in the pipeline? Curr Opin Pulmon Med 2004;10(3):197–203.
29. Ward P, Small I, Smith J, Suter P, Dutkowski R. Oseltamivir (Tamiflu) and its potential for use in the event of an influenza pandemic. J Antimicrob Chemother 2005;55(suppl 1):i5–i21.
30. Uyeki TM. Influenza diagnosis and treatment in children: a review of studies on clinically useful tests and antiviral treatment for influenza. Pediatr Infect Dis J 2003;22(2):164–177.
31. Kiso M, Mitamura K, Sakai-Tagawa Y, et al. Resistant influenza A viruses in Children treated with oseltamivir: descriptive study. Lancet 2004;364:759–765.
32. Abzug MJ. Presentation, diagnosis, and management of enterovirus infections in neonates. Paediatr Drugs 2004;6(1):1–10.
33. Abzug MJ, C.G., Bradley J, et al. National Institute of Allergy and Infectious Diseases Collaborative Antiviral Study Group. Double blind placebo controlled trial of pleconaril in infants with enteroviral meningitis. Pediatr Infect Dis J 2003;22(4):335–341.
34. Zerr DM, Frenkel LM. Advances in antiviral therapy. Curr Opin Pediatr 1999;11(1): 21–27.
35. Mattes FM, Hainsworth EG, Geretti AM, et al. A randomized, controlled trial comparing ganciclovir to ganciclovir plus foscarnet (each at half dose) for preemptive therapy of cytomegalovirus infection in transplant recipients. J Infect Dis 2004;189(8): 1355–1361.
36. Collaborative Antiviral Study Group. CASG 109: a phase II pharmacokinetic and pharmacodynamic evaluation of oral valganciclovir in neonates with symptomatic congenital CMV infection involving the central nervous system. 2005.

9
Host Genetic Susceptibility to Infection

Shamez N. Ladhani and Robert Booy

The risk of infection depends on complex interactions among the host, the pathogen, and the environment. Some pathogens, such as *Neisseria meningitidis* and *Streptococcus pneumoniae*, can cause serious life-threatening illness in healthy individuals, while others, such as *Pneumocystis carinii*, rely more on deficiencies in the host's immune system, for example due to chronic illness or immunosuppression, to cause serious infection. Moreover, the presentation and severity of illness vary considerably in different individuals exposed to the same organism. These differences result from variable virulence of different strains of the same pathogen and because of differences in the host's immune response (1–6). *N. meningitidis*, for example, can cause meningitis in some individuals, with a case fatality rate of around 5%, and septic shock in others, which has a case fatality rate of up to 40% (7).

Strong support for a host genetic basis for susceptibility to infection was provided by the research of Sorensen and colleagues (8). The authors identified all adoptees born between 1924 and 1926 from the Danish Adoption Register and followed them up to 1982. They determined the cause of death in the adoptees, and in their biologic and adoptive parents. They found that if a biologic parent died of infection before the age of 50 years, the child had a 5.81-fold (95% confidence interval [CI], 2.47–13.7) increased risk of also dying of infection, suggesting a strong genetic influence on the risk of death due to infection. The risk of death due to a cardiovascular or cerebrovascular event was also increased 4.5–fold (95% CI, 1.3–15.4) if a biologic parent also died of the same cause before the age of 50 years. On the other hand, the death of an adoptive parent due to infection or a vascular event did not confer an increased risk of death in the adopted child. Other twin studies have also shown a greater than twofold concordance in monozygotic compared with dizygotic twins for tuberculosis (9), leprosy (10), poliomyelitis (11), and hepatitis B (12). In respect to meningococcal disease, Haralambous and colleagues (13) studied 845 siblings of 443 white United Kingdom patients with meningococcal disease and found that 27 siblings, compared to an expected one case, contracted meningococcal disease. The sibling risk ratio (λS), calculated as the ratio of observed meningococcal disease cases among siblings of U.K. Caucasian cases to that expected, was 30.3, and, irrespective of whether siblings contracted meningococcal disease more than 1, 3, 6, 9, or 12 months after the index case, there was little variation in the λS (range: 8.2–11.9), suggesting that host genetic factors may contribute approximately one third of the total λS. This study demonstrated a strong association between genetic susceptibility and meningococcal disease.

Mendelian Inheritance and Susceptibility

Mendelian conditions that predispose to specific infections provide important clues for identifying the genes responsible and their role in susceptibility to infections. Mutations associated with mendelian inheritance, particularly recessive forms and dominant ones with near-complete penetrance, are often associated with a high risk of severe infection and death if not treated aggressively or prevented by bone marrow transplantation. The genetic basis of many inherited immunodeficiency syndromes has now been characterized. Common primary immunodeficiencies include disorders of humoral immunity (affecting B-cell differentiation or antibody production), T-cell function, combined B- and T-cell defects, phagocytic disorders, and complement deficiencies (14).

Severe combined immunodeficiency (SCID), for example, is characterized by an absence of T cells and all adaptive immunity. The first case of human SCID was described in 1950 (15). Children with SCID develop recurrent severe bacterial, viral, and fungal infections, with a high mortality rate within the first year of life if they do not receive bone marrow transplantation (16). The first genetic mutation responsible for SCID was identified in 1972 in the gene encoding adenosine deaminase, an enzyme required for detoxification of metabolic products within T cells (17). Since then, through completion of the Human Genome Project, advances in molecular biology and our understanding of the different immune pathways, mutations in at least 10 different genes have been shown to lead to development of SCID, through X-linked recessive or autosomal recessive inheritance, depending on the defect.

The most common mutation responsible for SCID occurs in the gene responsible for the γ chain of the interleukin-2 receptor (IL-2R), which is also shared by other interleukin receptors, including IL-4R, IL-7R, IL-9R, IL-15R, and IL-21R (18,19). Through understanding of the pathways involved in intracellular cytokine signaling, a mutation in the intracellular Janus kinase 3 (JAK3) signaling molecule that is activated by the IL-2R γ chain was also identified as a cause of SCID (20). Mutations in the genes encoding other molecules associated with development of the T-cell antigen receptor complex (including recombinase activating gene 1 [RAG1], RAG2, *Artemis*, CD3δ, and CD3ε) and CD45, a transmembrane protein tyrosine phosphatase that is essential for intracellular signal transduction through antigen receptors (21), have also been shown to lead to SCID (16,22). These gene products play an important role in T-cell development and function, and therefore affect activation and regulation of other cells within the immune system.

The genetic basis for other severe immunodeficiencies affecting T cells (such as CD40 ligand deficiency and hyper–immunoglobulin M [IgM] syndrome), B cells, neutrophils, and other cells of the immune system are continually being discovered (23–29). However, these mutations are rare and therefore unlikely to be responsible for the bulk of susceptibility to infection in the general population (30,31). Instead, alleles that are found more commonly in the general population but have minor effects on gene function are more likely to play an important role in explaining individual differences in susceptibility to infection.

Genetic mutations and polymorphisms are both differences in the genomic DNA sequences that occur naturally in a population. However, mutations are rare and, by definition, occur in less than 1% of the general population, while polymorphisms occur when the least common allele is found in at least 1% of the population. Single nucleotide polymorphisms (SNPs, commonly pronounced "snips"), which can be insertions, substitutions, or deletions, are single base differences that can be observed between individuals in a population at an average frequency of 1 per 300 to 1 per 500 base pairs (32,33). Within a gene, SNPs can occur (in order of increasing frequency) in introns (a noncoding sequence on the gene), the nontranslated (such as the promoter) region, and exons (a protein-coding genetic segment) (34). The SNPs in the intron region are unlikely to have a biologic effect, but they may be in linkage disequilibrium (two alleles at different genetic loci that occur together in an individual more often that would be expected by random chance) with another polymorphism in the same gene, which may be functionally important. The SNPs in the promoter region can alter binding affinity to different nuclear factors and, therefore, alter the rate of gene transcription and the amount of protein produced. The SNPs occurring within the 5'-upstream and 3'-downstream regions can affect the stability of messenger RNA (mRNA) or alter enhancer activity, thereby altering the efficiency of gene transcription or mRNA translation. The SNPs in the exon region often do not have functional consequences (silent SNPs) because they do not result in an amino acid change. In some cases, however, a SNP in the exon region can result in an amino acid substitution (nonsynonymous SNP) that can alter the structure or function of the resulting protein.

Polymorphisms in microsatellites may also be associated with increased risk of disease. Microsatellites are simple repetitive DNA sequences found throughout the human genome that tend to exhibit polymorphism in the number of repeats and are thus multiallelic (35). Although microsatellites themselves do not encode for protein products, they tend to occur in close proximity to the candidate genes and, because of this proximity, inheritance of certain microsatellite alleles is likely to occur simultaneously with functional polymorphisms within the candidate gene during meiosis, resulting in both the microsatellite repeat and the polymorphism being inherited from the same parent.

One of the earliest polymorphisms identified to have a role in susceptibility to infection was the β-globin gene responsible for sickle cell disease in people of African ancestry (36). An A to T substitution in the β-globin gene results in change from glutamic acid (GAG) to valine (GTG) at position 6, resulting in the production of hemoglobin S. Individuals carrying two copies of the hemoglobin S gene develop sickle cell disease, a blood condition that results in severe anemia and acute painful episodes associated with tissue hypoperfusion and ischemia. However, heterozygotes carrying a single copy of the hemoglobin S gene are strongly protected against severe malaria (37), probably by impairing entry into and growth of parasites in affected red cells (38). Other hemoglobin-opathies, such as α- and β-thalassemias (39) and glucose-6-phosphate dehy-drogenase deficiency (40) which, like sickle cell disease, are also more prevalent among Africans from malaria-endemic regions, have also been shown to confer protection against life-threatening malaria.

Studying Genetic Polymorphisms

Identification of the gene responsible in single-gene defect diseases has been relatively successful in terms of both speed and efficiency because of recent advances in genetic technology and the use of techniques such as linkage analy-sis and positional mapping. However, the study of conditions that are polygenic with nonmendelian inheritance, such as diabetes mellitus, atherosclerosis, and susceptibility to sepsis, is more difficult. There is often variable penetration of the genes involved, which are commonly at different loci, with a lack of family segregation. In addition, susceptibility to sepsis is compounded by a host of environmental risk factors, degree of exposure to the pathogen, and heteroge-neity of the organisms responsible.

Currently, the most common method of determining the contribution of different genetic polymorphisms in polygenic diseases involves studying can-didate genes that are known or suspected to play a role in disease pathogenesis. A higher frequency of any polymorphism identified in the candidate gene in individuals with the disease in question compared with sex- and ethnically-matched controls who do not have the disease would suggest a significant association. However, this association does not indicate causation and should be supported with a plausible biologic explanation along with in vitro and transgenic studies to determine how the polymorphism would affect the risk or severity of the disease. Many studies have examined the role of various gene mutations and polymorphisms in infections, but results can be difficult to compare because of differences in the case definitions used, heterogeneity within the control population, and the relatively small number of cases and controls in many studies.

With infection, genes that encode molecules associated with the immune system are those most likely to play an important role. The phylogenetically ancient system of innate immunity is considered to be the first-line defense against invading microbes and plays a vital role in the immediate response to pathogens. Unlike antibodies and T-cell receptors, which rely on somatic muta-tions, molecular participants of innate immunity are encoded in the genome. The innate system has evolved a range of mechanisms to recognize and attack foreign molecules through specialized pattern recognition receptors (PRRs) on cell membranes and within intracellular compartments, where they are able to distinguish self antigens from nonself. At least three different molecular systems play a vital role in the innate system, including Toll-like receptors on phagocytes, the complement system, and unique lineages of bone-marrow–derived cells that bear pattern recognition receptors on their cell surface. All these systems work together to alert the adaptive immune system through cytokine mediators and also have direct effects on other protective pathways such as the coagulation and fibrinolysis cascades. Genetic polymorphisms within key molecules involved in any of the pathways, therefore, may be important determinants of susceptibility to or severity of infection in individuals. These polymorphisms have been studied in a wide range of infections caused by bacteria (41–46), mycobacteria (47–50), viruses (46,51–56) and other organisms (57–62). This chapter focuses primarily on genetic susceptibility to bacterial infections. However many of the principles involved and limitations of published studies also apply to other infectious agents.

The Toll-Like Receptor Complex

Pattern recognition receptors recognize pathogen-associated molecular patterns (PAMPs), which are key molecules unique to different microbes. Lipopolysaccharide (LPS) or endotoxin is an important example of a pathogen-associated molecular pattern and is found on the outer membrane of Gram-negative bacterial cell walls (Fig. 9.1). Lipopolysaccharide consists of a highly variable polysaccharide (O-polysaccharide chain and R-core region) and a lipid component known as lipid A, which is responsible for the molecule's toxicity (63). Lipopolysaccharide is cleared both by nonimmunologic (through binding alkaline phosphatase and cholesterol) and immunologic mechanisms. The latter include binding to LPS-binding protein (LBP) and bactericidal/permeability increasing protein (BPI)—two highly conserved, structurally and functionally related lipid transfer proteins, whose genes are located on chromosome 10 (64,65). The BPI is a cationic protein produced by polymorphonuclear leukocytes that is cytotoxic to Gram-negative bacteria and also inhibits LPS-induced host cell responses (66). The LBP is produced constitutively by the liver. Binding of LBP to lipopolysaccharide is essential before it is recognized by the LPS receptor (cluster differentiation 14 [CD14]) on the surface of macrophages and monocytes (64). The LBP is also able to help bind whole Gram-negative bacteria to CD14, leading to phagocytosis and subsequent clearance of the bacteria (67). The concentrations of both BPI and LBP are increased in severe sepsis, suggesting that they have an important function as acute phase proteins (68).

Intravenous injection of a 21-kd modified N-terminal of recombinant BPI (rBPI21) has been shown to increase survival and decrease bacteremia in rats after intravenous injection of *Escherichia coli* (69). The rBPI21 also inhibited the rise in tumor necrosis factor-α (TNF-α) following intravenous challenge with

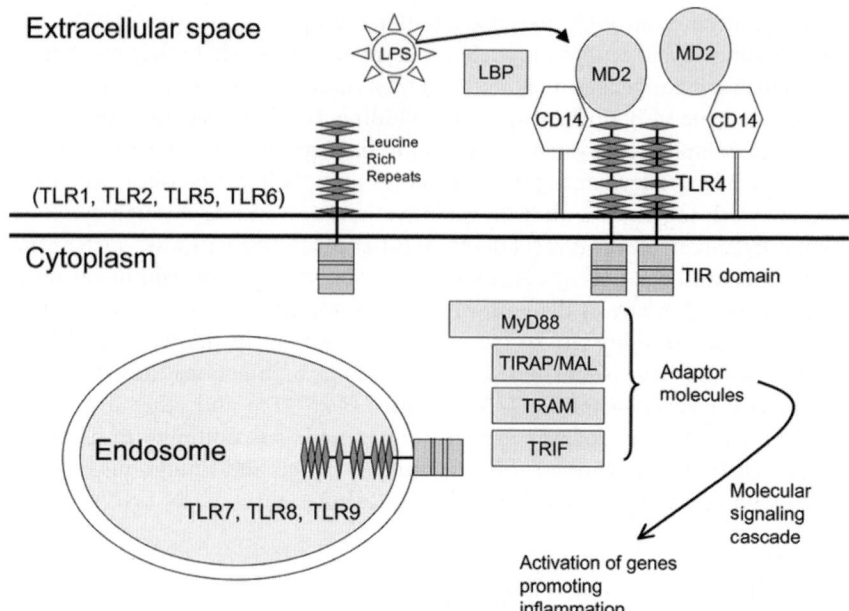

FIGURE 9.1. Human Toll-like receptors. TLR1, TLR2, TLR4, TLR5, and TLR6 are located on the cell surface, while TLR7, TLR8, and TLR9 are located inside endosomes. The location of TLR3 is uncertain. The extracytoplasmic domains of the TLRs contain leucine-rich repeats (flat diamonds) and the intracytoplasmic domains contain conserved domains known as the TIR domain. The recognition of lipopolysaccharide (LPS) from Gram-negative bacteria by TLR4 requires the presence of LPS-binding protein (LBP), cluster differentiation 14 (CD14), and MD2. Activation of TLR4 triggers a cascade of intracellular events involving a host of adaptor molecules such as MyD88, TIRAP, TRAM, and TRIF, and ultimately resulting in activation of genes that promote inflammation. (From Warren HS. Toll-like receptors. Crit Care Med 2005;33(12 suppl):S457–459, with permission.)

two strains of *E. coli*. In children with meningococcal sepsis, there was a trend toward more multiple severe amputations in those who received placebo compared with rBPI21 (15/203 [7.4%] vs. 6/190 [3.2%]; $p=.067$; odds ratio [OR], 2.5; 95% CI, 0.94–6.51), and fewer children given placebo had functional outcomes similar to that before illness 2 months later (126/190 [66.3%] vs. 136/176 [77.3%], $p=.019$) (70). Along similar lines, high concentrations of LBP such as those found in the acute phase response can block LPS-induced TNF-α release in murine macrophages in vitro, and inhibit LPS-mediated cytokine release, prevent hepatic failure, and increase survival in a murine model of bacteremia (71).

Lipopolysaccharide-Binding Protein–Bactericidal/Permeability Increasing Protein

Three biallelic polymorphisms have been identified in the BPI gene—Lys216Glu (A645G substitution), a PStI (T→C) polymorphism in intron 5, and a silent

TABLE 9.1. Clinical studies on lipopolysaccharide binding protein (LBP) and bactericidal/permeability increasing protein (BPI) polymorphisms

Country (reference)	Cases	No.	Controls	No.	SNP	Su/Se/Ou	Significance	Comments
LBP								
Germany (72)	Consecutive patients with sepsis	204	Healthy individuals	250	Cys98Gly allele	Su	0.35 vs. 0.25, p=0.02*	Males with sepsis had higher frequency of at least 1 allele (42% vs. 28%, p=0.02)
					Pro436Leu allele	Su	0.23 vs. 0.15, p=0.04*	G654C always associated with PstI (T→C) and Lys216Glu alleles
	Nonsurvivors	97	Survivors	107	Cys98Gly allele	Ou	0.32 vs. 0.37, p=NS	All 6 Cys98Gly homozygotes died
					Pro436Leu allele	Ou	0.16 vs. 0.29, p=NS	All 5 Pro436Leu homozygotes died
BPI								
Germany (72)	Consecutive patients with sepsis	204	Healthy individuals	250	Lys216Glu homozygous	Su	0.26 vs. 0.23, p=NS	G654C always associated with PstI (T→C) and Lys216Glu alleles
					G545C allele	Su	0.22 vs. 0.18, p=NS	
					PstI CC homozygous	Su	0.19 vs. 0.21, p=NS	
	Nonsurvivors	97	Survivors	107	Lys216Glu Homozygous	Ou	0.28 vs. 0.24, p=NS	
					G545C allele	Ou	0.13 vs. 0.30, p=0.0076*	
					PstI CC homozygous	Ou	0.21 vs. 0.17, p=NS	

*Significance levels calculated form raw data presented by the authors, who reported no significant difference between the two proportions.
SNP, single nucleotide polymorphism; Su/Se/Ou, susceptibility/severity/outcome; NS, not significant.

G545C variation—and two in the LBP gene (Cys98Gly and Pro436Leu) (Table 9.1). Hubacek and colleagues (72) examined these polymorphisms in 204 patients with sepsis and 250 healthy controls. The authors noted that the G545C silent mutation always occurred with the PstI (T→C) polymorphism and the Lys216Glu allele in the cases as well as the controls, suggesting that they were in linkage disequilibrium. Although the authors reported no significant difference in LBP genotypes between patients with sepsis and controls, analysis of their data suggests that carriers of both the Cys98Gly (35% vs. 25%, $p=.02$) and the Pro436Leu (23% vs. 15%, $p=.04$) alleles had a significantly higher risk of sepsis compared with healthy controls. In addition, the Pro436Leu allele was associated with increased survival (16% vs. 29%, $p=.052$). For BPI, there was no association between the three polymorphisms and the risk of sepsis, but the homozygous CC genotype at position 545 was associated with survival (13% vs. 30%, $p=.0076$) (Table 9.1). Gender analysis showed that Gly98 allele of LBP was more frequently found among male patients with sepsis compared with controls (42% vs. 28%, $p=.02$). A similar trend was reported with the Leu436 allele of LBP among males (26.7% vs. 16.3%, $p=.065$). However, these observed gender associations were only identified during post-hoc analysis and did not form part of the investigators' initial hypotheses; therefore, they must be interpreted with caution. On the other hand, the nine patients who were homozygote for either Gly98 ($n=6$) or Leu436 ($n=5$) were exclusively found among the 97 patients who died. Only one individual in the control group ($n=250$) had one of these rare homozygous genotypes. As with the BPI polymorphisms, the authors also found that the rare Leu436 allele was more frequently detected in individuals with the rare Gly98 allele, suggesting linkage disequilibrium. It should be noted that this study by Hubacek and colleagues (72) included patients with Gram-positive and Gram-negative sepsis, and both BPI and LBP only bind LPS from Gram-negative organisms. It is, therefore, possible that some of the negative findings reported may be due to inappropriate patient selection and/or a lack of power.

Cluster Differentiation 14

Cluster differentiation 14 (CD14) is a glycosylphosphatidylinositol-anchored membrane protein that recognizes a wide range of microbial products, including LPS from Gram-negative organisms, as well as peptidoglycans and lipoteichoic acid from Gram-positive organisms. CD14 has no transmembrane domain, and therefore cannot initiate intracellular signaling. However, binding of microbial products to CD14 is a vital step before they can be recognized by Toll-like receptors (73). Two soluble forms of CD14 (sCD14) also exist in plasma and are acute-phase proteins (74,75). The soluble forms of CD14 can bind the LPS-LBP and activate CD14-negative cells such as endothelial and epithelial cells (76). Overexpression of sCD14 in transgenic mice made them hypersensitive to LPS (77), while sCD14-deficient mice were insensitive to the effects of LPS (78). Increased levels of sCD14 have been shown to correlate with increased mortality in both Gram-positive and Gram-negative sepsis (76,79). It is possible that increased levels result in intense inflammation and activation of other cells such as endothelial and epithelial cells, which normally do not have membrane-associated CD14 molecules. This immune overactivation can be detrimental to the host and result in a worse outcome (80).

A genetic polymorphism has been identified in the CD14 promoter region and consists of a C to T transition 159 base pairs (bp) from the major transcription site, close to an important regulatory Sp1 transcription factor binding site (81–84). Individuals with the T allele have significantly increased circulating sCD14 and higher density of the monocyte CD14 receptors compared with carriers of the C allele (82–84). Transfection studies have shown that the T allele had higher promoter activity on gene expression than the C allele (84) and in vitro stimulation with LPS of monocytes bearing the homozygous TT genotype resulted in significantly higher levels of sCD14 and TNF-α compared with monocytes bearing the C allele (84).

Several studies have examined the role of CD14 polymorphisms in infections, but their results are difficult to compare because of differences in the case definitions used, the heterogeneity of control populations, and the small number of cases and controls in most studies (85,86) (Table 9.2). In a recent study of critically ill patients with systemic inflammatory response syndrome (SIRS), the homozygous TT promoter genotype was significantly associated with a positive blood culture (relative risk [RR], 1.4; $p < .02$), particularly with Gram-negative organisms (87). Systemic inflammatory response syndrome is considered to be due to overamplification of cytokines by immune cells, and patients with SIRS often progress to multiorgan failure and shock, which can result in death. In another study, the CD14 -159T allelic frequency (55% vs. 43%, $p = .012$) but not the TT genotype (31% vs. 21%, $p = .24$) was significantly higher in patients with septic shock. Similarly, the T allele frequency was higher among patients with septic shock who died compared with those who survived (65% vs. 42%, $p = .003$) (80). In a multiple logistic regression model, the homozygous CD14 -159TT genotype was independently associated with death (RR, 5.3; 95% CI, 1.2–22.5; $p = .02$). However, several other studies were unable to demonstrate increased risk of infection, sepsis, SIRS, or death associated with the CD14 T allele (85,86,88,89). It is of note that none of these studies measured soluble- or membrane-associated CD14 levels and their association with genotype, clinical disease, or outcome. Another study reported no significant difference in membrane-associated CD14 density, soluble CD14 levels, or TNF-α concentrations in healthy blood donors possessing the three different CD14 genotypes: CC, CT, and TT (90). Together, these results suggest that the CD14 polymorphism is not likely to have a major role in susceptibility, severity, or outcome of infection.

Toll-Like Receptors

Toll-like receptors (TLRs) recognize distinct pathogen-associated molecular patterns that have been evolutionarily conserved in specific classes of pathogens (Fig. 9.1) (91). Binding of specific microbial molecules to TLRs results in a cascade of events that eventually lead to production of reactive oxygen species

TABLE 9.2. Clinical studies on cluster differentiation 14 (CD14) polymorphisms

Country (reference)	Cases	No.	Controls	No.	SNP	Su/Se/Ou	Significance	Comments
Canada (87)	Positive blood cultures in critically ill patients with SIRS	127	Negative blood cultures	120	-159TT	Su	0.30 vs. 0.17, $p < .02$, RR = 1.4	Gram-negative infections associated with T allele (30% vs. 16%, $p < .03$)
France (80)	Nonsurvivors	84	Survivors	163	-159TT	Ou	0.26 vs. 0.22, $p =$ NS	
	White adults with septic shock	90	Healthy matched white controls	122	-159TT	Su	0.31 vs. 0.21, $p = .046$	
	Nonsurvivors of septic shock	50	Survivors	40	-159TT	Ou	0.40 vs. 0.20, $p = .008$	TT genotype associated with death in logistic regression, $p = .02$, OR = 5.3 (1.2–22.5)
U.S. (86)	SIRS in surgical patients admitted to intensive care unit	77	Unrelated healthy volunteers	39	-159TT	Su	0.22 vs. (data not given), $p =$ NS	
Germany (88)	Nonsurvivors of SIRS	12	Survivors	65	-159TT	Ou	(data not given), $p =$ NS	No difference is susceptibility between males and females
	Severe sepsis in adults	204	Controls (unknown source)	247	-159TT	Su	0.20 vs. 0.22, $p =$ NS	
	Nonsurvivors of severe sepsis	107	Survivors	97	-159TT	Ou	0.21 vs 0.18, $p =$ NS	
Germany (85)	Severe sepsis in adults with blunt trauma	14	No sepsis	44	-159TT	Su	0.29 vs. 0.16, $p =$ NS	
	Nonsurvivors of severe sepsis	6	Survivors	52	-159TT	Ou	0.33 vs. 0.17, $p =$ NS	
U.S. (89)	Severe sepsis in adults with severe burns	36	Mild or no sepsis	123	-159TT	Su/Se	0.083 vs. 0.22, $p =$ NS	

RR, relative risk; SIRS, systemic inflammatory response syndrome; SNP, single nucleotide polymorphism; Su/Se/Ou, susceptibility/severity/outcome; NS, not significant.

and upregulation of proinflammatory cytokines by NF-κB, a eukaryotic nuclear factor that plays an important role in inflammation, autoimmune response, cell proliferation, and apoptosis by regulating the expression of genes involved in these processes. At least 10 different TLRs have been identified and each interacts with different microbial cell wall products. TLR2 and TLR4 are of particular interest because they recognize cell wall components of Gram-positive and Gram-negative organisms, respectively. Appropriate ligand binding to either TLR2 or TLR4 results in activation of common intracellular pathways ultimately leading to activation of NF-κB and upregulation of proinflammatory cytokines, including TNF-α, IL-1, and IL-6.

TLR4

TLR4 is expressed on macrophages, endothelial cells, airway epithelia, smooth muscle cells, and, in small amounts, in most other tissues (92). It is a critical sensor for LPS, and binding of LPS to TLR4 results in activation of macrophages and monocytes and secretion of inflammatory cytokines (93). Activation of TLR4 requires binding to the LPS-LBP-CD14 complex and another molecule, MD2 (Fig. 9.1). The TLR4 in the mouse strain C3H/HeJ harbors a point mutation at Pro712His within exon 3 in the cytoplasmic domain that renders it nonfunctional (94), while the C57BL/10ScCR strain has a deletion of TLR4 (95). Both these strains of mice are at high risk for Gram-negative infection (96,97). Based on these animal studies, it was proposed that TLR4 mutations in humans could also be associated with an increased risk of Gram-negative sepsis.

Two co-segregating polymorphisms and a number of rare missense mutations have been identified in the human TLR4 gene. A common adenine for guanine substitution at nucleotide 896 from the start codon of the TLR4 gene (A896G) results in replacement of an aspartic acid residue with glycine at amino acid 299 (Asp299Gly) in the fourth exon of TLR4 and alters the extracellular domain of the receptor (86). The allelic frequency of the A896G substitution had been reported to be 6.6% and 7.9% in two United States white populations and 3.3% in a French Caucasian study (95). A co-segregating point mutation that results in a threonine to isoleucine substitution at amino acid position 399 (Thr399Ile) has also been reported. Initially, Arbour and colleagues (95) examined whether TLR4 polymorphisms were associated with the variability observed in airflow obstruction when different individuals are challenged with LPS. They found that seven (22.6%) of the LPS-hyporesponsive subjects had the co-segregating Asp299Gly and the Thr399Ile variants of TLR4 compared with only three LPS-responsive subjects (5.8%, $p = .029$). To ensure that other mutations were not responsible for the observed hyporesponsiveness, the authors sequenced the entire coding region and splice sites of the TLR4 gene and found only one other missense mutation (A137G leading to Try46Cys substitution), which was present in one LPS-hyporesponsive and one LPS-responsive subject, suggesting that this mutation did not have a role in responsiveness to LPS (95). In vitro studies showed that the Asp299Gly substitution was more effective than the TLR4 Thr399Ile substitution in reducing cell responsiveness to LPS. Furthermore, LPS responsiveness could be restored by transfection of epithelial cells and alveolar macrophages with vectors containing the wild-type genes (95). For the Asp299Gly substitution, it is speculated that replacement of the conserved Asp with Gly at position 299 causes disruption of the α-helical protein, resulting in a β-strand, which could affect ligand binding (95).

In a large cohort of 810 adults recruited randomly, the Asp299Gly polymorphism was associated with low levels of inflammatory mediators such as IL-6, C-reactive protein (CRP), and soluble vascular cell adhesion molecule 1 (VCAM-1), with an increased risk of severe bacterial infections (98) (Table 9.3). Similar results were reported in another study on individuals heterozygous for the Asp299Gly polymorphism, who had lower circulating inflammatory cytokines, acute phase reactants, and soluble adhesion molecules (92). In burns patients, carriage of the TLR4 A896G allele (Asp299Gly substitution) was significantly and independently associated with a 6.4-fold (95% CI, 1.8–23.2) increase in the risk of severe sepsis in 159 patients with severe burns affecting at least 20% total body surface area, after adjusting for age, burn size, ethnicity, and gender (89). Furthermore, the TLR4 polymorphism was particularly associated with an increased risk of severe sepsis in low-risk patients compared with high-risk patients, defined as those over the age of 50 years or having at least 30% burns surface area (unadjusted RR, 7.44 vs. 0.99). However, TLR4 polymorphisms were not associated with susceptibility or severity of infection in a U.S. study of 91 adults with septic shock (99). Similarly, TLR4 polymorphisms were not associated with development of SIRS (86) or sepsis (100) in two separate studies involving surgical patients. Interestingly, infections due to Gram-negative organisms occurred more frequently in patients with TLR4 polymorphisms compared with patients with wild-type TLR4 alleles in two of these studies (86,99). In patients with SIRS, there was an association between TLR polymorphisms and all-cause mortality at 28 days (36% vs. 11%, $p=.04$) (86) in one study and a trend toward increased risk of death in another study (19% vs. 5%, $p=.08$) (101). In keeping with the poor association between TLR4 polymorphisms and severe infection in many of these studies, a recent in vitro study reported no significant difference in monocyte CD14 density, monocyte count, concentrations of TNF-α, IL-6, IL-8, or endotoxin-induced cytokine synthesis in human whole blood between healthy heterozygous individuals and homozygous carriers of the wild-type allele, suggesting that heterozygosity for this TLR4 polymorphism may not be a major factor determining the cytokine response to LPS (102).

In meningococcal disease, the Asp299Gly/Thr399Ile co-segregating polymorphisms were not associated with susceptibility, severity or outcome in over 1000 patients in the U.K. (103) or with susceptibility to group A meningococcal meningitis in 252 Gambian children (104). In vitro studies have shown LPS-deficient mutants of *N. meningitidis* are still capable of transducing an inflammatory response, suggesting that the Gram-negative cell wall of *N. meningitidis* remains a potent inflammatory stimulant capable of utilizing signaling pathways

TABLE 9.3. Clinical studies on Toll-like receptor 4 (TLR4) polymorphisms

Country (reference)	Cases	No.	Controls	No.	SNP	Su/Se/Ou	Significance	Comments
Septic shock								
U.S. (99)	Adults with septic shock	91	Blood donors	73	A299G and T399I heterozygotes	Su	Combined: 0.12 vs. 0.11, $p=$NS. A299G: 0.055 vs. 0.0, $p=.05$	More Gram-negative infections in A299G (80% vs 35%, $p=.06$)
	Nonsurvivors	41	Survivors	50	A299G and T399I heterozygotes	Ou	Combined: 0.12 vs. 0.12, $p=$NS	Not associated with severity
Germany (100)	Adults with sepsis following major visceral bowel surgery	153	Surgical patients without sepsis	154	A299G	Su	0.065 vs. 0.012, $p=$NS	None were homozygous for GG and 84% of those with sepsis had polymicrobial infection
U.S. (89)	Nonsurvivors	62	Survivors	91	A299G	Ou	0.081 vs. 0.055, $p=$NS	
	Severe sepsis in adults with severe burns	36	Mild or no sepsis	123	A299G	Su/Se	0.19 vs. 0.089, $p=.08$	In logistic regression model, G allele was associated with 6.4-fold increase risk of severe sepsis
SIRS								
U.S. (86)	SIRS in surgical patients admitted to intensive care unit	77	Unrelated healthy volunteers	39	A299G and T399I (all had both polymorphisms)	Su	0.18 vs. 0.13%, $p=$NS (all heterozygous)	More Gram-negative infections among A299G (79% vs. 17%, $p=.004$)
	Nonsurvivors	12	Survivors	65	A299G and T399I	Ou	0.42 vs. 0.14, $p=.08$	28-day all cause mortality was assessed
U.K. (101)	Mortality in adults with SIRS	21	Survivors	58	A299G	Ou	0.19 vs. 0.05, $p=.08$; OR=4.3 (95% CI=0.9–2.12)	No association with severity
Meningococcal disease								
U.K. (103)	White patients with MD	1047	White blood donors	879	A299G	Su	0.065 vs. 0.059, $p=$NS	Not associated with age, serotype, or severity
Gambia (104)	Nonsurvivors	86	Survivors	961	A299G	Ou	0.067 vs. 0.041, $p=$NS	
	Children with group A meningococcal meningitis	252	251 matched child controls	251	A299G	Su	0.11 vs. 0.11, $p=$NS	No T399I polymorphisms identified
U.K. (106)	White adults and children with MD	220	White controls	283	Rare TLR4 variants	Su	0.064 vs. 0.0035, $p<.0001$, OR=27	
	Nonsurvivors	11	Survivors	186	Rare TLR4 variants	Ou	0.18 vs. 0.032, $p<.0001$	

MD, meningococcal disease; T399I, threonine/isoleucine polymorphism at position 399; Arg299Gly, arginine/glycine polymorphism at position 299; OR, odds ratio; 95% CI, 95% confidence interval; SIRS, systemic inflammatory response syndrome; SNP, single nucleotide polymorphism; Su/Se/Ou, susceptibility/severity/outcome; NS, not significant.

independent of those involved in LPS signaling (105). However, one study found a significant excess of relatively rare variants of TLR4 in ethnically white patients with meningococcal disease (106). The authors identified 14 rare missense mutations (including Asp299Gly and Thr399Ile), with allelic frequencies ranging from 0.3% to 5.3%, in 220 patients compared to only one in 283 unrelated white controls (OR, 27; $p<.0001$). Of note, only rare missense mutations were concentrated in the meningococcal group. The relatively more prevalent Asp299Gly and Thr399Ile substitutions, for example, were not significantly different in the cases (3.4%) compared with controls (5.3%) in the U.K. population sample ($p=.2$). The rare variants also showed a trend toward increased risk of death. The authors concluded that around 7.5% ($\pm3.7\%$) of meningococcal cases in white populations could be directly attributed to coding mutations in the TLR4 locus.

TLR2

TLR2, in contrast to TLR4, appears to be involved with infections due to gram-positive bacteria, such as *Staphylococcus aureus*, as well as *Borrelia burgdorferi* and *Treponema pallidum* (107). The human TLR2 protein is 784 amino acids in length. Residues 1 to 588 are speculated to form the ectodomain, 589 to 615 span the plasma membrane, and 616 to 784 comprise the cytoplasmic domain (106). TLR2 was initially shown to function as an LPS signal transducer when transfected into LPS nonresponder cell lines (108), and this activity was potentiated by CD14, the receptor that binds the LPS-LBP complex. However, C3H/HeJ mouse strains that have defective TLR4 but functional TLR2 remained profoundly hyporesponsive to LPS, suggesting that TLR4 was the major mammalian LPS signal transducer. Others subsequently showed that TLR2 is the major recognition molecule for lipoteichoic acid from the cell membrane of gram-positive organisms in a similar way to LPS from Gram-negative organisms and TLR4 (109,110). Furthermore, in an extensive analysis of TLR2 variants in patients with meningococcal disease, there was no significant association between any of the TLR2 mutations and susceptibility or outcome, thus providing further support that TLR2 is not a major receptor for LPS of *N. meningitidis* (106).

It is now recognized that commercial preparations of peptidoglycan used in earlier studies of TLR2 activation contained other cell wall components and that TLR2 was activated by these impurities (109,111). Like TLR4, TLR2 also requires the presence of CD14 for immune recognition (112,113). TLR2- and MyD88-deficient mice have an impaired response to *S. aureus* cell wall proteins, with higher mortality compared with wild-type mice when inoculated with *S. aureus* (114,115). TLR2 has also been shown to be the major mediator of macrophage activation in response to mycobacteria (116,117).

Four different polymorphisms in the TLR2 gene have been described in humans: two SNPs at Arg753Gln (=R753Q, due to G→A substitution) and Arg677Trp (=R677W, due to C→T substitution), a microsatellite GT repeat polymorphism about 100bp upstream of the translation start site in intron 2 (107,118,119) and a T-16933A polymorphism in the promoter region of the TLR2 gene identified in 23 healthy unrelated Caucasians. Both SNPs that code for amino acid substitutions are located in the C-terminus of the TLR2 and therefore are likely to affect signaling function of the molecule, rather than binding. The Arg residues at both sites (677 and 753) are highly conserved in all human and mice TLRs (118).

The Arg677Trp polymorphism has not been found among white probands (120). The Arg753Gln polymorphism was identified in 3% of healthy Caucasian blood donors. Transfection of 293T cells with either wild-type or mutant (Arg-753Trp) TLR2 showed that the response to LPS remained unaffected, but response to bacterial lipoproteins from *B. burgdorferi*, *T. pallidum*, and *Mycoplasma fermentans* was significantly reduced (107). High (>22) or low (<18) numbers of GT microsatellite repeats have been associated with lower promoter activity compared with medium (18 to 22) numbers of repeats (119). Using a statistical procedure, these GT repeats have been shown to be in significant linkage disequilibrium ($p < .001$) with the Arg753Gln polymorphism (121).

Only one study has assessed the association between the TLR2 T-16933A promoter polymorphism and infection (Table 9.4). This study reported that the AA genotype was significantly associated with an increased prevalence of sepsis (RR, 1.20; $p < .03$) and, more specifically, with Gram-positive infections (30% vs. 17%, $p < .04$), but not with positive blood cultures, septic shock, or mortality (87). In 69 patients with septic shock, the TLR2 Arg753Gln polymorphism occurred in two of 22 patients (9%) with Gram-positive septic shock compared to none of the other 47 patients with septic shock due to other organisms (107). Both patients were heterozygous for the Arg753Gln polymorphism and both had septic shock due to *S. aureus*. In a larger study of 420 consecutive white patients with microbiologically confirmed *S. aureus* infections, however, the Arg753Gln and microsatellite GT repeat polymorphisms were not associated with either susceptibility or *S. aureus*–attributable deaths (121). In this study, however, none of the patients had the homozygous Arg753Gln AA genotype and a recent in vitro study reported that only one wild-type allele is required for a full cytokine response to *S. aureus* lipoteichoic acid (122). Thus, the homozygous AA genotype may still be associated with increased susceptibility to Gram-positive infections but its low prevalence in the white population makes it unlikely to be an important risk factor for severe Gram-positive infections.

Heat Shock Proteins

Heat shock proteins (HSPs) are expressed in response to a variety of stress-inducing stimuli, including heat, ischemia, LPS, and other inflammatory mediators involved in the pathogenesis of severe sepsis (123,124). During cellular stress, HSPs help to ensure cellular survival by supporting degeneration of abnormal proteins (125,126). Some HSPs are expressed constitutively in

TABLE 9.4. Clinical studies on Toll-like receptor 2 (TLR2) polymorphisms

Country (reference)	Cases	No.	Controls	No.	SNP	Su/Se/Ou	Significance	Comments
Sepsis								
Canada (87)	Sepsis in critically ill patients with SIRS	178	No sepsis	59	-16933AA	Se	0.29 vs. 0.14, $p < .03$, RR=1.2	AA genotype associated with Gram-negative infections (30% vs. 17%, $p < .04$)
	Nonsurvivors	84	Survivors	153	-16933AA	Ou	0.26 vs. 0.25, p=NS	
Staphylococcal infections								
France (107)	Adults in intensive care with Gram-positive septic shock	22	Septic shock due to other organisms	69	A753G allele	Su	0.09 vs. 0.00, p=NS	Both patients with polymorphism had *S. aureus* septic shock
U.K. (121)	White patients with *S. aureus* infections	420	Umbilical cord of healthy white neonates	696	A753G allele	Su	0.05 vs. 0.05, p=NS	None of the patients were GG homozygotes
	Nonsurvivors	56	Survivors	364	A753G homozygous	Ou	0.95. 0.95, p=NS	
U.K. (121)	White patients with *S. aureus* infections	396	Umbilical cord of healthy white neonates	638	Low activity GT repeats	Su	0.27 vs. 0.28, p=NS	Low-activity alleles defined as <18 or >22 GT repeats
	Nonsurvivors	54	Survivors	342	Low activity GT repeats	Ou	0.23 vs. 0.27, p=NS	

Arg753Gln = Arginine/Glutamine polymorphism at position 753; RR, relative risk; SIRS, systemic inflammatory response syndrome; SNP, single nucleotide polymorphism; Su/Se/Ou, susceptibility/severity/outcome; NS, not significant.

unstressed cells where they play an important role in a number of fundamental biologic processes, including folding, assembly, and translocation of proteins across membranes (127). In addition, extracellular HSP70 (see below) utilizes both TLR2 and TLR4 to transduce a proinflammatory response by activating NF-κB and upregulating the expression of proinflammatory cytokines in human monocytes (128). Furthermore, HSP70 can upregulate both TLR2 and TLR4 during inflammation (129). During inflammation, HSPs protect cells from TNF-induced cytotoxicity (130,131). In a rat model of intraabdominal sepsis produced by cecal ligation and perforation, induction of HSP synthesis by thermal pretreatment reduced organ damage and enhanced survival (132). More recently, extracellular HSP70 levels from blood samples taken within 24 hours of admission to a pediatric intensive care unit from children with septic shock were significantly elevated compared with control patients (51.6 ng/mL vs. 8.1 ng/mL, respectively, $p=.0004$) (133).

The HSPs are divided into different families based on their molecular weight. Of these, the HSP70 family are the most conserved and best characterized. The genes for three proteins belonging to the HSP70 family—*HSP70-1*, *HSP70-2*, and *HSP70-HOM*—are located in a cluster of human leukocyte antigen (HLA) class III genes on chromosome 6, near the TNF locus. The *HSP70-1* and *HSP70-2* genes encode an identical heat-inducible protein product of 641 amino acids, while the intronless *HSP70-HOM* gene, whose 641 amino-acid protein is 90% homologous to the other two HSP70 proteins, is constitutively expressed at low levels and is not heat-inducible (134,135).

In a prospective study of 87 patients admitted to a surgical intensive care unit with severe sepsis, none of the HSP polymorphisms were associated with susceptibility, severity, or outcome (136). In another study, however, the wild-type HSP70-2 AA genotype was significantly associated with an increased risk of septic shock (OR, 3.5; 95% CI, 1.8–6.8; $p=.0005$) but not with death in a prospective cohort study of 343 adults with community-acquired pneumonia (137). In this study, there was significant linkage disequilibrium between the HSP70-2 AA and the TNF-α B2/B2 genotype ($p<.0001$), which was also associated with an increased risk of septic shock (OR, 2.7; 95% CI, 1.4–5.3; $p=.002$). In a logistic regression model including genetic as well as important clinical predictors of septic shock, however, only age ($p=.04$) and the HSP70-2 AA genotype ($p=.006$) remained significantly associated with an increased risk of septic shock.

Complement and Mannose-Binding Lectin

The complement system plays a critical role in the innate immune system and not only participates in the inflammatory process but also acts to modulate the adaptive immune response. The complement system was first identified as a heat-sensitive factor that "complemented" the effects of specific antibody to lyse bacteria and red blood cells (138). Over 30 different serum proteins and cell surface receptors are now recognized as part of the complement system. They act through complex interacting pathways to perform functions ranging from direct cell lysis to enhancing T- and B-cell responses (139). Like the TLRs, the complement system can be activated by pattern recognition receptors, such as mannose-binding lectin (MBL) and ficolins that recognize specific pathogen-associated molecular patterns.

The complement system can be activated by three different, but interacting pathways—classic, alternative, and lectin—that differ according to the nature of recognition, but merge to share a common final step in activating C3 (Fig. 9.2). The classic pathway is activated by C-reactive protein or antibody released in the humoral response. The alternative pathway is activated through interaction of C3 with properdin, factor B, and factor D to generate C3b. The lectin pathway is activated by recognition and binding of specific pathogen-associated molecular patterns by specific lectin proteins, including MBL, ficolin H, and ficolin L, These proteins are able to distinguish between self, nonself, and altered-self molecules through a carbohydrate recognition domain that can bind N-acetylglucosamine, fucose, mannose, and similar carbohydrates, which are commonly found on microbes. Deficiencies in components of the complement pathway, or of properdin, are known to significantly increase susceptibility

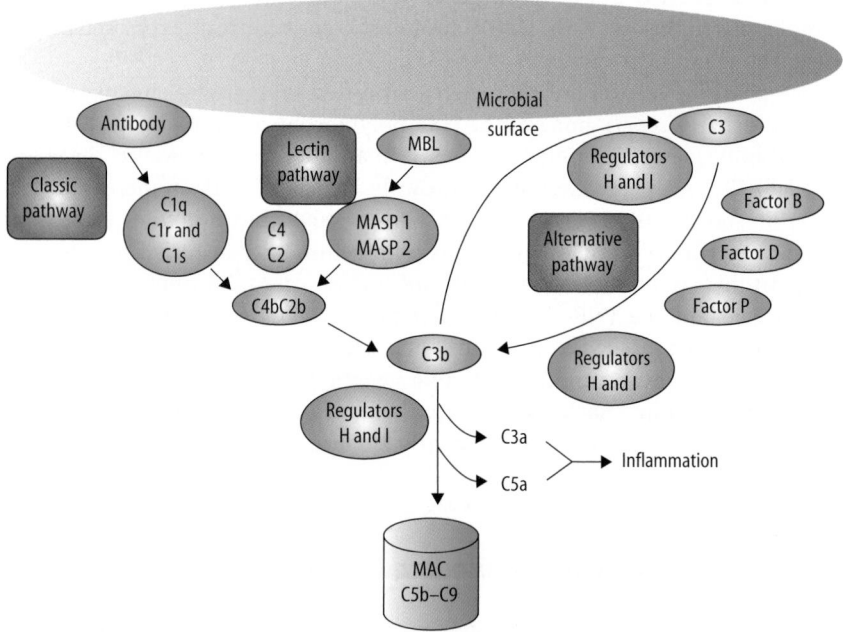

FIGURE 9.2. Complement activation through three different but interacting pathways, which lead to a common late pathway and generation of the membrane attack complex (MAC) and the C3a and C5a inflammatory mediators. (From Emonts M, Hazelzet JA, de Groot R, Hermans PW. Host genetic determinants of Neisseria meningitidis infections. Lancet Infect Dis 2003;3:565–577, with permission.)

to various infections, particularly meningococcal disease (140). On the other hand, excessive activation of the complement system in children with septic shock can lead to capillary leakage, more severe disease, and death (141). The estimated combined frequency of all complement deficiencies is 0.03% (140), with properdin deficiency being the single most common deficiency and accounting for around a third of cases, followed by C3 deficiency (142). Autosomal inherited deficiencies of C1, C2, C4, factor H, as well as components of the late complement pathways, including C5, C6, C7, C8, and C9, have also been reported (142). Deficiencies of C3, properdin, and components of the late pathway result in failure to form membrane attack complexes and increased susceptibility to recurrent meningococcal and other bacterial infections.

C3 plays a key role in the complement activation because all three complement pathways lead to activation of C3, resulting in the formation of C3a and C3b fragments (Fig. 9.2). C3a, together with C5a, has potent proinflammatory and chemoattractant properties, while C3b acts as an opsonin and, when bound to C3 convertase, forms C5 convertase, which produces C5a and C5b. C5b initiates the late components of the complement pathway, resulting in formation of the membrane attack complex, which creates pores in the bacterial cell membrane and facilitates phagocytosis.

Properdin is coded on the short arm of chromosome X and plays an important role in the alternative pathway leading to complement activation by stabilizing the C3 convertase C3b,Bb (143). Three different types of properdin deficiencies have been described. Type I deficiency is caused primarily by a mutation resulting in a premature stop codon in exon 4 to 6 and, therefore, absent properdin in plasma (144–146). Type II deficiency is characterized by low but detectable plasma levels and is caused by two distinct mutations— C2124T (Arg to Trp substitution) in exon 4 and G827A mutation intron 3 (145). In type III deficiency, properdin levels are normal but the protein in not functional (146). This is due to a single thymine to guanine mutation in exon 9, leading to substitution of tyrosine by an aspartic acid residue at position 387 (Tyr387Asp), which results in mutant protein being unable to stabilize the C3 convertase (146). In properdin deficiency, the increased risk of meningococcal disease is associated with insufficient C3 deposition on the surface of meningococci, thus resulting in insufficient phagocytosis. This can be reversed in vitro by adding properdin (147).

The rare complement mutations contribute little to influencing susceptibility to severe infections in the general population. The MBL deficiency (due to one or more polymorphisms), on the other hand, is relatively more common and of greater clinical significance. Mannose-binding lectin is a calcium-dependent C-type lectin and a member of the collectin family of proteins that includes collagen. It is an acute-phase protein produced by the liver and exhibits modest rises in serum levels after infection or trauma (148). It is an oligomer of polypeptide chains, with each chain composed of a collagen-like region linked to a carbohydrate recognition domain. In plasma, MBL exists in complex with serine proteases (also known as MBL-associated serine proteases, MASPs)—

MASP1 (149), MASP2 (150), MASP3 (151), and a smaller splice variant of MASP2 called MAp19 (152,153) or sMAP (154). When MBL binds to a fitting carbohydrate, the MASPs are cleaved into an A and a B chain and become active enzymes that can activate complement independent of antibody through cleavage of specific substrates. Activation of the complement cascade results in bacterial clearance, either by formation of complement-mediated membrane attack complexes on the bacterial membrane, opsonophagocytosis, or by activation of inflammatory cells (155).

The plasma concentration of MBL is determined by SNPs in the MBL gene *(mbl2)*, which comprise four exons. Exon 1 encodes a signaling peptide, a cysteine-rich region and part of the glycine-rich collagenous region and exon 4 encodes for the carbohydrate-recognition domain that adopts a globular formation. The *mbl1* gene is a pseudogene. At least three different SNPs have been identified in exon 1—B (codon 54, G34D), C (codon 57, G37D), and D (codon 52, R32C)—with A being the wild type (Fig. 9.3). The B variant occurs in around 25% of Eurasian populations, while the C variant is characteristic of sub-Saharan African population where it is present in around 50% of individuals. The D mutation is found in up to 14% of Caucasians, but is lower elsewhere.

Mutations in exon 1 result in disruption of the axial Gly-Xaa-Yaa pattern of the collagen region, resulting in distortion of the collagen helix. This dramatically reduces the formation of higher order oligomers, leading to enzymatic degradation and lower circulating levels of MBL. Around 33% of the population are heterozygotes for one of the codon variants and 5% are either homozygotes or heterozygotes for two different codons; the latter group is often referred to as functionally mutant homozygous for MBL deficiency (156,157). Concentrations of MBL in serum are about 20% lower in heterozygotes for any codon variant and are very low (typically <2%) or absent in functional mutant homozygotes (157,158).

As well as structural mutations, several SNPs have been described in the promoter region (158), including the H/L (−550), X/Y (−221), and P/Q (+4) loci of the MBL genes. The three loci are closely linked and four promoter haplotypes are commonly found (LXP, LYP, LYQ, and HYP). Of these, the LXP haplotype is associated with low levels of MBL. This combination occurs in about

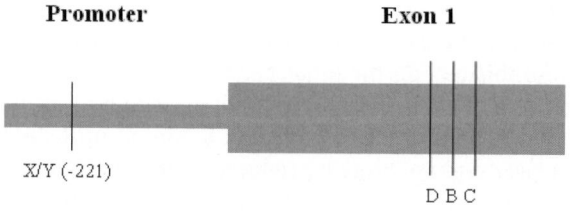

FIGURE 9.3. Common mannan-binding lectin (MBL) polymorphisms. The *mbl1* gene is a pseudogene; at least three different single nucleotide polymorphisms (SNPs) have been identified in exon 1: B (codon 54, G34D), C (codon 57, G37D), and D (codon 52, R32C); A is the wild type.

12% of the Caucasian population, who subsequently have very low MBL levels (159). The G-221C promoter polymorphism, which is present in about 40% of Europeans, is the most relevant noncoding polymorphism and has a smaller but detectable effect on MBL concentration in serum, with lower concentrations associated with the C allele compared with the G allele (also known as X and Y variants, respectively) (158).

Mannose-binding lectin deficiency was first linked with an opsonic dysfunction in children suffering from repeated infections and failure to thrive (160). Since then, MBL has been shown to play a major role in first-line defense against a range of different pathogens, and deficiency is associated with increased susceptibility to many infectious and autoimmune diseases. MBL may also play an important role in modulating disease severity, such as AIDS (161).

Summerfield and colleagues (162) studied the MBL codon variants in a cohort of 617 children with a range of different diagnoses admitted to one U.K. hospital and found that the combined frequency of MBL heterozygotes and homozygotes was significantly higher in 345 children with infection (42%) compared with 272 children with other diagnoses (24%) (OR, 2.4; 95% CI, 1.7–3.4; $p<.0001$) (Table 9.5). Furthermore, 13 of the 17 children with homozygous polymorphisms presented with severe infections, including six cases of septicemia. This difference remained statistically significant after correcting for ethnic variation in the study cohort. However, the broad definition of "infection" used by the authors makes the significance of the results difficult to interpret, particularly because there were no deaths (and therefore no association between the polymorphisms studied and mortality) reported in either cases or controls. In another study (163), the combined frequency of homozygous and heterozygous MBL codon variants was significantly higher in children admitted to the hospital with meningococcal disease compared with control children admitted to the same hospital with noninfectious illnesses (OR, 2.0; 95% CI, 1.3–3.0; $p=.001$). In a confirmatory community-based study involving 72 survivors of meningococcal disease and 110 healthy controls, the combined frequency of homozygous and heterozygous MBL codon variants was also higher in patients compared with controls (OR, 2.4; 95% CI, 1.2–246; $p=.008$). The population-attributable fraction of cases attributable to MBL variants was estimated to be 32% (homozygous 6%, heterozygous 26%).

In 272 adult Danish patients with SIRS, genotypically low MBL producers did not have an increased risk of SIRS when compared with 250 controls. However, within the cohort of patients with SIRS, low MBL producers had a significantly higher risk of sepsis, severe sepsis and septic shock ($p<.001$ for trend), as well as death (164). Low MBL production remained a significant and independent risk factor for death in a logistic regression model and was associated with infections due to both Gram-positive and Gram-negative organisms. In this study, increasing severity of sepsis was also associated with decreasing serum MBL levels ($p=.032$). On the other hand, a more recent study found that,

TABLE 9.5. Clinical studies on mannose-binding lectin (MBL) polymorphisms

Country (reference)	Cases	No.	Controls	No.	SNP	Su/Se/Ou	Significance	Comments
Infections								
U.K. (162)	Children of different ethnicities admitted to hospital with infection	345	Children admitted with noninfectious disease	272	Variant allele*	Su	0.42 vs. 0.24, $p<.0001$ OR=2.4, 95% CI=1.7–3.4	No association with the −221 promoter polymorphism
SIRS								
Canada (87)	Blood culture positive in critically ill patients with SIRS	113	Negative blood culture	109	MBL insufficiency***	Su	0.27 vs. 0.13. $p<.02$	No association with sepsis or septic shock
	Nonsurvivors of SIRS on day 28	76	Survivors	146	MBL insufficiency***	Ou	0.16 vs. 0.22, $p=NS$	No association with sepsis, septic shock or death
Respiratory infections								
Greenland (166)	Acute respiratory infections in MBL-sufficient children <2 years	13	Acute respiratory infections in MBL-insufficient children <2 years	239	MBL insufficiency***	Su	34 episodes in 1178 days at risk vs. 677 episodes in 28072 days at risk ($p<.001$) OR=2.1 (95% CI, 1.4–3.1)	
U.K. (156)	Patients with invasive pneumococcal disease	229	Adult volunteer donors	353	Variant Homozygotes****	Su	0.12 vs. 0.05, $p=.002$ (OR=2.6, 95% CI=1.4–4.8)	Heterozygotes for any codon not significant (0.32 vs. 0.35, $p=.98$)
U.K. (156)	Patients with invasive pneumococcal disease	108	Umbilical cord blood from healthy neonates	679	Variant Homozygotes****	Su	0.10 vs. 0.053, (OR=2.4, 95% CI=1.5–3.7)	This was a confirmatory study by same authors
Meningococcal disease								
U.K. (163)	Children hospitalized with MD	192	Children with noninfectious diseases	272	Homozygotes**		0.077 vs. 0.015, $p=.0006$ OR=6.5, 95% CI=2.0–27.2	Heterozygote frequency also higher in cases (0.30 vs. 0.22, $p=.02$)

U.K. (163)	Community-based study of children with MD	72	Healthy individuals	110	Homozygotes**		0.08 vs. 0.03, p=.06 (OR=4.5, 95% CI=0.9–29.1)	Heterozygote frequency also higher in cases (0.47 vs. 0.32, p=.02)
Children with malignancy								
U.K. (169)	Neutropenic episodes in children with malignancy on chemotherapy	60	No neutropenic episodes	36	Variant allele*	Su	0.62 vs. 0.67, p=NS	Median duration of febrile neutropenia double in variant group (20.5 vs. 10.0, p=.014)
Denmark (164)	SIRS in adult Danish patients	272	190 blood donors + 60 hospital staff members	250	Variant allele*	Su	0.44 vs. 0.37, p=NS	MBL variants associated with gram-positive and gram-negative infections
	Sepsis in patients with SIRS	197	No sepsis	75	Variant allele*	Su	0.51 vs. 0.27, p<.001	Decreasing serum MBL levels with increasing sepsis severity
	Nonsurvivors of SIRS	83	Survivors	189	Variant allele*	Ou	0.53 vs. 0.41, p=NS	MBL variants also associated with severity

*Variant allele: heterozygous or homozygous for any of the codons at positions 52, 54. or 57.

**Homozygotes: homozygotes for codons 52, 54 or 57 (52/52, 54/54 or 57/57) or double heterozygotes (52/54, 54/57 or 52/57).

***MBL insufficiency: XA/O and O/O (XA=wild-type allele with low MBL-producing -221 promoter polymorphism and O=heterozygotes for any of the codons at positions 52, 54 or 57).

****Variant Homozygotes: A/A group= YA/YA or YA/YA or XA/XA ; A/O group= YA/O or XA/O ; O/O group=variant allele.

MD, meningococcal disease; RR, relative risk; 95% CI, 95% confidence interval; SIRS, systemic inflammatory response syndrome; SNP, single nucleotide polymorphism; Su/Se/Ou, susceptibility/severity/outcome; NS, not significant.

although low MBL producers were more likely to have a positive blood culture (68% vs. 47%; $p<.02$; RR, 1.44), there was no association between the MBL genotype and the risk of clinical sepsis, septic shock, or death among 252 critically ill patients admitted to a mixed medical-surgical intensive care unit with SIRS (165).

Mannose-binding lectin polymorphisms were also studied in pneumococcal disease. Roy and colleagues (156) found that functionally homozygote polymorphisms were more prevalent in white adults and children with invasive pneumococcal disease compared to white, blood donor controls (12% vs. 5%; OR, 2.6; 95% CI, 1.4–4.8). However, neither individual heterozygous nor promoter polymorphisms (either alone or in combination with the MBL codon variants) was associated with susceptibility to infection or outcome. In a confirmatory study of 108 new cases with 679 healthy neonatal controls matched for ethnic origin and area of residence, the authors found the genotype frequencies among patients and controls were similar to their initial study, with an increased risk of pneumococcal infections in the homozygote group (10% vs. 5%, $p=.046$). When the results of the two studies were combined, individuals with functionally homozygote polymorphisms were 2.4 times more likely (95% CI, 1.5–3.7) to develop invasive pneumococcal disease. The attributable risk of MBL codon variants in the population studied was estimated to be 6.7%. The association between MBL polymorphisms and infections due to respiratory pathogens is further supported by Koch and colleagues (166), who followed a cohort 252 healthy children younger than 2 years of age in Greenland for 2 years. They found a 2.1-fold (95% CI, 1.4–3.1) increase in the relative risk of acute respiratory tract infections in low MBL producing children. This group (5%) included either functional homozygotes or heterozygotes with the low-MBL producing -221 promoter phenotype (X variant). The highest risk was found in children aged 6 to 17 months (OR, 2.92; 95% CI, 1.78–4.79), with no increased risk observed in children aged 18 to 23 months. This observation supports previous suggestions that MBL plays a significant role in immune defense in the vulnerable period between 6 and 18 months of age, when children are depleted of passively acquired maternal antibodies and the adaptive immune system is still immature (167,168). The population-attributable risk for acute respiratory infections was 7.2% for heterozygous or functionally homozygous alleles.

In children with malignancy receiving chemotherapy, although MBL concentrations were not associated with MBL polymorphisms and did not alter significantly during episodes of febrile neutropenia, children without any MBL mutations showed a doubling of MBL levels by day 7 ($p<.001$) with levels returning to preinfection levels by day 14 (169). The duration of febrile neutropenia in these children was half as long as children heterozygous or homozygous for the MBL codon variants (10.0 days vs. 20.5 days, $p=.014$), with children with the lowest MBL levels having the longest periods of febrile neutropenia ($p=.012$). The association between low MBL levels and increased risk of infection in patients with malignancy receiving chemotherapy is supported by another adult study, which found that patients with bacteremia or pneumonia had significantly lower serum MBL levels compared to those without infections ($p < .0001$) (170).

Fcγ Receptors

Antibody receptors are able to activate complement, facilitate phagocytosis, and mediate antibody-dependent cellular cytotoxicity, phagocytosis, superoxide generation, degranulation, cytokine production, and regulation of antibody production. Fcγ receptors (FcγR) recognize and bind the crystallizable fraction of the immunoglobulin. This is the nonvariable "trunk" of the immunoglobulin molecule to which are attached the two arms containing highly variable antigen receptor sites. The FcγR genes have been mapped within close proximity to the long arm of chromosome 1 (171). On leukocytes, they display considerable heterogeneity and are essential for host defense and immune regulation. The different FcγR subclasses differ in their ligand specificity and affinity through a combination of changes in primary structure, glycosylation, association with signaling molecules, and interaction with serine proteases.

Based on size, primary structure, monoclonal antibody reactivity, affinity of specific ligands, and cellular distribution patterns, three different classes of leukocyte FcγR are described in humans: FcγRI (CD64), FcγRII (CD32), and FcγRIII (CD16) (172). FcγRI is a high-affinity receptor for monomeric IgG1, IgG3, and IgG4, while FcγRII and FcγRIII are low-affinity receptors that interact only with complexed aggregate IgG. The efficacy of IgG-induced FcγR function displays interindividual heterogeneity due to genetic polymorphisms of three FcγR subclasses: FcγRIIa (CD32a), FcγRIIIa (CD16a), and FcγRIIIb (CD16b) (Fig. 9.4). FcγRIIIa is expressed on natural killer cells, monocytes, and macrophages (173). FcγRIIa and FcγRIIIb are expressed constitutively on neutrophils and exhibit structural and functional polymorphisms. Both receptors can bind IgG1 and IgG3 subclasses, but FcγRIIa is the only FcγR capable of binding IgG2, the isotype that dominates the immune response to encapsulated bacteria (174), as demonstrated by rare cases of selective IgG2 deficiency that present with recurrent acute otitis media and sinopulmonary infections (175,176).

Two allotypes of FcγRIIa, designated FcγRIIa R131 and FcγRIIa H131, depending on the presence of arginine or histidine at position 131 in exon 4, which encodes the extracellular IgG binding-domain of the receptor, have been described. Neutrophils bearing the FcγRIIa H/H genotype (high responders) bind IgG2 complexes more effectively and phagocytose IgG2-opsonized *N. meningitidis*, *Haemophilus influenzae*, streptococci, and *S. aureus* more efficiently than neutrophils bearing the FcγRIIa R/R genotype (low responders), while FcγRIIa H/R heterozygote neutrophils have intermediate efficacy (147,177–179). The FcγRIIa R/R genotype also binds IgG3 less efficiently (180).

The allotype distribution has marked ethnic variation (181). The FcγR H/H genotype in the healthy Japanese population is 60%, which coincides with a

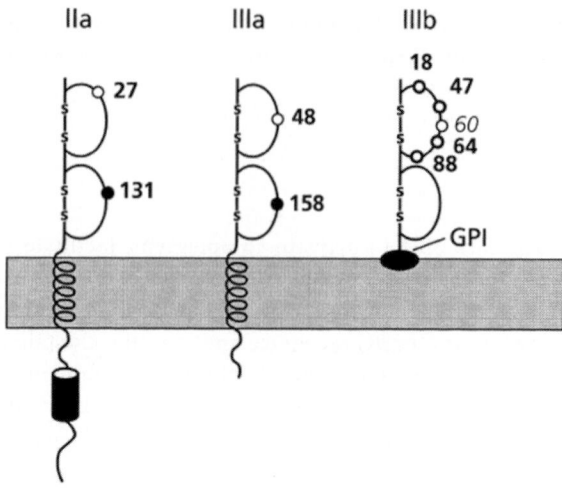

FIGURE 9.4. FcγR polymorphisms. FcγRIIa and FcγRIIIa both have one functional (closed circles) and one non-functional (small open circles) polymorphisms. The functional polymorphism in FcγRIIIb (depicted as a neutrophil antigen [NA] polymorphism in the text) is caused by four amino acid substitutions at positions 18, 47, 64, and 88 (small filled circles), which result in glycosylation differences that affect receptor affinity. (From van der Pol W, van de Winkel JG. IgG receptor polymorphisms: risk factors for disease. Immunogenetics 1998;48:222–232, with permission.)

very low incidence of meningococcal disease in Japan (three cases in >120 million inhabitants in 1995) (181). In Europe, the FcγRIIa H/H allotype in healthy individuals varies from 20% in the U.K. to 39% in Greece. The FcγRIIa polymorphism has also been associated with other diseases including heparin-induced thrombocytopenia, periodontitis, and systemic lupus erythematosus (179,182–185). The FcγRIIa, but not FcγRIIIa or FcγRIIIb, polymorphism, however, is in significant linkage disequilibrium with the IL-10 -1082 polymorphism (186).

A guanine to adenine nucleotide substitution at position 559 (G559A) of FcγRIIIa predicts either a valine or a phenylalanine at amino acid position 158 in the membrane-proximal, IgG-binding domain (FcγRIIIa -158F and -158V). These two alleles have gene frequencies of 0.57 and 0.43, respectively, in Europeans. Natural killer cells from homozygous FcγRIIIa V/V individuals bound more IgG than FcγRIIIa F/F cells and freshly isolated natural killer cells from FcγRIIIa V/V individuals carried significantly more cytophilic IgG than did natural killer cells from FcγRIIIa F/F individuals (187). Of note, FcγRIIIa is unique in its ability to induce TNF-α release by macrophages (188), and TNF-α levels are associated with outcome in various infectious diseases including meningococcal septicemia and meningitis (189–191). A second triallelic FcγRIIIa L/R/H polymorphism at position 48 has also been described, but has been shown to be in linkage disequilibrium with the FcγRIIIa 158F/V polymorphism (158F with the 48L allotype and 158V with 48H or 48R allotype; $p < .001$). Furthermore, the different abilities of the FcγRIIIa 158V/F polymorphisms to bind immunoglobulin have been shown to be unrelated to the FcγRIIIa 48H/R allotype.

FcγRIIIb deficiency is rare and usually identified in young healthy mothers upon analysis of a symptomatic neonatal neutropenia occurring in their newborns as a result of the formation of maternal anti-FcγRIIIb antibodies (192). Most individuals with FcγRIIIb deficiency have normal FcγRIIa phenotypes and are not particularly at risk of serious infections (192). FcγRIIIb has a neutrophil antigen (NA) polymorphism representing four amino acid substitutions in the membrane-distal immunoglobulin-like distal loop of the receptor. The FcγRIIIb NA1 allotype binds IgG1 and IgG3 immune complexes more efficiently than FcγRIIIb NA2 (186) and has stronger interaction with IgG-opsonized particles (177,193,194). Furthermore, IgG1-mediated phagocytosis of S. aureus, H. influenzae serotype b, and N. meningitidis is lower in leukocytes homozygous for FcγRIIIb NA2 (21% to 25%) than leukocytes homozygous for FcγRIIIb NA1 (177).

The FcγR polymorphisms were initially studied in individuals with deficiency of a component in the terminal pathway of complement activation (C5 to C9) (Table 9.6). These individuals are approximately 1000 times more susceptible to meningococcal infections compared with complement-sufficient individuals (140,195). In such patients, antibody-mediated lysis of meningococci through activation of the classical complement pathway, which is considered to be the major immune defense against meningococcal disease, is missing. These patients are unable to form membrane attack complexes, which are essential for damaging cell membranes and causing cell lysis (196). Therefore, antibody-mediated phagocytosis through the FcγR is likely to constitute a vital defense mechanism against meningococcal disease in this group of patients. Fijen and colleagues (197) first studied the FcγR polymorphisms in 15 patients from four families with C6 or C8 deficiency and found that a combination of the less efficient polymorphisms (FcγRIIa 131R/R and FcγRIIIb NA2/NA2 homozygotes) was more common in patients (six of eight cases) with a history of meningococcal disease compared with controls (one of seven cases) without a history of meningococcal disease (OR, 13.9; $p=.036$). No such association was observed in individuals with properdin deficiency (one of seven vs. none of eight cases), suggesting that antibody-mediated phagocytosis is particularly important in persons with terminal pathway of complement deficiency and that less efficient FcγR polymorphisms significantly increased the risk of meningococcal disease in these patients (147).

Subsequently, Platonov and colleagues (198) studied the FcγRIIa polymorphism in 29 Russian patients with terminal complement pathway deficiency and a history of meningococcal disease and found that the frequency of the homozygous FcγRIIa 131R/R genotype (17%) was similar to 107 complement-sufficient healthy blood donor controls (18%) ($p=.6$). However, the FcγRIIa 131R allele was associated with more severe meningococcal disease (14/31 vs. 1/18 severe episodes; OR, 14; $p<.01$). The authors also noted that the median age at first episode of meningococcal disease was significantly higher in patients

TABLE 9.6. Clinical studies on FcγR polymorphisms

Country (reference)	Cases	No.	Controls	No.	SNP	Su/Se/Ou	Significance	Comments
LCCD patients								
Netherlands (197)	History of MD in Dutch patients with LCCD	8	No history of MD in patients with LCCD	7	Combined FcγRIIa R131 and FcγRIIIb NA2 homozygous	Su	0.75 vs. 0.14, p=.036 OR=13.9, 95% CI=1.2–478	No association with age at first episode; no such association in patients with properdin deficiency
Russia (198)	Russian patients with LCCD and 63 episodes of MD	29	Russian blood donors	107	FcγRIIa R131 homozygous	Su	0.17 vs. 0.18, p=NS	RR patients developed first episode of MD at an older age
	Severe MD	15	Moderate MD	34	FcγRIIa R131 allele	Se	0.93 vs. 0.50, p<.01 OR=14	Children >10 years who were homozygous or heterozygous for the R131 allele were more likely to develop more severe and recurrent disease
Meningococcal disease								
Netherlands (180)	Children surviving fulminant meningococcal shock	25	Previous study in healthy white subjects	123	FcγRIIa R131 homozygous	Su	0.44 vs. 0.23, p=.028 OR=2.7, 95% CI=1.1–6.5	
Netherlands (186)	Patients with MD	50	Healthy controls	239	FcγRIIa R131 homozygous	Su	0.26 vs. 0.20, p=NS	
	First-degree relatives of patients with MD	183	Healthy controls	239	FcγRIIa R131 homozygous	Su	0.20 vs. 0.20, p=NS	
	Septic shock in patients with MD	18	No septic shock	32	FcγRIIa R131 homozygous	Se	0.17 vs. 0.34, p=NS	
	Septic shock in first-degree relatives of patients with MD	86	No septic sock	97	FcγRIIa R131 homozygous	Se	0.17 vs. 0.22, p=NS	

Country (ref)	Cases	N	Controls	N	Genotype	Su/Se	Result	Comment
Russia (199)	Russian patients with MD	98	Russian blood donors	107	FcγRIIa R131 homozygous	Su	0.32 vs. 0.18, $p<.06$ OR=1.9, 95% CI=0.9–4.1	R131/R131 homozygotes developed MD at an older age
	Severe MD: coma, shock, skin necrosis, neurologic sequelae	51	Nonsevere MD	47	FcγRIIa R131 homozygous	Se	0.41 vs. 0.21, $p<.02$	
	Severe complications of MD	38	No or mild MD complications	60	FcγRIIa R131 homozygous	Se	0.47 vs. 0.22, $p<.05$	
Spain (181)	Patients with MD	130	Blood donors	260	FcγRIIa R131 homozygous	Su	0.32 vs. 0.25, $p=NS$	
	Fulminant MD	13	Nonfulminant MD	117	FcγRIIa R131 homozygous	Se	0.61 vs. 0.29, $p=.04$ OR=3.9 (95% CI=1.0–16)	
	Meningococcal septicemia	44	Meningitis or mixed picture	86	FcγRIIa R131 homozygous	Se	0.50 vs. 0.23, $p=.004$ OR=3.3, 95% CI=1.4–7.8	
	Complications of MD	41	No complications	89	FcγRIIa R131 homozygous	Se	0.56 vs. 0.21, $p=.02$	
Netherlands (180)	Children surviving fulminant meningococcal shock	23	Previous study in healthy white subjects	3377	FcγRIIIb-NA2 homozygous	Su	0.30 vs. 0.45, $p=NS$	
Netherlands (186)	Patients with MD	50	Healthy controls	239	FcγRIIIb-NA2 homozygous	Su	0.50 vs. 0.38, $p=NS$	
	Septic shock in patients with MD	18	No septic shock	32	FcγRIIIb-NA2 homozygous	Se	(Data not given), $p=NS$	
	First-degree relatives of patients with MD	183	Healthy controls	239	FcγRIIIb-NA2 homozygous	Su	0.38 vs. 0.38, $p=NS$	
	Septic shock in first-degree relatives of patients with MD	86	No septic sock	97	FcγRIIIb-NA2 homozygous	Se	0.41 vs. 0.36, $p=NS$	

(Continued)

Table 9.6. Clinical studies on FcγR polymorphisms (Continued)

Country (reference)	Cases	No.	Controls	No.	SNP	Su/Se/Ou	Significance	Comments
Netherlands (186)	Patients with MD	50	Healthy controls	239	FcγRIIIa-158VV homozygous	Su	VV: 0.02 vs 0.11, p=NS FF: 0.46 vs. 0.41, p=NS	
	Septic shock in patients with MD	18	No septic shock	32	FcγRIIIa-158VV homozygous	Se	(Data not given), p=NS	
	First-degree relatives of patients with MD	183	Healthy controls	239	FcγRIIIa-158VV homozygous	Su	VV: 0.07 vs. 0.11, p=0.10 FF: 0.51 vs. 0.41, p=0.10	
	Septic shock in first-degree relatives of patients with MD	86	No septic sock	97	FcγRIIIa-158VV homozygous	Se	VV: 0.08 vs. 0.09, p=NS FF: 0.53 vs. 0.52, p=NS	V allele more prevalent in meningitis (38%) vs. sepsis + mixed (25%), p=.046
Respiratory infections								
U.S. (200)	Bacteremic pneumococcal pneumonia	42	Blood specimens from general medical clinics	136	FcγRIIa R131 homozygous	Su	0.50 vs. 0.29, p<.05	All four patients who died were homozygous for the FcγRIIa-R131/R131 polymorphism
	Nonbacteremic pneumococcal pneumonia	28	Blood specimens from general medical clinics	136	FcγRIIa R131 homozygous	Su	0.28 vs. 0.28, p=NS	
Netherlands (202)	Children with recurrent respiratory tract infections	48	Healthy adults	123	FcγRIIa R131 homozygous	Su	0.31 vs. 0.23, p=NS	H131 homozygotes were under-represented among cases (0.12 vs. 0.29, p=.01) No association with clinical presentation, severity, or frequency of infections

LCCD, late complement component deficiency; MD, meningococcal disease; RR, relative risk; 95% CI=95% confidence interval; SIRS, systemic inflammatory response syndrome; SNP, single nucleotide polymorphism; Su/Se/Ou, susceptibility/severity/outcome; NS, not significant.

with the homozygous FcγRIIa 131R/R genotype (17 years) compared with the heterozygous FcγRIIa 131R/H allotype (16 years) and the homozygous FcγRIIa 131H/H genotype (6 years) ($p<.05$). Patients carrying the FcγRIIa 131R allele were 3.3 times (95% CI, 1.0–12.0) more likely to contract meningococcal disease for the first time after the age of 10 years and twice (95% CI, 1.1–3.8) as likely to experience recurrent episodes after the age of 10 years.

In complement-sufficient individuals with meningococcal disease, the role of FcγRs is less clear (Table 9.6). The homozygous FcγRIIa 131R/R genotype was associated with susceptibility to meningococcal disease in two separate studies of 25 pediatric survivors of fulminant meningococcal septic shock (44% vs. 23%; OR, 2.7; 95% CI, 1.1–6.5; $p=.028$) (180) and 98 Slavic children with meningococcal disease (32% vs. 18%; $p=.02$) (199), but was not associated with meningococcal disease in two other studies involving 130 white, Spanish complement-normal patients (181), and 50 survivors of meningococcal disease, 183 first-degree relatives of patients with meningococcal disease, and 239 healthy controls (186). One of the studies reported that the FcγRIIa 131R/R genotype was more common in patients with septicemia (50% vs. 23%; OR, 3.3; 95% CI, 1.4–7.8; $p=.004$) (181), but this association was not confirmed in a larger study (186). The two studies that examined the association between FcγRIIa 131 polymorphisms and disease severity both reported that the FcγRIIa 131R/R genotype was more prevalent in patients with severe (OR, 4.7; 95% CI, 1.5–11.0; $p<.02$) (199) and fulminant (OR, 3.9; 95% CI, 1.0–16; $p=.04$) meningococcal disease (181), and those with severe complications of meningococcal disease (181,199). Furthermore, like patients with terminal complement pathway deficiency, the median age at disease onset in complement-sufficient patients was higher in FcγRIIa 131R/R homozygotes (18 years) compared with FcγRIIa 131H/R heterozygotes (7 years) or FcγRIIa 131H/H homozygotes (3½ years) (199). In this study, children older than 5 years with the homozygous FcγRIIa 131R/R genotype were 2.9 times (95% CI, 1.1–7.3; $p<.03$) more likely to develop meningococcal disease compared with FcγRIIa 131H/R heterozygotes or FcγRIIa 131H/H homozygotes. In a Spanish study, the FcγRIIa 131R/R genotype was found more frequently in patients older than 60 years (five of eight cases, 63%) compared with controls (two of 14 cases, 14%) (OR, 15; 95% CI, 1.1–232; $p=.03$).

Polymorphisms in the other FcγRs were not associated with meningococcal disease in two studies (180,186), although one of the studies found that the homozygous FcγRIIIa 158F/F genotype (0.51 vs. 0.41, $p=.042$) and a combination of the low-efficiency genotypes (FcγRIIa 131R/R, FcγRIIIa 158F/F, and FcγRIIIb NA2/NA2) were more common among relatives of patients with meningococcal disease compared with healthy controls (8% vs. 3%; OR, 2.6; 95% CI, 1.1–6.3; $p=.027$) (186). In this study, the FcγRIIIa 158V allele was more common among relatives of patients with meningitis compared with relatives of patients with sepsis ($p<.05$) (186). None of the studies contained enough patients with fatal meningococcal disease to confidently report any association between the FcγR polymorphisms and mortality.

FcγR polymorphisms have also been studied in patients with infections due to other encapsulated organisms. Yee and colleagues (200) reported that 50% of 42 patients with bacteremic pneumococcal pneumonia were homozygous for the FcγRIIa 131R/R genotype, compared to 28% of 28 American adults patients with nonbacteremic pneumonia ($p=.07$) and 29% of 136 controls ($p<.05$). Furthermore, all four of 42 patients with bacteremic pneumococcal pneumonia who died carried the homozygous FcγRIIa 131R/R genotype, suggesting that the FcγRIIa 131R/R genotype was associated not only with pneumococcal pneumonia but also with an increased risk of pneumococcal bacteremia and, possibly, death. Similarly, Yuan and colleagues (201) showed that the frequency of FcγRIIa 131R/R homozygosity was 43% in 63 children with invasive pneumococcal disease compared with 21% in 57 healthy blood donor controls ($p<.05$). In children with recurrent respiratory tract infections (six or more episodes in 1 year requiring six or more courses of antibiotics) and normal serum immunoglobulin levels, Sanders and colleagues (202) found that the FcγRIIa 131H/H genotype was significantly underrepresented (12.5% vs. 29%, $p=.01$) in the cases compared with controls. There was no association between the FcγR polymorphisms and clinical presentation, severity, or frequency of infections. However, all five children with invasive *H. influenzae* serotype b disease were homozygous for the FcγRIIIb NA2/NA2 genotype (202). The authors further reported that the superior IgG2-binding capacity of the FcγRIIa 131H/H genotype compared with the FcγRIIa R/R genotype became less significant when high levels of IgG2 were used in in vitro studies. They speculate that the FcγRIIa 131 polymorphism may be significant in young infants after they lose their protective maternal IgG at around 6 months of age and before they acquire their own IgG at around 18 months of age.

The Coagulation Pathway

Many studies have shown disturbances in the coagulation pathway in sepsis. The balance between procoagulant and anticoagulant properties of the host response is likely to determine whether disseminated intravascular coagulation, septic shock, and multiorgan failure occur. In fulminant meningococcal disease, there is activation of neutrophils, monocytes, and the coagulation and complement pathways (203–205), with upregulation of tissue factor expression on monocytes and endothelial cells (206,207) and a drop in levels of platelets, antithrombin III (208), protein C, and protein S (209,210). A high level of plasminogen activator inhibitor-1 (PAI-1) (205), which downregulates the fibrinolytic pathway (211), has also been reported. Acquired deficiencies of protein C and protein S have been associated with development of purpura fulminans after infection (212), while inherited deficiencies may cause neonatal purpura fulminans (213,214). However, deficiencies of these factors are rare (215) and therefore unlikely to be play an important role in influencing susceptibility to severe infections in the general population.

Factor V Leiden

A mutation from G to A at position 1691 in exon 10 of factor V Leiden results in a single amino acid substitution (R506Q), in turn resulting in loss of a cleavage site, thus preventing inactivation by activated protein C (216). This resistance to activated protein C is found in 8.8% of healthy Europeans (range 6.6% to 12.6%) and is a major abnormality of coagulation associated with an increased risk of venous thrombosis (217). Kondaveeti and colleagues (218) studied the factor V polymorphism in 259 children with meningococcal disease, 80 healthy controls, and 79 parents of children with fatal meningococcal disease and found no significant difference in the proportion of children with meningococcal disease with the factor V Leiden polymorphism (10%) compared with controls (9%) or parents of fatal cases (11%) (Table 9.7). These findings are consistent with a previous study that showed that factor V Leiden mutation was not more prevalent in parents of patients who died of meningococcal disease compared to controls (215). Of the survivors, however, children with the factor V Leiden polymorphism had significantly worse purpura fulminans, with five of 24 (21%) having complications (e.g., referral to plastic surgeon, skin grafting, or amputation) compared with 14 of 209 (7%) without the mutation (RR, 3.1; 95% CI, 1.2–7.9, p=.03).

Tissue-Type Plasminogen Activator and Plasminogen Activator Inhibitor-1

The fibrinolytic system counteracts the formation of microthrombi during infection by the release of tissue-type plasminogen activator (t-PA) (219), which is a serine protease that converts plasminogen into its active form, plasmin, which in turn promotes degradation of fibrin clots. In response, tissue plasminogen activator inhibitor 1 (PAI-1) is released, resulting in a decrease in t-PA activity and inhibition of fibrinolysis (211). PAI-1 is a 50-kd glycoprotein of the serine protease (SERPIN) family that acts as a rapid inhibitor of both tissue- and urinary-type plasminogen activator, the major proteolytic activators of plasminogen (220,221). PAI-1 is an acute-phase reactant produced by various cell types, including endothelial cells, hepatocytes, and platelets (222). Excessive PAI-1 levels can lead to a procoagulant state, and high PAI-1 levels have been associated with an adverse outcome in patients with sepsis (203) and meningococcal septic shock (204,205,223).

A polymorphism resulting in an insertion or deletion (I/D) of about 720 base pairs in intron h of the t-PA gene has been described and occurs with an allelic frequency of 0.5 (224). The functional significance of this polymorphism remains unknown, but it does not affect basal levels of t-Pa (225). In a study of 216 children with meningococcal disease, the t-PA polymorphism was not associated with susceptibility, mortality, or severity as determined by predicted risk of mortality (PRISM) scores, requirement for intensive care, frequency of septic shock, and risk of scarring, skin grafts, or amputations (226) (Table 9.8).

TABLE 9.7. Clinical studies on factor V Leiden polymorphisms on meningococcal diseases

Country (reference)	Cases	No.	Controls	No.	SNP	Su/Se/Ou	Significance	Comments
U.K. (218)	Children with MD	233	Healthy controls	80	G1691A allele	Su	0.10 vs. 0.09, p = NS	None of the patients were AA homozygous
	Purpura fulminans in children with MD	24	No purpura fulminans	209	G1691A allele	Se	0.21 vs. 0.07, RR = 3.1, p < .03	Complications: referral to plastic surgeon for skin grafting or amputation
	Nonsurvivors in a single center cohort	26	Survivors	158	G1691A allele	Ou	0.04 vs. 0.07, p = NS	
	Parents of nonsurvivors in a different cohort	79	Healthy controls	80	G1691A allele	Ou	0.12 vs. 0.09, p = NS	

MD, meningococcal disease; RR, relative risk; SNP, single nucleotide polymorphism; Su/Se/Ou, susceptibility/severity/outcome; NS, not significant.

In the PAI-1 gene, a common functional polymorphism exists with a single base-pair insertion (5G) or deletion (4G) at 675 bp upstream from the start of transcription in the promoter region of the PAI-1 gene (227). The presence of guanine at position -675 on the 5G allele is essential for binding of a transcriptase repressor to the PAI-1 promoter in vitro. Transfection of HepG2 cells with the 4G allele resulted in a sixfold increase in PAI-1 mRNA when stimulated with IL-1β (228). Individuals with the 4G/4G genotype have higher basal and inducible levels of PAI-1 than those with one or two copies of the 5G allele (228).

In a cohort of 175 children with meningococcal disease requiring intensive care in the U.K. and the Netherlands, median PAI-1 values were significantly higher in children with meningococcal disease compared with controls, and among children with meningococcal disease, levels were higher in those with sepsis compared with mixed disease or meningitis (223). The PAI-1 levels were also higher in children who died compared with those who survived. The homozygous 4G/4G genotype was not associated with susceptibility to infection but was associated with increased risk of death in the combined cohorts (RR, 2.0; 95% CI, 1.0–3.8; $p=.04$) (Table 9.8). Also, individuals with the homozygous 4G/4G genotype had significantly higher levels of PAI-1 compared with heterozygotes or 5G/5G homozygotes.

The same group repeated this study in a larger cohort of 510 patients with meningococcal disease and confirmed that the homozygous 4G/4G genotype was not associated with susceptibility to infection or clinical presentation, but was associated with severity of disease as determined by PRISM scores and the incidence of vascular complications in survivors (26.5% of 68 vs. 13.1% of 183 patients; RR, 2.4; 95% CI, 1.1–5.0; $p=.03$), as well as both predicted (41.1% in 4G/4G vs. 23.4% in 4G/5G and 19.0% in 5G/5G; $p=.02$) and actual mortality (28.4% in 4G/4G vs. 14.9% in 4G/5G and 5G/5G combined; RR, 1.9; 95% CI, 1.2–3.0; $p=.005$) (229). Logistic regression analysis showed a 40% (95% CI, 20–109%) and 91% (95% CI, 2–39%) reduction in the risk of dying if the patient carried the 4G/5G or 5G/5G alleles, respectively, compared with 4G/4G.

In another study of 80 patients with meningococcal disease, 183 first-degree relatives of patients with meningococcal disease (including 52 relatives of 16 patients who died), and 131 healthy white university student controls, there was no association with susceptibility to meningococcal infection or death, but the 4G/4G genotype was more prevalent in patients and relatives of patients with septic shock, such that carriers of the 4G/4G genotype had a sixfold increased risk of developing septic shock than meningitis (OR, 5.9; 95% CI, 1.9–18; $p=.001$) (230). A larger European study involving 347 children with meningococcal disease in 95 pediatric hospitals also found that the 4G/4G polymorphism was not associated with susceptibility when compared with 320 controls (cord blood from healthy, unrelated newborns) (27.3% vs. 28.8%; $p=.07$) (231). However, among children with meningococcal disease, the mortality rate was significantly higher (OR, 2.3; 95% CI, 1.0–5.1; $p=.037$) among patients with the 4G/4G genotype (12/90 died, 13%) compared with 4G/5G and 5G/5G genotypes (15/240 died, 6%). In the Central European cohort, the 4G/4G polymorphism

TABLE 9.8. Clinical studies on tissue-type plasminogen activator (t-PA) and tissue plasminogen activator inhibitor (PAI) polymorphisms among patients with meningo-coccal disease

Country (reference)	Cases	No.	Controls	No.	SNP	Su/Se/Ou	Significance	Comments
t-PA								
U.K. (226)	Children with MD of unknown ethnicity	216	Healthy controls—unknown source	103	D/D	Su	0.31 vs. 0.21, $p=$NS	
	Septicemia in patients with MD	103	Meningitis or mixed disease	112	D/D	Se	0.36 vs. 0.26, $p=$NS	
	Scarring, grafts, or amputations	23	No scarring, grafts, or amputations	193	D/D	Se	0.35 vs. 0.30, $p=$NS	
PAI								
Netherlands (230)	Patients with MD + first-degree relatives of patients with MD	50 + 183	White students aged 18–25 years	131	4G/4G	Su	0.26 and 0.26 vs. 0.27, $p=$NS	
	Septic shock in first-degree relatives of patients with MD	85	No septic shock in relatives	98	4G/4G	Se	0.36 vs. 0.17, $p=.001$ (compared with meningitis: OR$=5.9$, 95% CI$=1.9$–18)	
	First-degree relatives of 16 nonsurvivors of MD	52	Relatives of 45 survivors of MD	138	4G/4G	Ou	0.28 vs. 0.26, $p=$NS	
U.K. and Netherlands (223)	U.K. and Dutch children with MD	175	Friends of U.K. children with MD + healthy white Dutch infants	89 + 137	4G/4G	Su	0.27 vs. 0.26, $p=$NS	PAI-1 concentrations were significantly higher in 4G/4G

U.K. (229)	Sepsis in U.K. children with MD	92	No sepsis in children with MD	46	4G/4G	Se	0.27 vs. 0.22, p=NS
	Nonsurvivors among U.K. and Dutch children with MD	29	Survivors	146	4G/4G	Ou	0.41 vs. 0.23, p=.043 OR=2.0 (95% CI=1.0–3.8)
	Children with MD	405	Healthy unrelated Caucasian contact of MD	155	4G/4G	Su	0.27 vs. 0.31, p=NS
	Vascular complications in survivors*	42	No complications	209	4G/4G	Se	0.43 vs. 0.24, p=.01
	Nonsurvivors*	59	Survivors	251	4G/4G	Ou	0.46 vs. 0.27, p=.005 (RR=1.9)

*Severity and outcome studied in a single-centre U.K. cohort of 305 white children.
MD, meningococcal disease; RR, relative risk; 95% CI=95% confidence interval; SNP, single nucleotide polymorphism; Su/Se/Ou, susceptibility/severity/outcome; NS, not significant.

was also associated with development of sepsis (32.1% of 137 cases vs. 26.7% of 191 cases; OR, 2.2; 95% CI, 1.2–4.1; $p=.01$). This finding fits with current understanding of the pathophysiology of meningococcal disease because PAI-1 levels are significantly higher in patients with sepsis compared with meningitis (223). Furthermore, PAI-1 is an integral part of the coagulation pathway and is involved with development of disseminated intravascular coagulation, which plays an important role in the pathogenesis of sepsis but not meningitis (211,232). Thus, there appears to be a significant association among the 4G/4G polymorphism, higher plasma PAI-1 levels, development of sepsis, and worse outcome in meningococcal infections.

Thrombin-Activatable Fibrinolysis Inhibitor

Although PAI-1 is generally considered to be the major enzyme responsible for downregulation of fibrinolysis in sepsis, other antifibrinolytics such as the thrombin-activatable fibrinolysis inhibitor (TAFI) may also play an important role. Thrombin-activatable fibrinolysis inhibitor is a procarboxypeptidase that is activated by the thrombin-thrombomodulin complex (233). Activated TAFI (TAFIa) is a powerful antifibrinolytic that removes the carboxy-terminals of lysine and arginine residues from partially degraded fibrin, resulting in retardation of clot lysis through reduced plasminogen binding and activation (233). An inhibitor of TAFI has not been found, but TAFIa is intrinsically unstable with a half-life of only a few minutes (234,235). Patients with disseminated intravascular coagulation (236) and sepsis (237) have significantly lower levels of TAFI compared with controls, but similar levels are observed among septic patients who die compared with those who survive (237).

Plasma TAFI levels show a wide variation of up to fivefold in healthy individuals (237,238). This variation can partly be explained by polymorphisms in the coding region of the gene encoding the TAFI protein (239), two of which result in amino acid substitutions, including Thr147Ala (A505G substitution) and Thr325Ile (C1040T substitution) (240,241). The TAFI Thr147Ala substitution has little effect on the function of TAFI in vitro (240) and is in linkage disequilibrium with the TAFI Thr325Ile polymorphism (242,243). In contrast, activated TAFI-Ile325 has a longer half-life (15 minutes) than activated TAFI-Thr325 (8 minutes) at 37°C and 50% greater antifibrinolytic activity because of increased stability of the molecule (241,243).

The TAFI Thr325Ile polymorphism was studied in 50 patients with meningococcal disease, 138 first-degree relatives of 45 patients who survived, 52 first-degree relatives of 16 patients who died, and 212 controls, all of whom were recruited as part of a previous study on PAI-1 polymorphisms (230). There was no significant difference in the frequency of the homozygous TAFI-Ile325 polymorphism between controls (7.1%) and either survivors of meningococcal disease (4.0%) or relatives of patients with meningococcal disease (8.5%) (244). Patients whose parents were homozygous for the Ile/Ile genotype were 3.1 times more likely (95% CI, 1.0–9.5; $p=.03$) to die from meningococcal disease than healthy controls. They were also more likely to die when compared to patients whose parents carried other genotypes (OR, 2.7; 95% CI, 0.8–9.7; $p=0.14$), although this did not reach statistical significance. These results suggest that, like PAI-1, TAFI may also be associated with mortality in meningococcal disease, but larger studies are required to confirm this finding.

Angiotensin-Converting Enzyme

There is considerable evidence to support the existence of local renin-angiotensin systems in a number of human tissues, including leukocytes (245). Angiotensin-converting enzyme (ACE) is a key enzyme for the generation of angiotensin II from angiotensin I and also degrades bradykinin; both these molecules have multiple cellular effects resulting in activation of the proinflammatory response (246–248). Monocyte activation is associated with increased ACE expression (245), which drives autocrine cytokine synthesis (249), and paracrine tissue inflammatory responses (246,247).

The gene for ACE is located on chromosome 17q13 and contains a restriction fragment length polymorphism (RFLP) resulting in an insertion (I) or deletion (D) of a 2870-bp *alu* repeat sequence in intron 16 (250). It is believed that this intronic noncoding polymorphism is a marker for another genetic locus with more functional significance, but extensive haplotyping of the region was unable to identify the locus in the promoter region or a number of exons (251). Large interindividual differences in plasma ACE concentrations are found, but levels are similar in family members, suggesting a strong genetic influence (252). Among 80 healthy white individuals, the I/D polymorphism accounted for 47% of the variance in plasma ACE levels, being highest in those with the DD genotype (253). Plasma and T-cell ACE levels were 75% and 39% higher levels in those with the DD genotype (254). Studies that measured plasma ACE levels have not found any association with infectious diseases, probably because plasma ACE levels do not correlate with tissue levels (255). As a result, none of the studies of ACE polymorphisms measured plasma ACE levels in patients. Functional genetic polymorphisms have been identified in other renin-angiotensin-aldosterone system components including angiotensin receptors (256), bradykinin receptors (257), and angiotensinogen (258), but their association with infectious diseases has not been established.

In meningococcal disease, the ACE polymorphism was not associated with susceptibility in 110 white children compared with 841 healthy children from a DNA bank (259) (Table 9.9). However, the DD genotype was associated with more severe disease as determined by Glasgow Meningococcal Septicemia Prognostic Scoring, higher prevalence of intensive care admissions with longer intensive care stays, requirement for mechanical ventilation and inotropic support, and higher predicted risk of mortality (30% vs. 16%, $p=.01$) (259). Furthermore, five of 11 children who died (45%) had the DD genotype compared with 28 of 84 (33%) survivors requiring intensive care and one of 18 (6%) who were too well to be admitted to the intensive care unit ($p=.013$). However,

TABLE 9.9. Clinical studies on angiotensin-converting enzyme (ACE) polymorphisms

Country (reference)	Cases	No.	Controls	No.	SNP	Su/Se/Ou	Significance	Comments
U.K. (259)	White children with meningococcal disease	110	White children from DNA bank	841	DD	Su	0.31 vs. 0.24, p=NS	
	Requirement for intensive care	92	No requirement for intensive care	18	DD	Se	0.36 vs. 0.06, p=.011	DD patients had increased severity of illness scores and greater need for ventilation and inotropes
U.K. (255)	Nonsurvivors	11	Survivors	99	DD	Ou	0.45 vs. 0.29, p=NS	
	Adults with acute respiratory distress syndrome (ARDS)	96	Non-ARDS respiratory failure, CABG, healthy adults	88 + 174 + 1906	DD	Su	0.46 vs. 0.24, 0.25, 0.26 (p < .001 against all three control groups)	No difference in severity of illness scores
Canada (260)	Nonsurvivors	37	Survivors	59	DD	Ou	0.65 vs. 0.34, p < .02	
	Sepsis in low birth weight ventilated infants of different ethnicities	146	No sepsis	149	DD	Su	0.36 vs. 0.41, p=NS	

CABG, coronary artery bypass graft; SNP, single nucleotide polymorphism; Su/Se/Ou, susceptibility/severity/outcome; NS, not significant.

in a cohort of 295 mechanically ventilated very low birth weight (<1500 g) infants of different ethnic groups, the DD genotype was not associated with bloodstream infections, multiple infectious episodes, or mortality (260).

In the lungs, ACE has been shown to have effects on pulmonary vascular tone and permeability, fibroblast activity, and epithelial cell survival (261), all of which may play an important role in the pathogenesis of acute respiratory distress syndrome (ARDS). Individuals with the DD genotype were at increased risk of ARDS when compared to three different control groups: 88 white patients with non-ARDS respiratory failure with similar illness severity score (24%), 174 patients following coronary artery bypass grafting (25%), and 1906 individuals from the general population (26%) ($p < .001$ for each of the three control groups) (255) (Table 9.9). Within the ARDS group, the DD genotype was also associated with increased risk of death (65% vs. 34%, $p = .006$).

Cytokines

Cytokines regulate the intensity and duration of the host immune response and play an important role in mediating cell-to-cell communication. The host response to infection depends on a delicate balance between complex, well-timed, interacting proinflammatory and antiinflammatory cytokines. Although cytokines play a vital role in fighting infection, overzealous production can lead to deleterious effects. Patients who develop severe sepsis or those who die from sepsis, for example, have the highest levels of proinflammatory cytokines (262–264). However, clinical trials that have attempted to alter the septic cascade using either cytokines or agents that block specific cytokines have had a limited impact on improving the outcome of sepsis, with some studies showing an increase in mortality rate among patients receiving cytokine supplementation (265,266). There are several explanations for this observation. Redundance within the cytokine cascade, for example, makes the use of a single cytokine adjuvant or blocking agent unlikely to have a significant impact on the overall response. In addition, the timing of the intervention will also play an important role in determining optimum response, and this is difficult to standardize or measure in clinical trials. Finally, the host response to infection is highly heterogeneous. Recent studies have demonstrated that factors such as the timing, maximum levels, and duration of production of different cytokines vary considerably between different individuals, and many of these factors are controlled by specific polymorphisms within the cytokine genes (44,267,268).

TNF-Ligand Family

The TNF ligand family includes tumor necrosis factor-α (TNF-α) and TNF-β (269). Tumor necrosis factor-α has been identified as the proximal and central cytokine in the proinflammatory response that is associated with SIRS and multiple organ dysfunction syndrome (MODS) (270–272). Injection of TNF-α into experimental models produces profound shock—including hypotension, activation of the coagulation cascade, and organ dysfunction—that is similar to injection of endotoxin (273,274). The TNF-α levels are consistently high in patients with severe septic shock and inversely correlate with survival (262–264).

In contrast to TNF-α, which is expressed mainly by macrophages and consists of three identical subunits, TNF-β is expressed and released by T and B lymphocytes and is made up of a single lymphotoxin-α (LT-α) subunit and two lymphotoxin-β (LT-β) subunits (269). However, both TNF-α and TNF-β bind to the same TNF-receptors and invoke diverse biologic responses. The TNF locus is located on chromosome 6 within the major histocompatibility complex (MHC) class IV gene cluster. It consists of the functional gene for TNF-α, which is positioned between the LT-α gene and the LT-β gene. So far, at least nine polymorphisms and five microsatellites in the TNF locus have been characterized, some of which have been associated with susceptibility to infections.

Several polymorphisms in the promoter region of the TNF-α gene have been identified, including G-238A, G-244A, G-308A, G-376A, G-419C, and G-49A substitutions (275,276). Of these, the G-419C, G-244A, and G-49A polymorphisms are always associated with the G-308A polymorphism and the G-376A polymorphism is associated with the G-238A polymorphism (277). The rare TNF-α -308A allele, also known as TNF2, has direct effects on the *TNF*-α gene and is associated with a sixfold higher expression of both basal and induced mRNA for TNF-α, as well as higher serum levels of TNF-α in carriers (278). The study by Knight and colleagues (279) suggests that the presence of the TNF2 allele may increase *TNF*-α gene transcription through altering transcription factor (OCT-1) binding. However, other studies have been unable to demonstrate a difference in transcriptional regulation using reporter gene constructs and have, therefore, questioned whether the -308 locus is functionally important (280–282).

A genomic biallelic NcoI restriction fragment length polymorphism in the first intron of the *TNF-β/LT*-α gene was identified by the restriction fragments TNF-B1 (5.5 kilobase [kb]) and TNF-B2 (10.5 kb). This NcoI polymorphism correlates with a G252A substitution, resulting in an Asp26Thr amino acid substitution (283,284). The B2 allele, which corresponds to the less common *TNF-β/LT*-α A allele at position 252, has been shown to correlate with increased TNF-α concentrations in vivo (283,285). In vitro, phytohemagglutinin-stimulated monocytes from TNF-β/LT-α B1/B1 homozygous individuals showed significantly increased TNF-β/LT-α production, while monocytes from TNF-β/LT-α B2/B2 homozygous individuals produced significantly higher levels of IL-1β and TNF-α (284,286–288). The TNF-β/LT-α polymorphism is in significant linkage disequilibrium with the TNF-α -308 polymorphism so that TNF-β/LT-α 252A/A homozygosity occurred frequently among TNF-α -308GG homozygosity, which is associated with high TNF-α levels (284,289,290).

The TNF-α G-308A Polymorphism

Several studies have shown significant association between TNF-α polymorphisms and sepsis (Table 9.10). Mira and colleagues (276) studied all known TNF-α polymorphisms in 89 white French patients with septic shock and found that the TNF-α -308A allele was associated with septic shock (35/89, 39%) when compared with 87 healthy white French blood donors (16/87, 18%; $p=.002$). Within the septic shock group, the risk of death was also associated with the TNF-α -308A allele (25/48, 52% vs. 10/41, 24%, $p=.008$). In a logistic regression model, increasing age (OR, 1.46; 95% CI, 1.1–2.0) and TNF-α -308A allele (OR, 3.7; 95% CI, 1.4–10.2) were independently associated with death.

In 34 Belgian patients with early septic shock, 7/15 (47%) patients who died had the TNF-α -308A allele compared with 2/19 (11%) who survived ($p=.03$). In a multivariate model adjusted for severity of illness, the TNF-α -308A allele (but not high TNF-α levels, $p=0.3$), was independently associated with a 12-fold increase (95% CI, 1.4–96; $p=.02$) in the risk of death (291). Similarly, in the study by Gibot and colleagues (80) that evaluated the frequency of the C-159T promoter polymorphism in CD14 among 90 consecutive white French patients with septic shock, the investigators found that the TNF-α -308A allele was present in 26/50 (52%) patients who died compared with 10/40 (25%) who survived ($p=.009$). Moreover, 83% of the 12 patients with the combined TNF-α -308A allele and the rare homozygous CD14 -159T/T genotype (which were not in linkage disequilibrium) died. In a logistic regression model, this combination was independently associated with a 5.4-fold increased risk of death (95% CI, 1.1–26; $p<.03$). In another study, the TNF-α -308A/A homozygous genotype was also found to be more prevalent among 88 patients with MODS compared with 106 healthy controls (35% vs. 16%, $p<.001$) (292). However, there was no relationship between the polymorphism and plasma TNF-α levels ($p=.32$) or mortality ($p=.65$). On the other hand, in a much larger study involving 213 patients with severe sepsis or septic shock recruited from eight different intensive care units in England and Australia, there was no association between any of the TNF polymorphisms and either susceptibility or outcome when compared with 354 controls (293).

Several studies have also assessed the risk of sepsis among postoperative and posttrauma patients with the TNF-α polymorphisms. Tang and colleagues (294) studied 112 postoperative critically ill Taiwanese patients admitted to the surgical intensive care unit with SIRS and a definite focus of infection confirmed with a positive blood culture, of whom 42 (38%) developed septic shock. None of the patients were homozygous for the TNF-α -308AA genotype, but 12% were heterozygous compared with 5.1% of Taiwanese schoolchildren from a previous study ($p<.001$), suggesting that patients carrying this allele were more likely to require intensive care after surgical infection. Carriage of the TNF-α -308A allele was not associated with septic shock (50% of 26 vs. 34% of 86, $p>.05$) or death (62% of 26 vs. 48% of 86, $p>.05$). However, among 42

TABLE 9.10. Clinical studies on tumor necrosis factor-α (TNF-α) -308 polymorphisms

Country (reference)	Cases	No.	Controls	No.	SNP	Su/Se/Ou	Significance	Comments
Germany (280)	Postoperative sepsis in white Germans	80	White German blood donors	153	-308A allele	Su	0.17 vs 0.19, p=NS	
U.K. (299)	Nonsurvivors	41	Survivors	39	-308A allele	Ou	0.12 vs 0.24, p=NS	
	Children with severe, culture-proven MD	49	Children with nonsevere MD	49	-308A allele	Se	0.45 vs. 0.22, p=.02 RR=1.6 (95% CI=1.1–2.3)	
	Nonsurvivors of MD	18	Survivors	80	-308A allele	Ou	0.56 vs. 0.29, p=.03 RR=2.5 (95% CI=1.1–5.7)	
Netherlands (190)	Relatives of patients with MD	184	Blood donors	88	-308A allele	Su	0.41 vs. 0.43, p=NS	
	Relatives of 16 meningococcal nonsurvivors	52	Relatives of 50 survivors	138	-308A allele	Ou	0.43 vs. 0.41, p=NS	Low TNF-α producers had 10-fold increased risk of death
U.K. (297)	Nonsurvivors of MD	39	Survivors of MD	239	-308A allele	Ou	0.29 vs. 0.35, p=NS	
Taiwan (294)	Postoperative critically ill surgical patients with positive blood culture	112	Taiwanese children from a previous study	99	-308A allele	Su	0.12 vs. 0.051, p<.001	None of the patients had the -308AA homozygous genotype
France (276)	Septic shock	42	No septic shock	70	-308A allele	Se	0.31 vs. 0.19, p=NS	
	Nonsurvivors of septic shock	30	Survivors of septic shock	12	-308A allele	Ou	0.40 vs. 0.083, p<.05	Carriers of -308A allele had higher TNF-α levels
	White French patients with septic shock	89	White French blood donors	87	-308A allele	Se	0.39 vs. 0.18, p=.002	
U.S. (289)	Nonsurvivors of septic shock	48	Survivors of septic shock	41	-308A allele	Ou	0.52 vs. 0.24, p=.008	
	Septic shock in multiethnic patients with pneumonia	31	No septic shock in patients with pneumonia	249	-308A allele	Se	0.23 vs. 0.31, p=NS	
	Nonsurvivors of pneumonia	25	Survivors of pneumonia	255	-308A allele	Ou	0.32 vs. 0.29, p=NS	AA homozygous genotype also not associated with death

Population	Cases	n	Controls	n		Su/Se/Ou		Comments
France (80)	Nonsurvivors of septic shock in white French adults admitted to ICU	50	Survivors of septic shock	40	-308A allele	Ou	0.52 vs. 0.25, p=.009	This study included the CD14 polymorphism, and the combined genotypes had the worst outcome
U.S. (277)	Severe sepsis in severely injured adult trauma victims of multiethnic origin	37	No (n=55) or uncomplicated sepsis (n=60)	115	-308A allele	Se	0.43 vs. 0.17, p=.002	In a multivariate model, A-allele (p=.001) was associated with death
Belgium (291)	Nonsurvivors of severe trauma	19	Survivors of severe trauma	133	-308A allele	Ou	0.32 vs. 0.22, p=NS	
	Nonsurvivors of septic shock (? ethnic)	15	Survivors of septic shock	19	-308A allele	Ou	0.47 vs. 0.11, p=.02	In a multivariate model, the A allele (but not TNF-α levels) was associated with death
Germany (301)	Culture-proven invasive pneumococcal infection	69	Age-, sex-, and ethnicity-matched controls	50	-308A allele	Su	0.29 vs. 0.34, p=NS	
Germany (296)	Septic shock	13	No septic shock	56	-308A allele	Se	0.31 vs. 0.29, p=NS	
	Nonsurvivors	5	Survivors	64	-308A allele	Ou	0.20 vs. 0.30, p=NS	
	Severe sepsis in blunt trauma patients	14	No sepsis	56	-308A allele	Su	0.29 vs. 0.39, p=NS	
Ireland (300)	SIRS in patients with community-acquired pneumonia	74	No SIRS	38	-308A allele	Se	0.24 vs. 0.24, p=NS	No significant with increasing SIRS severity score
U.S. (89)	Survivors	11	Nonsurvivors	82	-308A allele	Ou	(Data not given), p=NS	
	Severe sepsis in adults with severe burns	36	Mild or no sepsis	123	-308 A allele	Su/Se	0.44 vs. 0.19, p=.002	In logistic regression model, A allele was associated with a 4.5-fold increased risk of severe sepsis

ICU, intensive care unit; MD, meningococcal disease; SIRS, systemic inflammatory response syndrome; OR, odds ratio; RR, relative risk; 95% CI, 95% confidence interval; SNP, single nucleotide polymorphism; Su/Se/Ou, susceptibility/severity/outcome; NS, not significant.

patients who developed septic shock, carriage of the TNF-α -308A allele was significantly associated with death (92% of 13 vs. 62% of 29 cases, $p<.05$). In this subgroup of patients, TNF-α -308A allele carriers had significantly higher TNF-α levels ($p<.05$). However, another study involving 80 German patients who developed postoperative sepsis was unable to find any association between the TNF-α -308 polymorphism and either the risk of infection or death when compared with healthy blood donors (280).

In 159 patients with severe burns affecting at least 20% of the total body surface area, carriage of the TNF-α -308A allele was independently associated with a 4.5-fold (95% CI, 1.7–12.0) increase in the risk of severe sepsis even after adjusting for age, burn size, ethnicity, and gender by multivariate logistic regression (89). In 173 ventilated very low birth weight infants of different ethnic origins, the TNF-α -308 polymorphism was not associated with late-onset bloodstream infections but mortality from sepsis was more than threefold higher in infants with the TNF-α -308A allele when compared with infants carrying the homozygous TNF-α -308GG genotype (6/23 vs. 4/59; $p=.026$) (295).

O'Keefe and colleagues (277) studied the TNF-α -308 polymorphism in an observational cohort study of 152 severely injured adult trauma victims of different ethnic origins admitted to a trauma center in the United States, of whom 24% developed sepsis. The TNF-α -308A allele was found more frequently in the 37 patients with severe sepsis (43%) compared with 115 patients with no ($n=55$) or uncomplicated ($n=60$) sepsis (17%, $p=.002$). This association remained when patients with severe sepsis were compared to those with uncomplicated sepsis only (50% of 12 vs. 18% of 66, $p=.016$). In a forward, stepwise multivariate, logistic regression model, only a high base deficit ≥6 mEq/L (OR, 3.9; 95% CI, 1.6–9.2), and carriage of the TNF-α -308A allele (OR, 4.6; 95% CI, 1.9–10.9; $p=.001$) were independently associated with increased risk of developing severe sepsis after trauma. The TNF-α -308A allele, however, was not associated with mortality (32% of 19 who died vs. 22% of 133 who survived, $p=.34$). In contrast, Majetschak and colleagues (296) found no association between the TNF-α -308 polymorphism and the risk of severe sepsis in 70 adults sustaining blunt trauma (0.29 vs. 0.36, $p=0.76$).

In meningococcal disease, the TNF-α -308 polymorphism was not associated with susceptibility to disease, severity or outcome among 276 English (297), 183 Irish (298), or 183 Dutch patients (190) with meningococcal disease, as well as 190 first-degree relatives of 61 patients with meningococcal disease (190). In an earlier study, however, the TNF-α -308A allele was associated with both severity of disease (45% vs. 22%; RR, 1.6; 95% CI, 1.1–2.3; $p=.02$) and outcome (56% vs. 29%; RR, 2.5; 95% CI, 1.1–5.7; $p=.03$) (299).

In community-acquired pneumonia, one study of 280 patients of different ethnic origins found that, although the TNF-α -308 polymorphism was not associated with either the risk of septic shock or death, there was a trend toward association between the TNF-α -308GG genotype and type II respiratory failure in a logistic regression model ($p=.03$) (289). Another study found no association between the TNF-α -308 polymorphism and development or severity of

SIRS, positive blood culture, or a fatal outcome among 93 patients with community-acquired pneumonia (300). The TNF-α polymorphism was also not associated with the risk of culture proven invasive pneumococcal infection, severe sepsis, or death among 69 hospitalized patients (301).

The TNF-α G-238A Polymorphism

The TNF-α -238 polymorphism was not associated with severe sepsis or death in three separate studies involving 89 French Caucasian adults with septic shock requiring intensive care (276), 213 English and Australian patients with severe sepsis or septic shock (293), and a cohort of 152 severely injured adult trauma victims (277) (Table 9.11). On the other hand, Westendorp and colleagues (190) found a trend toward increased TNF-α -238A allelic frequency among 52 relatives of 16 nonsurvivors (18%) compared with 138 relatives of 50 survivors (9%) of meningococcal disease ($p=.09$), but not when compared with 50 healthy blood donor controls (11%), suggesting that the polymorphism may be associated with increased risk of death in meningococcal disease.

The TNF-β/LT-α Polymorphism

Polymorphisms in the TNF-β/LT-α gene have usually been studied in conjunction with the other TNF polymorphisms. Most studies were performed in cohorts of patients following surgery or severe blunt trauma (Table 9.12). The two studies on adults with blunt trauma reported an increased risk of sepsis among individuals carrying the homozygous B2/B2 genotype, with odds ratios of 3.1 (95% CI, 1.4–6.6; $p=.004$) (285) and 11 (95% CI, 1.7–66) (296). Interestingly, the latter study found that homozygotes for the more common B1/B1 genotype were also at increased risk of developing sepsis (OR, 13; 95% CI, 1.8–95.5; $p=.014$) and patients homozygous for either B1 or B2 had a persistently higher cytokine-producing capacity during the first 4 to 8 days after trauma compared with heterozygotes (296).

In 40 critically ill patients admitted to a postoperative intensive care unit with severe sepsis, the homozygous B2/B2 genotype was associated with a significantly higher frequency of MODS, maximum multiple organ failure scores, and death (283). In a study of critically ill adults of different ethnic origins admitted to the intensive care unit with multiorgan dysfunction syndrome, the homozygous B2/B2 genotype was underrepresented among patients compared with healthy white controls (31% vs. 50%, $p=.06$) and there was a trend toward increased risk of death compared with carriers of the B1/B2 and B1/B1 genotypes (42% vs. 25%, $p=.10$) (292). Another study of 40 critically ill patients admitted to a postoperative intensive care unit with severe sepsis reported a higher incidence of MODS and maximum multiple organ failure scores among carriers of the homozygous B2/B2 genotype (283), and three studies confirmed the association between the homozygous B2/B2 genotype and death (136,283,302). In one of the studies, all eight patients with combined homozygous IL-1RN*2/2 (see below) and TNF-β/LT-α B2/B2 genotypes had multiple organ failure and

TABLE 9.11. Clinical studies on tumor necrosis factor-α (TNF-α) -238 polymorphisms

Country (reference)	Cases	No.	Controls	No.	SNP	Su/Se/Ou	Significance	Comments
Netherlands (190)	Relatives of meningococcal nonsurvivors	52	Relatives of 50 survivors and blood donors	138 and 50	-238A allele	Su	0.18 vs. 0.09 and 0.11 (died vs. survived: $p=.09$)	
France (276)	White French patients with septic shock admitted to ICU	89	Healthy white blood donors	87	-238A allele	Se	0.15 vs. 0.11, $p=$NS	
	Nonsurvivors of septic shock	48	Survivors of septic shock	41	-238A allele	Ou	0.12 vs. 0.17, $p=$NS	
U.S. (277)	Severe sepsis in severely injured adult trauma victims of multiethnic origin	37	No ($n=55$) or uncomplicated sepsis ($n=60$)	115	-238A allele	Se	0.08 vs. 0.11, $p=$NS	
	Nonsurvivors	19	Survivors	133	-238A allele	Ou	0.00 vs 0.09, $p=$NS	

ICU, intensive care unit; SNP, single nucleotide polymorphism; Su/Se/Ou, susceptibility/severity/outcome; NS, not significant.

died (302). On the other hand, the TNF-β/LT-α B2/B2 homozygous genotype was not associated with susceptibility, severity or outcome among 183 Irish patients with meningococcal disease when compared with 389 blood donor controls (298) or among 213 English and Australian patients admitted to an intensive care unit with severe sepsis or septic shock (293).

In adults with community-acquired pneumonia, the homozygous TNF-β/LT-α B2/B2 genotype was associated with septic shock in two studies involving 280 and 343 patients, with odds ratios of 3.6 (95% CI, 1.3–10.6) (289) and 2.7 (95% CI, 1.4–5.3) (137), respectively. This association remained significant after adjusting for other factors such as age, sex, ethnicity, clinical risk factors, and prior antibiotic exposure in one of the studies (289), but was lost in the second study (137). Another study involving 69 hospitalized patients with culture proven invasive pneumococcal infection reported no association between the TNF-β/LT-α B2/B2 genotype and the risk of infection compared with 50 controls, or the risk of septic shock among patients with proven infection (301). However, the numbers of patients in this study was relatively small and, thus, could have missed a significant finding. The TNF-β/LT-α polymorphism was not associated with death in any of the three studies (137,289,301).

Interleukin-1 Complex

The IL-1 family of cytokines, which includes IL-1α, IL-1β, and the IL-1 receptor antagonist (IL-1RA), plays an important role in the pathophysiologic responses to infection and inflammation, by mediating its own production and that of other proinflammatory cytokines (303–307). Along with TNF-α, IL-1α, and IL-1β are major inducers of early proinflammatory immune responses. They bind to IL-1 receptors on a variety of cells and initiate a cascade of events that lead to recruitment and activation of macrophages and neutrophils, vascular dilatation, and fever (308). In contrast, IL-1RA acts as a key antiinflammatory cytokine by regulating the activity of IL-1α and IL-1β through competitive combination with IL-1 receptors (309). Typically, the concentration of IL-1RA increases late during the course of inflammation so that the induced acute inflammation can terminate and does not become chronic and damage healthy tissues (310). In vivo, the IL-1RA/IL-1β molar ratio is considered to be the most important determinant of IL-1 activity, and a low ratio is associated with a heightened and prolonged proinflammatory immune response (311–313).

The genes for the IL-1 cytokine family are located within a cluster of human MHC on chromosome 2q13–21 within a 430-kb region (309,314). Genetic polymorphisms have been identified in all three IL-1 cytokines. The *IL-1α* gene has a C-889T promoter polymorphism, a +4845 polymorphism downstream from the transcription site, and a variable number of tandem repeats (VNTR) of 46bp within intron 6 (315–317). Although polymorphisms in the *IL-1α* gene are the least studied among the IL-1 family, they have been shown to correlate with serum IL-1α levels (318). The *IL-1β* gene has an AvaI C-511T promoter polymorphism, which is present in around 33% of the general white population

TABLE 9.12. Clinical studies on tumor necrosis factor-β (TNF-β) B2/B2 polymorphisms

Country (reference)	Cases	No.	Controls	No.	SNP	Su/Se/Ou	Significance	Comments
U.K. (292)	Critically ill adults with MODS	87	Unrelated healthy U.K. adults	30	B2/B2	Su	0.31 vs. 0.50, $p=.06$	No association between genotypes and plasma TNF levels
	Nonsurvivors of severe sepsis	21	Survivors	66	B2/B2	Ou	0.42 vs. 0.25, $p=0.10$	No difference when different combinations of IL-10 and TNF-β genotypes studied
U.S. (289)	Septic shock in adults with community acquired pneumonia	30	No septic shock	313	B2/B2*	Se	0.52 vs. 0.27, $p=.005$	Remained significant ($p=.03$) in logistic regression analysis; age-adjusted OR=3.6 (95% CI=1.3–10.7)
	Nonsurvivors of septic shock	22	Survivors	321	B2/B2	Ou	0.41 vs. 0.29, $p=NS$	Lost significance in logistic regression model
Germany (285)	Severe sepsis in postoperative patients after blunt trauma	53	No sepsis in postop patients after trauma	57	B2/B2	Se	0.64 vs. 0.37, $p=.004$	B2/B2 had higher TNF levels and more severe disease
Germany (302)	Nonsurvivors of severe sepsis in white German surgical ICU patients	47	Survivors of severe sepsis	46	B2 allele	Ou	0.74 vs. 0.46, $p=.0001$ OR=3.5	No linkage with IL-1; all eight with combined homozygous IL-1RA A2 and TNF-B2 genotypes died

Study	Phenotype	N	Comparison	N	Genotype	Su/Se/Ou	Statistics	Comments
U.S. (289)	Septic shock in multiethnic patients with pneumonia	31	No septic shock in patients with pneumonia	249	B2/B2	Se	0.52 vs. 0.27, $p=.01$	
Germany (283)	Nonsurvivors of pneumonia	25	Survivors of pneumonia	255	B2/B2	Ou	0.40 vs. 0.29, $p=$NS	
	Nonsurvivors of septic shock	23	Survivors of septic shock	17	B2/B2	Ou	0.65 vs. 0.12, $p<.005$	B2 polymorphism in linkage disequilibrium with HSP polymorphisms ($p<.01$)
	MODS (MOF score ≥4)	33	No MODS	7	B2/B2	Se	0.52 vs. 0.00, $p=.01$	
Germany (136)	Nonsurvivors of severe sepsis in surgical ICU	40	Survivors	47	B2/B2*	Ou	0.50 vs. 0.17, $p<.01$	
Germany (301)	Culture-proven invasive pneumococcal infection	69	Age-, sex-, and ethnicity-matched controls	50	B2/B2	Su	0.39 vs. 0.50, $p=$NS	
Germany (296)	Septic shock	13	No septic shock	56	B2/B2	Se	0.46 vs. 0.38, $p=$NS	
	Nonsurvivors	5	Survivors	64	B2/B2	Ou	0.40 vs. 0.41, $p=$NS	Overall, homozygotes more susceptible to severe sepsis compared to heterozygotes
	Severe sepsis in blunt trauma patients	14	No sepsis	56	B2/B2 B1/B1 Both	Su	0.64 vs. 0.39, $p=.01$ against B1/B2 0.29 vs. 0.14, $p=.01$ against B1/B2 0.93 vs. 0.54, $p=.008$ against B1/B2	

*Linkage disequilibrium between the HSP70-2 A/A polymorphism and TNF-B2/B2 ($p<.0001$) reported in this study.
HSP, heat shock protein; ICU, intensive care unit; MODS, multiple organ dysfunction syndrome; MOF score, multiple organ failure score; OR, odds ratio; SNP, single nucleotide polymorphism; Su/Se/Ou, susceptibility/severity/outcome; NS, not significant.

(319). This polymorphism is in 99.5% linkage disequilibrium with another T-31C promoter polymorphism, which blocks LPS binding of the transcription-initiation complex of IL-1β and impairs IL-1β transcription (319,320). This results in significantly lower levels of IL-1β secreted by LPS-stimulated monocytes from individuals homozygous for the rare allele compared with monocytes from individuals who were heterozygotic or homozygotic for the common allele (316). The *IL-1β* gene also has a TaqI C3954T polymorphism on exon 5 at amino acid 105 of the precursor form of IL-1, which is associated with four-fold increase in IL-1β secretion (316). The IL-1α −889 and IL-1β +3954 polymorphic sites have recently been shown to be in strong linkage disequilibrium (321). Studies using IL-1β–deficient mice found that response to LPS was similar to IL-1β–positive mice, suggesting that that IL-1β is not essential for the in vivo systemic response to LPS or that its role can be fulfilled by other cytokines with overlapping activities (322).

A polymorphic region within intron 2 of the *IL-1RA* gene *(IL-1RN*)* containing a variable number of tandem repeats (VNTR) of 86 bp has been identified. Five *IL-1RN** alleles have been reported and named according to the rank of frequencies in healthy individuals. Thus, alleles *1 to *5 (also termed A1 to A5 or RN1 to RN5) correspond to 4, 2, 5, 3, and 6 repeats of the 86 bp sequence with sizes of 410, 240, 500, 325, and 595 bp, respectively (315). Three potential motifs for DNA binding proteins are located in the 86-bp sequence, and it is possible that the number of repeats may influence gene transcription and protein synthesis (315). The *IL-1RN*2* allele, which is present in around 28% of the general white population, has recently been shown to be in 100% linkage disequilibrium with another polymorphism at position +2018 within exon 2 (315,323). The IL-1RN*2 polymorphism is associated with higher levels of IL-1RA (311,312,324,325), although some studies have report reduced levels with this allele (326,327). Mice lacking the *IL-1RN* gene, and therefore, the IL-1RA protein, have reduced body mass and lower IL-1 secretion in response to endotoxin, and are more susceptible to lethal endotoxemia than controls (328). On the other hand, overexpression of IL-1RA protects against lethal endotoxinemia in mice (328). In one clinical study, logistic regression analysis revealed that IL-1RA was the only cytokine whose plasma levels were of value in predicting mortality in 11 of 34 patients with sepsis (329). However, clinical trials testing recombinant IL-1RA could not demonstrate a clear benefit for septic patients (330,331).

In a study of 159 patients with severe burns affecting ≥20% total body surface area, the IL-1β T-31C polymorphism was not associated with an increased risk of severe sepsis (89). Similarly, IL-1β polymorphisms were not associated with sepsis in a cohort of 93 consecutive patients admitted to a surgical intensive care unit with severe sepsis (302). However, patients with sepsis had a higher frequency of the *IL-1RN*2* allele (37% vs. 24%; RR, 1.73; $p < .05$) and the homozygous *IL-1RN*2/2* genotype (14% vs. 7%, $p < .05$) compared with 261 healthy local blood donors. In this study, neither the IL-1RA nor the IL-1β polymorphism was associated with severity of infection or mortality.

The *IL-1RN*2* allele (41% vs 27%; OR, 1.79; *p*<.05) was also associated with sepsis in 60 consecutive Chinese patients when compared with 60 healthy volunteer controls (332). However, there was no association between any of the *IL-1α* VNTR alleles or the IL-1β C-511T polymorphism and the risk of sepsis. Among 16 patients who died, mortality was associated with more severe underlying disease, *Pseudomonas* sepsis, the homozygous *IL-1α*A2/A2* genotype (the A2 allele was defined as a 1200-bp fragment of the 46-bp tandem repeat) (25% vs. 2%, *p*=.02), the homozygous *IL-1β -511TT* genotype (81% vs. 7%, *p*<.001), and the homozygous *IL-1RN*2* genotype (31% vs. 5%, *p*=.01) in the univariate analysis. On the other hand, septic patients homozygous for the *IL-1α*A1/A1*, *IL-1β -511C/C*, or *IL-1RN*1/1* genotypes had a very low mortality (0–14%). Thus, the *IL-1RN*2* allele was associated with susceptibility to sepsis, while all three polymorphisms were associated with severity and death in this study.

In another study of 78 patients with severe sepsis, 56 patients with uncomplicated pneumonia and 130 unrelated ethnicity-matched healthy blood donors, no association was observed between polymorphisms in the *IL-1RN** gene and severe sepsis or pneumonia (327). However, the *IL-1RN*2/2* homozygous genotype was more frequently isolated from the 27 patients with severe sepsis who died compared with those who survived (37% vs. 6%; OR, 9.4; 95% CI, 2.31–38.1; *p*=.002). After adjusting for age and severity of illness, the *IL-1RN*2/2* homozygous genotype remained significantly associated with a 6.5-fold increase in death (95% CI, 1.0–41.5; *p*=.04). Furthermore, geometric mean plasma IL-1RA levels were significantly lower in the 27 sepsis patients who died compared to the 51 patients who survived (*p*<.001).

In adults and children with proven meningococcal disease, Read and colleagues (297) studied the IL-1 complex polymorphisms in 276 patients and found that only the IL-1β -511 polymorphism was significantly associated with death. Compared with heterozygotes, patients with the more common homozygous -511C/C genotype had a 3.4-fold (95% CI, 1.4–8.3; *p*<.001) increased risk of death (18% vs. 6% died), while those with the less common homozygous *IL-1β -511TT* genotype had a 7.4-fold (95% CI, 2.5–21.5; *p*<.001) increased risk of death (32.3% vs. 6% died). There was also a trend toward increased risk of death (17.3% vs. 11.3%) among carriers of the less common *IL-1RN +2018* allele (i.e., the *IL-1RN*2* allele). In a larger follow-up prospective study, the same investigators found no association between IL-1 polymorphisms and susceptibility to infection when compared with adult northern English blood donors (333). However, in a multivariable logistic regression model, mortality was independently associated with older age, infection with meningococcal serogroup C, homozygosity for the rare *IL-1β -511T/T* genotype, and carriage of the less common *IL-1RN +2018* allele (i.e., the *IL-1RN*2* allele).

These findings, however, were not replicated in an Irish study of 183 patients with meningococcal disease, which reported an increased susceptibility to infection among carriers of the *IL-1RN*2/2* homozygous genotype when compared with 389 Irish blood donors (14% vs. 8%, *p*=.033), but no association with severity of infection or mortality (298). This study also found no association between the IL-1β +3953 polymorphism and susceptibility, severity, or outcome among patients with meningococcal disease. In a separate study of 144 children with meningococcal disease, Carrol and colleagues (334) found that neither the *IL-1RN*2* allelic frequency (25% vs. 27%) nor the homozygous *IL-1RN*2/2* genotype (10% vs. 11%) was associated with disease when compared with 95 anonymous healthy blood donors. Instead, fewer children who had septic shock, severe disease, or required ventilation had the *IL-1RN*2* allele compared with those who did not, although none of these achieved statistical significance. Furthermore, there was no difference in IL-1RA concentrations among children with and without the *IL-1RN*2* allele.

Interleukin-6

Interleukin-6 (IL-6) is a pleiotropic cytokine with potent biologic effects, including T- and B-cell activation, induction of fever, and hepatic induction of acute-phase protein synthesis (335). Among the proinflammatory cytokines, IL-6 has been found most consistently in the circulation of patients with sepsis, occasionally up to 7500 times the normal level, particularly in patients with septic shock and those who subsequently died of sepsis (336–339). The expression of IL-6 is tightly regulated by several transcription factors, including nuclear factor-IL-6 (NF-IL-6) and signal transducer and activator of transcription 3/acute-phase response factor (STAT3/APRF) (340). Several functional polymorphisms in the IL-6 promoter region with cell type-specific regulation of IL-6 expression have been described, including G-597A, G-572C, A(n)-373T(n), and G-174C. These polymorphisms do not act independently of one another, and one polymorphism influences the functional effect of variation at other polymorphic sites. The presence of the G allele in the G-174C promoter polymorphism is associated with significantly higher levels of IL-6 in vitro and in healthy individuals (341). Healthy individuals homozygous for the -174G allele who received the *Salmonella typhi* vaccine had significantly higher plasma IL-6 values, but not IL-1β or TNF-α, after vaccination than did individuals homozygous for the C genotype ($p < .005$), suggesting that G-174C polymorphism in the promoter region of the IL-6 gene is functional in vivo, with an increased inflammatory response associated with the G allele (342).

Schluter and colleagues (343) studied the IL-6 G-174C polymorphism in 326 consecutive critically ill Caucasian German patients with a surgical intensive care unit stay of at least 3 days (Table 9.13). They found no difference in the frequency of the homozygous IL-6 -174GG genotype among 326 patients and 207 healthy sex-matched Caucasian German controls from another study (32% vs. 34%, $p = .83$), among the 95 patients who subsequently developed sepsis compared with 276 who did not (26% vs. 33%, $p = .28$), among the 45 patients with and 50 patients without severe sepsis in the sepsis subgroup (27% vs. 26%, $p = .94$), or among 34 septic patients who developed multiorgan failure compared with 16 patients who did not (21% vs. 21%, $p = .3$). On the other hand, the IL-6 polymorphism was associated with survival in patients with sepsis. Only 2/25 (8%) patients who died compared with 11/25 (44%) who survived

TABLE 9.13. Clinical studies on interleukin-6 (IL-6) G-174C polymorphisms

Country (reference)	Cases	No.	Controls	No.	SNP	Su/Se/Ou	Significance	Comments
Germany (343)	Sepsis in critically ill Caucasian German patients	95	No sepsis	276	-174GG	Su	0.26 vs. 0.34, p = NS	No association with mortality in patients without sepsis; median IL-6 levels higher in patients who died
	Severe sepsis	45	Sepsis not severe	50	-174GG	Se	0.26 vs. 0.33, p = NS	
	Nonsurvivors	25	Survivors	25	-174GG	Ou	0.08 vs. 0.44, p = .008 OR = 0.11, 95% CI = 0.02–0.57	in patients who died
Ireland (300)	SIRS in patients with community-acquired pneumonia	74	No SIRS	38	-174GG	Se	0.30 vs. 0.16, p = NS	No association with increasing SIRS severity score
	Nonsurvivors	11	Survivors	82	-174GG	Ou	(Data not given), p = NS	
U.S. (89)	Severe sepsis in adults with severe burns	36	Mild or no sepsis	123	-174GG	Su/Se	0.47 vs. 0.56, p = NS	

SIRS, systemic inflammatory response syndrome; OR, odds ratio; RR, relative risk; 95% CI, 95% confidence interval; SNP, single nucleotide polymorphism; Su/Se/Ou, susceptibility/severity/outcome; NS, not significant.

were GG homozygotes (OR, 0.11; 95% CI, 0.02–0.57; p=.008). In contrast to this finding, however, median IL-6 plasma levels were significantly *higher* in patients who died (749 vs. 210 pg/mL, p<.0001). The authors also found that there was no significant association between median or maximal plasma IL-6 concentrations and the IL-6 polymorphisms in sepsis. They therefore proposed that because the IL-6 promoter polymorphism is associated with higher plasma levels in healthy individuals (341) but not in patients with sepsis in their study, it is possible that the IL-6 polymorphisms may have an important role in long-term subliminal stimulation such as in chronic inflammatory disorders rather than acute sepsis.

In another study of 93 patients with community-acquired pneumonia, again, there was no significant difference in the IL-6 -174G allele or GG genotype and development or severity of SIRS, positive blood culture, or a fatal outcome (300). Similarly, this polymorphism was not associated with severe sepsis in 159 patients with severe burns affecting ≥20% total body surface area (p=.35) (89). On the other hand, a recent Irish study reported that the IL-6 -174GG homozygous genotype was associated with both severity of infection (41% vs. 26%, p=.037) and a fatal outcome (52% vs. 29%; p=.023; OR, 2.64; 95% CI, 1.12–6.22) among 183 patients with meningococcal disease (298).

In a recent study, Watanabe and colleagues (344) speculated that IL-6 levels in critically ill patients may be associated not only with IL-6 promoter polymorphisms but also with polymorphisms of other proinflammatory cytokines, such as TNF-α and IL-1β. These cytokines interact with each other at different levels during an inflammatory response. The authors studied 150 critically ill Japanese patients and found very high levels of IL-6 (>10,000 pg/mL) in 30 patients. All measures of severity of illness, as well as TNF-α and IL-1β levels, were higher in this subgroup. In addition, there was significant positive correlation between maximum IL-6 and TNF-α (r=0.659, p<.001), and between maximum IL-6 and IL-1β (r=0.521, p<.001) levels. The distribution of IL-6, IL-1β, and TNF-α polymorphisms in the 150 patients was not different when compared to 150 healthy Japanese blood donors. However, when the 30 patients with very high IL-6 levels were compared with the other 120 patients, the allelic frequencies of TNF-α -308A (6.7% vs. 1.7%, p=.054), IL-1β -511T (58.3% vs. 41.3%, p=.018), and alleles other than IL-1RN*1 (18.3% vs. 6.2%, p=.008) were significantly higher in the former group. Interestingly, in this study, all patients were homozygous for the IL-6 GG genotype at both G-174C and G-596A sites, suggesting that these polymorphisms were not responsible for the high IL-6 levels. Instead, plasma IL-6 levels were more likely to be influenced by other cytokines and their polymorphisms. It is possible that the levels of other cytokines may also be controlled in a similar manner.

Interleukin-10

Interleukin-10 is a potent antiinflammatory cytokine that downregulates the potentially harmful effects of proinflammatory cytokines (345,346). It is produced mainly by monocytes and acts to downregulate proinflammatory cytokines such as IL-1β, IL-6, IL-8, and TNF-α, which are produced by T-helper cells. Interleukin-10 also inhibits MHC class II expression, resulting in impaired bacterial clearance (347), and influences the adaptive immune response by downregulating monocyte HLA-DR expression by intracellular sequestration (348). Interleukin-10 knockout mice have a higher lethality due to septic shock, possibly because of an unrestricted proinflammatory cytokine response (349). In septic shock, serum levels of IL-10 are increased and associated with a higher mortality (350–353). Furthermore, nonsurvivors of sepsis have persistently raised levels of IL-10 while survivors show decreasing IL-10 levels over time (341). However, excess IL-10 can induce immunosuppression in bacterial sepsis (354) and can increase the risk of severe infection and death by impairing bacterial clearance (347,355). Thus, high IL-10 production may protect against SIRS but may result in immunosuppression and an increased risk of infection.

A genetic component is considered to determine between 50% and 75% of variation in IL-10 production (190,356). The IL-10 gene has been mapped to chromosome 1q31–32 and at least 23 SNPs have been reported (http://bris.ac.uk/pathandmicro/services/GAI/cytokine4.html). At least two dinucleotide CA-repeat microsatellites (−1151 bp and −3978 bp from the transcription start site and named *IL10.G* and *IL10.R*, respectively) and three promoter polymorphisms (G-1082A, C-819T, and C-592A) upstream from the transcription start site have been shown to influence IL-10 expression (357–362). The three promoter polymorphisms occur within putative transcription factor binding sites that affect IL-10 expression (361,363). The C-819T polymorphism is always found with the C-592A polymorphism (360,364,365). Thus, only four possible haplotypes of the three polymorphisms can occur: GCC, ACC, GTA, and ATA. In Europeans, the GGC prevalence is approximately 50%, while in Asians it is less than 5%; the GTA haplotype is extremely rare (366).

Stimulated mononuclear cells from patients homozygous for the IL-10 -1082GG genotype have higher transcriptional activity and secrete higher levels of IL-10 (360,367). Similarly, stimulated whole blood from IL-10 -1082GG homozygous patients produced significantly higher amounts of IL-10 compared with IL-10 -1082A/A homozygotes (301), although others have not been able to reproduce these results (368,369). Stimulated whole blood from healthy volunteers carrying the homozygous IL-10 -592C/C genotype also produced significantly higher IL-10 compared with the IL-10 -592AA genotype (368). When the combined haplotypes were transiently infected into cells, the GCC haplotype showed significantly increased transcriptional activity compared with ACC, which in turn had increased transcriptional activity compared with ATA (370).

In 116 Chinese patients, there was a significant association between sepsis and carriage of at least one IL-10 -1082G allele (60% vs. 50%; $p < .05$; OR, 1.5; 95% CI, 1.0–3.0), which is associated with high IL-10 production, but not the homozygous IL-10 -1082GG genotype (27% vs. 31%, $p = 0.5$) (371) (Table 9.14).

TABLE 9.14. Clinical studies on interleukin-10 (IL-10) polymorphisms

Country (reference)	Cases	No.	Controls	No.	SNP	Su/Se/Ou	Significance	Comments
Ireland (300)	SIRS in patients with community acquired pneumonia	74	No SIRS	38	-1082 GG	Se	0.37 vs. 0.26, p=NS	Significant association with increasing SIRS severity score: 18% for SIRS2, 36% for SIRS3 and 50% for SIRS3 (p<.05)
	Nonsurvivors	11	Survivors	82		Ou	0.82 vs. 0.51, p=.01 OR=4.3 (1.4–13.2)	
Scotland (368)	Critically ill adult patients admitted to ICU with sepsis	31	No sepsis	36	-592C/C	Su	0.66 vs. 0.65, p=NS	CC homozygotes had the highest LPS-stimulated IL-10 levels in monocytes
	Critically ill adult patients admitted to ICU with sepsis	31	No sepsis	36	-1082–GG	Su	0.32 vs. 0.22, p=NS	Not associated with IL-10 release, development of sepsis or outcome
	Nonsurvivors	22	Survivors	45	-592C/C	Ou	0.76 vs. 0.43, p=.04	Outcome measured for all critically ill patients, irrespective of sepsis
	Nonsurvivors	22	Survivors	45	-1082 GG	Ou	(Data not given), p=NS	
Germany (301)	White Germans with invasive pneumococcal infection	69	Matched unrelated white orthopedic patients	50	-1082 GG	Su	0.23 vs. 0.26, p=NS	
	Septic shock in patients with invasive pneumococcal infection	13	No septic shock	56	-1082 GG	Se	0.54 vs. 0.16, p=.024 OR=6.1 (95% CI=1.4–27.2)	IL-10 levels not associated with septic shock

Study	Group	n	Comparison	n	SNP/genotype	Su/Se/Ou	Result	Comments
U.K. (292)	Nonsurvivors	5	Survivors	64	-1082 GG	Ou	0.60 vs. 0.20, p=.04	IL-10 levels not associated with death
	Critically ill adults of different ethnicities with MODS	88	Healthy controls	303	GCC/GCC homozygous haplotype	Su	0.06 vs. 0.30, p<.001	Intermediate producers over-represented (67% vs. 42%) among MODS patients
China (371)	Nonsurvivors	31	Survivors	57	GCC/GCC homozygous haplotype	Ou	0.065 vs. 0.053, p=NS	IL-10 levels not associated with genotype or death
	Severe sepsis in Chinese adults	116	Ethnicity-matched blood donors	141	-1082 G allele	Su	0.60 vs. 0.50, p<.05, OR=1.5(1.0–3.0)	More G/A heterozygotes among cases compared with controls (66% vs. 40%, p<.05)
	Nonsurvivors	?	Survivors	?	-1082 G allele	Ou	0.50 vs. 0.50, p=NS	
China (371)	Severe sepsis in Chinese adults	116	Ethnicity-matched blood donors	141	-592 CC	Su	0.61 vs. 0.65, p=NS	No association between haplotypes and susceptibility/outcome
	Nonsurvivors	?	Survivors	?	-592 CC	Ou	(Data not given), p=NS	

ICU, intensive care unit; MODS, multiple organ dysfunction syndrome; ?, not reported by authors; SIRS, systemic inflammatory response syndrome; OR, odds ratio; RR, relative risk; 95% CI, 95% confidence interval; SNP, single nucleotide polymorphism; Su/Se/Ou, susceptibility/severity/outcome; NS, not significant.

The IL-10 -592 and IL-10 -819 polymorphisms, which are in linkage disequilibrium, were also not associated with severe sepsis, and haplotype analysis did not show any significant differences between patients and controls. Furthermore, none of the polymorphisms was associated with death. In contrast, another study involving 67 consecutive critically ill Caucasian patients admitted to the intensive care unit found no association between any of the IL-10 polymorphisms and subsequent development of sepsis (368). Instead, patients who subsequently developed sepsis had significantly *lower* admission IL-10 levels compared with those who did not develop sepsis ($p=.001$). Furthermore, patients with the homozygous IL-10 -592C/C genotype, which was associated with significantly higher LPS-stimulated IL-10 levels, were more likely to survive irrespective of whether they developed sepsis or not. In a separate study involving adults with multiorgan dysfunction syndrome, those IL-10 polymorphisms resulting in high IL-10 production (the GCC homozygous haplotype) were significantly underrepresented (6% vs. 30%, $p<.001$) in the patient group compared with 303 healthy controls, while intermediate producers (GGC/ACC or GCC/ATA heterozygotes) were overrepresented (67% vs. 42%, $p<.001$) (292). However, there was no significant difference in median plasma IL-10 levels ($p=.35$) or mortality between the low, intermediate, and high IL-10 producers (33%, 36%, and 40%, respectively; $p=.96$) (292).

In meningococcal disease, the IL-10 -1082GG and the IL-10 -592C/C homozygous genotype were not associated with susceptibility, severity of infection, or outcome in 183 patients when compared with 389 Caucasian Irish blood donors in a recent study (298) (Table 9.14). Instead, the IL-10 -1082A/A homozygous genotype was associated with severity of infection when 76 patients with severe meningococcal disease were compared with 107 cases of mild disease (29% vs. 13%, $p=.0078$; OR, 2.7; 95% CI, 2.3–3.6).

In patients with community-acquired pneumonia, the IL-10 -1082G allele ($p=.02$ for trend) and the IL-10 -1082GG genotype ($p<.05$) were both significantly associated with increasing severity of SIRS (300). The IL-10 -1082G allele was also associated with mortality; 82% of the 11 patients who died had the G allele compared with 51% of those who survived (OR, 4.3, 95% CI, 1.4–13.2; $p=.01$). This association remained significant after adjusting for age, sex, smoking, illness severity, and presence of chronic obstructive pulmonary disease. In another study of 69 hospitalized white German patients with culture proven, community-acquired invasive pneumococcal infection, although the homozygous IL-10 -1082GG genotype was not associated with susceptibility to invasive pneumococcal infection (23% vs. 26%, $p=$NS), it was associated with an increased risk of septic shock (54% vs. 16%; OR, 6.1; 95% CI, 1.4–27.2; $p=.024$) and there was a trend toward increased risk of death (60% of 5 cases vs. 20% of 64 cases, $p=.076$). However, serum IL-10 levels were not associated with severe infection or septic shock. Thus, there is a poor correlation among IL-10 genotypes, IL-10 levels, and clinical outcome in patients with sepsis. However, genotypes resulting in high IL-10 production are associated with severity of pneumococcal infections and death.

Interferon-γ

Interferon-γ (IFN-γ) is a 34-kd multifunctional potent proinflammatory cytokine produced endogenously by T lymphocytes, monocytes, and natural killer cells, and it promotes naive T-cell differentiation to the T-helper-1 phenotype, upregulates MHC class II expression, and increases secretion of other proinflammatory cytokines including IL-1 and TNF-α (372,373). In clinical studies, the use of IFN-γ as an adjuvant in preventing infections in severely injured patients demonstrated mixed results; clinically significant reduction in the rate of infection were not consistently observed (374–376).

The gene for IFN-γ is located on chromosome 12 and contains at least two functionally important polymorphisms. A CA-repeat microsatellite sequence in the noncoding intron 1 region has been associated with susceptibility to and severity of rheumatoid arthritis in Canadians (377). The 12 CA-repeat microsatellite allele (termed allele 2) has been associated with production of higher concentrations of IFN-γ in vitro (378,379). In addition, an A874T SNP at the 5' end of the CA repeat region in the first intron of the INF-γ gene has been absolutely correlated with the presence or absence of the 12 CA-repeat microsatellite allele 2 (380). This T to A polymorphism coincides with a putative NF-κB binding site, which might have functional consequences for the transcription of the human IFN-γ gene. The AA genotype has been associated with lower IFN-γ levels in healthy individuals and patients with tuberculosis (381). Stassen and colleagues (382) studied the CA microsatellite repeat polymorphism in 61 adults patients with severe trauma, of whom 49% developed sepsis (Table 9.15). The presence of allele 2 (=12 CA repeats) was associated with increased risk of sepsis (62% vs. 44%; $p=0.06$; OR, 2.09; 95% CI, 1.02–4.30).

Interferon-γ-Receptor 1

Mutations in the INF-γ-receptor 1 (IFN-γ-R1) gene on chromosome 6 have been associated with severe and unremitting mycobacterial infections (383,384). Most of the mutations reported are nonsense mutations resulting in absence of receptor expression or missense mutations affecting the binding affinity of the receptor. Davis and colleagues (385) studied polymorphisms in the microsatellite region near the IFN-γ-R1 gene (termed D6S471) and the risk of serious infection in 38 patients with major trauma in order to determine whether IFN-γ-R1 has a role in susceptibility to severe infection. They identified three alleles (designated alphabetically as A, B, and C depending on the distance traveled during on the gel electrophoresis) and five genotypes (AA, BB, CC, AB, and AC) for D6S471. The AA genotype was associated with increased risk of infection (42% of the 24 infected cases vs. 0% of 14 uninfected cases, $p=.004$), while the BB genotype was protective (21% vs. 57%, $p=.028$). Indeed, all 10 patients with the AA genotype developed major infection. However, no associations have

TABLE 9.15. Clinical studies on interferon-γ (IFN-γ) polymorphisms

Country (reference)	Cases	No.	Controls	No.	SNP	Su/Se/Ou	Significance	Comments
U.S. (382)	Severe sepsis in adults patients with severe trauma (mixed ethnic)	30	No sepsis	31	Allele 2	Su	0.62 vs. 0.44, p = .06, OR = 2.1 (95% CI, 1.0–4.3)	Allele 2 = twelve CA repeats
U.S. (385)	Major infection in adults with severe trauma	24	No infection	14	AA genotype	Su	1.00 vs 0.00, p = .004	
	Major infection in adults with severe trauma	24	No infection	14	BB genotype	Su	0.21 vs. 0.57, p = .03	

OR, odds ratio; 95% CI, 95% confidence interval; SNP, single nucleotide polymorphism; Su/Se/Ou, susceptibility/severity/outcome; NS, not significant.

been found between the microsatellite repeat and any of the known polymorphisms within the IFN-γ-R1 gene. The functional significance of the genotype
variations in D6S471, therefore, remains to be determined.

Discussion

The last few decades have seen a dramatic increase in our understanding of the
mechanisms by which the host immune system responds to microbial invasion.
We now understand that a favorable host response to infection relies on a delicate balance of multiple immune response pathways, where either under- or
overactivation of any one of the pathways may be detrimental to the host.
Genetic polymorphisms within key immune pathways are likely to alter this
balance and, therefore, affect the overall host immune response. However,
published studies on polymorphisms within any single gene have reported only
modest effects (if any) for each locus (odds ratios of 1.5–2.5). Instead, it is more
likely that genetic predisposition to complex diseases such as sepsis is likely to
require, in most cases, the presence of multiple mutations or polymorphisms
in different genes within the same individual in order to significantly increase
the risk of infection or severe disease (147,198).

Most of the studies on genetic susceptibility to infection published so far have
examined only one or at most a few preselected candidate genes that are known
or suspected to play a role in the pathogenesis of sepsis. It is, therefore, not
surprising that the results of such studies are so heterogeneous—very few
genetic polymorphisms have consistently shown a significant association in
different studies. As a result, there is increasing skepticism about the value of
association study designs in the detection of genetic variations contributing to
complex diseases. This problem is compounded by the fact that the results of
different studies are often difficult to compare because of both methodologic
and biologic variations. Methodologic problems include small sample sizes,
marginal statistical significance, poor selection of control groups, genotyping
complexity (the MBL haplotype, for example, contains three codon variants and
three promoter polymorphisms), an unexpectedly low frequency of homozygotes in the control group, ethnic heterogeneity, and lack of Hardy-Weinberg
equilibrium in the control genotypes (156,162). The selection of proper controls
is particularly important in order to avoid bias that may arise due to differences
in age, sex, ethnicity, medical treatments, and so on. For example, certain MBL
polymorphisms may increase the risk of acute respiratory tract infections in
children aged 6 to 17 months, who have relatively low immunoglobulin levels,
but not in older children (166). In addition, the sample size of the study has to
be sufficiently large to detect even modest effects of the polymorphism being
studied. This is particularly important in the current era where, with the rapid
progress in genetic technology, multiple genes can now be studied simultaneously and, therefore, the number of patients with a particular combined haplotype would be relatively low (87,298,302,386).

In spite of the recent advances, however, our understanding of the immune system, the different pathways involved, and the complex interactions between the different pathways remains deficient. For example, we know that TLR4 is important for LPS signaling, but *N. meningitidis* can induce proinflammatory cytokine responses through pathways that are independent of CD14 and TLR4, indicating that LPS is not the sole mediator of *N. meningitidis*–induced inflammation (105,387,388). This sort of redundancy in the different immune pathways would also explain the lack of success with cytokine therapy in sepsis, where it is now clear that an effective immune response requires an appropriately timed and well-balanced pro- and antiinflammatory cytokine response. Thus, supplementing or blocking one particular cytokine is unlikely to have a major impact on the overall immune response.

In addition, the functional significance of the polymorphisms for many immune genes is still poorly understood, with many studies providing conflicting results for both in vivo and in vitro effects of the polymorphism being studied. With TLR4, for example, monocytes heterozygous for either of the two polymorphisms have been shown to exhibit the same response to purified LPS as the wild-type alleles, while plasma concentrations of TNF-α, IL-6, and IL-8 were not significantly different between heterozygous individuals and homozygous carriers of the wild-type allele (102). These results suggest that the TLR4 polymorphisms may only be markers for mutations in other immune-related genes (389). Similarly, a recent study was unable to find any significant correlation between different cytokine gene polymorphisms and in vitro production of the corresponding cytokine and, following an extensive review of the literature, the authors concluded that discrepancies in the population studied, the cellular sources from which the cytokines were released and in the in vitro incubation protocols made it impossible to compare different studies on the association between cytokine polymorphisms and levels (390).

As a result of the numerous problems associated with case-control association studies, and with the multiple functions of most genes being almost entirely unknown, genome-wide association studies are now considered to be the way forward in understanding the genetic components of complex multifactorial diseases, such as sepsis. Advances in genotyping technology have progressed so rapidly in the last few years that it is now possible to perform whole genome association studies, which have been especially productive because they remove the constraints of biologic candidacy. Although immune-related genes are most likely to play an important role in the host immune response to infection, it is nevertheless striking to note that many alleles currently known to influence susceptibility to infection relate more to the route of organism entry to the cell, such as the Duffy protein and susceptibility to *Plasmodium vivax* malaria (391), and the hospitality of the cell's biochemical environment once inside the cell, such as glucose-6-phosphate dehydrogenase deficiency, the thalassemias, and various hemoglobinopathies in the case of malaria (392), than to interindividual variability in the vigor of the innate or adaptive immune response. Genome-wide linkage analysis is already being used to study genetic susceptibility to infection. Recent studies, for example, have identified significant linkage between markers on chromosomes 15q and Xq and tuberculosis in Gambian adults (393) and between chromosome 22q12 and kala-azar, a life-threatening protozoal disease caused by *Leishmania* parasites (394). Current genotyping technology allows for hundreds of thousands of polymorphisms to be studied in several thousand genes at a time. The results of such studies will inevitably improve our understanding of the role of the host's genetic makeup in susceptibility to, and severity of, infection. Identification of key genetic polymorphisms could eventually lead to bedside assessment of individual immune response genotype and allow tailoring of drugs and doses to individual patients based on their genetic makeup (395).

Conclusion

Population studies have shown that host genetic variability plays an important part in determining susceptibility to and severity of infection. Genetic polymorphisms within key immune response genes are able to influence the clinical presentation, severity, and outcome of sepsis by altering the ability to recognize and respond to pathogens, as well as manipulating the intensity of the subsequent inflammatory response. So far, published studies aimed at understanding genetic susceptibility to infection have often been limited to one or a few preselected candidate genes, usually involving relatively small sample sizes and poorly selected controls. Recent advances in the genotyping technology now allow for whole genome-wide association studies, which should provide invaluable insight into the pathogenesis of complex polygenic diseases including sepsis. Understanding the interaction between the host genetic makeup and susceptibility to infection may lead to development of more accurate bedside prognostic tools for patients with severe infections and allow for patient-specific targeted therapy in the near future.

References

1. Bucheton B, Kheir MM, El-Safi SH, et al. The interplay between environmental and host factors during an outbreak of visceral leishmaniasis in eastern Sudan. Microbes Infect 2002;4:1449–1457.
2. Modiano D, Petrarca V, Sirima BS, et al. Different response to Plasmodium falciparum malaria in west African sympatric ethnic groups. Proc Natl Acad Sci U S A 1996;93:13206–13211.
3. Stead WW, Senner JW, Reddick WT, Lofgren JP. Racial differences in susceptibility to infection by Mycobacterium tuberculosis. N Engl J Med 1990;322:422–427.
4. Ibrahim ME, Lambson B, Yousif AO, et al. Kala-azar in a high transmission focus: an ethnic and geographic dimension. Am J Trop Med Hyg 1999;61:941–944.
5. Lanciers S, Hauser B, Vandenplas Y, Blecker U. The prevalence of Helicobacter pylori positivity in asymptomatic children of different ethnic backgrounds living in the same country. Ethn Health 1996;1:169–173.

6. Jeannel D, Garin B, Kazadi K, Singa L, deThe G. The risk of tropical spastic para-paresis differs according to ethnic group among HTLV-I carriers in Inongo, Zaire. J Acquir Immune Defic Syndr 1993;6:840–844.

7. Emonts M, Hazelzet JA, de Groot R, Hermans PW. Host genetic determinants of Neisseria meningitidis infections. Lancet Infect Dis 2003;3:565–577.

8. Sorensen TI, Nielsen GG, Andersen PK, Teasdale TW. Genetic and environmental influences on premature death in adult adoptees. N Engl J Med 1988;318:727–732.

9. Comstock GW. Tuberculosis in twins: a re-analysis of the Prophit survey. Am Rev Respir Dis 1978;117:621–624.

10. Chakravarti MR, Vogel F. A Twin Study on Leprosy, vol 1. Stutthart: Thieme, 1973.

11. Herndon CN, Jennings RG. A twin family study on susceptibility to poliomyelitis. Am J Hum Genet 1951;3:17.

12. Lin TM, Chen CJ, Wu MM, et al. Hepatitis B virus markers in Chinese twins. Anti-cancer Res 1989;9:737–741.

13. Haralambous E, Weiss HA, Radalowicz A, Hibberd ML, Booy R, Levin M. Sibling familial risk ratio of meningococcal disease in UK Caucasians. Epidemiol Infect 2003;130:413–418.

14. Simonte SJ, Cunningham-Rundles C. Update on primary immunodeficiency: defects of lymphocytes. Clin Immunol 2003;109:109–118.

15. Glanzmann E, Riniker P. Essentielle Lymphocytophtose. Ein neues Krankeitsbild aus der Sauglingspathologie. Ann Paediat 1950;174:1–5.

16. Buckley RH. Molecular defects in human severe combined immunodeficiency and approaches to immune reconstitution. Annu Rev Immunol 2004;22:625–655.

17. Giblett ER, Anderson JE, Cohen F, Pollara B, Meuwissen HJ. Adenosine-deaminase deficiency in two patients with severely impaired cellular immunity. Lancet 1972;2:1067–1069.

18. Noguchi M, Nakamura Y, Russell SM, et al. Interleukin-2 receptor gamma chain: a functional component of the interleukin-7 receptor. Science 1993;262:1877–1880.

19. Puck JM, Deschenes SM, Porter JC, et al. The interleukin-2 receptor gamma chain maps to Xq13.1 and is mutated in X-linked severe combined immunodeficiency, SCIDX1. Hum Mol Genet 1993;2:1099–1104.

20. Russell SM, Tayebi N, Nakajima H, et al. Mutation of Jak3 in a patient with SCID: essential role of Jak3 in lymphoid development. Science 1995;270:797–800.

21. Irie-Sasaki J, Sasaki T, Penninger JM. CD45 regulated signaling pathways. Curr Top Med Chem 2003;3:783–796.

22. Buckley RH. The multiple causes of human SCID. J Clin Invest 2004;114:1409–1411.

23. Ferrari S, Plebani A. Cross-talk between CD40 and CD40L: lessons from primary immune deficiencies. Curr Opin Allergy Clin Immunol 2002;2:489–494.

24. Doffinger R, Patel S, Kumararatne DS. Human immunodeficiencies that predispose to intracellular bacterial infections. Curr Opin Rheumatol 2005;17:440–446.

25. Lawrence T, Puel A, Reichenbach J, et al. Autosomal-dominant primary immuno-deficiencies. Curr Opin Hematol 2005;12:22–30.

26. Bonilla FA, Geha RS. Primary immunodeficiency diseases. J Allergy Clin Immunol 2003;111:S571–S581.

27. Candotti F, Notarangelo L, Visconti R, O'Shea J. Molecular aspects of primary immunodeficiencies: lessons from cytokine and other signaling pathways. J Clin Invest 2002;109:1261–1269.

28. Buckley RH. Primary cellular immunodeficiencies. J Allergy Clin Immunol 2002;109:747–757.
29. Champi C. Primary immunodeficiency disorders in children: prompt diagnosis can lead to lifesaving treatment. J Pediatr Health Care 2002;16:16–21.
30. Kalman L, Lindegren ML, Kobrynski L, et al. Mutations in genes required for T-cell development: IL7R, CD45, IL2RG, JAK3, RAG1, RAG2, ARTEMIS, and ADA and severe combined immunodeficiency: HuGE review. Genet Med 2004; 6:16–26.
31. Lindegren ML, Kobrynski L, Rasmussen SA, et al. Applying public health strategies to primary immunodeficiency diseases: a potential approach to genetic disorders. MMWR Recomm Rep 2004;53:1–29.
32. Brookes AJ. The essence of SNPs. Gene 1999;234:177–186.
33. Cardon LR, Bell JI. Association study designs for complex diseases. Nat Rev Genet 2001;2:91–99.
34. Stephens JC, Schneider JA, Tanguay DA, et al. Haplotype variation and linkage disequilibrium in 313 human genes. Science 2001;293:489–493.
35. Epplen C, Santos EJ, Maueler W, van Helden P, Epplen JT. On simple repetitive DNA sequences and complex diseases. Electrophoresis 1997;18:1577–1585.
36. Cooke GS, Hill AV. Genetics of susceptibility to human infectious disease. Nat Rev Genet 2001;2:967–977.
37. Allison AC. Protection afforded by sickle-cell trait against subtertian malarial infection. Br Med J 1954;4857:290–294.
38. Pasvol G, Weatherall DJ, Wilson RJ. Cellular mechanism for the protective effect of haemoglobin S against P. falciparum malaria. Nature 1978;274:701–703.
39. Flint J, Hill AV, Bowden DK, et al. High frequencies of alpha-thalassaemia are the result of natural selection by malaria. Nature 1986;321:744–750.
40. Ruwende C, Khoo SC, Snow RW, et al. Natural selection of hemi- and heterozygotes for G6PD deficiency in Africa by resistance to severe malaria. Nature 1995;376:246–249.
41. Dahmer MK, Randolph A, Vitali S, Quasney MW. Genetic polymorphisms in sepsis. Pediatr Crit Care Med 2005;6:S61–S73.
42. Lin MT, Albertson TE. Genomic polymorphisms in sepsis. Crit Care Med 2004;32:569–579.
43. Bayley JP, Ottenhoff TH, Verweij CL. Is there a future for TNF promoter polymorphisms? Genes Immun 2004;5:315–329.
44. van Deventer SJ. Cytokine and cytokine receptor polymorphisms in infectious disease. Intensive Care Med 2000;26(suppl 1):S98–102.
45. Schroder NW, Diterich I, Zinke A, et al. Heterozygous Arg753Gln polymorphism of human TLR-2 impairs immune activation by Borrelia burgdorferi and protects from late stage Lyme disease. J Immunol 2005;175:2534–2540.
46. Anastassopoulou CG, Kostrikis LG. The impact of human allelic variation on HIV-1 disease. Curr HIV Res 2003;1:185–203.
47. Bellamy R. Genetic susceptibility to tuberculosis. Clin Chest Med 2005;26:233–246, vi.
48. Newport MJ, Nejentsev S. Genetics of susceptibility to tuberculosis in humans. Monaldi Arch Chest Dis 2004;61:102–111.
49. Fitness J, Floyd S, Warndorff DK, et al. Large-scale candidate gene study of tuberculosis susceptibility in the Karonga district of northern Malawi. Am J Trop Med Hyg 2004;71:341–349.

50. Fitness J, Tosh K, Hill AV. Genetics of susceptibility to leprosy. Genes Immun 2002;3:441–453.

51. Kaslow RA, Dorak T, Tang JJ. Influence of host genetic variation on susceptibility to HIV type 1 infection. J Infect Dis 2005;191(suppl 1):S68–S77.

52. Thursz M. Pros and cons of genetic association studies in hepatitis B. Hepatology 2004;40:284–286.

53. Wilson J, Rowlands K, Rockett K, et al. Genetic variation at the IL10 gene locus is associated with severity of respiratory syncytial virus bronchiolitis. J Infect Dis 2005;191:1705–1709.

54. Tal G, Mandelberg A, Dalal I, et al. Association between common Toll-like receptor 4 mutations and severe respiratory syncytial virus disease. J Infect Dis 2004;189: 2057–2063.

55. Gentile DA, Doyle WJ, Zeevi A, et al. Cytokine gene polymorphisms moderate illness severity in infants with respiratory syncytial virus infection. Hum Immunol 2003;64:338–344.

56. Thursz MR, Thomas HC. Host factors in chronic viral hepatitis. Semin Liver Dis 1997;17:345–350.

57. Troye-Blomberg M. Genetic regulation of malaria infection in humans. Chem Immunol 2002;80:243–252.

58. Choi EH, Nutman TB, Chanock SJ. Genetic variation in immune function and susceptibility to human filariasis. Expert Rev Mol Diagn 2003;3:367–374.

59. Kwiatkowski D. Genetic susceptibility to malaria getting complex. Curr Opin Genet Dev 2000;10:320–324.

60. Burt RA. Genetics of host response to malaria. Int J Parasitol 1999;29:973–979.

61. Hill AV. Genetic susceptibility to malaria and other infectious diseases: from the MHC to the whole genome. Parasitology 1996;112(suppl):S75–S84.

62. Blackwell JM. Genetic susceptibility to leishmanial infections: studies in mice and man. Parasitology 1996;112(suppl):S67–S74.

63. Ulevitch RJ, Tobias PS. Receptor-dependent mechanisms of cell stimulation by bacterial endotoxin. Annu Rev Immunol 1995;13:437–457.

64. Schumann RR, Leong SR, Flaggs GW, et al. Structure and function of lipopolysaccharide binding protein. Science 1990;249:1429–1431.

65. Gray PW, Corcorran AE, Eddy RL Jr, Byers MG, Shows TB. The genes for the lipopolysaccharide binding protein (LBP) and the bactericidal permeability increasing protein (BPI) are encoded in the same region of human chromosome 20. Genomics 1993;15:188–190.

66. Elsbach P, Weiss J. Role of the bactericidal/permeability-increasing protein in host defence. Curr Opin Immunol 1998;10:45–49.

67. Grunwald U, Fan X, Jack RS, et al. Monocytes can phagocytose Gram-negative bacteria by a CD14–dependent mechanism. J Immunol 1996;157:4119–4125.

68. Froon AH, Dentener MA, Greve JW, Ramsay G, Buurman WA. Lipopolysaccharide toxicity-regulating proteins in bacteremia. J Infect Dis 1995;171:1250–1257.

69. Ammons WS, Kohn FR, Kung AH. Protective effects of an N-terminal fragment of bactericidal/permeability-increasing protein in rodent models of gram-negative sepsis: role of bactericidal properties. J Infect Dis 1994;170:1473–1482.

70. Levin M, Quint PA, Goldstein B, et al. Recombinant bactericidal/permeability-increasing protein (rBPI21) as adjunctive treatment for children with severe meningococcal sepsis: a randomised trial. rBPI21 Meningococcal Sepsis Study Group. Lancet 2000;356:961–967.

71. Lamping N, Dettmer R, Schroder NW, et al. LPS-binding protein protects mice from septic shock caused by LPS or gram-negative bacteria. J Clin Invest 1998;101:2065–2071.

72. Hubacek JA, Stuber F, Frohlich D, et al. Gene variants of the bactericidal/permeability increasing protein and lipopolysaccharide binding protein in sepsis patients: gender-specific genetic predisposition to sepsis. Crit Care Med 2001;29:557–561.

73. Wright SD, Ramos RA, Tobias PS, Ulevitch RJ, Mathison JC. CD14, a receptor for complexes of lipopolysaccharide (LPS) and LPS binding protein. Science 1990; 249:1431–1433.

74. Durieux JJ, Vita N, Popescu O, et al. The two soluble forms of the lipopolysaccharide receptor, CD14: characterization and release by normal human monocytes. Eur J Immunol 1994;24:2006–2012.

75. Bas S, Gauthier BR, Spenato U, Stingelin S, Gabay C. CD14 is an acute-phase protein. J Immunol 2004;172:4470–4479.

76. Landmann R, Reber AM, Sansano S, Zimmerli W. Function of soluble CD14 in serum from patients with septic shock. J Infect Dis 1996;173:661–668.

77. Ferrero E, Jiao D, Tsuberi BZ, et al. Transgenic mice expressing human CD14 are hypersensitive to lipopolysaccharide. Proc Natl Acad Sci U S A 1993;90:2380–2384.

78. Haziot A, Ferrero E, Lin XY, Stewart CL, Goyert SM. CD14–deficient mice are exquisitely insensitive to the effects of LPS. Prog Clin Biol Res 1995;392:349–351.

79. Burgmann H, Winkler S, Locker GJ, et al. Increased serum concentration of soluble CD14 is a prognostic marker in gram-positive sepsis. Clin Immunol Immunopathol 1996;80:307–310.

80. Gibot S, Cariou A, Drouet L, Rossignol M, Ripoll L. Association between a genomic polymorphism within the CD14 locus and septic shock susceptibility and mortality rate. Crit Care Med 2002;30:969–973.

81. Zhang DE, Hetherington CJ, Tan S, et al. Sp1 is a critical factor for the monocytic specific expression of human CD14. J Biol Chem 1994;269:11425–11434.

82. Hubacek JA, Rothe G, Pit'ha J, et al. C(-260)→T polymorphism in the promoter of the CD14 monocyte receptor gene as a risk factor for myocardial infarction. Circulation 1999;99:3218–3220.

83. Baldini M, Lohman IC, Halonen M, Erickson RP, Holt PG, Martinez FD. A polymorphism in the 5' flanking region of the CD14 gene is associated with circulating soluble CD14 levels and with total serum immunoglobulin E. Am J Respir Cell Mol Biol 1999;20:976–983.

84. Ripoll L, Collet JP, Barateau V. A novel CD14 gene polymorphism that determines variable monocyte activation is associated with the risk of myocardial infarction in young adults. Circulation 1999;18(suppl 1):I821.

85. Heesen M, Bloemeke B, Schade U, Obertacke U, Majetschak M. The -260 C→T promoter polymorphism of the lipopolysaccharide receptor CD14 and severe sepsis in trauma patients. Intensive Care Med 2002;28:1161–1163.

86. Agnese DM, Calvano JE, Hahm SJ, et al. Human toll-like receptor 4 mutations but not CD14 polymorphisms are associated with an increased risk of gram-negative infections. J Infect Dis 2002;186:1522–1525.

87. Sutherland AM, Walley KR, Russell JA. Polymorphisms in CD14, mannose-binding lectin, and Toll-like receptor-2 are associated with increased prevalence of infection in critically ill adults. Crit Care Med 2005;33:638–644.

88. Hubacek JA, Stuber F, Frohlich D, et al. The common functional C(-159)T polymorphism within the promoter region of the lipopolysaccharide receptor CD14 is

not associated with sepsis development or mortality. Genes Immun 2000;1:405–407.

89. Barber RC, Aragaki CC, Rivera-Chavez FA, Purdue GF, Hunt JL, Horton JW. TLR4 and TNF-alpha polymorphisms are associated with an increased risk for severe sepsis following burn injury. J Med Genet 2004;41:808–813.

90. Heesen M, Blomeke B, Schluter B, Heussen N, Rossaint R, Kunz D. Lack of association between the -260 C→T promoter polymorphism of the endotoxin receptor CD14 gene and the CD14 density of unstimulated human monocytes and soluble CD14 plasma levels. Intensive Care Med 2001;27:1770–1775.

91. Cook DN, Pisetsky DS, Schwartz DA. Toll-like receptors in the pathogenesis of human disease. Nat Immunol 2004;5:975–979.

92. Zarember KA, Godowski PJ. Tissue expression of human Toll-like receptors and differential regulation of Toll-like receptor mRNAs in leukocytes in response to microbes, their products, and cytokines. J Immunol 2002;168:554–561.

93. Erroi A, Fantuzzi G, Mengozzi M, et al. Differential regulation of cytokine production in lipopolysaccharide tolerance in mice. Infect Immun 1993;61:4356–4359.

94. Poltorak A, He X, Smirnova I, et al. Defective LPS signaling in C3H/HeJ and C57BL/10ScCr mice: mutations in Tlr4 gene. Science 1998;282:2085–2088.

95. Arbour NC, Lorenz E, Schutte BC, et al. TLR4 mutations are associated with endotoxin hyporesponsiveness in humans. Nat Genet 2000;25:187–191.

96. Henneke P, Golenbock DT. Innate immune recognition of lipopolysaccharide by endothelial cells. Crit Care Med 2002;30:S207–S213.

97. Akira S. Toll-like receptors and innate immunity. Adv Immunol 2001;78:1–56.

98. Kiechl S, Lorenz E, Reindl M, et al. Toll-like receptor 4 polymorphisms and atherogenesis. N Engl J Med 2002;347:185–192.

99. Lorenz E, Mira JP, Frees KL, Schwartz DA. Relevance of mutations in the TLR4 receptor in patients with gram-negative septic shock. Arch Intern Med 2002;162:1028–1032.

100. Feterowski C, Emmanuilidis K, Miethke T, et al. Effects of functional Toll-like receptor-4 mutations on the immune response to human and experimental sepsis. Immunology 2003;109:426–431.

101. Child NJ, Yang IA, Pulletz MC, et al. Polymorphisms in Toll-like receptor 4 and the systemic inflammatory response syndrome. Biochem Soc Trans 2003;31:652–653.

102. Heesen M, Bloemeke B, Kunz D. The cytokine synthesis by heterozygous carriers of the Toll-like receptor 4 Asp299Gly polymorphism does not differ from that of wild type homozygotes. Eur Cytokine Netw 2003;14:234–237.

103. Read RC, Pullin J, Gregory S, et al. A functional polymorphism of toll-like receptor 4 is not associated with likelihood or severity of meningococcal disease. J Infect Dis 2001;184:640–642.

104. Allen A, Obaro S, Bojang K, et al. Variation in Toll-like receptor 4 and susceptibility to group A meningococcal meningitis in Gambian children. Pediatr Infect Dis J 2003;22:1018–1019.

105. Ingalls RR, Lien E, Golenbock DT. Membrane-associated proteins of a lipopolysaccharide-deficient mutant of Neisseria meningitidis activate the inflammatory response through toll-like receptor 2. Infect Immun 2001;69:2230–2236.

106. Smirnova I, Mann N, Dols A, et al. Assay of locus-specific genetic load implicates rare Toll-like receptor 4 mutations in meningococcal susceptibility. Proc Natl Acad Sci U S A 2003;100:6075–6080.

107. Lorenz E, Mira JP, Cornish KL, Arbour NC, Schwartz DA. A novel polymorphism in the toll-like receptor 2 gene and its potential association with staphylococcal infection. Infect Immun 2000;68:6398–6401.

108. Yang RB, Mark MR, Gray A, et al. Toll-like receptor-2 mediates lipopolysaccharide-induced cellular signalling. Nature 1998;395:284–288.

109. Travassos LH, Girardin SE, Philpott DJ, et al. Toll-like receptor 2-dependent bacterial sensing does not occur via peptidoglycan recognition. EMBO Rep 2004;5: 1000–1006.

110. Lotz S, Aga E, Wilde I, et al. Highly purified lipoteichoic acid activates neutrophil granulocytes and delays their spontaneous apoptosis via CD14 and TLR2. J Leukoc Biol 2004;75:467–477.

111. Takeda K, Akira S. Toll receptors and pathogen resistance. Cell Microbiol 2003;5:143–153.

112. Gupta D, Kirkland TN, Viriyakosol S, Dziarski R. CD14 is a cell-activating receptor for bacterial peptidoglycan. J Biol Chem 1996;271:23310–23316.

113. Cleveland MG, Gorham JD, Murphy TL, Tuomanen E, Murphy KM. Lipoteichoic acid preparations of gram-positive bacteria induce interleukin-12 through a CD14-dependent pathway. Infect Immun 1996;64:1906–1912.

114. Takeuchi O, Hoshino K, Akira S. Cutting edge: TLR2-deficient and MyD88-deficient mice are highly susceptible to Staphylococcus aureus infection. J Immunol 2000;165:5392–5396.

115. Takeuchi O, Hoshino K, Kawai T, et al. Differential roles of TLR2 and TLR4 in recognition of gram-negative and gram-positive bacterial cell wall components. Immunity 1999;11:443–451.

116. Underhill DM, Ozinsky A, Hajjar AM, et al. The Toll-like receptor 2 is recruited to macrophage phagosomes and discriminates between pathogens. Nature 1999; 401:811–815.

117. Bochud PY, Hawn TR, Aderem A. Cutting edge: a Toll-like receptor 2 polymorphism that is associated with lepromatous leprosy is unable to mediate mycobacterial signaling. J Immunol 2003;170:3451–3454.

118. Kang TJ, Chae GT. Detection of Toll-like receptor 2 (TLR2) mutation in the lepromatous leprosy patients. FEMS Immunol Med Microbiol 2001;31:53–58.

119. Yim JJ, Ding L, Schaffer AA, Park GY, Shim YS, Holland SM. A microsatellite polymorphism in intron 2 of human Toll-like receptor 2 gene: functional implications and racial differences. FEMS Immunol Med Microbiol 2004;40:163–169.

120. Schroder NW, Hermann C, Hamann L, Gobel UB, Hartung T, Schumann RR. High frequency of polymorphism Arg753Gln of the Toll-like receptor-2 gene detected by a novel allele-specific PCR. J Mol Med 2003;81:368–372.

121. Moore CE, Segal S, Berendt AR, Hill AV, Day NP. Lack of association between Toll-like receptor 2 polymorphisms and susceptibility to severe disease caused by Staphylococcus aureus. Clin Diagn Lab Immunol 2004;11:1194–1197.

122. von Aulock S, Schroder NW, Traub S, et al. Heterozygous toll-like receptor 2 polymorphism does not affect lipoteichoic acid-induced chemokine and inflammatory responses. Infect Immun 2004;72:1828–1831.

123. Christians ES, Yan LJ, Benjamin IJ. Heat shock factor 1 and heat shock proteins: critical partners in protection against acute cell injury. Crit Care Med 2002;30: S43–S50.

124. Deitch EA, Beck SC, Cruz NC, de Maio A. Induction of heat shock gene expression in colonic epithelial cells after incubation with Escherichia coli or endotoxin. Crit Care Med 1995;23:1371–1376.

125. Riezman H. Why do cells require heat shock proteins to survive heat stress? Cell Cycle 2004;3:61–63.

126. Imai J, Yashiroda H, Maruya M, Yahara I, Tanaka K. Proteasomes and molecular chaperones: cellular machinery responsible for folding and destruction of unfolded proteins. Cell Cycle 2003;2:585–590.

127. Hendrick JP, Hartl FU. The role of molecular chaperones in protein folding. FASEB J 1995;9:1559–1569.

128. Asea A, Rehli M, Kabingu E, et al. Novel signal transduction pathway utilized by extracellular HSP70: role of toll-like receptor (TLR) 2 and TLR4. J Biol Chem 2002;277:15028–15034.

129. Zhou J, An H, Xu H, Liu S, Cao X. Heat shock up-regulates expression of Toll-like receptor-2 and Toll-like receptor-4 in human monocytes via p38 kinase signal pathway. Immunology 2005;114:522–530.

130. Kusher DI, Ware CF, Gooding LR. Induction of the heat shock response protects cells from lysis by tumor necrosis factor. J Immunol 1990;145:2925–2931.

131. Jaattela M, Wissing D, Bauer PA, Li GC. Major heat shock protein hsp70 protects tumor cells from tumor necrosis factor cytotoxicity. EMBO J 1992;11:3507–3512.

132. Villar J, Ribeiro SP, Mullen JB, Kuliszewski M, Post M, Slutsky AS. Induction of the heat shock response reduces mortality rate and organ damage in a sepsis-induced acute lung injury model. Crit Care Med 1994;22:914–921.

133. Wheeler DS, Fisher LE Jr, Catravas JD, Jacobs BR, Carcillo JA, Wong HR. Extracellular hsp70 levels in children with septic shock. Pediatr Crit Care Med 2005;6:308–311.

134. Milner CM, Campbell RD. Structure and expression of the three MHC-linked HSP70 genes. Immunogenetics 1990;32:242–251.

135. Milner CM, Campbell RD. Polymorphic analysis of the three MHC-linked HSP70 genes. Immunogenetics 1992;36:357–362.

136. Schroeder S, Reck M, Hoeft A, Stuber F. Analysis of two human leukocyte antigen-linked polymorphic heat shock protein 70 genes in patients with severe sepsis. Crit Care Med 1999;27:1265–1270.

137. Waterer GW, ElBahlawan L, Quasney MW, Zhang Q, Kessler LA, Wunderink RG. Heat shock protein 70-2+1267 AA homozygotes have an increased risk of septic shock in adults with community-acquired pneumonia. Crit Care Med 2003;31: 1367–1372.

138. Bordet J, Gengou O. Sur l'existence de substances sensibilisatrices dans la plupart des serum antimicrobiens. Ann Inst Pasteur 1901;15:289–302.

139. Carroll MC. The complement system in regulation of adaptive immunity. Nat Immunol 2004;5:981–986.

140. Figueroa JE, Densen P. Infectious diseases associated with complement deficiencies. Clin Microbiol Rev 1991;4:359–395.

141. Hazelzet JA, de Groot R, van Mierlo G, et al. Complement activation in relation to capillary leakage in children with septic shock and purpura. Infect Immun 1998;66:5350–5356.

142. Fijen CA, Kuijper EJ, te Bulte MT, Daha MR, Dankert J. Assessment of complement deficiency in patients with meningococcal disease in The Netherlands. Clin Infect Dis 1999;28:98–105.

143. Densen P, Weiler JM, Griffiss JM, Hoffmann LG. Familial properdin deficiency and fatal meningococcemia. Correction of the bactericidal defect by vaccination. N Engl J Med 1987;316:922–926.
144. Spath PJ, Sjoholm AG, Fredrikson GN, et al. Properdin deficiency in a large Swiss family: identification of a stop codon in the properdin gene, and association of meningococcal disease with lack of the IgG2 allotype marker G2m(n). Clin Exp Immunol 1999;118:278–284.
145. Westberg J, Fredrikson GN, Truedsson L, Sjoholm AG, Uhlen M. Sequence-based analysis of properdin deficiency: identification of point mutations in two phenotypic forms of an X-linked immunodeficiency. Genomics 1995;29:1–8.
146. Fredrikson GN, Westberg J, Kuijper EJ, et al. Molecular characterization of properdin deficiency type III: dysfunction produced by a single point mutation in exon 9 of the structural gene causing a tyrosine to aspartic acid interchange. J Immunol 1996;157:3666–3671.
147. Fijen CA, Bredius RG, Kuijper EJ, et al. The role of Fcgamma receptor polymorphisms and C3 in the immune defence against Neisseria meningitidis in complement-deficient individuals. Clin Exp Immunol 2000;120:338–345.
148. Thiel S, Holmskov U, Hviid L, Laursen SB, Jensenius JC. The concentration of the C-type lectin, mannan-binding protein, in human plasma increases during an acute phase response. Clin Exp Immunol 1992;90:31–35.
149. Matsushita M, Fujita T. Activation of the classical complement pathway by mannose-binding protein in association with a novel C1s-like serine protease. J Exp Med 1992;176:1497–1502.
150. Thiel S, Vorup-Jensen T, Stover CM, et al. A second serine protease associated with mannan-binding lectin that activates complement. Nature 1997;386:506–510.
151. Dahl MR, Thiel S, Matsushita M, Fujita T, et al. MASP-3 and its association with distinct complexes of the mannan-binding lectin complement activation pathway. Immunity 2001;15:127–135.
152. Schwaeble W, Dahl MR, Thiel S, Stover C, Jensenius JC. The mannan-binding lectin-associated serine proteases (MASPs) and MAp19: four components of the lectin pathway activation complex encoded by two genes. Immunobiology 2002;205:455–466.
153. Stover CM, Thiel S, Lynch NJ, Schwaeble WJ. The rat and mouse homologues of MASP-2 and MAp19, components of the lectin activation pathway of complement. J Immunol 1999;163:6848–6859.
154. Takahashi M, Endo Y, Fujita T, Matsushita M. A truncated form of mannose-binding lectin-associated serine protease (MASP)-2 expressed by alternative polyadenylation is a component of the lectin complement pathway. Int Immunol 1999;11:859–863.
155. Turner MW. The role of mannose-binding lectin in health and disease. Mol Immunol 2003;40:423–429.
156. Roy S, Knox K, Segal S, et al. MBL genotype and risk of invasive pneumococcal disease: a case-control study. Lancet 2002;359:1569–1573.
157. Lipscombe RJ, Sumiya M, Hill AV, et al. High frequencies in African and non-African populations of independent mutations in the mannose binding protein gene. Hum Mol Genet 1992;1:709–715.
158. Madsen HO, Garred P, Thiel S, et al. Interplay between promoter and structural gene variants control basal serum level of mannan-binding protein. J Immunol 1995;155:3013–3020.

159. Madsen HO, Satz ML, Hogh B, Svejgaard A, Garred P. Different molecular events result in low protein levels of mannan-binding lectin in populations from southeast Africa and South America. J Immunol 1998;161:3169–3175.

160. Super M, Thiel S, Lu J, Levinsky RJ, Turner MW. Association of low levels of mannan-binding protein with a common defect of opsonisation. Lancet 1989;2: 1236–1239.

161. Garred P, Madsen HO, Balslev U, et al. Susceptibility to HIV infection and progression of AIDS in relation to variant alleles of mannose-binding lectin. Lancet 1997;349:236–240.

162. Summerfield JA, Sumiya M, Levin M, Turner MW. Association of mutations in mannose binding protein gene with childhood infection in consecutive hospital series. BMJ 1997;314:1229–1232.

163. Hibberd ML, Sumiya M, Summerfield JA, Booy R, Levin M. Association of variants of the gene for mannose-binding lectin with susceptibility to meningococcal disease. Meningococcal Research Group. Lancet 1999;353:1049–1053.

164. Garred P, Strom J, Quist L, Taaning E, Madsen HO. Association of mannose-binding lectin polymorphisms with sepsis and fatal outcome, in patients with systemic inflammatory response syndrome. J Infect Dis 2003;188:1394–1403.

165. Sutherland AM, Russell JA. Issues with polymorphism analysis in sepsis. Clin Infect Dis 2005;41(suppl 7):S396–S402.

166. Koch A, Melbye M, Sorensen P, et al. Acute respiratory tract infections and mannose-binding lectin insufficiency during early childhood. JAMA 2001;285:1316–1321.

167. Koch A, Melbye M, Sorensen P, et al. [Acute respiratory tract infections and mannose-binding lectin insufficiency in small children.] Ugeskr Laeger 2002;164: 5635–5640.

168. Turner MW, Super M, Singh S, Levinsky RJ. Molecular basis of a common opsonic defect. Clin Exp Allergy 1991;21(suppl 1):182–188.

169. Neth O, Hann I, Turner MW, Klein NJ. Deficiency of mannose-binding lectin and burden of infection in children with malignancy: a prospective study. Lancet 2001;358:614–618.

170. Peterslund NA, Koch C, Jensenius JC, Thiel S. Association between deficiency of mannose-binding lectin and severe infections after chemotherapy. Lancet 2001; 358:637–638.

171. van der Pol WL, van de Winkel JG. [Immunology in clinical practice. X. IgG receptors: structure, function and immunotherapy.] Ned Tijdschr Geneeskd 1998;142: 335–340.

172. Ravetch JV, Kinet JP. Fc receptors. Annu Rev Immunol 1991;9:457–492.

173. Van Der Pol W, van de Winkel JG. IgG receptor polymorphisms: risk factors for disease. Immunogenetics 1998;48:222–232.

174. Warmerdam PA, van de Winkel JG, Vlug A, Westerdaal NA, Capel PJ. A single amino acid in the second Ig-like domain of the human Fc gamma receptor II is critical for human IgG2 binding. J Immunol 1991;147:1338–1343.

175. Insel RA, Anderson PW. Response to oligosaccharide-protein conjugate vaccine against Haemophilus influenzae b in two patients with IgG2 deficiency unresponsive to capsular polysaccharide vaccine. N Engl J Med 1986;315:499–503.

176. Umetsu DT, Ambrosino DM, Quinti I, Siber GR, Geha RS. Recurrent sinopulmonary infection and impaired antibody response to bacterial capsular polysaccharide antigen in children with selective IgG-subclass deficiency. N Engl J Med 1985; 313:1247–1251.

177. Bredius RG, Fijen CA, de Haas M, et al. Role of neutrophil Fc gamma RIIa (CD32) and Fc gamma RIIIb (CD16) polymorphic forms in phagocytosis of human IgG1- and IgG3-opsonized bacteria and erythrocytes. Immunology 1994;83:624–630.
178. Sanders LA, Feldman RG, Voorhorst-Ogink MM, et al. Human immunoglobulin G (IgG) Fc receptor IIA (CD32) polymorphism and IgG2-mediated bacterial phagocytosis by neutrophils. Infect Immun 1995;63:73–81.
179. Sanders LA, van de Winkel JG, Rijkers GT, et al. Fc gamma receptor IIa (CD32) heterogeneity in patients with recurrent bacterial respiratory tract infections. J Infect Dis 1994;170:854–861.
180. Bredius RG, Derkx BH, Fijen CA, et al. Fc gamma receptor IIa (CD32) polymorphism in fulminant meningococcal septic shock in children. J Infect Dis 1994;170: 848–853.
181. Domingo P, Muniz-Diaz E, Baraldes MA, et al. Associations between Fc gamma receptor IIA polymorphisms and the risk and prognosis of meningococcal disease. Am J Med 2002;112:19–25.
182. Burgess JK, Lindeman R, Chesterman CN, Chong BH. Single amino acid mutation of Fc gamma receptor is associated with the development of heparin-induced thrombocytopenia. Br J Haematol 1995;91:761–766.
183. Yamamoto K, Kobayashi T, Grossi S, et al. Association of Fcgamma receptor IIa genotype with chronic periodontitis in Caucasians. J Periodontol 2004;75: 517–522.
184. Duits AJ, Bootsma H, Derksen RH, et al. Skewed distribution of IgG Fc receptor IIa (CD32) polymorphism is associated with renal disease in systemic lupus erythematosus patients. Arthritis Rheum 1995;38:1832–1836.
185. Salmon JE, Millard S, Schachter LA, et al. Fc gamma RIIA alleles are heritable risk factors for lupus nephritis in African Americans. J Clin Invest 1996;97:1348–1354.
186. van der Pol WL, Huizinga TW, Vidarsson G, et al. Relevance of Fcgamma receptor and interleukin-10 polymorphisms for meningococcal disease. J Infect Dis 2001;184:1548–1555.
187. Koene HR, Kleijer M, Algra J, et al. Fc gammaRIIIa-158V/F polymorphism influences the binding of IgG by natural killer cell Fc gammaRIIIa, independently of the Fc gammaRIIIa-48L/R/H phenotype. Blood 1997;90:1109–1114.
188. Abrahams VM, Cambridge G, Lydyard PM, Edwards JC. Induction of tumor necrosis factor alpha production by adhered human monocytes: a key role for Fcgamma receptor type IIIa in rheumatoid arthritis. Arthritis Rheum 2000;43:608–616.
189. Waage A, Halstensen A, Espevik T. Association between tumour necrosis factor in serum and fatal outcome in patients with meningococcal disease. Lancet 1987;1:355–357.
190. Westendorp RG, Langermans JA, Huizinga TW, Verweij CL, Sturk A. Genetic influence on cytokine production in meningococcal disease. Lancet 1997;349: 1912–1913.
191. Booy R, Nadel S, Hibberd M, Levin M, Newport MJ. Genetic influence on cytokine production in meningococcal disease. Lancet 1997;349:1176.
192. de Haas M, Kleijer M, van Zwieten R, Roos D, von dem Borne AE. Neutrophil Fc gamma RIIIb deficiency, nature, and clinical consequences: a study of 21 individuals from 14 families. Blood 1995;86:2403–2413.
193. Salmon JE, Edberg JC, Kimberly RP. Fc gamma receptor III on human neutrophils. Allelic variants have functionally distinct capacities. J Clin Invest 1990;85: 1287–1295.

194. Salmon JE, Edberg JC, Brogle NL, Kimberly RP. Allelic polymorphisms of human Fc gamma receptor IIA and Fc gamma receptor IIIB. Independent mechanisms for differences in human phagocyte function. J Clin Invest 1992;89:1274–1281.

195. Platonov AE, Beloborodov VB, Vershinina IV. Meningococcal disease in patients with late complement component deficiency: studies in the U.S.S.R. Medicine (Baltimore) 1993;72:374–392.

196. Wurzner R, Orren A, Lachmann PJ. Inherited deficiencies of the terminal components of human complement. Immunodefic Rev 1992;3:123–147.

197. Fijen CA, Bredius RG, Kuijper EJ. Polymorphism of IgG Fc receptors in meningococcal disease. Ann Intern Med 1993;119:636.

198. Platonov AE, Kuijper EJ, Vershinina IV, et al. Meningococcal disease and polymorphism of FcgammaRIIa (CD32) in late complement component-deficient individuals. Clin Exp Immunol 1998;111:97–101.

199. Platonov AE, Shipulin GA, Vershinina IV, Dankert J, van de Winkel JG, Kuijper EJ. Association of human Fc gamma RIIa (CD32) polymorphism with susceptibility to and severity of meningococcal disease. Clin Infect Dis 1998;27:746–750.

200. Yee AM, Phan HM, Zuniga R, Salmon JE, Musher DM. Association between FcgammaRIIa-R131 allotype and bacteremic pneumococcal pneumonia. Clin Infect Dis 2000;30:25–28.

201. Yuan FF, Wong M, Pererva N, et al. FcgammaRIIA polymorphisms in Streptococcus pneumoniae infection. Immunol Cell Biol 2003;81:192–195.

202. Sanders LA, van de Winkel JG, Rijkers GT, et al. Fc gamma receptor IIa (CD32) heterogeneity in patients with recurrent bacterial respiratory tract infections. J Infect Dis 1994;170:854–861.

203. Paramo JA, Perez JL, Serrano M, Rocha E. Types 1 and 2 plasminogen activator inhibitor and tumor necrosis factor alpha in patients with sepsis. Thromb Haemost 1990;64:3–6.

204. Brandtzaeg P, Joo GB, Brusletto B, Kierulf P. Plasminogen activator inhibitor 1 and 2, alpha-2-antiplasmin, plasminogen, and endotoxin levels in systemic meningococcal disease. Thromb Res 1990;57:271–278.

205. Kornelisse RF, Hazelzet JA, Savelkoul HF, et al. The relationship between plasminogen activator inhibitor-1 and proinflammatory and counterinflammatory mediators in children with meningococcal septic shock. J Infect Dis 1996;173:1148–1156.

206. Gregory SA, Morrissey JH, Edgington TS. Regulation of tissue factor gene expression in the monocyte procoagulant response to endotoxin. Mol Cell Biol 1989;9:2752–2755.

207. Osterud B, Flaegstad T. Increased tissue thromboplastin activity in monocytes of patients with meningococcal infection: related to an unfavourable prognosis. Thromb Haemost 1983;49:5–7.

208. Lammle B, Tran TH, Ritz R, Duckert F. Plasma prekallikrein, factor XII, antithrombin III, C1(-)-inhibitor and alpha 2-macroglobulin in critically ill patients with suspected disseminated intravascular coagulation (DIC). Am J Clin Pathol 1984;82:396–404.

209. Powars D, Larsen R, Johnson J, et al. Epidemic meningococcemia and purpura fulminans with induced protein C deficiency. Clin Infect Dis 1993;17:254–261.

210. Leclerc F, Hazelzet J, Jude B, et al. Protein C and S deficiency in severe infectious purpura of children: a collaborative study of 40 cases. Intensive Care Med 1992;18:202–205.

211. Suffredini AF, Harpel PC, Parrillo JE. Promotion and subsequent inhibition of plasminogen activation after administration of intravenous endotoxin to normal subjects. N Engl J Med 1989;320:1165–1172.

212. Levin M, Eley BS, Louis J, Cohen H, Young L, Heyderman RS. Postinfectious purpura fulminans caused by an autoantibody directed against protein S. J Pediatr 1995;127:355–363.

213. Gomez E, Ledford MR, Pegelow CH, Reitsma PH, Bertina RM. Homozygous protein S deficiency due to a one base pair deletion that leads to a stop codon in exon III of the protein S gene. Thromb Haemost 1994;71:723–726.

214. Marciniak E, Wilson HD, Marlar RA. Neonatal purpura fulminans: a genetic disorder related to the absence of protein C in blood. Blood 1985;65:15–20.

215. Westendorp RG, Reitsma PH, Bertina RM. Inherited prethrombotic disorders and infectious purpura. Thromb Haemost 1996;75:899–901.

216. Bertina RM, Koeleman BP, Koster T, et al. Mutation in blood coagulation factor V associated with resistance to activated protein C. Nature 1994;369:64–67.

217. Rees DC, Cox M, Clegg JB. World distribution of factor V Leiden. Lancet 1995;346:1133–1134.

218. Kondaveeti S, Hibberd ML, Booy R, Nadel S, Levin M. Effect of the Factor V Leiden mutation on the severity of meningococcal disease. Pediatr Infect Dis J 1999;18:893–896.

219. Levi M, Ten Cate H, van der Poll T, van Deventer SJ. Pathogenesis of disseminated intravascular coagulation in sepsis. JAMA 1993;270:975–979.

220. Ny T, Sawdey M, Lawrence D, Millan JL, Loskutoff DJ. Cloning and sequence of a cDNA coding for the human beta-migrating endothelial-cell-type plasminogen activator inhibitor. Proc Natl Acad Sci U S A 1986;83:6776–6780.

221. Pannekoek H, Veerman H, Lambers H, et al. Endothelial plasminogen activator inhibitor (PAI): a new member of the Serpin gene family. EMBO J 1986;5:2539–2544.

222. Ryan MP, Kutz SM, Higgins PJ. Complex regulation of plasminogen activator inhibitor type-1 (PAI-1) gene expression by serum and substrate adhesion. Biochem J 1996;314 (Pt 3):1041–1046.

223. Hermans PW, Hibberd ML, Booy R, et al. 4G/5G promoter polymorphism in the plasminogen-activator-inhibitor-1 gene and outcome of meningococcal disease. Meningococcal Research Group. Lancet 1999;354:556–560.

224. Ludwig M, Wohn KD, Schleuning WD, Olek K. Allelic dimorphism in the human tissue-type plasminogen activator (TPA) gene as a result of an Alu insertion/deletion event. Hum Genet 1992;88:388–392.

225. Miura O, Sugahara Y, Nakamura Y, Hirosawa S, Aoki N. Restriction fragment length polymorphism caused by a deletion involving Alu sequences within the human alpha 2-plasmin inhibitor gene. Biochemistry 1989;28:4934–4938.

226. Kondaveeti S, Hibberd ML, Levin M. The insertion/deletion polymorphism in the t-PA gene does not significantly affect outcome of meningococcal disease. Thromb Haemost 1999;82:161–162.

227. Eriksson P, Kallin B, van 't Hooft FM, Bavenholm P, Hamsten A. Allele-specific increase in basal transcription of the plasminogen-activator inhibitor 1 gene is associated with myocardial infarction. Proc Natl Acad Sci U S A 1995;92:1851–1855.

228. Dawson SJ, Wiman B, Hamsten A, Green F, Humphries S, Henney AM. The two allele sequences of a common polymorphism in the promoter of the plasminogen

activator inhibitor-1 (PAI-1) gene respond differently to interleukin-1 in HepG2 cells. J Biol Chem 1993;268:10739–10745.

229. Haralambous E, Hibberd ML, Hermans PW, Ninis N, Nadel S, Levin M. Role of functional plasminogen-activator-inhibitor-1 4G/5G promoter polymorphism in susceptibility, severity, and outcome of meningococcal disease in Caucasian children. Crit Care Med 2003;31:2788–2793.

230. Westendorp RG, Hottenga JJ, Slagboom PE. Variation in plasminogen-activator-inhibitor-1 gene and risk of meningococcal septic shock. Lancet 1999;354: 561–563.

231. Geishofer G, Binder A, Muller M, et al. 4G/5G promoter polymorphism in the plasminogen-activator-inhibitor-1 gene in children with systemic meningococcaemia. Eur J Pediatr 2005;164:486–490.

232. Zenz W, Muntean W, Zobel G, Grubbauer HM, Gallistl S. Treatment of fulminant meningococcemia with recombinant tissue plasminogen activator. Thromb Haemost 1995;74:802–803.

233. Bajzar L, Morser J, Nesheim M. TAFI, or plasma procarboxypeptidase B, couples the coagulation and fibrinolytic cascades through the thrombin-thrombomodulin complex. J Biol Chem 1996;271:16603–16608.

234. Boffa MB, Bell R, Stevens WK, Nesheim ME. Roles of thermal instability and proteolytic cleavage in regulation of activated thrombin-activable fibrinolysis inhibitor. J Biol Chem 2000;275:12868–12878.

235. Marx PF, Hackeng TM, Dawson PE, Griffin JH, Meijers JC, Bouma BN. Inactivation of active thrombin-activable fibrinolysis inhibitor takes place by a process that involves conformational instability rather than proteolytic cleavage. J Biol Chem 2000;275:12410–12415.

236. Watanabe R, Wada H, Watanabe Y, et al. Activity and antigen levels of thrombin-activatable fibrinolysis inhibitor in plasma of patients with disseminated intravascular coagulation. Thromb Res 2001;104:1–6.

237. Zeerleder S, Schroeder V, Hack CE, Kohler HP, Wuillemin WA. TAFI and PAI-1 levels in human sepsis. Thromb Res 2006;118:205–212.

238. Chetaille P, Alessi MC, Kouassi D, Morange PE, Juhan-Vague I. Plasma TAFI antigen variations in healthy subjects. Thromb Haemost 2000;83:902–905.

239. Bouma BN, Marx PF, Mosnier LO, Meijers JC. Thrombin-activatable fibrinolysis inhibitor (TAFI, plasma procarboxypeptidase B, procarboxypeptidase R, procarboxypeptidase U). Thromb Res 2001;101:329–354.

240. Zhao L, Morser J, Bajzar L, Nesheim M, Nagashima M. Identification and characterization of two thrombin-activatable fibrinolysis inhibitor isoforms. Thromb Haemost 1998;80:949–955.

241. Schneider M, Boffa M, Stewart R, Rahman M, Koschinsky M, Nesheim M. Two naturally occurring variants of TAFI (Thr-325 and Ile-325) differ substantially with respect to thermal stability and antifibrinolytic activity of the enzyme. J Biol Chem 2002;277:1021–1030.

242. Henry M, Aubert H, Morange PE, et al. Identification of polymorphisms in the promoter and the 3' region of the TAFI gene: evidence that plasma TAFI antigen levels are strongly genetically controlled. Blood 2001;97:2053–2058.

243. Brouwers GJ, Vos HL, Leebeek FW, et al. A novel, possibly functional, single nucleotide polymorphism in the coding region of the thrombin-activatable fibrinolysis inhibitor (TAFI) gene is also associated with TAFI levels. Blood 2001;98:1992–1993.

244. Kremer Hovinga JA, Franco RF, Zago MA, Ten CH, Westendorp RG, Reitsma PH. A functional single nucleotide polymorphism in the thrombin-activatable fibrinolysis inhibitor (TAFI) gene associates with outcome of meningococcal disease. J Thromb Haemost 2004;2:54–57.

245. Lazarus DS, Aschoff J, Fanburg BL, Lanzillo JJ. Angiotensin converting enzyme (kininase II) mRNA production and enzymatic activity in human peripheral blood monocytes are induced by GM-CSF but not by other cytokines. Biochim Biophys Acta 1994;1226:12–18.

246. Guba M, Steinbauer M, Buchner M, et al. Differential effects of short-term ace- and AT1-receptor inhibition on postischemic injury and leukocyte adherence in vivo and in vitro. Shock 2000;13:190–196.

247. Weber KT. Fibrosis, a common pathway to organ failure: angiotensin II and tissue repair. Semin Nephrol 1997;17:467–491.

248. Yamamoto T, Wang L, Shimakura K, Sanaka M, Koike Y, Mineshita S. Angiotensin II-induced pulmonary edema in a rabbit model. Jpn J Pharmacol 1997;73:33–40.

249. Constantinescu CS, Goodman DB, Hilliard B, Wysocka M, Cohen JA. Murine macrophages stimulated with central and peripheral nervous system myelin or purified myelin proteins release inflammatory products. Neurosci Lett 2000;287:171–174.

250. Tiret L, Rigat B, Visvikis S, et al. Evidence, from combined segregation and linkage analysis, that a variant of the angiotensin I-converting enzyme (ACE) gene controls plasma ACE levels. Am J Hum Genet 1992;51:197–205.

251. Keavney B, McKenzie CA, Connell JM, et al. Measured haplotype analysis of the angiotensin-I converting enzyme gene. Hum Mol Genet 1998;7:1745–1751.

252. Cambien F, henc-Gelas F, Herbeth B, et al. Familial resemblance of plasma angiotensin-converting enzyme level: the Nancy Study. Am J Hum Genet 1988; 43:774–780.

253. Rigat B, Hubert C, Henc-Gelas F, Cambien F, Corvol P, Soubrier F. An insertion/deletion polymorphism in the angiotensin I-converting enzyme gene accounting for half the variance of serum enzyme levels. J Clin Invest 1990;86:1343–1346.

254. Costerousse O, Allegrini J, Lopez M, Henc-Gelas F. Angiotensin I-converting enzyme in human circulating mononuclear cells: genetic polymorphism of expression in T-lymphocytes. Biochem J 1993;290(pt 1):33–40.

255. Marshall RP, Webb S, Bellingan GJ, et al. Angiotensin converting enzyme insertion/deletion polymorphism is associated with susceptibility and outcome in acute respiratory distress syndrome. Am J Respir Crit Care Med 2002;166:646–650.

256. Bonnardeaux A, Davies E, Jeunemaitre X, et al. Angiotensin II type 1 receptor gene polymorphisms in human essential hypertension. Hypertension 1994;24:63–69.

257. Braun A, Kammerer S, Bohme E, Muller B, Roscher AA. Identification of polymorphic sites of the human bradykinin B2 receptor gene. Biochem Biophys Res Commun 1995;211:234–240.

258. Caulfield M, Lavender P, Farrall M, et al. Linkage of the angiotensinogen gene to essential hypertension. N Engl J Med 1994;330:1629–1633.

259. Harding D, Baines PB, Brull D, et al. Severity of meningococcal disease in children and the angiotensin-converting enzyme insertion/deletion polymorphism. Am J Respir Crit Care Med 2002;165:1103–1106.

260. John BR, Loggins J, Yanamandra K. Angiotensin converting enzyme insertion/deletion polymorphism does not alter sepsis outcome in ventilated very low birth weight infants. J Perinatol 2005;25:205–209.

261. Kiely DG, Cargill RI, Wheeldon NM, Coutie WJ, Lipworth BJ. Haemodynamic and endocrine effects of type 1 angiotensin II receptor blockade in patients with hypoxaemic cor pulmonale. Cardiovasc Res 1997;33:201–208.

262. Debets JM, Kampmeijer R, van der Linden MP, Buurman WA, van der Linden CJ. Plasma tumor necrosis factor and mortality in critically ill septic patients. Crit Care Med 1989;17:489–494.

263. Waage A, Brandtzaeg P, Halstensen A, Kierulf P, Espevik T. The complex pattern of cytokines in serum from patients with meningococcal septic shock. Association between interleukin 6, interleukin 1, and fatal outcome. J Exp Med 1989;169: 333–338.

264. Tang GJ, Kuo CD, Yen TC, et al. Perioperative plasma concentrations of tumor necrosis factor-alpha and interleukin-6 in infected patients. Crit Care Med 1996;24:423–428.

265. Deans KJ, Haley M, Natanson C, Eichacker PQ, Minneci PC. Novel therapies for sepsis: a review. J Trauma 2005;58:867–874.

266. Zeni F, Freeman B, Natanson C. Anti-inflammatory therapies to treat sepsis and septic shock: a reassessment. Crit Care Med 1997;25:1095–1100.

267. Cox ED, Hoffmann SC, DiMercurio BS, et al. Cytokine polymorphic analyses indicate ethnic differences in the allelic distribution of interleukin-2 and interleukin-6. Transplantation 2001;72:720–726.

268. Bidwell J, Keen L, Gallagher G, et al. Cytokine gene polymorphism in human disease: on-line databases. Genes Immun 1999;1:3–19.

269. Bazzoni F, Beutler B. The tumor necrosis factor ligand and receptor families. N Engl J Med 1996;334:1717–1725.

270. Bone RC. Toward a theory regarding the pathogenesis of the systemic inflammatory response syndrome: what we do and do not know about cytokine regulation. Crit Care Med 1996;24:163–172.

271. Goris RJ. MODS/SIRS: result of an overwhelming inflammatory response? World J Surg 1996;20:418–421.

272. Pinsky MR. Organ-specific therapy in critical illness: interfacing molecular mechanisms with physiological interventions. J Crit Care 1996;11:95–107.

273. Tracey KJ, Beutler B, Lowry SF, et al. Shock and tissue injury induced by recombinant human cachectin. Science 1986;234:470–474.

274. Strieter RM, Kunkel SL, Bone RC. Role of tumor necrosis factor-alpha in disease states and inflammation. Crit Care Med 1993;21:S447–S463.

275. Wilson AG, di Giovine FS, Duff GW. Genetics of tumour necrosis factor-alpha in autoimmune, infectious, and neoplastic diseases. J Inflamm 1995;45:1–12.

276. Mira JP, Cariou A, Grall F, et al. Association of TNF2, a TNF-alpha promoter polymorphism, with septic shock susceptibility and mortality: a multicenter study. JAMA 1999;282:561–568.

277. O'Keefe GE, Hybki DL, Munford RS. The G→A single nucleotide polymorphism at the –308 position in the tumor necrosis factor-alpha promoter increases the risk for severe sepsis after trauma. J Trauma 2002;52:817–825.

278. Wilson AG, di Giovine FS, Blakemore AI, Duff GW. Single base polymorphism in the human tumour necrosis factor alpha (TNF alpha) gene detectable by NcoI restriction of PCR product. Hum Mol Genet 1992;1:353.

279. Knight JC, Udalova I, Hill AV, et al. A polymorphism that affects OCT-1 binding to the TNF promoter region is associated with severe malaria. Nat Genet 1999;22:145–150.

280. Stuber F, Udalova IA, Book M, et al. -308 tumor necrosis factor (TNF) polymorphism is not associated with survival in severe sepsis and is unrelated to lipopolysaccharide inducibility of the human TNF promoter. J Inflamm 1995;46:42–50.

281. Brinkman BM, Zuijdeest D, Kaijzel EL, Breedveld FC, Verweij CL. Relevance of the tumor necrosis factor alpha (TNF alpha) -308 promoter polymorphism in TNF alpha gene regulation. J Inflamm 1995;46:32–41.

282. Abraham LJ, Kroeger KM. Impact of the -308 TNF promoter polymorphism on the transcriptional regulation of the TNF gene: relevance to disease. J Leukoc Biol 1999;66:562–566.

283. Stuber F, Petersen M, Bokelmann F, Schade U. A genomic polymorphism within the tumor necrosis factor locus influences plasma tumor necrosis factor-alpha concentrations and outcome of patients with severe sepsis. Crit Care Med 1996;24:381–384.

284. Messer G, Spengler U, Jung MC, et al. Polymorphic structure of the tumor necrosis factor (TNF) locus: an NcoI polymorphism in the first intron of the human TNF-beta gene correlates with a variant amino acid in position 26 and a reduced level of TNF-beta production. J Exp Med 1991;173:209–219.

285. Majetschak M, Flohe S, Obertacke U, et al. Relation of a TNF gene polymorphism to severe sepsis in trauma patients. Ann Surg 1999;230:207–214.

286. Pociot F, Molvig J, Wogensen L, et al. A tumour necrosis factor beta gene polymorphism in relation to monokine secretion and insulin-dependent diabetes mellitus. Scand J Immunol 1991;33:37–49.

287. Fugger L, Morling N, Ryder LP, et al. NcoI restriction fragment length polymorphism (RFLP) of the tumor necrosis factor (TNF alpha) region in four autoimmune diseases. Tissue Antigens 1989;34:17–22.

288. Molvig J, Pociot F, Baek L, et al. Monocyte function in IDDM patients and healthy individuals. Scand J Immunol 1990;32:297–311.

289. Waterer GW, Quasney MW, Cantor RM, Wunderink RG. Septic shock and respiratory failure in community-acquired pneumonia have different TNF polymorphism associations. Am J Respir Crit Care Med 2001;163:1599–1604.

290. Bouma G, Crusius JB, Oudkerk PM, et al. Secretion of tumour necrosis factor alpha and lymphotoxin alpha in relation to polymorphisms in the TNF genes and HLA-DR alleles. Relevance for inflammatory bowel disease. Scand J Immunol 1996; 43:456–463.

291. Appoloni O, Dupont E, Vandercruys M, Andriens M, Duchateau J, Vincent JL. Association of tumor necrosis factor-2 allele with plasma tumor necrosis factor-alpha levels and mortality from septic shock. Am J Med 2001;110:486–488.

292. Reid CL, Perrey C, Pravica V, Hutchinson IV, Campbell IT. Genetic variation in proinflammatory and anti-inflammatory cytokine production in multiple organ dysfunction syndrome. Crit Care Med 2002;30:2216–2221.

293. Gordon AC, Lagan AL, Aganna E, et al. TNF and TNFR polymorphisms in severe sepsis and septic shock: a prospective multicentre study. Genes Immun 2004; 5:631–640.

294. Tang GJ, Huang SL, Yien HW, et al. Tumor necrosis factor gene polymorphism and septic shock in surgical infection. Crit Care Med 2000;28:2733–2736.

295. Hedberg CL, Adcock K, Martin J, Loggins J, Kruger TE, Baier RJ. Tumor necrosis factor alpha—308 polymorphism associated with increased sepsis mortality in ventilated very low birth weight infants. Pediatr Infect Dis J 2004;23: 424–428.

296. Majetschak M, Obertacke U, Schade FU, et al. Tumor necrosis factor gene poly-morphisms, leukocyte function, and sepsis susceptibility in blunt trauma patients. Clin Diagn Lab Immunol 2002;9:1205–1211.

297. Read RC, Camp NJ, di Giovine FS, et al. An interleukin-1 genotype is associated with fatal outcome of meningococcal disease. J Infect Dis 2000;182:1557–1560.

298. Balding J, Healy CM, Livingstone WJ, et al. Genomic polymorphic profiles in an Irish population with meningococcaemia: is it possible to predict severity and outcome of disease? Genes Immun 2003;4:533–540.

299. Nadel S, Newport MJ, Booy R, Levin M. Variation in the tumor necrosis factor-alpha gene promoter region may be associated with death from meningococcal disease. J Infect Dis 1996;174:878–880.

300. Gallagher PM, Lowe G, Fitzgerald T, et al. Association of IL-10 polymorphism with severity of illness in community acquired pneumonia. Thorax 2003;58:154–156.

301. Schaaf BM, Boehmke F, Esnaashari H, et al. Pneumococcal septic shock is associ-ated with the interleukin-10-1082 gene promoter polymorphism. Am J Respir Crit Care Med 2003;168:476–480.

302. Fang XM, Schroder S, Hoeft A, Stuber F. Comparison of two polymorphisms of the interleukin-1 gene family: interleukin-1 receptor antagonist polymorphism con-tributes to susceptibility to severe sepsis. Crit Care Med 1999;27:1330–1334.

303. Boraschi D, Tagliabue A. The interleukin-1 receptor family. Vitam Horm 2006;74:229–254.

304. Boraschi D, Bossu P, Macchia G, Ruggiero P, Tagliabue A. Structure-function relationship in the IL-1 family. Front Biosci 1996;1:d270–d308.

305. Dinarello CA. Interleukin-1. Dig Dis Sci 1988;33:25S-35S.

306. Dinarello CA. Proinflammatory cytokines. Chest 2000;118:503–508.

307. Arend WP. The balance between IL-1 and IL-1Ra in disease. Cytokine Growth Factor Rev 2002;13:323–340.

308. Dinarello CA. Biology of interleukin 1. FASEB J 1988;2:108–115.

309. Dinarello CA. Biologic basis for interleukin-1 in disease. Blood 1996;87:2095–2147.

310. Granowitz EV, Santos AA, Poutsiaka DD, et al. Production of interleukin-1–receptor antagonist during experimental endotoxaemia. Lancet 1991;338:1423–1424.

311. Wilkinson RJ, Patel P, Llewelyn M, et al. Influence of polymorphism in the genes for the interleukin (IL)-1 receptor antagonist and IL-1beta on tuberculosis. J Exp Med 1999;189:1863–1874.

312. Hurme M, Santtila S. IL-1 receptor antagonist (IL-1Ra) plasma levels are co-ordinately regulated by both IL-1Ra and IL-1beta genes. Eur J Immunol 1998; 28:2598–2602.

313. van Deuren M. Kinetics of tumour necrosis factor-alpha, soluble tumour necrosis factor receptors, interleukin 1–beta and its receptor antagonist during serious infections. Eur J Clin Microbiol Infect Dis 1994;13(suppl 1):S12–S16.

314. Nicklin MJ, Weith A, Duff GW. A physical map of the region encompassing the human interleukin-1 alpha, interleukin-1 beta, and interleukin-1 receptor antago-nist genes. Genomics 1994;19:382–384.

315. Tarlow JK, Blakemore AI, Lennard A, et al. Polymorphism in human IL-1 receptor antagonist gene intron 2 is caused by variable numbers of an 86-bp tandem repeat. Hum Genet 1993;91:403–404.

316. Pociot F, Molvig J, Wogensen L, Worsaae H, Nerup J. A TaqI polymorphism in the human interleukin-1 beta (IL-1 beta) gene correlates with IL-1 beta secretion in vitro. Eur J Clin Invest 1992;22:396–402.

317. van den Velden PA, Reitsma PH. Amino acid dimorphism in IL1A is detectable by PCR amplification. Hum Mol Genet 1993;2:1753.
318. Shirodaria S, Smith J, McKay IJ, Kennett CN, Hughes FJ. Polymorphisms in the IL-1A gene are correlated with levels of interleukin-1alpha protein in gingival crevicular fluid of teeth with severe periodontal disease. J Dent Res 2000;79:1864–1869.
319. di Giovine FS, Takhsh E, Blakemore AI, Duff GW. Single base polymorphism at -511 in the human interleukin-1 beta gene (IL1 beta). Hum Mol Genet 1992;1:450.
320. El-Omar EM, Carrington M, Chow WH, et al. Interleukin-1 polymorphisms associated with increased risk of gastric cancer. Nature 2000;404:398–402.
321. Campos MI, Santos MC, Trevilatto PC, Scarel-Caminaga RM, Bezerra FJ, Line SR. Evaluation of the relationship between interleukin-1 gene cluster polymorphisms and early implant failure in non-smoking patients. Clin Oral Implants Res 2005;16:194–201.
322. Fantuzzi G, Zheng H, Faggioni R, et al. Effect of endotoxin in IL-1 beta-deficient mice. J Immunol 1996;157:291–296.
323. Cox A, Camp NJ, Nicklin MJ, di Giovine FS, Duff GW. An analysis of linkage disequilibrium in the interleukin-1 gene cluster, using a novel grouping method for multiallelic markers. Am J Hum Genet 1998;62:1180–1188.
324. Andus T, Daig R, Vogl D, et al. Imbalance of the interleukin 1 system in colonic mucosa–association with intestinal inflammation and interleukin 1 receptor antagonist (corrected) genotype 2. Gut 1997;41:651–657.
325. Danis VA, Millington M, Hyland VJ, Grennan D. Cytokine production by normal human monocytes: inter-subject variation and relationship to an IL-1 receptor antagonist (IL-1Ra) gene polymorphism. Clin Exp Immunol 1995;99:303–310.
326. Tountas NA, Casini-Raggi V, Yang H, et al. Functional and ethnic association of allele 2 of the interleukin-1 receptor antagonist gene in ulcerative colitis. Gastroenterology 1999;117:806–813.
327. Arnalich F, Lopez-Maderuelo D, Codoceo R, et al. Interleukin-1 receptor antagonist gene polymorphism and mortality in patients with severe sepsis. Clin Exp Immunol 2002;127:331–336.
328. Hirsch E, Irikura VM, Paul SM, Hirsh D. Functions of interleukin 1 receptor antagonist in gene knockout and overproducing mice. Proc Natl Acad Sci U S A 1996;93:11008–11013.
329. Arnalich F, Garcia-Palomero E, Lopez J, et al. Predictive value of nuclear factor kappaB activity and plasma cytokine levels in patients with sepsis. Infect Immun 2000;68:1942–1945.
330. Fisher CJ Jr, Dhainaut JF, Opal SM, et al. Recombinant human interleukin 1 receptor antagonist in the treatment of patients with sepsis syndrome. Results from a randomized, double-blind, placebo-controlled trial. Phase III rhIL-1ra Sepsis Syndrome Study Group. JAMA 1994;271:1836–1843.
331. Opal SM, Fisher CJ Jr, Dhainaut JF, et al. Confirmatory interleukin-1 receptor antagonist trial in severe sepsis: a phase III, randomized, double-blind, placebo-controlled, multicenter trial. The Interleukin-1 Receptor Antagonist Sepsis Investigator Group. Crit Care Med 1997;25:1115–1124.
332. Ma P, Chen D, Pan J, Du B. Genomic polymorphism within interleukin-1 family cytokines influences the outcome of septic patients. Crit Care Med 2002;30:1046–1050.

333. Read RC, Cannings C, Naylor SC, et al. Variation within genes encoding interleukin-1 and the interleukin-1 receptor antagonist influence the severity of meningococcal disease. Ann Intern Med 2003;138:534–541.

334. Carrol ED, Mobbs KJ, Thomson AP, Hart CA. Variable number tandem repeat polymorphism of the interleukin-1 receptor antagonist gene in meningococcal disease. Clin Infect Dis 2002;35:495–497.

335. Borden EC, Chin P. Interleukin-6: a cytokine with potential diagnostic and therapeutic roles. J Lab Clin Med 1994;123:824–829.

336. Hack CE, de Groot ER, Felt-Bersma RJ, et al. Increased plasma levels of interleukin-6 in sepsis. Blood 1989;74:1704–1710.

337. Schluter B, Konig B, Bergmann U, Muller FE, Konig W. Interleukin 6—a potential mediator of lethal sepsis after major thermal trauma: evidence for increased IL-6 production by peripheral blood mononuclear cells. J Trauma 1991;31:1663–1670.

338. Calandra T, Gerain J, Heumann D, Baumgartner JD, Glauser MP. High circulating levels of interleukin-6 in patients with septic shock: evolution during sepsis, prognostic value, and interplay with other cytokines. The Swiss-Dutch J5 Immunoglobulin Study Group. Am J Med 1991;91:23–29.

339. Patel RT, Deen KI, Youngs D, Warwick J, Keighley MR. Interleukin 6 is a prognostic indicator of outcome in severe intra-abdominal sepsis. Br J Surg 1994;81:1306–1308.

340. Akira S. IL-6–regulated transcription factors. Int J Biochem Cell Biol 1997;29:1401–1418.

341. Fishman D, Faulds G, Jeffery R, et al. The effect of novel polymorphisms in the interleukin-6 (IL-6) gene on IL-6 transcription and plasma IL-6 levels, and an association with systemic-onset juvenile chronic arthritis. J Clin Invest 1998;102:1369–1376.

342. Bennermo M, Held C, Stemme S, et al. Genetic predisposition of the interleukin-6 response to inflammation: implications for a variety of major diseases? Clin Chem 2004;50:2136–2140.

343. Schluter B, Raufhake C, Erren M, et al. Effect of the interleukin-6 promoter polymorphism (-174 G/C) on the incidence and outcome of sepsis. Crit Care Med 2002;30:32–37.

344. Watanabe E, Hirasawa H, Oda S, Matsuda K, Hatano M, Tokuhisa T. Extremely high interleukin-6 blood levels and outcome in the critically ill are associated with tumor necrosis factor- and interleukin-1–related gene polymorphisms. Crit Care Med 2005;33:89–97.

345. van der Poll T, Marchant A, van Deventer SJ. The role of interleukin-10 in the pathogenesis of bacterial infection. Clin Microbiol Infect 1997;3:605–607.

346. Cohen MC, Cohen S. Cytokine function: a study in biologic diversity. Am J Clin Pathol 1996;105:589–598.

347. van der Poll T, Marchant A, Keogh CV, Goldman M, Lowry SF. Interleukin-10 impairs host defense in murine pneumococcal pneumonia. J Infect Dis 1996;174:994–1000.

348. Fumeaux T, Pugin J. Role of interleukin-10 in the intracellular sequestration of human leukocyte antigen-DR in monocytes during septic shock. Am J Respir Crit Care Med 2002;166:1475–1482.

349. Latifi SQ, O'Riordan MA, Levine AD. Interleukin-10 controls the onset of irreversible septic shock. Infect Immun 2002;70:4441–4446.

350. Zanotti S, Kumar A, Kumar A. Cytokine modulation in sepsis and septic shock. Expert Opin Investig Drugs 2002;11:1061–1075.

351. Gogos CA, Drosou E, Bassaris HP, Skoutelis A. Pro- versus anti-inflammatory cytokine profile in patients with severe sepsis: a marker for prognosis and future therapeutic options. J Infect Dis 2000;181:176–180.

352. Doughty L, Carcillo JA, Kaplan S, Janosky J. The compensatory anti-inflammatory cytokine interleukin 10 response in pediatric sepsis-induced multiple organ failure. Chest 1998;113:1625–1631.

353. Monneret G, Finck ME, Venet F, et al. The anti-inflammatory response dominates after septic shock: association of low monocyte HLA-DR expression and high interleukin-10 concentration. Immunol Lett 2004;95:193–198.

354. Steinhauser ML, Hogaboam CM, Kunkel SL, Lukacs NW, Strieter RM, Standiford TJ. IL-10 is a major mediator of sepsis-induced impairment in lung antibacterial host defense. J Immunol 1999;162:392–399.

355. Doughty LA, Kaplan SS, Carcillo JA. Inflammatory cytokine and nitric oxide responses in pediatric sepsis and organ failure. Crit Care Med 1996;24:1137–1143.

356. Reuss E, Fimmers R, Kruger A, Becker C, Rittner C, Hohler T. Differential regulation of interleukin-10 production by genetic and environmental factors–a twin study. Genes Immun 2002;3:407–413.

357. Eskdale J, Gallagher G. A polymorphic dinucleotide repeat in the human IL-10 promoter. Immunogenetics 1995;42:444–445.

358. Eskdale J, Kube D, Gallagher G. A second polymorphic dinucleotide repeat in the 5' flanking region of the human IL10 gene. Immunogenetics 1996;45:82–83.

359. Eskdale J, Kube D, Tesch H, Gallagher G. Mapping of the human IL10 gene and further characterization of the 5' flanking sequence. Immunogenetics 1997;46:120–128.

360. Turner DM, Williams DM, Sankaran D, Lazarus M, Sinnott PJ, Hutchinson IV. An investigation of polymorphism in the interleukin-10 gene promoter. Eur J Immunogenet 1997;24:1–8.

361. Lazarus M, Hajeer AH, Turner D, et al. Genetic variation in the interleukin 10 gene promoter and systemic lupus erythematosus. J Rheumatol 1997;24:2314–2317.

362. Gibson AW, Edberg JC, Wu J, Westendorp RG, Huizinga TW, Kimberly RP. Novel single nucleotide polymorphisms in the distal IL-10 promoter affect IL-10 production and enhance the risk of systemic lupus erythematosus. J Immunol 2001;166:3915–3922.

363. Kube D, Platzer C, von Knethen A, et al. Isolation of the human interleukin 10 promoter. Characterization of the promoter activity in Burkitt's lymphoma cell lines. Cytokine 1995;7:1–7.

364. Koss K, Satsangi J, Fanning GC, Welsh KI, Jewell DP. Cytokine (TNF alpha, LT alpha and IL-10) polymorphisms in inflammatory bowel diseases and normal controls: differential effects on production and allele frequencies. Genes Immun 2000;1:185–190.

365. D'Alfonso S, Rampi M, Rolando V, Giordano M, Momigliano-Richiardi P. New polymorphisms in the IL-10 promoter region. Genes Immun 2000;1:231–233.

366. Opdal SH. IL-10 gene polymorphisms in infectious disease and SIDS. FEMS Immunol Med Microbiol 2004;42:48–52.

367. Miura Y, Thoburn CJ, Bright EC, Chen W, Nakao S, Hess AD. Cytokine and chemokine profiles in autologous graft-versus-host disease (GVHD): interleukin 10 and interferon gamma may be critical mediators for the development of autologous GVHD. Blood 2002;100:2650–2658.

368. Lowe PR, Galley HF, Abdel-Fattah A, Webster NR. Influence of interleukin-10 polymorphisms on interleukin-10 expression and survival in critically ill patients. Crit Care Med 2003;31:34–38.

369. Fijen JW, Tulleken JE, Hepkema BG, van der Werf TS, Ligtenberg JJ, Zijlstra JG. The influence of tumor necrosis factor-alpha and interleukin-10 gene promoter polymorphism on the inflammatory response in experimental human endotoxemia. Clin Infect Dis 2001;33:1601–1603.

370. Crawley E, Kay R, Sillibourne J, Patel P, Hutchinson I, Woo P. Polymorphic haplotypes of the interleukin-10 5' flanking region determine variable interleukin-10 transcription and are associated with particular phenotypes of juvenile rheumatoid arthritis. Arthritis Rheum 1999;42:1101–1108.

371. Shu Q, Fang X, Chen Q, Stuber F. IL-10 polymorphism is associated with increased incidence of severe sepsis. Chin Med J (Engl) 2003;116:1756–1759.

372. Boehm U, Klamp T, Groot M, Howard JC. Cellular responses to interferon-gamma. Annu Rev Immunol 1997;15:749–795.

373. Lammas DA, Casanova JL, Kumararatne DS. Clinical consequences of defects in the IL-12–dependent interferon-gamma (IFN-gamma) pathway. Clin Exp Immunol 2000;121:417–425.

374. Polk HC Jr, Cheadle WG, Livingston DH, et al. A randomized prospective clinical trial to determine the efficacy of interferon-gamma in severely injured patients. Am J Surg 1992;163:191–196.

375. Dries DJ, Jurkovich GJ, Maier RV, et al. Effect of interferon gamma on infection-related death in patients with severe injuries. A randomized, double-blind, placebo-controlled trial. Arch Surg 1994;129:1031–1041.

376. Mock CN, Dries DJ, Jurkovich GJ, Maier RV. Assessment of two clinical trials: interferon-gamma therapy in severe injury. Shock 1996;5:235–240.

377. Khani-Hanjani A, Lacaille D, Hoar D, et al. Association between dinucleotide repeat in non-coding region of interferon-gamma gene and susceptibility to, and severity of, rheumatoid arthritis. Lancet 2000;356:820–825.

378. Pravica V, Asderakis A, Perrey C, Hajeer A, Sinnott PJ, Hutchinson IV. In vitro production of IFN-gamma correlates with CA repeat polymorphism in the human IFN-gamma gene. Eur J Immunogenet 1999;26:1–3.

379. Dufour C, Capasso M, Svahn J, et al. Homozygosis for (12) CA repeats in the first intron of the human IFN-gamma gene is significantly associated with the risk of aplastic anaemia in Caucasian population. Br J Haematol 2004;126:682–685.

380. Pravica V, Perrey C, Stevens A, Lee JH, Hutchinson IV. A single nucleotide polymorphism in the first intron of the human IFN-gamma gene: absolute correlation with a polymorphic CA microsatellite marker of high IFN-gamma production. Hum Immunol 2000;61:863–866.

381. Lopez-Maderuelo D, Arnalich F, Serantes R, et al. Interferon-gamma and interleukin-10 gene polymorphisms in pulmonary tuberculosis. Am J Respir Crit Care Med 2003;167:970–975.

382. Stassen NA, Leslie-Norfleet LA, Robertson AM, Eichenberger MR, Polk HC Jr. Interferon-gamma gene polymorphisms and the development of sepsis in patients with trauma. Surgery 2002;132:289–292.

383. Dorman SE, Picard C, Lammas D, et al. Clinical features of dominant and recessive interferon gamma receptor 1 deficiencies. Lancet 2004;364:2113–2121.

384. Dorman SE, Holland SM. Interferon-gamma and interleukin-12 pathway defects and human disease. Cytokine Growth Factor Rev 2000;11:321–333.

385. Davis EG, Eichenberger MR, Grant BS, Polk HC Jr. Microsatellite marker of interferon-gamma receptor 1 gene correlates with infection following major trauma. Surgery 2000;128:301–305.

386. Ahrens P, Kattner E, Kohler B, et al. Mutations of genes involved in the innate immune system as predictors of sepsis in very low birth weight infants. Pediatr Res 2004;55:652–656.

387. Sprong T, van der Ley P, Steeghs L, et al. Neisseria meningitidis can induce proinflammatory cytokine production via pathways independent from CD14 and toll-like receptor 4. Eur Cytokine Netw 2002;13:411–417.

388. Sprong T, Stikkelbroeck N, van der Ley P, et al. Contributions of Neisseria meningitidis LPS and non-LPS to proinflammatory cytokine response. J Leukoc Biol 2001;70:283–288.

389. Erridge C, Stewart J, Poxton IR. Monocytes heterozygous for the Asp299Gly and Thr399Ile mutations in the Toll-like receptor 4 gene show no deficit in lipopolysaccharide signalling. J Exp Med 2003;197:1787–1791.

390. Warle MC, Farhan A, Metselaar HJ, et al. Are cytokine gene polymorphisms related to in vitro cytokine production profiles? Liver Transpl 2003;9:170–181.

391. Rios M, Bianco C. The role of blood group antigens in infectious diseases. Semin Hematol 2000;37:177–185.

392. Richer J, Chudley AE. The hemoglobinopathies and malaria. Clin Genet 2005; 68:332–336.

393. Bellamy R, Beyers N, McAdam KP, et al. Genetic susceptibility to tuberculosis in Africans: a genome-wide scan. Proc Natl Acad Sci U S A 2000;97:8005–8009.

394. Bucheton B, Abel L, El-Safi S, et al. A major susceptibility locus on chromosome 22q12 plays a critical role in the control of kala-azar. Am J Hum Genet 2003; 73:1052–1060.

395. Valdimarsson H, Stefansson M, Vikingsdottir T, et al. Reconstitution of opsonizing activity by infusion of mannan-binding lectin (MBL) to MBL-deficient humans. Scand J Immunol 1998;48:116–123.

10
Nosocomial Infections in the Pediatric Intensive Care Unit

Xavier Sáez-Llorens and Octavio Ramilo

Nosocomial infections (NIs) are caused by microbial agents or their toxins acquired while the patient is hospitalized and clinically manifested by local or systemic host inflammatory responses. For several reasons, the pediatric intensive care unit (PICU) is one of the most frequent and important hospital locations for the development of NI. Patients admitted to the PICU often require use of invasive procedures and ventilatory support, and exhibit some degree of immune suppression due to young age, underlying disease, chronic stress, steroid use, and lack of mobility. The presence of congenital anomalies that disrupt anatomic barriers and the increased susceptibility to viral pathogens (e.g., varicella, respiratory syncytial virus [RSV], rotavirus) also contribute to increased risk of infection in the PICU (1,2). In addition, the extent of physical contact between patients and health care workers is greater and more intimate, particularly during feeding and diapering activities. Broad-spectrum antibiotics are given frequently to critically ill children, allowing selective pressure on microbial genes that facilitates the development or selection of drug-resistant organisms, which are more difficult to treat and control.

The overall mortality attributable to the various nosocomial infections within the PICU has been estimated to be between 10% and 15% (3,4). Infections acquired in the PICU are associated with an increased risk of death, with a relative risk of 3.4 (95% confidence interval [CI], 1.5–7.6) (5). The type of patient, underlying disease, number of organ systems affected, frequent use of invasive therapies, and presence of multiresistant pathogens contribute to this high risk. Besides case-morbidity and case–fatality rates associated with nosocomial infections, it has been estimated that the direct costs of and future wages lost because of these infections amount to approximately $4 billion annually in the United States (6). Additionally, many prospective payment systems refuse to cover the additional reimbursement entailed as a consequence of treating a nosocomial infection (7,8). It is believed that at least one third of all nosocomial infections could be prevented through stringent implementation of established strategies from hospitals´ infection control programs (9).

Epidemiology

In 1986, data on nosocomial infections from PICUs and neonatal ICUs were added to the National Nosocomial Infections Surveillance (NNIS) system lead by the Centers for Disease Control (CDC). In 1997, the CDC established the Pediatric Prevention Network (PPN) to evaluate nosocomial infections at children´s hospitals. Information from PICUs is derived from community, university, and independent children's hospitals in the United States. Most published national incidence figures of pediatric nosocomial infections are generated from NNIS and PPN sources.

In contrast to data gathered at adult ICUs, where urinary tract infections are the most common hospital-acquired NIs, primary bloodstream infections (28%), pneumonia (21%), and urinary tract infections (15%) are the most frequent NIs in the PICU according to the NNIS system information (Table 10.1) (10). The mean overall rate was 6.1 infections per 100 patients, or 14.1 per 1000 patient-days. A report of PPN collected data from 20 PICUs indicated a median NI rate of 13.9 per 1000 patient-days, and the most frequent sites of infection were also bloodstream, lower respiratory tract, urinary tract, and skin and soft tissue (11). These U.S. data differ from a recent multicenter European study in which the incidence of NIs at several PICUs was 23.5% and pneumonias, followed by bacteremia, urinary infections, and postsurgical wound infections, were the most common identified primary sites (12). In Panama, a prospective study of 4095 episodes of nosocomial infection in a tertiary pediatric hospital during the period 1996 to 2002 revealed frequencies of 40% for the pulmonary site (ventilator-related and viral respiratory infections), 26% for the bloodstream compartment, 14% for postsurgical areas, and 7% for the urinary tract

TABLE 10.1. Distribution of nosocomial infections by site in pediatric intensive care units

Site of infection	Totals	
	Number	Percentage
Bloodstream	3139	28.0
Pneumonia*	2283	20.4
Urinary tract	1691	15.1
Lower respiratory tract	1316	11.8
Surgical area	819	7.3
Ear, eye, nose, throat	716	6.4
Gastrointestinal tract	520	4.6
Skin/soft tissue	365	3.3
Cardiovascular system	222	2.0
Central nervous system	94	0.8

From the National Nosocomial Infections Surveillance (NNIS) System, U.S. (1990–1999).
*Ventilatory-associated infection.

site. The average annual incidence of nosocomial infection in the PICU was 13.1% (13).

Many factors predispose PICU patients to acquisition of nosocomial infections. Because these factors can vary among institutions within a single country and even more between different countries, differences in surveillance methods, incidences, and predominant sites of infections can be easily explained. Length of stay, types of patients managed, infection control strategies, and use of invasive devices within a particular PICU are variables logically associated with development of nosocomial infections. In addition, young age, prolonged antimicrobial therapy, histamine receptor-2 blockade, and parenteral nutrition are associated with higher rates of PICU nosocomial infections (10,14). Children younger than 5 years of age, particularly those of less than 1 year, have the highest incidence of hospital-acquired infections. The most common organisms isolated from PICU-acquired infections include coagulase-negative staphylococci, enterococci, *Staphylococcus aureus*, *Enterobacter cloacae*, *Candida* species, *Pseudomonas aeruginosa*, *Klebsiella pneumoniae*, *Acinetobacter* spp., and certain viruses, but their predominance depends on the infection site (3,5,13).

Sites of Infection

The most common sites for nosocomial infections in PICU subjects are the bloodstream, respiratory tree, urinary tract, and postsurgical areas. Other sites of infection include conjunctiva, ears, sinuses, and distant tissues seeded by bacteremic episodes.

Bloodstream Infections

Bacteremias are the most frequent nosocomial infections in children admitted to many critical care units. A major contributing factor is the presence of intravascular devices, especially central venous catheters (CVCs). These catheters are used to administer medications and total parenteral nutrition (TPN), and for clinical monitoring. Unfortunately, much of the current concepts on epidemiology, pathogenesis, and resulting morbidity and mortality of catheter-related bloodstream infections emerges mainly from data collected in adult ICUs. The NNIS system found that CVC-associated bloodstream infections in pediatric patients were among the highest of all recorded rates of nosocomial infections, with a mean rate of 7.6 per 1000 catheter-days (15). Only mean rates observed in neonatal ICUs, which manage very low birth weight infants, were higher (i.e., 11.3 per 1000 catheter-days). Children hospitalized in critical care areas are more likely to develop a bloodstream infection if they have a CVC or an arterial catheter, or receive TPN (5).

Catheter insertion areas influence the likelihood of developing a bloodstream infection. Areas of skin with a greater density of colonizing flora seem to be at a higher risk. In adults, CVCs inserted at subclavian vein sites tend to have the lowest risk of bloodstream infection, whereas those at jugular and femoral sites have the highest (16). The risk is low with peripheral venous catheters.

The manufactured material and type of catheter also seem to impact the probability of developing nosocomial infection. Nontunneled CVCs made of polyvinyl chloride or polyethylene are associated with high infection rates, whereas those manufactured with polytetrafluoroethylene or polyurethane have lower risk. Tunneled (e.g., Broviac, Hickman, BARD), implantable, and peripherally inserted CVCs have lower infectious complications than nontunneled catheters (17). Nontunneled catheters are the most frequent devices used at PICUs. Tunneled, implantable, and peripherally inserted CVCs are preferably used for high-risk children subjected to transplantation or prolonged use of therapeutic drugs for cancer and chronic medical conditions (18). In addition to catheter-related bacteremias, other complications include phlebitis and infections located within exit-site areas, tunnel, or device pocket.

The pathogenesis of intravascular catheter-related infections has been studied extensively. Contamination of intravenous fluids is now rarely responsible for bloodstream infections because of implementation of infection control measures. Introduction of microbes from contaminated skin at the time of catheter insertion or thereafter during daily manipulation of the catheter hub are the most common ways involved in the development of infection (18).

Pulmonary Infections

Although nosocomial viral infections, most notably caused by RSV, influenza, parainfluenza, and adenoviruses, can be acquired during hospitalization, particularly in pediatric institutions, most lung infectious processes developed at the PICU refer to ventilator-associated pneumonia. It is estimated that less than 5% of nosocomial pneumonias acquired in the PICU, especially in developed countries, are caused by viruses (3,10).

Ventilator-associated pneumonia is a common problem in PICUs and is usually the second most frequent nosocomial infection reported in critical care units. In a recent prospective cohort study, the pooled mean rate of ventilator-associated pneumonia was 11.6 per 1000 ventilator-days, whereas similar data gathered by the NNIS revealed a frequency of 6 per 1000 (19,20). Children younger than 1 year of age were most affected. Mechanical ventilation was found to be the major risk factor associated with lower respiratory tract infections, with a relative risk of 3.9 (95% CI, 2.2–6.8) (5). Patients had been in the PICU for a mean period of 9 days before developing ventilator-associated pneumonia (20). Other risk factors included immunodeficiency, treatment with immunosuppressive drugs, use of prolonged neuromuscular blockade, admission for major respiratory failure, presence of tracheotomy, use of histamine receptor-2 blockers, and high initial predicted risk of mortality pediatric risk of mortality (PRISM) scores.

Urinary Tract Infections

Involvement of the urinary tract is the third most common nosocomial infection in PICUs. More than 90% of hospital-acquired urinary infections occur in catheterized children (21). In noncatheterized patients, commensal periurethral flora, immunologic and structural factors, and frequent voiding play an important role in avoiding urinary tract infection. Antibiotic use, fecal incontinence typical of young age, immunodeficiency, unrecognized urostasis, and presence of congenital urinary reflux increase the risk (22).

In catheterized patients, recognized pathways through which bacteria gain access into the bladder include extraluminal migration through the periurethral mucus sheath (especially seen in females), contamination of the catheter lumen when the drain junction is disconnected, and contamination of the drainage bag through the outflow valve with subsequent ascending migration of bacteria (23). There is some evidence that the use of sealed catheter junctions or antibiotic prophylactic therapy during catheterization can reduce probability of nosocomial urinary infection, but cost, adverse drug reactions, and emergence of antibiotic-resistant perineal flora are important issues against their rationale (9).

Surgical Infections

Postoperative children are an important subset of the PICU population. Neurosurgical, cardiothoracic, orthopedic, abdominal, and solid-organ transplant patients are at high risk of developing nosocomial infections. Postoperative wound infections account for roughly 7% of all nosocomial infections in PICU patients (24). These infections are more prevalent in patients subjected to urgent surgeries than in those undergoing elective procedures (9).

The rates of surgical-site infections detected within the PICU are likely lower than expected because critically ill children have usually a short stay in this unit, and development of infection can occur several days after surgical procedures. Because wound classification was devised to predict the degree of microbial contamination of the injured skin, the type of wound is a powerful predictor of the likelihood of surgical-site infection (25). In addition, age, severity of illness, duration of preoperative hospital stay, immunologic and clinical status of the patient, and duration of surgery contribute to risk of infection (26).

Of all early nosocomial infections occurring at the PICU after neurosurgery, those involving ventriculoperitoneal shunts (VPS) are most prevalent (10). Most VPS infections develop within 2 weeks of surgery. Currently, the incidence of infection associated with VPS is between 5% and 10% (27). Young age, underlying disease, CVC placement, use of TPN, tracheotomy, prior therapy with broad-spectrum antibiotics, and presence of organisms in the cerebrospinal fluid (CSF) are all associated with increased risk for VPS infection (28,29).

The postoperative cardiothoracic patient is common within the PICU. Approximately 4% to 7% of postoperative heart children develop wound infections, depending on surgery type and need for invasive devices (30,31). If the sternum has to be opened emergently, the probability of infection increases up to 25% (32). Postoperative wound infections after cardiac surgery are more frequent in patients with young age, longer period of ventilation, longer preoperative stay, and longer postoperative PICU hospitalization (31).

Definitions and Diagnosis

A nosocomial infection is traditionally defined as any infection not present or incubated at the time of the patient's admission (33). Differentiation between microbial colonization and infection is of paramount importance to reach a proper diagnosis and avoid liberal and unnecessary use of antimicrobial treatment. Because patients managed at the PICU are subjected to multiple invasive procedures and artificial devices (e.g., vascular lines, pressure-monitoring transducers, urinary tract catheters, intracranial pressure sensors, dialysis devices, respiratory therapy equipment), clear definitions are critical to rule out colonization rather than infection.

Potential catheter-associated bloodstream infections should be evaluated with a minimum of two blood cultures taken before institution of initial or new antimicrobial therapy, including at least one blood sample drawn by venipuncture and another obtained through the catheter central line (34). Meticulous terminology guidelines to standardize detection and reporting of catheter-related bacteremia are described in Table 10.2.

Methods commonly used to diagnose pneumonia in the community setting, such as chest auscultation, sputum examination, and thorax radiography, have poor precision for the diagnosis of nosocomial pneumonia in mechanically ventilated patients (25). Auscultation often is hindered by sounds of the ventilation system, and a variety of underlying pulmonary conditions (e.g., bronchopulmonary dysplasia, adult respiratory distress syndrome, cystic fibrosis, fluid overload) may produce sounds indistinguishable from those present in pneumonia. Cultures of tracheal aspirates may be misleading because the endotracheal tube often is colonized with potential pathogens, especially in patients ventilated for more than a few days (35). Accordingly, it is important not to overinterpret the presence of a positive endotracheal tube culture as evidence of nosocomial pneumonia.

The isolation of *Candida* species from cultures of respiratory secretions obtained through endotracheal intubation or bronchoalveolar lavages in immunocompetent patients managed at the PICU is a frequent therapeutic decision challenge for intensivists and infectious disease specialists. There is a poor correlation between the presence of *Candida* and histologic evidence of fungal pneumonia in lung biopsy evaluations or in postmortem studies (36–38). In addition, there is very low association of mucosal colonization with *Candida* and posterior development of systemic candidiasis (39).

Finally, the presence of new radiographic findings consistent with pneumonia may be extraordinarily difficult to assess in patients with underlying lung disease or those recovering from thoracic or complicated cardiac surgery. Bronchoscopic techniques, such as quantitative culture of protected brush specimens and protected bronchoalveolar lavage, offer greater sensitivity and specificity in diagnosing ventilator-associated pneumonia, but these methods are more invasive, difficult to perform safely in severely ill patients, and have not been properly studied in children (25,40). Table 10.3 describes published guidelines aimed to standardize definitions and procedures to diagnose ventilator-associated pneumonia in PICU patients.

Diagnosis of nosocomial infections, other than catheter or ventilator related, is usually more straightforward. Urinary tract infections are diagnosed based on urine analysis and bacterial colony counts. For an adequate diagnosis, urine sampling should be obtained by catheterization or suprapubic tap because bag-collected specimens are usually contaminated by microbial colonizers of peri-anal areas. Urine catheters maintained in place for several days become frequently colonized by nosocomial flora. Thus, proper diagnosis of urinary infections in catheterized patients requires careful assessment of clinical findings and urine analysis of inflammatory markers (33). The presence of *Candida* species in the urine is common among hospitalized patients, particularly those receiving prolonged antibacterial therapy and subjected to urinary catheterization. Fortunately, asymptomatic candiduria is usually associated with low morbidity and systemic complications, particularly in immunocompetent hosts even without specific antifungal treatment (41,42). Central nervous system

TABLE 10.2. Diagnostic criteria for infections related to intravascular catheters

Infection type	Diagnostic criteria
Catheter colonization	Growth of a microorganism from a culture of the catheter tip, subcutaneous catheter segment, or catheter hub
Phlebitis	Induration or inflammatory signs around the catheter exit site
Exit-site infection	Inflammatory signs within 2 cm of the catheter exit site, with or without fever or purulent exudate emerging from exit site
Tunnel infection	Inflammatory signs >2 cm from the exit site, along the subcutaneous tract of a tunneled catheter
Pocket infection	Infected fluid in the subcutaneous pocket of a totally implantable intravascular device, often associated with inflammatory signs over the pocket; occasionally there is spontaneous rupture and drainage of pus or necrosis of the overlying skin
Catheter-related bloodstream infection	Bacteremia or fungemia in a patient who has an intravascular device and ≥1 positive blood culture obtained from peripheral vein and clinical manifestations of infection; confirmation requires one of the following: a positive catheter culture with same microbe species and antibiogram as that isolated from a peripheral vein culture or simultaneous quantitative cultures of blood samples with a ratio of ≥5:1 (CVC: peripheral) and differential time to positivity (i.e., blood from CVC positive at least 2 hours earlier than blood taken from peripheral vein)

Modified from Mermel et al. (19).

TABLE 10.3. Centers for Disease Control (CDC) definitions for ventilator-associated nosocomial pneumonia in children

Criteria for children older than 1 year of age*	Criteria for children 1 year of age or younger*

1. Rales or dullness to percussion on physical examination of chest and any of the following:
  a. New onset of purulent sputum or change in character of sputum
  b. Organism isolated from blood culture
  c. Isolation of pathogen from specimen obtained by transtracheal aspirate, bronchial brushing, or biopsy
 	
2. New or progressive chest x-ray infiltrate, consolidation, cavitation, or pleural effusion and any of the following:
  a. New onset of purulent sputum or change in character of sputum
  b. Organism isolated from blood culture
  c. Isolation of pathogen from specimen obtained by transtracheal aspirate, bronchial brushing, or biopsy
  d. Virus isolation or antigen detection in respiratory secretions
  e. Positive IgM or fourfold IgG increase in paired serology for pathogen
  f. Positive histopathology of pneumonia
	1. Two of the following: apnea, tachypnea, bradycardia, wheezing, rhonchi, or cough, and any of the following:
	  a. Increased respiratory secretions
	  b. New onset of purulent sputum or change in character of sputum
	  c. Organism isolated from blood culture
	  d. Isolation of pathogen from specimen obtained by transtracheal aspirate, bronchial brushing, or biopsy
	  e. Virus isolation or antigen detection in respiratory secretions
	  f. Positive IgM or fourfold IgG increase in paired serology for pathogen
	  g. Positive histopathology of pneumonia
	
	2. New or progressive chest x-ray infiltrate, consolidation, or pleural effusion, and any of the following:
	  a. Increased respiratory secretions
	  b. New onset of purulent sputum or change in character of sputum
	  c. Organism isolated from blood culture
	  d. Isolation of pathogen from specimen obtained by transtracheal aspirate, bronchial brushing, or biopsy
	  e. Virus isolation or antigen detection in respiratory secretions
	  f. Positive IgM or fourfold IgG increase in paired serology
	  g. Positive histopathology of pneumonia

*Either criteria 1 or 2 must be met for diagnosing nosocomial pneumonia in children.

(CNS) infections depend on the isolation of bacteria and presence of abnormal inflammatory indices in CSF samples. Echocardiographic, clinical findings, and positive blood cultures document the presence of endocarditis. Diagnosis of nosocomial sinusitis relies on clinical manifestations and x-ray findings. Post-surgical wound infections are diagnosed by Gram stains and cultures of exudates.

Etiologic Organisms

Coagulase-negative staphylococci, *S. aureus*, enterococci, gram-negative aerobic bacilli (e.g., species of *Enterobacter*, *Pseudomonas*, and *Klebsiella*), and *Candida* species (e.g., *C. albicans* and others) are the leading pathogens causing catheter-associated infections. Coagulase-negative staphylococci account for roughly 40% of all bloodstream infections in PICUs, whereas gram-negative bacilli are implicated in 25%, and fungi in approximately 10% (3,5,10,43).

Gram-negative aerobic bacilli such as *Pseudomonas aeruginosa*, *Enterobacter cloacae*, *Klebsiella pneumoniae*, and *Staphylococcus aureus* are usually the organisms most commonly associated with ventilator-associated pneumonias (3,5,10). In recent years, many PICUs are facing problems with the emergence of multiple-resistant bacterial pathogens. Strains of *Pseudomonas*, *Acineto-bacter*, *Klebsiella*, *Enterobacter*, and *Stenotrophomonas maltophilia* have developed resistance to most β-lactam antibiotics and aminoglycosides (18,43). Methicillin-resistant *S. aureus* (MRSA) has also emerged as an important etiologic agent. Thus, the effectiveness of empiric antimicrobial therapy for these patients is now more difficult to predict. Nosocomial viral pneumonia is mainly caused by RSV, but influenza viruses can also be involved. Accordingly, annual influenza vaccination of health personnel should be mandatory (44,45).

Escherichia coli, enterococci, *Pseudomonas*, *Klebsiella*, and *Candida* account for the majority of isolates implicated in nosocomial urinary infections at the PICU (3,21,43). Long-term complications of these infections are persistent fever, pyelonephritis, and secondary bacteremia, or sepsis. In contrast to adults, mortality caused by nosocomial urinary tract infection is fortunately rare in children (9).

The pathogens reported from surgical-site infections differ according to the type of procedure. *P. aeruginosa* and *S. aureus* are commonly identified after gastrointestinal tract surgery. *S. aureus* is the most frequent pathogen reported after chest and cardiovascular surgery, followed by coagulase-negative staphylococci (3,43).

The most common bacterium isolated from VPS is coagulase-negative *Staphylococcus*, which accounts for 50% to 75% of infections (3,28). These staphylococcal strains produce a mucoid substance that enhances adherence to smooth surfaces and protects against lysozymal activity (44). *S. aureus* is another important pathogen, responsible for 5% to 15% of early VPS infections. Both types of staphylococci are thought to infect the catheter at the time of insertion through a colonized skin. Gram-negative enteric bacilli are less common and account for 5% to 15% of all cases. These gram-negative bacterial infections usually occur because of abnormalities at the distal end of the catheter, their onset is often delayed, and frequently they are associated with bowel perforation (44).

Episodes of nosocomial gastroenteritis are caused by viruses (e.g., rotavirus, adenoviruses, enteroviruses) and by *Clostridium difficile* (3). Sinusitis and otitis are caused by gram-negative bacilli, particularly *P. aeruginosa* and *Enterobacter*, and by *S. aureus*. Etiologic agents of endocarditis include coagulase-negative staphylococci, *S. aureus*, enterococci, aerobic gram-negative bacilli, and *Candida* species (3,43).

Microorganisms causing surgical-site infections are those usually present as colonizers of the injured skin before or after the surgical procedure.

Gram-positive cocci, notably *S. aureus*, followed by enterococci, coagulase-negative staphylococci, and occasionally *S. pyogenes*, are the most frequent isolates. Gram-negative bacilli of various types account for 30% to 40% of causative pathogens. *Candida* species are identified in roughly 5% of surgical-site infections. Rarely, *Bacteroides fragilis* and other anaerobic bacteria are isolated from infected wounds, but proper cultures for these organisms are seldom performed.

Identification of the pathogen causing nosocomial infection is extremely important both for guiding specific antimicrobial therapy and for assessing prognosis. A recent nationwide study conducted in 49 U.S. hospitals by the Surveillance and Control of Pathogens of Epidemiologic Importance (SCOPE) study group evaluated the crude mortality associated with specific microorganisms causing nosocomial infections in adult and pediatric ICU and non-ICU wards (43). Infections caused by *Candida* species, enterococci, *Pseudomonas aeruginosa*, and *Acinetobacter baumannii* were associated with higher case-fatality rates than those caused by other gram-negative and gram-positive bacteria. The mortality risk was almost half as low for infections attributable to coagulase-negative staphylococci.

Antimicrobial Management

Because the spectrum of etiologic organisms causing nosocomial infections varies according to the numerous factors affecting patients managed at the PICU, empiric antimicrobial therapy should be based on the severity of clinical disease, the type and site of infection, the nature of the underlying morbidity, and knowledge of the relative frequency and local susceptibility patterns of hospital-acquired pathogens. In most situations, empiric treatment should include an agent effective against gram-positive bacteria, such as nafcillin, oxacillin, or vancomycin, and an agent effective against most gram-negative bacteria, including *Pseudomonas*, such as ceftazidime or cefepime, with or without an aminoglycoside (46–48). In institutions where infection with MRSA is common, the use of vancomycin as initial therapy is appropriate. Unless renal or ototoxicity is a major concern, gentamicin is generally equivalent to third- generation cephalosporins against gram-negative rods, is synergistic with ampicillin and vancomycin against enterococci, and is much less costly. Combination of the cephalosporin with an aminoglycoside is commonly used when infection with a resistant gram-negative rod is suspected. Empiric antifungal therapy can be initiated in situations in which suspicion of fungemia is very high (i.e., a severely ill patient who is colonized with *Candida* or a neutropenic subject who is not responding to ongoing broad-spectrum antibacterial therapy). Once culture information becomes available, the treatment regimen can be tailored to specific pathogens isolated, or discontinued if no infection is identified. This is essential to avoid prolonged use of unnecessary antibiotics that may lead to increase resistance among the nosocomial pathogens in the PICU.

Substantial evidence indicates that most uncomplicated bloodstream infections associated with central venous catheters can be treated effectively without removing the catheter (34,47). Treatment of fungemia without catheter removal, however, has a relatively low success rate and is associated with higher mortality and complications (34,49). Consideration of catheter removal should also be given with difficult-to-treat bacteria, such as multiresistant enterococci and gram-negative bacilli. In addition, catheters should be removed immediately if evidence of embolic phenomena, septic thrombophlebitis, or endocarditis is present. Persistently positive blood cultures despite the administration of antimicrobial therapy, or recrudescence of infection shortly after therapy is completed, should prompt removal of catheter. Biofilm production that allows microbial adherence to the catheter wall and difficult bacterial contact with antimicrobial drugs facilitates persistent growth of coagulase-negative staphylococci in repeated blood cultures. Because the pathogenicity of these staphylococcal species is low, a few days of vancomycin therapy alone can be attempted before considering catheter removal (50,51).

Few data exist regarding the optimal duration of therapy for bloodstream infection if the catheter remains in place, but experience suggests that 10 to 14 days after the last positive culture result is usually adequate. If the catheter is removed, shorter courses of therapy (5 to 7 days) are appropriate for uncomplicated infections, especially those caused by less virulent pathogens such as coagulase-negative staphylococci (25).

Empiric antimicrobial treatment for nosocomial pneumonia in a mechanically ventilated patient should be guided by Gram stain of the endotracheal aspirate. Once culture information is available, the treatment regimen can be tailored accordingly. Prolonged treatment of patients in whom the diagnosis of pneumonia is questionable should be avoided because it often leads to endotracheal colonization with antimicrobial-resistant bacteria (25). The duration of treatment has not been studied, but the recommendation is usually about 10 days to treat uncomplicated cases.

For other nosocomial infections, empiric therapy should also be guided by Gram stain of infected urine, exudates, or drained purulent material and by epidemiologic data generated periodically on etiologies and bacterial susceptibility patterns of PICU-acquired infections at the corresponding institution (25,52).

Treatment of nosocomial *Candida* infections warrants specific comments. Isolation of *Candida* from normally sterile fluids (e.g., blood, CSF, joint or pleural fluids) or abscesses requires antifungal therapy. Amphotericin B or its lipid formulations is still the initial drug of choice for catheter-related candidemia or systemic candidiasis (53). New potent antifungal drugs such as caspofungin and voriconazole are already commercially available but these are usually reserved for resistant fungi, particularly by strains of *Candida* other than *C. albicans* (54). Diagnosis of ventilatory-associated *Candida* pneumonia in immunocompetent patients is very challenging because the presence of *Candida* in respiratory secretions usually denotes simple colonization, and no clear association has been demonstrated with histologic evidence of lung infection or with development of systemic fungal disease (36–38). In general, therefore, antifungal treatment is not advised. Asymptomatic candiduria usually does not require therapy. In patients with symptoms, abnormal urine analysis, or persistent urine isolation of *Candida* after catheter removal, a short 5-day treatment with fluconazole is commonly recommended (55).

Preventive Measures

Important general principles for reduction of nosocomial infections within critical care units include proper area spacing to avoid patient crowding, adequate health personnel-to-patient ratios, and optimal methods of infection control policies.

Area Spacing

The location and design of a PICU is an important part of infection control success. Ideally, each patient should be physically separated from other patients, with sinks available between patients to remind staff and to facilitate hand-washing before and after contact with other patients. Experts have suggested 300 to 400 square feet of patient-care space per patient and additional space for storage, utility, and ancillary services (56).

Recently, the American Academy of Architecture for Health published guidelines on the design and construction of critical care units (57). These units require special space and equipment allocations to provide adequate patient management. In addition to privacy, atmosphere, and spatial design, special considerations were given to the number and location of hand-washing stations. Proper hand-washing remains the single most effective strategy to decrease the occurrence and spread of nosocomial infections within the PICU.

Staffing

High patient-to-nurse ratios also contribute to development of PICU-acquired nosocomial infections. Ratios of more than 1.5 patients per nurse are significantly associated with increased rates of lower respiratory infections (5).

Isolation

Cohort isolation may be required during outbreaks periods when infected or colonized patients are in contact with infected or colonized staff personnel. Several specific isolation procedures are recommended because of the different types of patients managed at the PICU and of the different etiologic pathogens that can be involved (56). Accordingly, specific guidelines should be implemented for neonates, immunodeficiency patients, children with cardiopulmonary diseases, postsurgical patients, and when viruses (RSV, influenza, varicella zoster, rotavirus), bacteria (multiresistant nosocomial agents, *Mycobacteria*, pertussis), or fungi (species of *Candida*) are suspected to be circulating within the PICU (58).

Isolation of specific patient populations also plays a role in limiting the spread of nosocomial agents. Each ICU should have at least one airborne-infection isolation room (57).

Hand-Washing

Hand-washing remains the most important single method of interrupting the occurrence and transmission of hospital pathogens within the PICU (59,60). Several studies have documented a substantial failure rate of hospital personnel to wash their hands at critical-care units. Adequate and convenient hand-washing facilities should be available and strict hand-washing policies established and enforced for all individuals entering the unit. Hands are colonized with both a permanent and a transient flora. In contrast to transient flora, the permanent flora is generally not removed with routine hand-washing techniques, but these organisms can be significantly reduced in number or inactivated by some antibacterial solutions (61).

At least one hand-washing station, equipped with hands-free operable controls, should be provided for every three patient beds in an open area floor (57). Additionally, there should be another station in each patient room and at nursing and medication locations. Because adherence to hand-washing worsens as work load increases, current efforts are directed to the use of alcohol disinfectants that take less time than traditional methods of soap, water, and towels, are cheaper in the whole context of readiness, and are apparently more effective to reduce resident hand microbial flora (62).

Gown and Gloves

Gowns traditionally have been used in the past in the PICU, but these clothes offer unproven advantages in interrupting transmission or microorganisms in critical care settings. Several studies have shown no change in infection and colonization rates when gowns are added to hand-washing methods (56). Some experts believe that gown use can reduce the perception of the importance of hand-washing by health personnel. Gowns, therefore, should be worn for specific isolation instances and for contact with selected type of patients.

Strict gown and glove use can modestly reduce rates of nosocomial infections but are not more effective than strict hand-washing and are associated with poor compliance (62). These precautions can be important in selected subsets of patients such as solid-organ transplant recipients and immunodeficiency subjects.

Environmental Cultures

Routine environmental culturing for bacterial contamination is only indicated in the setting of an investigation for a particular reservoir during potential outbreaks of infection (56). Verification of sterile procedures in formula preparation and equipment maintenance may mandate routine surveillance culturing.

Traffic and Visits

Traffic through the PICU should be limited to essential staff and family members. Congested areas, such as nurses' station, should be separated from patient care and storage space. Visiting policies should require that all visitors be well, preferably with verbal screening, and not recently exposed to highly communicable infections (56). This is especially critical during the viral respiratory season. Hand-washing policies should be also enforced in these persons.

Housekeeping

Routine housekeeping of the PICU is difficult in times of high census, but it should remain a priority. Daily wet mopping of the floor and daily dusting of the shelves, light fixtures, and ventilation ducts with a damp cloth should be performed (56). Every 1 to 2 months, the walls should be scrubbed with a phenolic or quaternary ammonium germicide. Cleaning that has the potential of dispersing dust should not be done when patients with open wounds are in the rooms. The nursing station, medication area, phones, computers, and medical charts should be wiped with an antiseptic cleaning solution at least daily (56).

Rational Use of Antibiotics

Published evidence supports the notion that rationalizing the use of empiric antimicrobial agents ameliorates the development of bacterial resistance in nosocomial pathogens, reduces secondary infection caused by opportunistic microbes such as fungi and enterococci, and decreases costs (63–65). Because patients at the PICU are critically ill, however, empiric therapy should be broad enough to cover a wide list of potential causative microorganisms. Accordingly, initial antibiotic regimens should be based on data generated by a continuous epidemiologic surveillance of nosocomial microbial agents circulating in each PICU.

Preoperative prophylactic antibiotics can minimize or at least retard the degree of microbial contamination of the surgical site and plausibly reduce rates of postsurgical infections (66,67). Unfortunately, most studies evaluating the potential usefulness of antimicrobial prophylaxis have been conducted in adults. Although a consensus about the effectiveness of this preventive strategy still remains elusive, many clinicians follow practices routinely performed in adults. A single dose of a prophylactic antibiotic should be administered within 2 hours before making the surgical incision. Administration of a second dose is usually not recommended unless the surgical procedure is prolonged for more than 4 to 6 hours.

Antifungal prophylaxis to prevent mucosal *Candida* colonization in patients receiving broad-spectrum antibacterial agents and subjected to mechanical ventilation is still a controversial issue (68–70). Although some neonatologists recommend fluconazole prophylaxis for ventilated very low birth weight infants to potentially reduce rates of systemic candidiasis (71), clear evidence supporting this concept is lacking and many concerns exist about the future development of fungal resistance to azole compounds.

Specific Measures

Guidelines for the prevention, diagnosis, and management of catheter-related infections have been published (16,19). The recommended preventive strategies are listed in Table 10.4. Although many of these strategies have been studied only in adults, most pediatric intensivists and infectious disease experts support adherence to these recommendations. Recommendations for the prevention of catheter-related bacteremia include rigorous attention to aseptic techniques for catheter insertion and care. After hand-washing and gloves wearing, an iodine or 2% chlorhexidine solution should be applied to catheter insertion site. There is no evidence to suggest that the use of topical antimicrobial ointments under catheter dressings decreases infection rates. Dressings should be changed every other day. Catheters should be removed as soon as they become useless, the insertion site becomes purulent, or catheter sepsis is suspected.

Routine replacement of arterial and central venous catheters is not recommended. Infusion sets should be changed every 72 hours unless lipid or blood products are used, in which case they should be changed every 24 hours. Multilumen catheters are associated with an increased risk of nosocomial bactere-

TABLE **10.4.** Strategies for the prevention of catheter-related bloodstream infections

- Removing catheters when no longer needed
- Placement of catheters by well-trained staff personnel
- Achievement of adequate patient-to-nurse ratios
- Use polytetrafluoroethylene or polyurethane catheters
- Minimal use of open stopcock ports
- Enforce hand-washing and maximal sterile barrier precautions during catheter insertions
- Skin antisepsis with 2% chlorhexidine
- Use of transparent or gauze dressings
- Replacement of pulmonary artery catheters at least every 7 days
- Replacement of intravenous administration sets every 72 to 96 hours; if used for lipid emulsions and blood products, replace every 24 hours
- Use of antibiotic/antiseptic-impregnated catheters, antibiotic lock prophylaxis, mupirocin ointment at insertion site, systemic antibiotic prophylaxis, or anticoagulants in catheters are yet of unproven benefit or concern

TABLE **10.5.** Strategies to prevent ventilator-associated pneumonia in children

- Enforce hand-washing, glove use, and standard precautions techniques
- Use sterile water in ventilator humidifiers
- Minimize use of H2-blockers if feasible
- Increase use of oral, rather than nasal, intubation
- Place patients in a semirecumbent rather than supine position if possible
- Change mechanical ventilator breathing circuits no more frequently than every 48 hours
- Disinfect handheld medication nebulizers between patients
- Disinfect and sterilize reusable equipment
- Cohorting of patients infected with potentially transmissible viruses and multiresistant pathogens
- Periodic draining and discarding any condensate that collects in the tubing of a mechanical ventilator
- Use sterile single-use catheters for open-suction procedures
- Selective decontamination of the digestive tract, routine use of sucralfate, administration of intermittent feedings to lower stomach pH, and use of bacterial filters on ventilator circuits are yet of unproven benefit

mia. Arterial line flush solution should be changed every 24 to 48 hours and the entire system changed every 48 hours with nondisposable transducers and every 96 hours with disposable transducers.

The usefulness of impregnated antimicrobial agents on catheters to prevent nosocomial infections in PICUs has not been elucidated yet. The data on the effect of central venous catheters coated with chlorhexidine-silver sulfadiazine or minocycline-rifampin combinations have been reviewed, and it was found that both modalities significantly reduced rates of catheter-related bloodstream infections when compared with unmedicated catheters (72,73). Unfortunately, these studies have not involved any pediatric patients. The long-term impact of these catheters on antimicrobial resistance is of great concern among many infectious disease authorities. Specific measures such as antibiotic rotation, selective decontamination of the gastrointestinal tract to reduce incidence of ventilator-associated pneumonias, and the routine use of antibiotic-impregnated catheters to reduce risk of bloodstream infections are currently being evaluated in critically ill pediatric patients.

Although bloodstream infections are the most common nosocomial problem in the PICU, ventilator-associated pneumonias have the highest mortality rate of up to 20%. Thus, prevention of ventilator-associated pneumonia is a critical task of infection control teams and intensivists. Measures commonly used to prevent ventilator-associated pneumonias include elevating the head of the bed to 30 degrees, avoiding contact between respiratory secretions and health care providers with barrier precautions, removing nasogastric and endotracheal tubes as soon as possible, reducing unnecessary reintubation, using oral intubation, maintaining adequate pressure in endotracheal tube cuffs, avoiding gastric overdistention, and sterilizing reusable breathing circuits and humidifiers. The CDC has published guidelines for the reduction of nosocomial lung infections (74). These and other recommendations are listed in Table 10.5. More studies are needed, however, to evaluate the potential benefits of these preventive measures in the pediatric population.

References

1. Pollack, MM, Yeh TS, Ruttiman UE, et al. Evaluation of pediatric intensive care. Crit Care Med 1984;12:376–383.
2. Crone RK. Pediatric and neonatal intensive care. Can Janaest 1988;35:S30–S33.
3. Banerjee SN, Grohskopf LA, Sinkowitz-Cochran RL, Jarvis WR; National Nosocomial Infections Surveillance System; Pediatric Prevention Network. Incidence of pediatric and neonatal intensive care unit-acquired infections. Infect Control Hosp Epidemiol 2006;27(6):561–570.
4. Millikan J, Tait GA, Ford-Jones EL, et al. Nosocomial infections in a pediatric intensive care unit. Crit Care Med 1988;16:233–237.
5. Grohskopf LA, Sinkowitz-Cochran RL, Garret DO, et al. A national point-prevalence survey of pediatric intensive care unit-acquired infections in the Unites States. J Pediatr 2002;140:432–438.
6. Weinstein RA. Nosocomial Infection update. Emerg Infect Dis 1998;4:416–420.
7. Haley RW, Schaberg DR, Crossley KB, et al. Extra charges and prolongation of stay attributable to nosocomial infections: a prospective interhospital comparison. Am J Med 1981;70:50–58.
8. Haley RW, White JW, Culver DH, et al. The financial incentive for hospitals to prevent nosocomial infections under the prospective payment systems. JAMA 1987;257:1677–1684.
9. Stein F, Trevino R. Nosocomial infections in the pediatric intensive care unit. Pediatr Clin North Am 1994;41:1245–1257.
10. Richards MJ, Edwards JR, Culver DH, et al. Nosocomial infections in pediatric intensive care units in the United States. Pediatrics 1999;103:e39.
11. Stover BH, Shulman ST, Bratcher DF, et al. Nosocomial infection rates in US children's hospitals neonatal and pediatric intensive care units. Am J Infect Control 2001;29:152–157.
12. Raymond J, Aujard Y, and the European Study Group. Nosocomial infection in pediatric patients: a European multicenter prospective study. Infect Control Hosp Epidemiol 2000;21:260–263.
13. Suman O and Sáez-Llorens X. Infecciones nosocomiales en un hospital de tercer nivel. Pediatr Panama 2003;32:13–19.
14. Sing-Naz N, Sprague BM, Patel KM, et al. Risk factors for nosocomial infections in critically ill children: a prospective study. Crit Care Med 1996;24:875–878.
15. Centers for Disease Control and Prevention National Nosocomial Infections Suveillance (NNIS) System report: data summary from January 1992–June 2001, issued in August 2001. Am J Infect Control 2001;6:404–421.
16. Centers for Disease Control and Prevention. Guidelines for the prevention of intravascular catheter-related infections. MMWR 2002;51(RR-10):1–32.
17. Mermel LA. Prevention of intravascular catheter-related infections. Ann Intern Med 2000;132:391–402.
18. Rowin ME, Patel VV, Christenson JC. Pediatric intensive care unit nosocomial infections: epidemiology, sources and solutions. Crit Care Clin 2003;19:1–2.
19. Mermel LA, Farr BM. Sheretz RJ, et al. Guidelines for the management of intravascular catheter-related infections. Clin Infect Dis 2001;32:1249–1272.
20. Elward AM, Warren DK, Fraser VJ. Ventilator-associated pneumonia in pediatric intensive care unit patients: risk factors and outcomes. Pediatrics 2002;109:758–764.

21. Lohr JA, Downs SM, Dudley S, et al. Hospital-acquired urinary tract infections in the pediatric patient: a prospective study. Pediatr Infect Dis J 1994;13:8–12.
22. Langley JM, Hanakowski M, Leblanc JC. Unique epidemiology of nosocomial urinary tract infections in children. Am J Infect Control 2001;29:94–98.
23. Meares EM. Current patterns in nosocomial urinary tract infections. Urology 1991;37:9–12.
24. Miliken J, Tait GA. Ford-Jones L, et al. Nosocomial infections in the pediatric intensive care unit. Crit Care Med 1988;16:233–237.
25. Huskins WC, Goldmann DA. Nosocomial infection. In: Feigin RD, Cherry J, Demmler GJ, Kaplan S, eds. Textbook of Pediatric Infectious Diseases, 5th ed. Philadelphia: Saunders, 2004:2874–2925.
26. Culver D, Horan TC, Gaynes R, et al. Surgical wound infection rates by wound class, operative procedure, and patient risk index. National Nosocomial Infections Surveillance System. Am J Med 1991;91:S152–157.
27. Mayhall CG, Archer NH, Lamb VA, et al. Ventriculostomy-related infections: a prospective epidemiologic study. N Engl J Med 1984;310:553–559.
28. Yogev R. Cerebrospinal fluid shunt infections: a personal view. Pediatr Infect Dis J 1985;4:113–118.
29. Filka J, Huttova M, Tuharsky J, et al. Nosocomial meningitis in children after ventriculoperitoneal shunt insertion. Acta Paediatr 1999;88:576–578.
30. Dagan O, Cox PN, Ford-Jones L, et al. Nosocomial Infections following cardiovascular surgery: Comparison of two periods, 1987 vs. 1992. Crit Care Med 1999; 27:104–108.
31. Mehta PA, Cunningham CK, Colella CB, et al. Risk factors for sternal wound and other infections in pediatric cardiac surgery patients. Pediatr Infect Dis J 2000;19:1000–1004.
32. Pollock EM, Ford-Jones L, Rebeyka I, et al. Early Nosocomial infections in pediatric cardiovascular surgery patients. Crit Care Med 1990;18:378–384.
33. Garner JS, Jarvis WR, Emori TG, et al. CDC definitions for nosocomial infections. Am J Infect Control 1988;16:128–140.
34. Mermel LA, Farr BM, Sherertz RJ, et al. Guidelines for the management of intravascular catheter-related infections. Clin Infect Dis 2001;32:1249–1272.
35. Golden SE, Shehab ZM, Bjelland JC, et al. Microbiology of endotracheal aspirates in intubated pediatric intensive care unit patients: correlations with radiographic findings. Pediatr Infect Dis J 1987;6:665–669.
36. Wright WL, Wenzel RP. Nosocomial Candida. Epidemiology, transmission, and prevention. Infect Dis Clin North Am 1997;11:411–425.
37. el-Ebiary M, Torres A, Fabregas N, et al. Significance of the isolation of Candida species from respiratory samples in critically ill, non-neutropenic patients. An immediate post-mortem histologic study. Am J Respir Crit Care Med 1997;156: 583–590.
38. Palabiyikoglu I, Oral M, Tulunay M. Candida colonization in mechanically ventilated patients. J Hosp Infect 2001;47:239–242.
39. Rello J, Esandi ME, Diaz E, et al. The role of Candida sp isolated from bronchoscopic samples in nonneutropenic patients. Chest 1998;114:146–149.
40. Mayhall CG. Ventilator-associated pneumonia or not? Contemporary diagnosis. Emerg Infect Dis 2001;7:200–204.
41. Alvarez-Lerma F, Nolla-Salas J, len C, et al. Candiduria in critically ill patients admitted to intensive care medical units. Intensive Care Med 2003;29:1069–1076.

42. Sobel JD, Lundstrom T. Management of candiduria. Curr Urol Rep 2001; 2:321–325.
43. Wisplinghoff H, Bischoff T, Tallent SM, et al. Nosocomial bloodstream infection in US hospitals: analysis of 24,179 cases from a Prospective Nationwide Surveillance Study. Clin Infect Dis 2004;39:309–317.
44. Holladay RC, Campbell GD. Nosocomial viral pneumonia in the intensive care unit. Clin Chest Med 1995;16:121–133.
45. Oliveira EC, Lee B, Colice GL. Influenza in the intensive care unit. J Intensive Care Med 2003;18:80–91.
46. Fridkin SK, Steward CD, Edwards JR, et al. Surveillance of antimicrobial use and antimicrobial resistance in United States hospitals: project ICARE phase 2. Project Intensive Care Antimicrobial Resistance Epidemiology (ICARE) hospitals. Clin Infect Dis 1999;29:245–252.
47. Wiener ES. Catheter sepsis: The central venous line Achilles´ heel. Semin Pediatr Surg 1995;4:207–214.
48. Meyer E, Schwab F, Jonas D, Rueden H, Gastmeier P, Daschner FD. Surveillance of antimicrobial use and antimicrobial resistance in intensive care units (SARI): antimicrobial use in German intensive care units. Intensive Care Med 2004; 30:1089–1096.
49. Dato VM, Dajani AS. Candidemia in children with central venous catheters. Role of catheter removal and amphotericin B therapy. Pediatr Infect Dis J 1990;9:309–314.
50. Schulin T, Voss A. Coagulase-negative staphylococci as a cause of infections related to intravascular prosthetic devices. Clin Microbiol Infect 2001;7:S1–7.
51. Rello J, Ochagavia A, Sabanes E, et al. Evaluation of outcome of intravenous catheter-related infections in critically ill patients. Am J Respir Crit Care Med 2000; 162:1027–1030.
52. Singh N, Yu VL. Rational empiric antibiotic prescription in the ICU. Clinical research is mandatory. Chest 2000;117:1496–1499.
53. Lewis RE, Klepser ME. The changing face of nosocomial candidemia: epidemiology, resistance, and drug therapy. Am J Health Syst Pharm 1999;56:525–533.
54. Rapp RP. Changing strategies for the management of invasive fungal infections. Pharmacotherapy 2004;24:S4–28.
55. Kicklighter SD, Springer SC, Cox T, Hulsey TC, Turner RB. Fluconazole for prophylaxis against candidal rectal colonization in the very low birth weight infant. Pediatrics 2001;107:293–298.
56. Donowitz LG. The critical care patient. In: Donowitz LG, ed. Hospital-Acquired Infection in the Pediatric Patient. Baltimore: Williams & Wilkins, 1988:323–327.
57. American Institute of Architects Academy of Architecture for Health. Guidelines for Design and Construction for Hospitals and Health Care Facilities. Dallas: Dallas Facilities Guidelines Institute, 2001:24–32.
58. O'Connell NH, Humphreys H. Intensive care unit design and environment factors in the acquisition of infection. J Hosp Infect 2000;45:255–262.
59. Gauthier M. Nosocomial infections in the pediatric intensive care unit: etiology and prevention. Crit Care Med 1993;21:S315–316.
60. Farr BM. Infection control in intensive care units: modern solutions. Curr Opin Infect Dis 1993;6:520–525.
61. Zaragoza M, Salles M, Gomez J. Handwashing with soap or alcoholic solutions? A randomized clinical trial of its effectiveness. Am J Infect Control 1999;27:258–261.

62. Slota M, Green M, Farley A, et al. The role of gown and glove isolation and strict handwashing in the reduction of nosocomial infection in children with solid organ transplants. Crit Care Med 2001;29:405–412.

63. Sáez-Llorens X, Castrejón MM, Castaño E, et al. Impact of an antibiotic restriction policy on hospital expenditures and bacterial susceptibilities: a lesson from a pediatric institution in a developing country. Pediatr Infect Dis J 2000;19:200–206.

64. White AC, Atmar RL, Wilson J, et al. Effects of requiring prior authorization for selected antimicrobials: expenditures, susceptibilities, and clinical outcomes. Clin Infect Dis 1997;25:230–239.

65. Geissler A, Gerbeaux P, Granier I, et al. Rational use of antibiotics in the intensive care unit: impact on microbial resistance and costs. Intensive Care Med 2003;29:49–54.

66. American Academy of Pediatrics: Antimicrobial prophylaxis in pediatric surgical patients. In: Pickering LK, ed. 2000 Red Book: Report of the Committee on Infectious Diseases, 25th ed. Elk Grove Village, IL: American Academy of Pediatrics, 2000:730–735.

67. Dellinger EP, Gross PA, Barrett TL, et al. Quality standard for antimicrobial prophylaxis in surgical procedures. The Infectious Diseases Society of America. Infect Control Hosp Epidemiol 1994;15:182–188.

68. Garrelts JC, Schroeder TR, Harrison PB. Impact of fluconazole administration on outcomes in critically ill patients. Ann Pharmacother 2004;38:1588–1592.

69. Pelz RK, Hendrix CW, Swoboda SM, et al. Double-blind placebo-controlled trial of fluconazole to prevent candidal infections in critically ill surgical patients. Ann Surg 2001;233:542–548.

70. Calandra T, Marchetti O. Clinical trials of antifungal prophylaxis among patients undergoing surgery. Clin Infect Dis 2004;39(suppl 4):S185–192.

71. McGuire W, Clerihew L, Austin N. Prophylactic intravenous antifungal agents to prevent mortality and morbidity in very low birth weight infants. Cochrane Database Syst Rev 2004;(1):CD003850.

72. Crnich CJ and Maki DG. The promise of novel technology for the prevention of intravascular device-related bloodstream infection. Pathogenesis and short-term devices. Clin Infect Dis 2002;34:1232–1242.

73. Darouiche RR, O'Raad I, Heard SO, et al. A comparison of two antimicrobial-impregnated central venous catheters. N Engl J Med 1999;340:1–8.

74. Centers for Disease Control (CDC). Guidelines for prevention of nosocomial pneumonia. MMWR 1997;46 (RR-1):1–79.

11
Infections in the Immunocompromised Patient in the Pediatric Intensive Care Unit

Karyn Moshal, Olaf Neth, David Cubitt, and Nigel Klein

Over the last decade there have been remarkable advances in the treatment of childhood disease. However, many of the conditions, and the therapeutic modalities employed in their treatment, are associated with immunodeficiency. As a result, an increasing population of children are at risk from frequent, rare, and severe infections, some of which will require admission to the intensive care unit. In clinical practice, optimal management relies heavily on the appreciation of the specific infectious susceptibilities associated with specific immunodeficiency states, and obtaining a rapid and accurate diagnosis of the offending organism. This chapter discusses the major infectious processes that occur in some of the more common primary and secondary immunodeficiencies, addresses the effective utilization of modern molecular techniques for diagnosing and monitoring infection in these populations of patients, and discusses some of the novel treatment modalities now employed in their management.

The Size of the Problem

It is difficult to provide a true estimate of how many of the patients admitted to the pediatric intensive care unit (PICU) are truly immunodeficient. The number of children admitted with a genetically determined immune defect or a profound secondary deficiency may be less than 10%. However, if patients with more subtle immune defects, such those that occur in premature neonates, postoperatively, and in children with mild immunosuppression/immunodeficiency, are included, the numbers will be much higher. This chapter concentrates on the severe defects but also addresses the more numerous but less dramatic problems faced in the other categories.

Immunity and Age

The age at presentation can be very informative. An initial presentation of severe opportunistic infection requiring PICU admission is often the first clue to the underlying diagnosis. Infants with a severe combined or T-cell immune deficiency usually present in the first few months. Typical infections are *Pneumocystis jinoveci* pneumonia, cytomegalovirus (CMV) pneumonitis, pneumonitis due to respiratory syncytial virus (RSV), disseminated enteroviral infection, and invasive fungal infections. Severe viral infections including those due to Epstein-Barr virus (EBV) can also be seen in this population of patients, but these patients may also develop EBV-associated X-linked lymphoproliferative disease. Leukocyte adhesion deficiency may also present with life-threatening bacterial infections.

Children presenting between the ages of 6 months and 5 years are more likely to have an antibody disorder. Such children present once placentally transferred maternal immunoglobulin G (IgG) has declined. Patients with antibody deficiencies, complement deficiency, or asplenia are more likely to present with infections due to encapsulated bacteria such as *Haemophilus influenzae* type B, *Neisseria meningitidis*, or *Streptococcus pneumonia*. Children with chronic mucocutaneous candidiasis (CMC) and phagocytic disorders such as chronic granulomatous disease (CGD) typically present in early life with recurrent candida and staphylococcal infections. Life-threatening infections of the liver and lungs by both bacteria and fungi usually occur later in childhood in CGD.

Children requiring admission to intensive care for a first infectious insult are less likely to have an underlying severe immune defect. However, if the infection is unusual, for example PCP, or particularly severe, or on the background of a history of frequent but minor infections, the child should be screened for primary and secondary immunodeficiencies.

Severe Immunodeficiency

Bone Marrow Transplant Patients

Bone marrow transplant (BMT) patients are susceptible to infections before, during, and after the procedure. Danger arises not just from the acquisition of infection during the period when immune defenses are depleted, but also from reactivation of latent infections, and from the sometimes overwhelming immune reconstitution that can accompany the recovery phase. In the first month after transplant, before reingraftment, patients are most susceptible to infections caused by both gram-negative and gram-positive bacterial infections and fungal infections. However, it is patients with graft versus host disease, largely due to therapeutic immunosuppression, who are particularly susceptible to severe CMV pneumonitis.

Children undergoing BMT who are admitted to the PICU have a particularly poor prognosis. The reasons for this are complex and largely beyond the scope of this chapter. Two thirds of children are admitted with either respiratory distress or sepsis, and in many cases it is the persistence of infection as a result of the immune deficiency that ultimately proves fatal. Such patients require prolonged mechanical ventilation, and children who have an associated pneumonic infection do particularly poorly. The most commonly isolated pathogens in this group are CMV, RSV, adenovirus, aspergillus, and PCP, with a number of children being co-infected with more than one pathogen. Overall only 56% survive to discharge (1).

Fungal infections are particularly problematic in the BMT population and can cause severe and disseminated disease. *Aspergillus* and *Candida* spp. are the most common fungal pathogens. Recognition of the dangers of infection and the institution of fungal prophylaxis as well as preemptive treatment as part of the routine care of children undergoing BMT has reduced, but not eliminated, the number of fungal infections (2). In addition to this, advances in treatment, with the introduction of new classes of antifungal agents, has improved the prognosis for these children.

CMV is one of the herpes group of viruses, and infections are ubiquitous in the population. CMV usually causes trivial or asymptomatic disease in the immunocompetent host, but can cause severe disease in the immunocompromised. This manifests predominantly as respiratory disease, but also as hepatitis, enteritis, and choreoretinitis in this patient population. Although not all children are infected prior to being transplanted, and particularly in the younger children, there are many dangers relating to either the development of primary infection, or reactivation of latent virus in the patients who are CMV positive prior to transplantation. The CMV status of the donor and whether this is concordant with the CMV status of the patient is also a risk factor in the development of severe CMV disease.

Solid Organ Transplants

Children receiving solid organ transplants, as with BMT patients, are at risk from infection both before and after the transplant. The susceptibilities of these patients and the organisms causing infection are similar to those receiving BMT. There are, however, key differences:

1. Solid organ transplant recipients are usually less immunosuppressed than BMT patients, and are not at risk of immune reconstitution syndrome and its associated inflammatory and infective complications. However, they are at risk of postsurgical wound infections and surgery related complications.

2. Infection of the transplanted organ due to latent or colonizing organisms, present either in the donor or recipient, can occur and cause invasive disease in the context of immunosuppression. Children with cystic fibrosis receiving lung and heart-lung transplants are often colonized with *Pseudomonas* spp. Those colonized with *Burkholderia cepacia* are particularly at risk of developing disease that is difficult to treat, as it is highly resistant. This is an independent poor prognostic factor in lung transplantation (3,4).

3. Solid organ transplant recipients are at risk of reactivation of latent infections, such as CMV. Unlike the BMT patients who are most likely to develop pneumonitis, CMV disease depends on the sites where the virus is latent and on the organ that has been transplanted. Lung, heart-lung, and liver transplant patients are most vulnerable to systemic disease, and also to infection that can precipitate rejection and increase vulnerability to other infections such as fungal infections (5). Heart and heart-lung transplant recipients are particularly vulnerable to fungal infection in the first few months posttransplant and have a high mortality. Candidal infections occur most commonly in liver and lung transplant patients. Invasive *Aspergillus* infections account for almost half of all invasive fungal infections in lung transplant patients, and, when causing disease in liver transplant patients, occur soon after transplant (6).

4. Parvovirus is emerging as a potentially important cause of infection in heart transplant patients.

Oncologic Patients

More than 1 in 600 children develops a malignancy in the first 15 years of life in the developed world. Survival in children with cancer has increased dramatically during the past four decades (7). This progress is due not only to advances in specific oncologic therapies and supportive care, but also to improvement in the management of oncologic emergencies. Cancer patients comprise about 4% of PICU admissions and do well overall (8).

Pancytopenia secondary to bone marrow replacement or chemotherapy may result in hemorrhage, anemia, and susceptibility to infection. As granulocyte counts fall, the frequency, duration, and severity of infections dramatically increase. This is particularly marked when the neutrophil count falls below 500 cells per microliter, but occurs with low lymphocyte counts as well (9,10). Infections are worse during relapse of the underlying disease, and the failure of leukocytes to recover following an infection is associated with a poor prognosis. This is largely determined by both the underlying disease and the potency of chemotherapy.

Febrile neutropenia is defined as a decrease in the absolute neutrophil count (ANC) coupled with a temperature >38°C for more than 4 hours, or on two occasions at least 4 hours apart, or >38.5°C on one occasion. The prompt initiation of antibiotic therapy in febrile neutropenic patients has decreased the mortality rate for gram-negative infection.

Life-threatening emergencies when patients have severe neutropenia include typhlitis and perirectal abscess, and require immediate full supportive care including the administration of granulocyte colony-stimulating factor (G-CSF). The choice of antibiotics depends on the predominant organisms and antibiotic sensitivity patterns.

Initial empiric treatment for febrile neutropenia consists of a β-lactam antibiotic and an aminoglycoside, plus a glycopeptide if a coagulase-negative staphylococci or enterococcus are isolated, or if the child has an endoprosthesis or a tunnel infection and initial therapy is unsuccessful (9,11).

The treatment of cancer has become more intensive and is associated with more severe oral mucositis and diarrhea. Damage to mucosal barriers increases the risk of infection and may encourage translocation of colonizing gram-positive flora. In addition, patients with cancer are usually fitted with indwelling central venous catheters, which may also explain the increasing number of staphylococcal infections. Selection pressure on both colonizing and environmental pathogens occurs, and as most antimicrobial regimes are weighted against gram-negative bacteria, this may also contribute to the increasing incidence of isolation of gram-positive pathogens. Early empirical therapy may limit the culture of causative pathogens.

Recently the spectrum of pathogens has begun to change, with the emergence of more gram-negative, mycobacterial, and fungal infections. This is likely to be due to a combination of variable use of quinolone prophylaxis, an increase in quinolone resistance, and multidrug-resistant pathogens (8). In addition to these issues, other factors leading to susceptibility to infections in this patient group include the type of underlying oncologic disease, intensity of therapy (high dose and stem cell transplant), the degree and duration of neutropenia (including impaired functioning), the disruption of normal barriers (skin, respiratory, gastrointestinal, and genitourinary tract) and the nutritional status of the patient (malnutrition affects lymphocyte, neutrophil, and mononuclear cell function and the complement system).

Minor Immunodeficiency and the Pediatric Intensive Care Unit

Background

Primary immunodeficiencies have a prevalence of approximately 1 in 20,000, and advances in the care of serious acquired immune defects have reduced the proportion of children requiring PICU admission. In contrast, minor immunodeficiencies such as those caused by genetic polymorphisms within the innate immune system, and as a result of transient acquired immunoparalysis, are less severe but much more common. As such, they may be more important quantitatively in influencing the susceptibility of children to infections, both as reasons for admission to the PICU and in acquiring infections while in the PICU for other reasons.

The Innate Immune System and Susceptibility to Infection

It has become increasingly apparent that some individuals suffer from more infections than others. One of the reasons appears to be due to polymorphisms in the innate immune system (Table 11.1). The best understood and investigated defect of innate immunity is mannose-binding lectin (MBL) deficiency (12). Mannose-binding lectin is a circulating liver-derived plasma protein that

TABLE 11.1. Defects in innate immunity and their association with infections

Immune defects	Pathogen susceptibility
Neutrophils	Bacteria: gram positive and gram negative
	Fungi: *Candida, Aspergillus*
Complement system	Bacteria: gram positive and gram negative
	Fungi: *Pneumocystis jiroveci*
	Parasites: Cryptosporidium
Mannose-binding lectin	Bacteria: gram positive and gram negative, *M. tuberculosis*
	Viruses: HIV, IAV, HSV
	Fungi: *Pneumocystis jiroveci, Candida, Aspergillus*
	Parasites: *Trypanosoma cruzi, Cryptosporidium parvum, Plasmodium falciparum*
Defensins	Bacteria: gram positive and gram negative
	Fungi: Yeast
	Viruses: Adenoviruses

HIV, human immunodeficiency virus; IAV, influenza A virus; HSV, herpes simplex virus.

recognizes repeating arrays of sugars on the surface of many bacteria, fungi, viruses, and parasites. Studies of consecutive and prospective series of children have shown that MBL deficiency predisposes to infectious illness including meningococcal disease, pneumococcal disease, mycoplasma infections, and herpes virus infections.

Recently it has been shown that MBL deficiency is also associated with increased severity of sepsis and increased incidence of systemic inflammatory response syndrome (SIRS) (13,14). The reasons are unclear, but is likely to be due to both an increased susceptibility to infection and an increased inflammatory response to the infectious stimulus (Fig. 11.1).

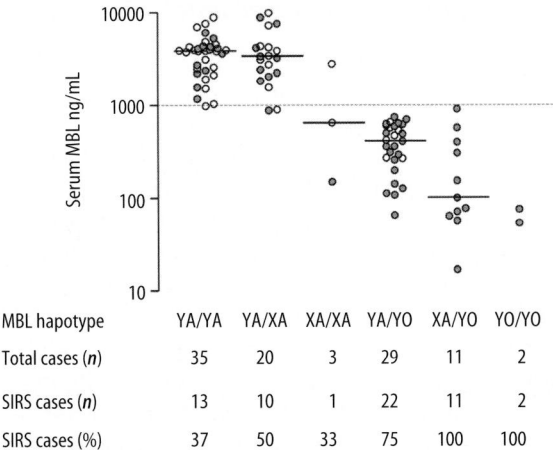

MBL hapotype	YA/YA	YA/XA	XA/XA	YA/YO	XA/YO	YO/YO
Total cases (*n*)	35	20	3	29	11	2
SIRS cases (*n*)	13	10	1	22	11	2
SIRS cases (%)	37	50	33	75	100	100

FIGURE 11.1. Systemic inflammatory response syndrome (SIRS) in relation to mannose-binding lectin (MBL) serum levels. YA/YA individuals have the highest MBL levels and YO/YO have the lowest serum MBL levels. Filled circles denote cases that developed SIRS, open circles the cases that did not. Patients with profound MBL deficiency are much more likely to develop SIRS (13).

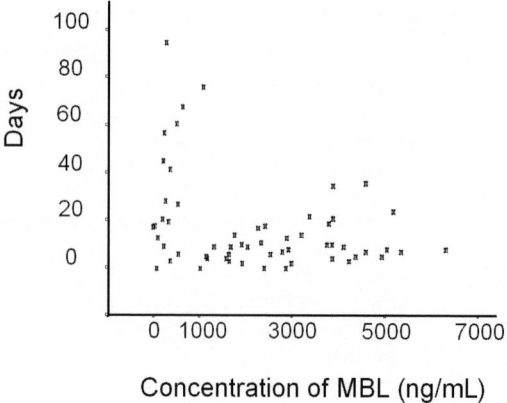

Concentration of MBL (ng/mL)

Figure 11.2. Duration of febrile neutropenia in relationship to MBL serum levels. Patients with low MBL levels are more likely to have prolonged episodes of febrile neutropenia (15).

Polymorphisms in innate immune components such as MBL or human Toll-like receptors may also influence the rate of infections in the context of an underlying immune deficiency. For example, Figure 11.2 shows that children with cancer and low MBL levels were more likely to suffer from prolonged episodes of febrile neutropenia than those with high MBL levels (15). An MBL deficiency was also associated with more severe infections and increased risk of admission to the PICU (16,17).

Acquired Immunoparalysis and Nosocomial Infection

There are increasing concerns about the high rate of hospital-acquired infections. In the PICU, nosocomial infections may occur in 20% of patients, and, perhaps most worryingly, PICU patients are more likely to harbor bacteria that are multiply antibiotic resistant. In the last decade it has been recognized that one reason why PICU patients may be particularly susceptible to nosocomial infection is that they are often in a state of immunoparalysis. This occurs as a result of an overcompensated antiinflammatory response to an initial inflammatory insult such as infection, trauma, and surgery (Fig. 11.3). In this state, the patient is said to have *acquired immunoparalysis*, and is unable to produce an adequate immune response to a new threat (e.g., nosocomial infection). The proinflammatory/antiinflammatory balance is indicated by monocyte expression of major histocompatibility complex (MHC) class II, which is reduced in the antiinflammatory state. When monocytes are stimulated ex vivo with lipopolysaccharide (LPS), they fail to produce high levels of tumor necrosis factor-α (TNF-α). This is in part regulated by interleukin-10 (IL-10). The expression of monocyte MHC class II correlates well with this hyporesponsiveness to LPS stimulation. The latter state appears to predict the onset of infection some days

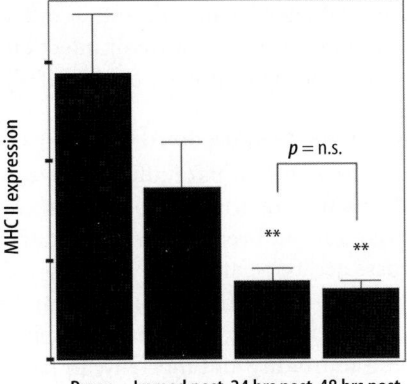

Figure 11.3. Monocyte MHC class II expression following major abdominal surgery (18). All patients show evidence of immunoparalysis and are at increased risk of nosocomial infection.

before its onset (Fig. 11.4). A number of studies are looking at ways to modulate this state to try and reduce the rates of hospital acquired infections.

Diagnosing Infection in the Pediatric Intensive Care Unit

The following factors are to be considered in all immunocompromised patients:

1. In addition to the opportunistic infections associated with their conditions, immunocompromised patients are susceptible to seasonal and endemic pathogens and are at least as likely as the healthy population to be infected with

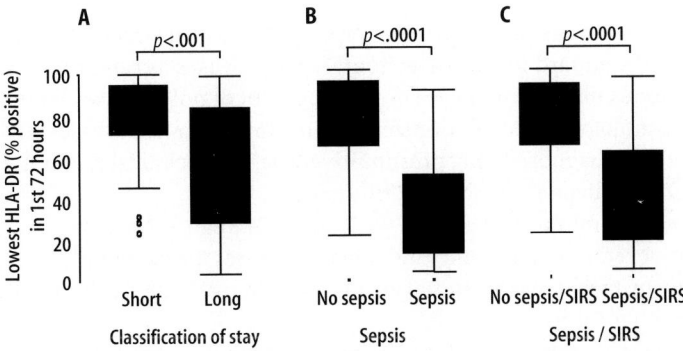

Figure 11.4. Children who underwent cardiac surgery for correction of congenital cardiac defects had a greater chance of developing sepsis if the expression of their monocyte human leukocyte antigen (HLA)-DR expression dropped below 60% in the first 72 hours after surgery (19).

them. However, these pathogens can present a different clinical picture in these patients. It is important to be aware of infectious contacts and other risk factors, and to consider their presence even if the clinical picture is atypical.

2. Seasonal viral infections include, starting in the spring through to late winter, varicella zoster virus (VZV); parainfluenza 1, 2, and 3; enteroviruses; RSV; influenza A and B; and rotavirus. Adenoviruses are endemic and occur year round; however, sporadic outbreaks of particular strains do occur. Adenoviruses and enteroviruses are associated with high morbidity and can result in death due to multiorgan failure or infection of the central nervous system (20). With the aid of molecular techniques, it has been established that rhinoviruses are a significant cause of morbidity and mortality in patients undergoing allogeneic stem cell transplantation (21,22).

3. Reactivation or primary infection with herpes viruses (CMV, EBV, herpes simplex virus [HSV], VZV, human herpes virus type 6 [HHV6]) are significant risk factors for morbidity and mortality, although the morbidity and mortality are decreased by prophylaxis and preemptive treatment early in the infective/reactivation process (23).

4. Geographically circumscribed, environmental, and zoonotic infections also occur. Toxoplasmosis, rare in the United Kingdom, is an important cause of severe infection in immunocompromised patients elsewhere in the world, where it is endemic.

5. Presentation of unusual pathogens can also be atypical and cause more severe disease than in the immunocompetent patient. Meticulous history taking, which addresses animal contacts, travel, and unpasteurized food, is important and can yield crucial information. These points are often not prioritized with extremely ill patients in the intensive care environment.

Diagnostic Techniques

Diagnostic techniques are improving rapidly. The use of viral culture, although still the gold standard for the detection of many viruses, is rapidly being superseded by molecular technology. The development of polymerase chain reaction (PCR) technology has revolutionized diagnostic virology. Diseases that previously could be diagnosed only presumptively based on clinical findings can now be definitively diagnosed often within hours.

The use of multiplex, real-time PCR with Taqman probes has been introduced in several centers, and this enables viruses to be rapidly detected in eluates from throat swabs and also provides an estimate of the viral load in blood or other fluids.

Molecular technology has also been developed to detect and identify bacterial and fungal DNA (24). This is particularly important in immunocompromised patients. They are often on numerous antibiotics, making reliance on conventional blood culture technology impossible. They are also susceptible to infection with fastidious organisms that grow poorly on conventional culture media. These patients' clinical condition seldom allows time to wait for results of conventional culture techniques in order to start on appropriate treatment.

The application of new diagnostic technology allows early appropriate treatment, which may result in improved patient survival.

Viral Load

The number of infecting or latent viral particles, or "viral load," can now be measured using molecular techniques. Active replication of the herpes viruses in particular is an important measure of developing disease. Increasing viral load over time definitively demonstrates this. However, the technology is still relatively new, and the viral load that correlates with active disease is still being defined and is different for each virus.

The development of disease is also linked to the presence or absence of different immune cell populations. Severe viral disease in these patients can be prevented, both with the use of prophylactic agents, as well as with early treatment intervention by tracking viral load over time (25).

Application of regular monitoring of latent viruses by real-time PCR and the use of preemptive treatment enable appropriate use of antiviral agents or other therapeutic modalities, such as antilymphocyte monoclonal antibodies (e.g., anti CD20 antibody), for EBV-driven lymphoproliferative disease.

An example is infection with parvovirus B19, an important cause of aplasia in patients undergoing stem cell transplantation, chemotherapy, and solid organ transplantation. During an acute aplastic crisis, vast numbers of virus particles may be present in the serum that can be detected by electron microscopy, but PCR is the method of choice for diagnosis (Fig. 11.5).

Real-Time Polymerase Chain Reaction

The use of real-time PCR has revolutionized the diagnosis and monitoring of viral infections. Tests can be multiplexed, enabling simultaneous detection and quantification of several different viral genomes within hours of receipt of clinical samples (26).

Routine monitoring of high-risk patients enables more appropriate use of antiviral agents and a movement away from prophylaxis to preemptive treatment, once viral loads start rising and exceeding clinically significant thresholds.

A further advantage of these techniques is that they provide information about the efficacy of treatment regimens. This may be particularly important in immunosuppressed patients following transplantation, when it is often difficult to distinguish between graft versus host disease and the effect of viral infection.

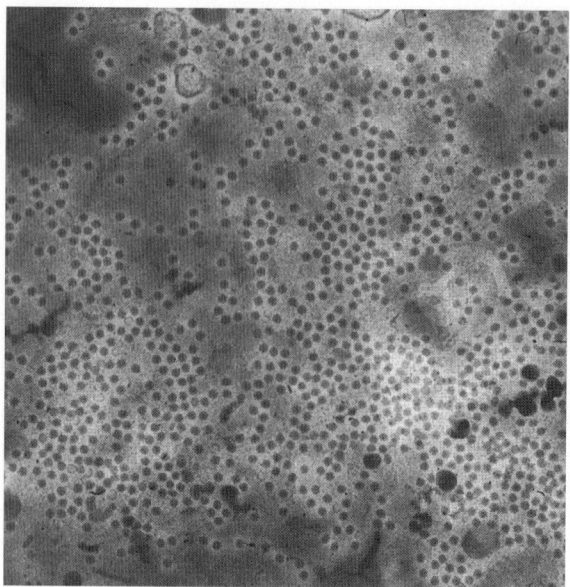

FIGURE 11.5. Parvovirus B19 in the serum of a patient undergoing an aplastic crisis.

The use of real-time PCR to monitor a patient who is developing EBV post-transplant lymphoproliferative disease, and the efficacy of treatment with anti-CD20 antibody in clearing the infection, is illustrated in Figure 11.6.

Respiratory Tract Infections

Immune-deficient children frequently first present to hospital with severe respiratory tract infections that are often associated with viruses or *Pneumocystis jiroveci*. Respiratory syncytial virus and parainfluenza 3 infections have

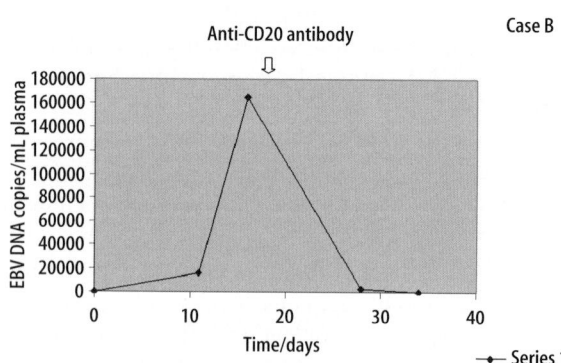

FIGURE 11.6. Epstein-Barr virus (EBV) clearance by treatment with anti-CD20 antibody.

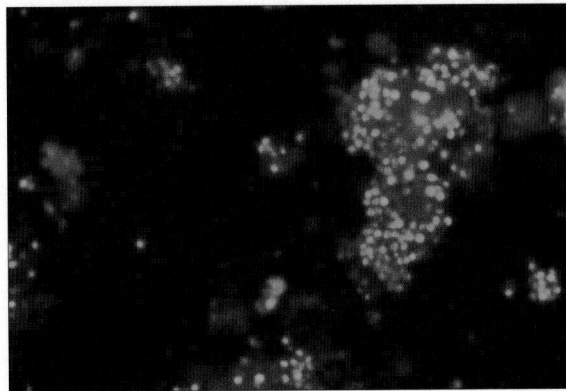

Figure 11.7. *Pneumocystis jiroveci* oocysts in a bronchoalveolar patient in a patient with severe combined immunodeficiency.

been associated with high mortality rates in patients undergoing bone marrow transplantation. A rapid diagnosis can be obtained within a few hours by obtaining a nasopharyngeal aspirate or bronchoalveolar lavage and then examining fixed cells on a multispot slide for the presence of viral inclusions or oocysts using fluorescein isothiocyanate (FITC) conjugated monoclonal antibodies specific for RSV; metapneumovirus; parainfluenza 1, 2, and 3; influenza A and B; adenovirus; and *Pneumocystis* (Fig. 11.7).

Cytomegalovirus early antigen can be detected by infecting cell monolayers, grown on glass coverslips, and examining them for the presence of viral inclusions using a monoclonal antibody specific for detection of early antigen fluorescent foci (DEAFF) test.

Enteric Virus Infections

Immunocompromised and immunodeficient patients are often infected with one or more enteric viruses (e.g., rotavirus, adenovirus, norovirus, sapovirus, astrovirus) (27). These viruses are often present in enormous numbers ($>10^8$/g feces), are excreted for prolonged periods of time, and therefore pose a significant risk to other patients if strict enteric precautions are not applied.

Negative-staining fecal extracts and examination by electron microscopy (Fig. 11.8) provide a rapid method of detection (<2 hours) but has a threshold of detection of approximately 1 to 10 million viruses/g. Application of reverse-transcriptase PCR (RT-PCR) has been shown to be far more sensitive, but is comparatively slow and requires the use of many different sets of primers. It is the method of choice for detection of entero- and noroviruses.

16S Ribosomal Polymerase Chain Reaction

Immunocompromised children often receive antibacterial prophylaxis and frequently receive empiric antibiotic therapy when they are unwell. Additionally,

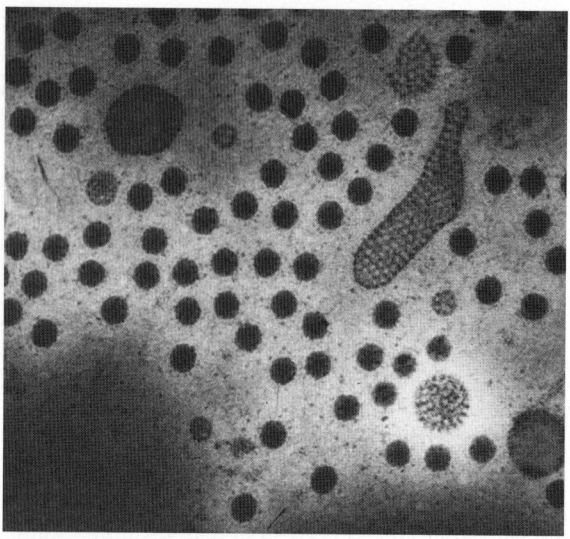

Figure 11.8. Rotavirus and astrovirus in a fecal sample from a patient with X-linked SCID.

they are susceptible to infection with opportunistic and fastidious organisms. All these factors increase the difficulty in isolating organisms causing disease, which in turn makes targeted treatment more difficult and treatment regimes more complicated, and increases morbidity.

16S ribosomal PCR is a new molecular technique that, when applied to sterile fluids, such as blood, cerebrospinal fluid, and joint, pleural, and peritoneal fluid, is a valuable tool in identifying the presence of bacterial infection. The PCR technology is sensitive and specific in identifying single infecting agents. 16S ribosomal PCR is an assay that is based on the fact that bacterial ribosomal DNA consists of highly conserved regions shared by all bacterial species, interspersed with regions that are genus or species specific, allowing identification of almost any bacterial organism, but particularly useful in identifying those that either do not grow in culture or are difficult to isolate due to concurrent antibiotic therapy. Once bacterial ribosomal DNA has been isolated from sterile tissue using primers targeted at these conserved regions and amplified using conventional PCR techniques, it can then be sequenced and the bacteria identified (24).

Treatment

New Antifungal Agents and Combined Therapy

New antifungal agents, both new classes and new drugs in existing classes, have been developed, which have changed the prognosis of children with severe disseminated fungal infections (28). The availability of a number of drugs suitable for use in disseminated infections has not only increased choice, but also allowed the use of combined therapy, the standard approach to the treatment of severe bacterial and viral infections, to be used in fungal infections too.

The two recent advances in fungal therapy are the introduction of voriconazole and caspofungin, the latter being the first of a new class of drug, the echinocandins.

Echinocandins

The echinocandins are a novel class of antifungal agents whose action inhibits synthesis of fungal wall products needed for maintaining osmotic integrity of the cell wall and important in cell division and growth. They have been approved for use as third-line agents in the treatment of fungal infections, but their main utility is in their use as adjunctive therapy in combination with either voriconazole or liposomal amphotericin (29).

The echinocandins are fungicidal against all *Candida* spp, and fungistatic against *Aspergillus* spp. They also have some activity against PCP, although they are not used routinely for PCP.

The echinocandins are available only as intravenous agents, but have a long half-life (10 to 15 hours), which is dose related. This means they can be given once daily. They are protein bound and well distributed in the tissues. They penetrate the central nervous system (CNS), but only achieve reasonable levels in the cerebrospinal fluid of patients with active CNS disease. They are metabolized by the liver.

Caspofungin is well tolerated. Side effects are mainly gastrointestinal disturbances, headaches, and raised liver transaminases. There are few drug interactions. Unfortunately, the main interactions are with chemotherapeutic agents used in oncology treatment. Levels also need to be monitored when used with drugs that induce drug clearance or are mixed inducers/inhibitors.

Voriconazole

This is one of the new triazoles, approved for therapy in the United States and Europe. It has excellent efficacy against both yeasts and molds, and is rapidly becoming the first-line antifungal agent of choice in severe invasive infection (28–30).

One of the major advantages of voriconazole is that it is available in both oral and intravenous preparations, is well absorbed orally, and has excellent cerebrospinal fluid and tissue penetration. It has a half-life of 6 hours and is metabolized in the liver. It is well tolerated and has few adverse effects. These fall into four separate groups: abnormal liver function; skin rashes; dose-related visual disturbances; and confusion or hallucinations, which are rare.

Voriconazole does have significant drug interactions, and when administering it with other medication the need for dosage adjustment of all drugs being given must be considered.

New Antiviral Agents/New Uses for Old Antiviral Agents

The HIV pandemic heralded a new era in viral diagnostic technology, the development of new antiviral agents, and a reevaluation of antiviral agents already in use.

Ribavirin

Ribavirin has long been used in the treatment of severe RSV infection in premature infants, those with underlying immunodeficiencies, and chronic lung disease. It is active against hepatitis C and the hemorrhagic fever viruses. It is being used increasingly either as monotherapy or in conjunction with cidofovir in the treatment of severe adenovirus infection in transplant patients (23).

Cidofovir

Cidofovir is a broad-spectrum antiviral agent. It is used primarily for the treatment of CMV disease, both in the immunocompromised patient where ganciclovir is less effective and in patients with ganciclovir-resistant strains of CMV. It has activity against other herpes viruses, and also is active against adenovirus, which causes severe diseases and can be fatal in transplant patients. Cidofovir is particularly useful in patients co-infected with both these viruses. The major adverse effect is nephrotoxicity (25).

Oral Antiviral Agents

Valacyclovir

Acyclovir was one of the earliest developed antiviral agents. It is active against HSV 1 and 2 and VZV. Its activity against other herpes viruses is limited and variable. It is available in intravenous, oral, and topical formulations; however, oral bioavailability is low, of the order of 15% to 30%, and lower than this in immunocompromised patients. Additionally, the half-life is short.

Valacyclovir is the prodrug of acyclovir. It has enhanced oral bioavailability, making it a useful alternative oral agent, both for treatment and prophylaxis in the immunocompromised patient. It has been shown to reduce the risk of CMV viremia and therefore is a useful prophylactic agent in patients at risk for CMV as well as varicella and herpes simplex infections (31).

Valganciclovir

Ganciclovir is a broad-spectrum antiherpetic agent. However, its main utility is its activity against CMV. Oral bioavailability is poor. Valganciclovir, the prodrug of ganciclovir, as with valacyclovir, is well absorbed when used orally, with a high bioavailability of the active form. This makes it a potentially useful drug to be used as prophylaxis in the immunocompromised patient. This is a useful adjunctive therapeutic measure, as the morbidity and mortality related to CMV disease in immunocompromised patients, particularly transplant patients, is high (31).

Conclusion

Children are now surviving from diseases that until recently were considered to be untreatable. However, although frequently successful at rectifying the underlying defect, the treatment of many of these conditions renders patients at considerable risk of severe and sometimes-atypical infections. Optimal care of such patients requires a good knowledge of potential infectious complications, strategies for infection prevention, a proactive program of early pathogen detection, and an effective multidisciplinary approach to the management of established infections. Although congenital or an established acquired immunodeficiency is the most likely reason for immunocompromised patients to be admitted to intensive care units, it is being increasingly recognized that immunocompetent children admitted to hospital or intensive care also have a higher risk of developing infection. This is not just because of the bacterial flora present in hospital environments, and is not directly related to the patient's underlying condition. It does appear to be influenced by polymorphisms in the innate immune system and other factors such as major, and even minor, surgery. Therapeutic measures to prevent or reduce the risks of nosocomial infection are under investigation and are likely to be increasingly important in the context of increasing antibiotic resistance and ever more complex medical procedures.

References

1. Jacobe S, Hassan A, Veys P, Mok Q. Outcome of children requiring admission to the intensive care unit after bone marrow transplantation. Crit Care Med 2003;31(5):1299–1305.
2. Brown JMY. Fungal infections in bone marrow transplant patients. Curr Opin Infect Dis 2004;17:347–352.
3. Whiteford ML, Wilkinson JD, McColl JH, et al. Outcome of Burkholderia (Pseudomonas) cepacia colonisation in children with cystic fibrosis following a hospital outbreak. Thorax 1995;50(11):1194–1198.
4. Snell GI, de Hoyos A, Krajden M, et al. Pseudomonas cepacia in lung transplant recipients with cystic fibrosis. Chest 1993;103(2):466–471.
5. Fishman JA, Patience C. Xenotransplantation: infectious risk revisited. Am J Transplant 2004;4(9):1383–1390.
6. Singh N. Fungal infections in the recipients of solid organ transplantation. Infect Dis Clin North Am 2003;17:113–134.
7. Stiller C. Aetiology and epidemiology. In: Pinkerton CR, Plowman PN, eds. Paediatric Oncology: Clinical Practice and Controversies, 2nd ed. London: Chapman and Hall, 1997:3–21.
8. Lanzkowsky P. Supportive care and management of oncological emergencies. In: Manual of Pediatric Hematology and Oncology, 4th ed. New York: Elsevier, 2005:695–748.

9. Bodey GP, Buckley M, Sathe YS, Freireich EJ. Quantitative relationships between circulating leukocytes and infection in patients with acute leukaemia. Ann Intern Med 1966;64:328–340.

10. Viscoli C, Castagnola E. Factors predisposing cancer patients to infection. Cancer Treat Res 1995;79:1–30.

11. Haupt R, Romanengo M, Fears T, Viscoli C, Castagnola E. Incidence of septicaemias and invasive mycoses in children undergoing treatment for solid tumours: a 12-year experience at a single Italian institution. Eur J Cancer 2001;37:2413–2419.

12. Turner MW. The role of mannose-binding lectin in health and disease. Mol Immunol 2003;40:423–429.

13. Fidler KJ, Wilson P, Davies JC, Turner MW, Peters MJ, Klein NJ. Increased incidence and severity of the systemic inflammatory response syndrome in patients deficient in mannose-binding lectin. Intensive Care Med 2004;30:1438–1445.

14. Garred P, J Storm J, Quist L, Taaning E, Madsen HO. Association of mannose-binding lectin polymorphisms with sepsis and fatal outcome, in patients with systemic inflammatory response syndrome. J Infect Dis 2003;188:1394–1403.

15. Neth O, Hann I, Turner MW, Klein NJ. Deficiency of mannose binding lectin and burden of infection in children with malignancy: a prospective study. Lancet 2001;358:614–618.

16. Peterslund NA, Koch C, Jensenius JC, Thiel S. Association between deficiency of mannose-binding lectin and severe infections after chemotherapy. Lancet 2001;358:637–638.

17. Horiuchi T, Gondo H, Miyagawa H, et al. Association of MBL gene polymorphisms with major bacterial infection in patients treated with high-dose chemotherapy and autologous PBSCT. Genes Immun 2005;6:162–166.

18. McHoney M, Klein NJ, Eaton S, Pierro A. Decreased monocyte class II MHC expression following major abdominal surgery in children is related to operative stress. Pediatr Surg Int 2006;22(4):330–334.

19. Allen ML, Peters MJ, Goldman A, et al. Early postoperative monocyte deactivation predicts systemic inflammation and prolonged stay in pediatric cardiac intensive care. Crit Care Med. 2003;30(5):1140–1145.

20. Howard DS, Phillips GL II, Reece DE, et al. Adenovirus Infections in hematopoietic stem cell transplant recipients. Clin Infect Dis 1999;9;29(6):1494–1501.

21. Ghosh S, Champlin R, Couch R, et al. Rhinovirus infections in the myelosuppressed adult blood and marrow transplant recipients. Clin Infect Dis 1999;29(3):533–535.

22. vanElden LJR, van Kraaij MGJ, Nijhaus M, et al. Polymerase chain reaction is more sensitive than viral culture and antigen testing for the detection of respiratory viruses in adults with haematological cancers and pneumonia. Clin Infect Dis 2002;34:177–183.

23. Ljungman P. Prevention and treatment of viral infections in stem cell transplant recipients. Br J Haematol 2002;118:44–57.

24. Harris KA, Hartley JC. Development of broad-range 16S rDNA PCR for use in the routine diagnostic clinical microbiology service. J Med Microbial 2003;52:685–691.

25. Kampmann B, Cubitt D, Walls T, et al. Improved outcome for children with disseminated adenoviral infection following allogeneic stem cell transplantation. Br J Haematol 2005;130:595–603.

26. Gunson RN, Collins TC, Carman WF. Real time RT-PCR detection of 12 respiratory viral infections in four triplex reactions. J Clin Virol 2005;33:341–344.

27. Gallimore CI, Cubitt WD, Richards AF, Gray JJ. Diversity of enteric viruses detected in patients with gastroenteritis in a tertiary referral paediatric hospital. J Med Virol 2004;73:443–449.

28. Groll AH, Gea-Banacloche JC, Glasmacher A, Just-Nuebling G, Maschmeyer G, Walsh TJ. Clinical pharmacology of antifungal compounds. Infect Dis Clin North Am 2003;17(1):159–191.

29. Barnes PD, Marr KA. Aspergillosis: spectrum of disease, diagnosis and treatment. Infect Dis Clin North Am 2006;20:545–561.

30. Steinbach WJ, Walsh TJ. Mycoses in pediatric patients. Infect Dis Clin North Am 2006;20:662–678.

31. Inouye RT, Panther LA, Hay CM, Hammer SM. Antiviral agents. In: Richman DD, Whitley RJ, Hayden FG, eds. Clinical Virology, 2nd ed. New York: ASM Press, 2002.

12
Infants and Children with Human Immunodeficiency Virus

Steven B. Welch and E.G. Hermione Lyall

Epidemiology

Worldwide over 40 million people are estimated to be infected with human immunodeficiency virus (HIV) (1), with 640,000 newly infected children in 2004, the majority living in sub-Saharan Africa. By contrast, pediatric HIV infection is relatively rare in Europe and North America, with only about 200 new cases diagnosed in children in the United States in 2003 (2), and a cumulative total of almost 1500 cases reported to the National Survey of HIV in Pregnancy and Childhood in the United Kingdom (3). In the 1990s, children with HIV made up 3% of admissions to the pediatric intensive care unit (PICU) in London (4), but 15% of admissions in Durban, South Africa (5).

Clinical Features of Children Presenting with HIV

Human immunodeficiency virus is a human retrovirus that principally infects CD4-positive T-helper lymphocytes (CD4 cells). The vast majority of children acquire infection perinatally. Destruction of CD4 cells leads to increased susceptibility to infection, and the clinical manifestations of HIV are due to complications of infection and the direct effects of HIV. Clinical progression occurs at a variable rate, leading to a spectrum of clinical presentations. The rate of progression and severity of infection determine which children will be in the more severe categories likely to present to PICU. They also determine the longer term likelihood of survival.

Up to 20% of children born with HIV infection present with severe symptoms or die in infancy (6). Infants presenting with severe disease are known as fast progressors, and they are more likely to be born to mothers who have advanced HIV disease (7). Whether their poor prognosis is related to a greater inoculum of HIV, earlier infection, a less effective immune response, the acquisition of immune escape mutants, or a combination of the above is not completely understood. The mononucleosis-like seroconversion illness of primary HIV described in some adults does not occur in perinatally infected infants. This pattern of early progression of disease in infancy, with severe immunodeficiency and opportunistic infection, leads to the majority of admissions of HIV-infected children to PICU (4).

The most common severe opportunistic infection is *Pneumocystis* pneumonia (PcP), caused by *pneumocystis jiroveci* (previously known as *P. carinii*) (8). Other patterns of presentation in infancy include recurrent respiratory infections; failure to thrive, with or without chronic diarrhea; hepatosplenomegaly and lymphadenopathy; recurrent oral candidiasis, and encephalopathy. Human immunodeficiency virus enters the central nervous system (CNS) during primary infection via the microglial cells, and a neurotoxic process is set in motion. Infants with HIV encephalopathy have signs of motor dysfunction resembling children with other causes of cerebral palsy. Imaging of the CNS in infancy often demonstrates vasculopathy of the basal ganglia, and generalized atrophy is a later finding. Effective treatment of the HIV infection, although it may prevent further deterioration, cannot reverse CNS damage.

Older children who present with HIV may have had mild symptoms for many years without HIV being diagnosed. They may present with recurrent mild infections (upper respiratory tract infections, otitis media, sinusitis, skin infections, lymphadenitis), or they may present with one or two episodes of more serious infection (e.g., pneumonia, meningitis, osteomyelitis). Children may also present with more severe episodes of common childhood infections, such as chickenpox, and may take longer to recover from such infections. Following chickenpox, recurrent or multidermatomal shingles may occur. Infections may be accompanied by hepatosplenomegaly and lymphadenopathy, or problems of growth and weight gain. Human immunodeficiency virus should be considered in any family where one or more members are presenting with tuberculosis (TB). Older children may also have developmental problems such as pubertal delay. They may also have more subtle cognitive dysfunction, reduced concentration, and expressive language delay with poor school performance.

Lymphoid interstitial pneumonitis (LIP) occurs in up to 20% of children with HIV, and is a condition characterized by chronic lymphoid infiltrates within the lungs. It is often symptomless, being only evident on chest radiography, although children with LIP may have more frequent chest infections and recurrent wheezy symptoms. Bronchiectasis can be a long-term consequence of LIP, with recurrent infections. The chest x-ray (CXR) findings are nonspecific with widespread nodular infiltrates, often associated with hilar lymphadenopathy. Radiologically the differential diagnosis includes infections such as miliary TB, although children with miliary TB are usually very unwell compared to the relative lack of symptoms in children with LIP. Lymphoid interstitial pneumonitis is rare in very young infants and tends to present from the end of the first year of life. Children with LIP usually also have hepatosplenomegaly, lymphadenopathy, and often parotitis. In any child who presents with bilateral chronic, painless parotitis, HIV is the most likely diagnosis.

Classification of HIV Disease in Children

The severity of HIV infection can be assessed clinically by the types of complications present, immunologically based on numbers of CD4 cells, and virologically based on the plasma HIV viral load. Immunologic and virologic assessment can also be used to predict the likelihood of future clinical deterioration.

The current Centers for Disease Control (CDC) classification system of HIV infection used for children under the age of 13 years was revised in 1994 prior to the availability of measurement of HIV plasma viremia (9). This system is based on clinical signs and symptoms, which are assigned to four categories: N (none); A (mild); B (moderate); and C (severe) (Table 12.1). An immunologic score between 1 (no suppression) and 3 (severe suppression) is derived from the age-related CD4-positive lymphocyte count (CD4 count) (Table 12.2). Opportunistic infections and other conditions associated with an adult AIDS diagnosis are all category C. The majority of children with HIV admitted to PICU are likely to have a category C diagnosis.

TABLE 12.1. Symptom categories for children with HIV

Category N: not symptomatic
No signs or symptoms considered to be due to HIV, or only one of the conditions listed in category A

Category A: mildly symptomatic
Two or more of the conditions listed below, but none of the conditions listed in categories B or C
    Hepatomegaly   Splenomegaly
    Dermatitis   Parotitis
    Lymphadenopathy ($\geq$0.5 cm at more than two sites; bilateral = one site)
    Recurrent or persistent upper respiratory infection, sinusitis, otitis media

Category B: moderately symptomatic
Symptomatic conditions other than those listed for category A or C that are attributed to HIV
Including:
Anemia, neutropenia, thrombocytopenia, persisting >30 days
Bacterial meningitis, pneumonia, or sepsis (single episode)
Candidiasis, oropharyngeal, persisting 2 months in children >6 months of age
Cardiomyopathy
CMV infection, with onset before 1 month of age
Diarrhea, recurrent or chronic
Hepatitis
Herpes simplex virus (HSV) stomatitis, recurrent (more than two episodes in 1 year)
HSV bronchitis, pneumonitis, or esophagitis with onset before 1 month of age
Herpes zoster (shingles) involving at least two distinct episodes or more than one dermatome
Leiomyosarcoma
Lymphoid interstitial pneumonitis (LIP)
Neuropathy
Nocardiosis
Persistent fever >30 days
Toxoplasmosis, onset before 1 month of age
Varicella, disseminated

(Continued)

TABLE **12.1.** *Continued*

Category C: severely symptomatic

Any condition listed in the 1987 surveillance case definition of AIDS, with the exception of LIP

Bacterial infections, serious, multiple or recurrent, (any combination of at least two culture confirmed infections within a 2-year period), of the following types: septicemia, pneumonia, meningitis, bone or joint infection, abscess of an internal organ or body cavity (excluding otitis media; skin/mucosal abscesses; catheter-related infections).

Candidiasis, esophageal or pulmonary

CMV disease with onset >1 month of age (at a site other than liver, spleen, lymph nodes)

Coccidioidomycosis, disseminated

Cryptococcus, extrapulmonary

Cryptosporidiosis or isosporiasis with diarrhea >30 days

Encephalopathy (at least one of the following progressive findings present for at least 2 months in the absence of a concurrent illness other than HIV infection): failure to attain or loss of developmental mile stones or intellectual ability (verified by standard psychological tests); impaired brain growth or acquired microcephaly demonstrated by head circumference measurements or brain atrophy on neuroimaging; acquired symmetrical motor deficit, with two or more: paresis, abnormal reflexes, ataxia, or gait disturbance

Histoplasmosis, disseminated

HSV with mucocutaneous ulceration for >30 days, or bronchitis, pneumonitis, esophagitis, of any duration in a child over 1 month of age

Kaposi's sarcoma

Lymphoma, primary in brain

Lymphoma, small noncleaved cell (Burkitt's), or immunoblastic or large cell of B-cell or unknown immunophenotype

Mycobacterium tuberculosis, disseminated or extrapulmonary

Mycobacterium, other species, disseminated (at a site other than the lungs or in addition to lungs, skin, or cervical or hilar lymph nodes)

Pneumocystis carinii pneumonia

Progressive multifocal leukoencephalopathy

Salmonella (nontyphoid) septicemia, recurrent

Toxoplasmosis of the brain with onset after 1 month of age

Wasting syndrome in the absence of a concurrent illness other than HIV, that could explain the following:

Persistent weight loss >10% of base line, or downward crossing of at least two of the following percentile lines on the weight for age chart in a child >1 year of age (95th, 75th, 50th, 25th, 5th), or

Less than 5th percentile on the weight for height chart on two consecutive measurements >30 days apart, plus either chronic diarrhea or persistent fever, also >30 days

TABLE **12.2.** Immune categories for children's with HIV, based on age-specific $CD4^+$ T-lymphocyte counts and percentages of total lymphocytes

	Age of child					
	<12 months		1–5 years		6–12 years	
Immune category	μL	(%)	μL	(%)	μL	(%)
No suppression 1	≥1500	(≥25)	≥1000	(≥25)	≥500	(≥25)
Moderate suppression 2	750–1,499	(15–24)	500–999	(15–24)	200–499	(15–24)
Severe suppression 3	<750	(<15)	<500	(<15)	<200	(<15)

Assessment of the CD4 count in any child must be in relation to the appropriate count for age. The 50th percentile CD4 count at age 6 months is 3000×10^6/L, compared to 1000×10^6/L at 6 years, by which time the CD4 count range approaches that of adults (10,11). For each child the CD4 count will vary, and is often depressed with intercurrent infections. This parameter, therefore, should ideally be measured when the child is in a stable clinical condition. The percentage of total lymphocytes that are CD4-positive (CD4 percentage) varies less with age and other factors than does the absolute count, and can be a useful measure of immune function in children, but may be misleading if the total lymphocyte count is very low. The CD4 count may be less predictive of symptomatic disease in young infants, and infants with HIV and severe PcP have rarely presented with normal CD4 counts.

Plasma viral load data from prospective cohorts followed from birth, in the pre–combination therapy era, demonstrate the difference in response to primary HIV infection in the relatively immune incompetent infant compared to adults. Within 4 to 8 weeks of birth a peak viremia is reached in HIV-infected infants, which may take several years to decline to a steady level. The peak viremia is higher and the decline much slower than seen in newly infected adults, where HIV will decline to the steady level within 2 to 4 months (12). Infants with rapidly progressive disease in the first year of life generally have higher levels of viremia in the first 2 months than do those who do not become symptomatic until later. The HIV plasma viral load has also been measured in cohorts of children presenting with symptoms of disease. The relative risk of death was 2.1 times greater if the presenting HIV RNA was >100,000 copies per milliliter (13).

The PENTA Calculator: Risk of HIV Progression According to CD4 Count and Plasma HIV RNA, Without Combination Treatment

Both the baseline CD4 count and the plasma viral load are independently predictive of progression of HIV disease in children. In one cohort, if the CD4 percentage dropped below 15%, the relative risk of death was 2.8 (95% confidence interval [CI] 1.6–4.9%). In a time-independent model, the relative risk of death per five-point decrease in CD4 percentage was 1.3 (95% CI 1.2–1.5) (12).

Parents of children with HIV can now be given a good estimate of the risk of progression of disease in an untreated child, according to the age of presentation, CD4 count, and viral load (14). In a large meta-analysis of nearly 4000 children from Europe and the U.S., the above data have been collated to give risks of progression to AIDS or death at different ages (Fig. 12.1). From this meta-analysis, in children over 2 years of age, the 12-month risk of developing AIDS was 6% for a CD4 $\geq$20%, increased to 18% with a CD4 percentage of 10%, and 34% with a CD4 percentage of 5%. The annual risk of death increased from <2% for CD4 percentage $\geq$10%, to 12% with a CD4 percentage of 5%. For children over 6 months of age, progression to AIDS or death increased sharply for viral loads over 10^5 copies/mL. At 2 years of age the risk of progressing to AIDS was 5% with a viral load <10^5 copies/mL, 24% at 10^6 copies/mL, and 66% at 10^7

Probability of death within 12 months

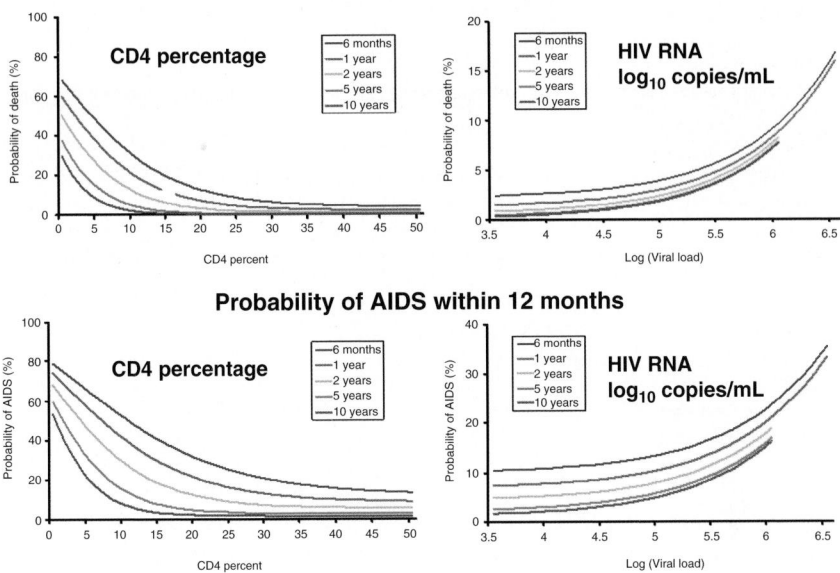

FIGURE 12.1. Risks of progression to AIDS or death at different ages.

copies/mL. These data have been used to generate a computer program, the Pediatric European Network for the Treatment of AIDS (PENTA) calculator. For a child of less than 13 years the program can give an estimated risk of AIDS or death in the following 6 to 12 months (15).

Presentation of HIV in the Pediatric Intensive Care Unit

Children whose HIV has progressed to an advanced stage are at risk of severe complications that may require admission to the PICU. The most common problem is acute respiratory failure, which in Europe accounts for 46% to 77% of PICU admissions (4,16). Respiratory failure frequently presents in previously undiagnosed, rapidly progressing infants. It is usually due to PcP, often with further co-infecting pathogens. Respiratory failure may also present in older children, or in those already known to have HIV, especially if their disease is advanced. Failure of any organ system may occur in HIV, resulting in PICU admission. Some reasons for PICU admission are listed in Table 12.3.

Diagnosis and Management of Respiratory Failure

Infants Not Previously Diagnosed with HIV

Most infants in respiratory failure will not have a previous diagnosis of HIV infection. In developed countries, especially during the winter, such infants are

TABLE 12.3. Reasons for admission to PICU with HIV

Respiratory
PCP
CMV pneumonitis
Pneumonitis due to common respiratory viruses (respiratory syncytial virus, influenza, parainfluenza, adenovirus)
Bacterial pneumonia
Tuberculosis
LIP (rarely)
Airway obstruction

Cardiovascular
Cardiomyopathy

Neurologic
HIV encephalopathy
Encephalopathy due to other causes
Bacterial meningitis
Cryptococcal meningitis
Cerebral toxoplasmosis

Gastrointestinal
HIV enteropathy
Gastroenteritis
Acute abdomen
Hepatitis and liver failure
Pancreatitis

Renal
HIV nephropathy
Renal failure
Hyponatremia

Severe infection
Sepsis
Disseminated mycobacterial infection
Disseminated varicella

Immune reconstitution

Iatrogenic
Complications of antiretroviral drugs

Malignancy
Lymphoma
Kaposi's sarcoma

commonly referred to the PICU with a diagnosis of respiratory failure due to bronchiolitis. The possibility of an underlying immune deficiency should be considered in any infant who responds poorly to treatment, who has epidemiologic risk factors, who has a history of previous recurrent infections or failure to thrive, or who has hepatosplenomegaly, widespread lymphadenopathy, parotitis, severe oral thrush, or abnormal neurologic signs. Evidence of interstitial pneumonitis on CXR should also prompt suspicion, but is not always present.

Once the possibility of immune deficiency has been raised, the first priority remains treatment of the respiratory failure, specifics of which are not discussed here. Details of HIV testing are given below, but until the diagnosis is confirmed, other immune deficiencies such as severe combined immunodeficiency (SCID) remain possible. Children with SCID require irradiated blood products because of the risk of engraftment of transfused leukocytes; children with HIV do not. However, it is important to use irradiated blood products until SCID is excluded and HIV is confirmed.

A laboratory diagnosis of the cause of the respiratory failure is required to guide antimicrobial treatment. A comparison of HIV-infected and uninfected children with respiratory failure in South Africa showed that, while tuberculosis and other bacterial pneumonias were equally common in each group, PcP and cytomegalovirus (CMV) pneumonitis occurred almost exclusively in HIV-infected infants, who were also significantly more likely to be infected with multiple organisms (5). The pattern is similar in developed countries, but with a much lower incidence of tuberculosis (4).

Common causes of respiratory failure in HIV are listed in Table 12.4. Blind treatment would require prolonged courses of multiple potentially toxic drugs. Laboratory confirmation or exclusion of the presence of specific pathogens allows rationalization of therapy, thus reducing the risk of side effects. Examination of samples obtained noninvasively from the upper airway is not sufficiently sensitive to exclude important conditions such as PcP (17,18). Open lung biopsy or percutaneous needle aspiration may be used, but the most commonly used technique is bronchoalveolar lavage (BAL), which may be performed either bronchoscopically or blindly by instillation of sterile saline into the endotracheal tube and aspiration of the sample by deep suction. Staff members carrying out a BAL should take appropriate precautions to reduce their risk of exposure to HIV and respiratory pathogens (see below). The sample obtained at BAL should be sent to the laboratory for investigations as listed in Table 12.4. It is important to establish a working relationship with the appropriate laboratories so that results can be obtained as quickly as possible. If there is any delay,

TABLE 12.4. Diagnosis of the cause of respiratory failure in HIV

Organism	Laboratory investigation
Conventional bacterial pathogens (*Streptococcus pneumoniae, Staphylococcus aureus, Haemophilus influenzae, Klebsiella, Moraxella catarrhalis*)	Gram stain and culture
Pneumocystis jiroveci	Silver staining or immunofluorescence
Cytomegalovirus	Immunofluorescence/PCR/culture
Respiratory viruses (respiratory syncytial virus, influenza, parainfluenza, adenovirus)	Immunofluorescence/PCR/culture
Mycobacterium tuberculosis and other mycobacteria	Ziehl-Nielsen or auramine stain and mycobacterial culture
Fungi	Microscopy and culture

it may be necessary to treat blindly with multiple antimicrobials, and discontinue specific treatments if negative laboratory results subsequently become available.

Respiratory Failure in Older Children

Older children, and those already known to have HIV infection and who develop respiratory failure, are likely to have a similar range of pathogens as in infants. They may be more likely to have reactivated PcP than primary infection. The issue of confirming the diagnosis in order to treat rationally is the same as in infants, and a BAL is usually required. In a child with known HIV and deteriorating respiratory function who is not yet requiring mechanical ventilation, it can be difficult to determine the optimal time to perform a BAL, as the procedure itself may cause respiratory deterioration and result in mechanical ventilation becoming necessary (4).

Older children may often be symptomatic from LIP, but it is a rare cause of respiratory failure and PICU admission.

Causes of Respiratory Failure in Infants and Children with HIV

Pneumocystis Pneumonia

Asymptomatic infection with *P. jiroveci* is extremely common in immunocompetent individuals, but in immunocompromised children it carries a high mortality, and defines category C (severe) HIV infection. In a series of over 40 admissions of children with HIV infection to PICU in London, PcP accounted for 59% of cases of lower respiratory tract infection (4). Rapidly progressing HIV-infected infants often present with primary PcP, most commonly at age 3 to 6 months (16,19,20).

The infection is usually confined to the lungs, and causes respiratory failure without associated systemic sepsis. In children with HIV and PcP, there are usually large numbers of organisms in the alveoli, but very little exudate. Infiltrates of plasma cells greatly thicken the alveolar walls (17). The clinical presentation is of a nonproductive cough, low-grade fever, respiratory distress and progressive hypoxia, and respiratory failure. In adults and older children, there may be a prolonged history, but in infants disease progression is more rapid, and the majority of infants with HIV and PcP progress to respiratory failure requiring mechanical ventilation.

The typical CXR changes of PcP are that of an interstitial infiltrate, but this may also be due to viral pneumonitis, and PcP may present with other patterns, such as generalized "white-out" or lobar consolidation. Serum lactate dehydrogenase is often elevated, but diagnosis of PcP requires identification of the organism in the laboratory. This is done by staining of BAL-obtained secretions with methenamine silver or toluidine blue O, or by immunofluorescence.

The first choice antibiotic for treatment of PcP is high-dose trimethoprim-sulfamethoxazole (20 mg/kg/day of trimethoprim, 100 mg/kg/day of sulfamethoxazole, in four divided doses) for 3 weeks. Side effects include rash, neutropenia, renal dysfunction or gastrointestinal side effects, but treatment should be continued unless the reaction is severe. Alternatives include nebulized or intravenous pentamidine, which is more likely to cause severe side effects than is trimethoprim-sulfamethoxazole, and may interact with antiretroviral drugs to increase the risk of pancreatitis. Atovaquone has been used to treat moderately severe PcP in adults, but there is little experience of its use on PICU.

Adjunctive steroid therapy has been shown to be beneficial in trials in adults with PcP, reducing both the requirement for mechanical ventilation and the mortality (21); there are no such trials in children. Several small case series and comparisons with historical controls suggest benefit (22–24), but an analysis of cases of PcP in the U.K. up to 1998 showed no evidence of improved survival in children treated with corticosteroids, although the treatment was not randomized or controlled (25). In our center, children with confirmed PcP requiring mechanical ventilation are treated with steroids. There are concerns about the effect of corticosteroids on possible co-infection with CMV, which is common. In adults treated for PcP with steroids, outcome is worse in those co-infected with CMV, irrespective of other parameters of HIV infection (26). Unless a child is known not to be co-infected with CMV, it is prudent to start ganciclovir treatment for presumed CMV infection, when steroids are used as adjunctive therapy for PcP, while awaiting confirmation of the child's CMV status (see below).

Surfactant treatment has been used in children ventilated for PcP, but despite showing short-term improvements in ventilatory requirements, there are no data to show improvement in outcome (27), and it is not a routine part of treatment.

Pneumocystis pneumonia remains a serious condition with a high mortality. In Cape Town, children with HIV and PcP had a mortality of 44%, almost double that of children with HIV and other causes of pneumonia (28). However, the use of steroids and better delivery of intensive care do appear to result in some improvement in outcome. In London, mortality from PcP in the PICU has fallen from 27% between 1992 and 1997, to 21% between 1998 and 2002 (4).

Further, children who survived PcP in the PICU often did not survive to hospital discharge due to their advanced HIV disease (29). Improved antiretroviral treatment has changed this. Data from both the U.K. and the U.S. show improved median survival from diagnosis of PcP from 1 to 8 months before 1993 to 14 to 19 months between 1993 and 1998 (19,25,30).

Pneumocystis pneumonia and mechanical ventilation do cause significant lung damage, and children who survive their PICU admission often remain tachypneic and hypoxic for a considerable time afterward. They should be started on prophylaxis to prevent recurrence of PcP, using trimethoprim-sulfamethoxazole, dapsone, or atovaquone. This significantly reduces the rate of PcP recurrence (31). Secondary prophylaxis has been used lifelong, but is probably not necessary following adequate immune reconstitution with restoration of normal numbers of CD4 cells. Primary PcP prophylaxis is also used in all children known to have HIV infection and reduced CD4 cell count.

Cytomegalovirus Pneumonitis

Cytomegalovirus is a herpes virus that usually causes asymptomatic infection in immunocompetent children. By adulthood, 40% to 80% of people in developed countries and almost 100% in less developed countries have serologic evidence of previous infection (32). Following primary infection with CMV, latency is established and subsequent intermittent asymptomatic shedding of virus is common. In children with HIV, CMV can cause an interstitial pneumonitis similar in presentation to PcP, and co-infection with both pathogens is common. Cytomegalovirus may be detected by immunofluorescence, but finding the virus in urine or upper respiratory secretions may represent asymptomatic shedding, and is not diagnostic of CMV organ disease. Finding CMV in a specimen obtained at BAL is more useful in diagnosing CMV pneumonitis, but it is often necessary to start treatment in acutely ill children before confirming the diagnosis, especially if CMV co-infection is suspected in children being started on steroids for PcP. Serial quantitative CMV blood polymerase chain reaction (PCR) provides the best guide to monitoring treatment.

Cytomegalovirus may cause progressive multisystem disease. In data from the U.K., one third of HIV-positive children with CMV pneumonitis had involvement of at least one other organ system, and half of these children had CMV retinitis (25). This may be difficult to treat and may result in blindness (33). Cytomegalovirus may also cause meningoencephalitis, hepatitis, severe gastrointestinal disease, and bone marrow suppression. All children diagnosed with CMV pneumonitis should have detailed funduscopy to look for retinitis, as well as cranial imaging.

The first-choice therapy for CMV infection is intravenous ganciclovir, which carries the risk of additional bone marrow suppression when used together with trimethoprim-sulfamethoxazole. Alternatives include foscarnet and cidofovir, which also have significant side effects. Unlike older children (34,35), the optimal dosing regimens for treatment of CMV in children with HIV are not certain, and rapid metabolism in infancy may make therapeutic levels particularly difficult to achieve (36). Cytomegalovirus is a chronic infection, and treatment controls CMV viremia but may not eradicate it. As with PcP, prophylactic treatment may be required.

Other Causes of Respiratory Failure

In addition to opportunistic infections, children with HIV are also more prone to bacterial pneumonia. Tuberculosis, nontuberculous mycobacteria, common respiratory viruses such as respiratory syncytial virus (RSV), influenza or adenovirus, and fungal infections may all cause respiratory failure in children with HIV. In addition, noninfective causes such as upper airway obstruction due to lymphadenopathy, and HIV- or drug-related myocarditis may contribute to respiratory failure. The treatment of these conditions does not differ from their treatment in non–HIV-infected children, and requires supportive intensive care and appropriate antimicrobials as indicated.

Nonrespiratory Causes of Pediatric Intensive Care Unit Admission

The direct effects of HIV or of its associated infections may affect any organ system, and result in admission to PICU. Causes are listed in Table 12.3. Neurologic complications are important, but cryptococcal meningitis and cerebral toxoplasmosis are less common in children than in adults.

Currently, admission to PICU because of complications of antiretroviral treatment is rare, but as the numbers of children treated increase, and they survive longer, it is possible that admissions due to iatrogenic complications may increase. Complications of antiretroviral drugs are listed in Table 12.5.

TABLE 12.5. Antiretroviral classes of drugs and major side effects

Drug classes	Early side effects (usually within first 2–3 months)	Later side effects (accumulate over time usually >6 months)
Nucleoside reverse transcriptase inhibitors (NRTIs) Zidovudine Lamivudine Didanosine Abacavir Emtricitabine Stavudine Nucleotide RTI Tenofovir	*Common* Nausea; vomiting; diarrhea; headache; anemia; neutropenia; hepatic dysfunction *Rare* Pancreatitis (especially didanosine and stavudine); potentially fatal hypersensitivity reaction in 5% to abacavir (very rare in Africans), usually within first 6 weeks of treatment; do not restart drug if hypersensitivity has occurred; renal toxicity with tenofovir	Mitochondrial toxicity (worst with stavudine > zidovudine > didanosine); lactic acidosis, hepatic steatosis (especially didanosine and stavudine); peripheral neuropathy; myopathy; cardiomyopathy; lipoatrophy (fat loss in face and limbs) with stavudine; possible bone demineralization and renal toxicity with tenofovir
Nonnucleoside reverse transcriptase inhibitors (NNRTIs) Nevirapine Efavirenz	Nevirapine—rash in up to 16% (Stevens-Johnson syndrome or life-threatening rash seen in 0.3%); liver toxicity, increased risk if prior hepatitis B/C Efavirenz—rash in up to 10% (but rarely severe, Stevens-Johnson syndrome very rare); altered lipids; wide range of central nervous system problems, often resolve in 2–4 weeks	Fat redistribution: central fat accumulation and peripheral lipoatrophy; insulin resistance with hyperglycemia; osteonecrosis, osteopenia/ osteoporosis
Protease inhibitors (PIs) Lopinavir Ritonavir Saquinavir Nelfinavir Atazanivir Fos-amprenavir	Gastrointestinal upset: vomiting, diarrhea, abdominal pain; hyperlipidemia (elevated triglyceride and cholesterol); jaundice with atazanivir	

Note: Children have fewer adverse drug reactions than do adults.

Drugs causing pancreatitis may be more likely to result in PICU admission. Children who present late with advanced HIV infection may also develop severe complications of immune reconstitution after starting antiretroviral treatment, as their inflammatory response to previously tolerated pathogens increases, and it is quite conceivable that such children could require admission to PICU.

It is also worth noting that because of their condition and previous illness, a proportion of PICU admissions are elective postsurgical admissions (4).

Testing for HIV on the Pediatric Intensive Care Unit

Requesting an HIV Test

Many children, especially infants with PcP, are not known to be HIV infected before admission to the PICU, and HIV testing is likely to be performed while the child is critically ill. Testing a child for HIV is difficult for most families under any circumstances, but is especially stressful while the child has a life-threatening illness. The approach to obtaining consent is therefore particularly important.

Usually HIV is suspected when a child presents with a severe or unusual infection likely to be due to underlying immunodeficiency. Certain associated factors, such as country of origin or maternal intravenous drug use, may make HIV more likely in one infant, whereas parental consanguinity may make congenital immunodeficiency more likely in another. As far as possible, an HIV test should be considered normal and offered along with other tests relevant to the child's condition. However, when asking parents for consent to do an HIV test, certain important points should be made:

1. The HIV test is part of routine immune investigation in all infants/children where immunodeficiency is suspected, whatever the family's origin, and all parents are asked to consent to the test.

2. As the majority of infants/children with HIV infection are vertically infected, a positive HIV antibody test in the child implies a definite positive test in the mother, and the possibility of positivity in other family members. The family should be reassured that testing and treatment for other members is also available.

3. An HIV diagnosis is not the "death sentence" that many family members (and some doctors) believe, but is a treatable, although not currently curable, infection. Children and adults with access to treatment and care now have a good life expectancy.

4. Unfortunately, HIV still remains a stigmatized diagnosis in many communities. Families should be assured that appropriate confidentiality will be maintained regarding the diagnosis. Building trust for a long-term relationship with the family is very important at this early stage.

The majority of families give consent to HIV testing, and wish to know the results as soon as possible. Some families have difficulty confronting this diagnosis and may take longer to accept HIV testing in this very difficult situation. Usually, with the input of the multidisciplinary team, it is possible over time to build up trust so that the child can be tested and then receive appropriate care. Very rarely where the parents continue to refuse HIV testing and this goes against the best interest of the child, then judicial consent for intervention may be sought.

Laboratory Diagnosis of HIV

Children 18 Months of Age and Over

Up to 18 months of age, anti-HIV antibody in the child's blood may be of transplacental maternal origin and therefore is not diagnostic of HIV infection in the child (37,38). Beyond this age, HIV infection can be diagnosed, as in adults, by detection of anti-HIV antibody. Current antibody tests are highly sensitive and specific, but a positive result should always be confirmed on a repeat sample. Rapid point of care tests can give a result within 15 to 20 minutes, but again should be confirmed with a formal laboratory test (Table 12.6).

Infants Younger than 18 Months of Age

The gold standard test for HIV infection in infancy is HIV DNA PCR on peripheral blood lymphocytes (39). This test amplifies HIV proviral DNA integrated in the genome of the host lymphocytes. As most infants are infected with HIV in the peripartum period, HIV DNA is not amplified from all infected infants at birth. Within the first weeks of life the sensitivity of the test increases rapidly, and by 3 months of age nearly 100% of non–breast-fed HIV-infected infants will be HIV DNA PCR positive. In view of the genomic diversity of HIV, and to avoid a false-negative result in the infant, a maternal sample should always be

TABLE 12.6. Testing children for HIV: age-appropriate tests

| Age of child | Diagnosis of HIV infection | | If HIV infected, establish level of HIV disease progression |
	Serology	Genomic amplification	Viral parameters
≥18 months	HIV antibody test positive	Not necessary	HIV plasma viral load (RNA copies/mL) CD4 count
<18 months	HIV antibody test positive with a "category C" condition in the infant makes an HIV diagnosis highly likely	HIV DNA PCR positive (confirm that the maternal virus can be amplified to avoid false negative results)	HIV plasma viral load (RNA copies/mL) CD4 count

amplified with the first infant sample to confirm that the primers used can detect the maternal virus. If a maternal virus cannot be detected by the HIV DNA PCR used, then a different primer set or a different method of genomic amplification should be used.

If an infant or another family member presents with signs or symptoms of HIV disease, then the infant should have an HIV DNA PCR test. The result of the infant's test, whether negative or positive, should be confirmed by a repeat test. It is not usually necessary to carry out other surrogate or less sensitive diagnostic tests (e.g., HIV p24 antigen, immunoglobulin G concentration, or CD4 count) unless there is a concern about the sensitivity of the HIV DNA PCR, or PCR is not available.

Even if the mother has had a negative HIV antibody test in early pregnancy, she may still be infected later in pregnancy or during breast-feeding if she has unprotected sex. If her infant presents with signs or symptoms consistent with HIV, then testing should still be undertaken. There is an increased risk of infection of the infant during primary maternal infection as the level of maternal HIV viremia is very high for the first few weeks during seroconversion.

In the PICU, where the infant has evidence of an opportunistic infection (e.g., PcP), an HIV antibody result can be obtained within hours, whereas the HIV DNA PCR result may take several days. Although the genomic result is required to confirm whether the infant has HIV, the combination of category C clinical disease and HIV antibody makes underlying HIV infection highly likely.

Prevention of Cross-Infection with HIV in the Pediatric Intensive Care Unit

Primary Prevention

All children admitted to the PICU should be treated as potentially infectious for all blood-borne viruses. Universal precautions should include the covering of any open wounds by staff, wearing of gloves when handling body fluids, safe use and disposal of all sharps, the use of goggles to protect the eyes when performing any procedure likely to cause splashing, such as endotracheal suction, BAL, or flushing of blocked intravenous lines, safe portering of specimens to the laboratory, and safe handling of specimens within the laboratory. These precautions should be adopted for all patients irrespective of their known HIV status.

Postexposure Prophylaxis

If any member of the staff or the family suffers a needlestick injury or other exposure from a patient with known or suspected HIV, an urgent assessment of the individualized risk for this contact should be made. Postexposure prophylaxis (PEP) with antiretroviral therapy is effective at reducing the risk of transmission (40). Each hospital's occupational health department should have a policy in place for the drug regimen PEP to be used for suspected wild-type virus, and an arrangement for consultation at all hours with rapid access to the PEP. Occupational health clinicians or their deputies should be available 24 hours to see affected staff members immediately after a possible exposure, assess the risk of transmission, and advise the staff members so that they can make an informed decision about the risks and benefits of taking PEP, and of checking baseline and subsequent serology. It may be appropriate to start PEP while awaiting the results of serology or PCR testing of the patient, following obtaining consent. In patients with known resistant virus, consideration should be given to devising, in advance, a suggested effective regimen for PEP in the event of an occupational or accidental exposure.

Long-Term Survival for Children with HIV in the Era of Combination Therapy

Excellent guidelines have been drawn up for the treatment of children with HIV (41,42). All children presenting with a category C illness, whatever the CD4 count or viral load, should start treatment as soon as possible. The latest PENTA guidelines (2004) use data from the HIV Paediatric Prognostic Markers Collaborative Study (HPPMC) cohort, and advise treatment according to CD4 count/viral load, with the aim of maintaining the 1-year risk of progression to AIDS at <10% and risk of death at <5%. There is an important balance to strike here between treating too early and too late. Treatments may have significant short- and long-term side effects, and perfect adherence is difficult for children to maintain over years. Poor adherence leads to development of viral resistance and the need for further more complicated regimes. Treatment regimens are generally made up of at least three drugs, usually from two of the classes of antiretroviral agents (Tables 12.7 and 12.8).

Since the advent of effective combination antiretroviral therapy in 1997, both mortality and morbidity for children with HIV have altered dramatically. This has been demonstrated in data from nearly 1000 children in the U.K. Collaborative HIV Pediatric Study (CHIPS) cohort (30). Mortality declined from 9.3 per

TABLE **12.7.** When to start treatment in children with HIV

	Clinical category	CD4 count	Viral load (copies/mL)
Infants	B / C *	<30–35%	>1,000,000
1–3 years	C	<20%	>250,000
4–8 years	C	<15%	>250,000
9–12 years	C	<15%	>250,000
13–17 years	C	200–350	—

*Some experts treat all infants, as it is clinically very difficult to identify who will progress rapidly or develop encephalopathy.

TABLE 12.8. What antiretrovirals to start with in children with HIV

Infants
Either two nucleoside reverse transcriptase inhibitors (NRTI) + one protease inhibitor (PI)
Or two NRTI + one nonnucleoside reverse transcriptase inhibitors (NNRTI)
Children
Either two NRTI + one PI
Or two NRTI + one NNRTI

Dual NRTI recommended include zidovudine + lamivudine or didanosine; lamivudine + abacavir; didanosine + lamivudine; stavudine is not recommended for first-line therapy.
PIs recommended include lopinavir + ritonavir boost, felfinavir.
NNRTIs recommended: nevirapine and efavirenz (there is no efavirenz dose for children <3 years of age or <13 kg).

100 child years in 1997 to 2 per 100 child years in 2001–2002. Over this time, progression to AIDS also declined threefold and admissions to hospital by 80%. The only group in which there was little improvement in outcome was in infants, where deaths from presenting illnesses occurred before antiretroviral therapy could begin. This emphasizes the importance of antenatal diagnosis of maternal HIV, to enable uptake of interventions to reduce the risk of perinatal infection (e.g., antiretroviral therapy, planned cesarean section, and avoidance of breast-feeding).

Conclusion

At the beginning of the HIV epidemic, the mortality of children with PcP in the PICU was extremely high (84% to 100%). In the absence of antiretroviral treatment, the small number who did leave the PICU often died within the following year (29). Other causes of admission also had high mortality, and many questioned the appropriateness of admitting children with HIV to the PICU. In less developed countries, mortality in the PICU remains high and the debate still goes on (5,43,44), although it is likely to change as antiretroviral treatment becomes more widely available.

In developed countries it is clear that the mortality in the PICU of children with HIV is improving, although conditions such as PcP continue to have significant mortality. What is beyond dispute is the vastly improved outcome of children who survive to be discharged from the PICU. There should now be no debate about the appropriateness of intensive care for children presenting with HIV or likely HIV, in the developed world, and withdrawal of intensive care from children with severe respiratory failure should be based solely on the manageability of the respiratory failure itself and not on a judgment regarding quality and prognosis of subsequent survival.

Despite advances in treatment, there remain a small number of often older children whose HIV has progressed to a very advanced stage, and who may have complications of HIV such as malignancy. If these children with end-stage HIV require PICU admission, an individualized assessment of their prognosis, based on both the prognosis and treatment of their complication and the further treatability of their HIV, should be undertaken involving the family and the PICU and HIV multidisciplinary teams.

References

1. www.UNAIDS.org.
2. www.cdc.gov/hiv/stats/2003SurveillanceReport.pdf.
3. www.hpa.org.uk/infections/topics_az/hiv_and_sti/publications/annual2004/fop_3_ hiv.pdf.
4. Cooper S, Lyall H, Walters S, et al. Children with human immunodeficiency virus admitted to a paediatric intensive care unit in the United Kingdom over a 10-year period. Intensive Care Med 2004;30:113–118.
5. Jeena PM, Coovadia HM, Bhagwanjee S. Prospective, controlled study of the outcome of human immunodeficiency virus-1 antibody-positive children admitted to an intensive care unit. Crit Care Med 1996;24:963–967.
6. European Collaborative Study. Hospitalization of children born to human immunodeficiency virus-infected women in Europe. Pediatr Infect Dis J 1997;16: 1151–1156.
7. Blanche S, Tardieu M, Duliege A, et al. Longitudinal study of 94 symptomatic infants with perinatally acquired human immunodeficiency virus infection. Evidence for a bimodal expression of clinical and biological symptoms. Am J Dis Child 1990;144: 1210–1215.
8. Stringer JR, Beard CB, Miller RF, Wakefield AE. A new name (Pneumocystis jiroveci) for pneumocystis from humans. Emerg Infect Dis 2002;8. from:URL:http://www.cdc. gov/ncidod/EID/vol8no9/02–0096.htm.
9. Centers for Disease Control and Prevention. 1994 Revised Classification system for human immunodeficiency virus infection in children less than 13 years of age. MMWR Morb Mortal Wkly Rep 1994;43:1–17.
10. European Collaborative Study. Age-related standards for T lymphocyte subsets based on uninfected children born to human immunodeficiency virus 1-infected women. The European Collaborative Study. Pediatr Infect Dis J 1992;11: 1018–1026.
11. Comans-Bitter WM, de Groot R, van den Beemd R, et al. Immunophenotyping of blood lymphocytes in childhood. Reference values for lymphocyte subpopulations. J Pediatr 1997;130:388–393.
12. Shearer WT, Quinn TC, LaRussa P, et al. Viral load and disease progression in infants infected with human immunodeficiency virus type 1. Women and Infants Transmission Study Group. N Engl J Med 1997;336:1337–1342.
13. Mofenson LM, Korelitz J, Meyer WA 3rd, et al. The relationship between serum human immunodeficiency virus type 1 (HIV-1) RNA level, CD4 lymphocyte percent, and long-term mortality risk in HIV-1-infected children. National Institute of Child Health and Human Development Intravenous Immunoglobulin Clinical Trial Study Group. J Infect Dis 1997;175:1029–1038.
14. Dunn D, HIV Paediatric Prognostic Markers Collaborative Study Group. Short-term risk of disease progression in HIV-1-infected children receiving no antiretroviral therapy or zidovudine monotherapy: a meta-analysis. Lancet 2003;362:1595–1596.
15. http://www.ctu.mrc.ac.uk/penta/trials.htm.

16. Casanova Roman M, Rios Hurtado J, Garcia Martin FJ, Milano Manso G, Martinez Valverde A. Ingresos por sida en cuidados intensivos pediatricos. An Esp Pediatr 2000;52:537–541.
17. Hughes WT. Current status of laboratory diagnosis of Pneumocystis carinii pneumonitis. CRC Crit Rev Clin Lab Sci 1975;6:145–170.
18. Shelhamer JH, Gill VJ, Quinn TC, et al. The laboratory evaluation of opportunistic pulmonary infections. Ann Intern Med 1996;124:585–599.
19. Simonds RJ, Oxtoby MJ, Caldwell MB, Gwinn ML, Rogers MF. Pneumocystis carinii pneumonia among US children with perinatally acquired HIV infection. JAMA 1993;270:470–473.
20. Zar HJ, Dechaboon A, Hanslo D, Apolles P, Magnus KG, Hussey G. Pneumocystis carinii pneumonia in South African children infected with human immunodeficiency virus. Pediatr Infect Dis J 2000;19:603–607.
21. National Institutes of Health–University of California. Consensus Statement on the use of corticosteroids as adjunctive therapy for pneumocystis pneumonia in the acquired immunodeficiency syndrome. N Engl J Med 1990;323:1500–1504.
22. Sleasman JW, Hemenway C, Klein AS, Barrett DJ. Corticosteroids improve survival of children with AIDS and Pneumocystis carinii pneumonia. Am J Dis Child 1993; 147:30–34.
23. Bye MR, Cairns-Bazarian AM, Ewig JM. Markedly reduced mortality associated with corticosteroid therapy of Pneumocystis carinii pneumonia in children with acquired immunodeficiency syndrome. Arch Pediatr Adolesc Med 1994;148:638–641.
24. McLaughlin GE, Virdee SS, Schleien CL, Holzman BH, Scott GB. Effect of corticosteroids on survival of children with acquired immunodeficiency syndrome and Pneumocystis carinii-related respiratory failure. J Pediatr 1995;126:821–824.
25. Williams AJ, Duong T, McNally LM, et al. Pneumocystis carinii pneumonia and cytomegalovirus infection in children with vertically acquired HIV infection. AIDS 2001;15:335–339.
26. Jensen A-MB, Lundgren JD, Benfield T, Nielsen TL, Vestbo J. Does cytomegalovirus predict a poor prognosis in pneumocystis carinii pneumonia treated with corticosteroids? Chest 1995;108:411–414.
27. Marriage SC, Underhill H, Nadel S. Use of natural surfactant in an HIV-infected infant with Pneumocystis carinii pneumonia. Intensive Care Med 1996;22:611–612.
28. Zar HJ, Apolles P, Argent A, et al. The etiology and outcome of pneumonia in human immunodeficiency virus-infected children admitted to intensive care in a developing country. Pediatr Crit Care Med 2001;2:108–112.
29. Cooper M, Jacobe S, Novelli V, Petros A. Outcome of HIV-positive children with Pneumocystis carinii pneumonia requiring intensive care. Clin Intensive Care 2002;13:85–87.
30. Gibb DM, Duong T, Tookey PA, et al. National Study of HIV in Pregnancy and Childhood Collaborative HIV Paediatric Study. Decline in mortality, AIDS, and hospital admissions in perinatally HIV-1 infected children in the United Kingdom and Ireland. Br Med J 2003;327:1019.
31. Centers for Disease Control and Prevention. 1995 revised guidelines for prophylaxis against pneumocystis carinii pneumonia for children infected with or perinatally exposed to human immunodeficiency virus. MMWR Morb Mortal Wkly Rep 1995; 44:1–11.
32. Zaia JA. Epidemiology and pathogenesis of cytomegalovirus disease. Semin Hematol 1990;27:1–4.

33. Wren SME, Fielder AR, Bethell D, et al. Cytomegalovirus retinitis in infancy. Eye 2004;18:389–392.
34. Frenkel LM, Capparelli EV, Dankner WM, et al. Pediatric AIDS Clinical Trial Group. Oral ganciclovir in children: pharmacokinetics, safety, tolerance, and antiviral effects. J Infect Dis 2000;182:1616–1624.
35. Kimberlin DW. Antiviral therapy for cytomegalovirus infections in pediatric patients. Semin Pediatr Infect Dis 2002;13:22–30.
36. Williams A, Lyall H, Tudor Williams G, et al. Proceedings of the European Society for Paediatric Infectious Disease, 2000. Noordwijk, The Netherlands.
37. European Collaborative Study. Children born to women with HIV-1 infection: natural history and risk of transmission. European Collaborative Study. Lancet 1991;337:253–260.
38. Blanche S, Rouzioux C, Moscato ML, et al. A prospective study of infants born to women seropositive for human immunodeficiency virus type 1, HIV Infection in Newborns French Collaborative Study Group. N Engl J Med 1989;320:1643–1648.
39. Owens DK, Holodniy M, McDonald TW, Scott J, Sonnad S. A meta-analytic evaluation of the polymerase chain reaction for the diagnosis of HIV infection in infants. JAMA 1996;275:1342–1348.
40. Centers for Disease Control and Prevention. Updated U.S. Public Health Service Guidelines for the Management of Occupational Exposures to HBV, HCV and HIV and Recommendations for Postexposure Prophylaxis. MMWR Morb Mortal Wkly Rep 2001;50:1–52.
41. Sharland M, Blanche S, Castelli G, Ramos J, Gibb DM; PENTA Steering Committee. PENTA guidelines for the use of antiretroviral therapy, 2004. HIV Med 2004;5(suppl 2):61–86.
42. http://aidsinfo.nih.gov/guidelines/default_db2.asp?id=51).
43. Notterman DA. Acquired immunodeficiency syndrome, Pneumocystis carinii pneumonia, and futility. Crit Care Med 1996;24:907–909.
44. Thirsk ER, Kapongo MC, Jeena PM, et al. HIV-exposed infants with acute respiratory failure secondary to acute lower respiratory infections managed with and without mechanical ventilation. South Afr Med J 2003;93:617–620.

13
Life-Threatening Tropical Infections

Kathryn Maitland and Bridget Wills

Global travel movements have increased tremendously over the last 40 years and are still increasing. In the 1960s the numbers of international tourist arrivals worldwide were less than 100 million. Between 1990 and 2000 the average annual growth in international tourist arrivals was 4.3% and by 2002 the worldwide figure had risen to 715 million (1,2). Globally, infectious diseases rank as the second highest cause of death after cardiovascular diseases, and in low-income countries they remain responsible for up to 45% of deaths. During the 20th century a combination of increasing prosperity, improvements in education, public health and sanitation, and the introduction of effective immunization programs resulted in deaths from infectious disease becoming a relatively rare occurrence in most rich nations. However, in parallel with the recent rise in foreign travel, the risks of encountering infectious diseases that do not occur or are uncommon in the country of residence are now increasing. In addition, increases in the numbers of legal and illegal economic migrants, as well as in refugees seeking asylum from wars or political unrest, mean that increasing numbers of children from low-income countries are becoming resident in countries with a different disease profile. Not only is the number of unvaccinated or inadequately vaccinated children at risk of acquiring diseases thought to have been controlled locally likely to rise, but also these children may present to medical care with unfamiliar tropical diseases acquired in their country of origin.

When a child presents with a possible travel-associated or tropical illness, it is important to take a detailed travel and exposure history. Important points to focus on include details of the endemicity of diseases or presence of other hazards in the countries traveled to or in the country of origin; a full vaccination history including any specific vaccinations received prior to travel; whether malaria chemoprophylaxis was taken correctly, if indicated; whether specific measures were employed to prevent insect bites and whether bites were known to have occurred; and whether other pre-travel advice regarding drinking water and consumption of street food was adhered to. For recent immigrants, details of the type of housing, standard of sanitation, and exposure to possible animal vectors in the country of origin may also be relevant.

Many parasitic, viral, and bacterial diseases may be encountered, a large proportion of them acquired via the bite of infected mosquitoes, ticks, sand flies, tsetse flies, or other arthropods. Malaria is much the most important arthropod-borne disease globally and is a significant risk to travelers. Although largely preventable by effective malaria chemoprophylaxis if prescribed and taken correctly, prophylaxis is not 100% effective. Other important parasitic diseases in terms of worldwide morbidity and mortality include trypanosomiasis, leishmaniasis, and lymphatic filariasis, but presentation of these disorders is rarely acute.

Among the arthropod-borne viral (arboviral) diseases, dengue is the most significant human infection. In recent years it has become endemic in many cities and urban areas in the tropics and is a frequent cause of serious disease. Although it has been reported in a number of travelers, mainly from Asia, it is thought to be underreported by most surveillance systems in the developed world. In contrast to dengue, most other arboviral diseases are primarily zoonotic. Severe human infections are relatively rare and are usually characterized by encephalitis, the most prevalent example worldwide being Japanese encephalitis virus (JEV) infection. Effective vaccines are available for some arboviral infections, including JEV, but the prospects for a dengue vaccine remain limited at present.

Arthropod-borne bacterial infections include Lyme disease, rickettsial infections, and plague. Although most of these diseases are seen following travel to tropical countries, some, such as Lyme disease, are associated with travel to specific geographic locations in Europe and the continental United States. Other bacterial infections may also be associated with very specific exposure. For meningococcal disease, the most significant travel risk is in Muslim pilgrims returning from the Hajj, in Mecca, in whom outbreaks of serogroup W135 have been reported. Leptospirosis may be contracted while traveling abroad, most often associated with certain recreational activities (e.g., water rafting in Thailand) (2).

The first section of this chapter focuses on the diagnosis and management of several important arthropod-borne infections: falciparum malaria and the two closely related arboviral diseases, dengue and Japanese encephalitis. We provide a comprehensive approach to the management of severe and complicated disease, but details of prophylaxis and prevention are not addressed. The second section discusses vaccine-preventable diseases that remain relatively common in the tropics but are now rarely seen in the developed world. The third section considers some of the new viral infections that have emerged in Asia in recent years and pose a serious threat to global health.

Arthropod-Borne Infections

Malaria

Epidemiology

Malaria is one of the most common and important parasite diseases worldwide. Over a third of the world's population (2 billion people) live in malaria-endemic areas, with 1 billion people estimated to carry parasites at any one time (3).

The greatest burden of malaria falls on sub-Saharan Africa (SSA), where there are an estimated 200 to 450 million children infected with malaria parasites each year. Malaria results in between 1 and 2.7 million deaths annually; however, over 90% of the world's malaria deaths occur in SSA, almost entirely in children younger than 5 years of age (4). There are four species of malaria that naturally infect humans, yet mortality is almost exclusively due to *Plasmodium falciparum*. *P. falciparum* is the commonest species throughout the tropics and subtropics, but *P. vivax* has the widest geographical range; it is prevalent in many temperate zones, but also in the subtropics and tropics. *P. malariae* is patchily present over the same geographical range as *P. falciparum* but is much less common; and *P. ovale* is found chiefly in tropical Africa. Measures to eradicate malaria have been largely ineffective. During the late 1950s and 1960s coordinated mass action, particularly with the use of the pesticide DDT, witnessed great achievements in many areas of the world, but only limited successes were achieved in Africa. A recent, more rational approach to malaria control has focused on the provision of insecticide-impregnated bed nets and access to early treatment. Nevertheless, globally malaria is on the increase. The resurgence of malaria in most tropical countries equates with an increased risk to travelers. Throughout the world, many countries are reporting an increasing number of cases of imported malaria, largely due to the great increase in long-distance travel and immigration (5–7). In the U.K., for example, although the total number of reported cases of imported malaria has remained around 2000 per year from 1979 to 2002, major changes in the pattern of imported malaria has occurred over this period. There has been a steady rise in the number and proportion of the potentially lethal falciparum malaria among these cases, from 17% in 1977 to 77% by 2001. Approximately 13% of these cases were in children younger than 15 years of age (2). Most cases of falciparum malaria were among travelers of African ethnic origin who were visiting friends and relatives in highly malarious areas but had taken no chemoprophylaxis (2).

Transmission

Natural transmission of malaria infection occurs through exposure to the bite of infective female *Anopheles* mosquitoes. Anophelines bite between dusk and dawn (whereas *Aedes* and some *Culices* mosquitoes tend to bite during the day and do not transmit malaria). Congenital infection in endemic areas is uncommon and usually manifests as a transient parasitemia, whereas disease risks are rare. Infection, however, may also be transmitted accidentally; this occurs not infrequently as a result of blood transfusion when the donor harbors malaria parasites. Drug addicts using the same hypodermic needle have also been known to infect one another (8). Cases of malaria have also been described in inhabitants living near airports ("airport malaria") who have been inoculated by infective mosquitoes from malarious areas (9).

In naturally acquired infection, the mosquito injects sporozoites into the subcutaneous tissues, and within approximately 30 minutes of inoculation these sporozoites invade parenchymal cells of the liver. The pre-erythrocytic stage lasts about 6 to 16 days before hepatic schizonts rupture, releasing many thousands of merozoites, which in turn target and invade red blood cells. During the incubation period, defined as the time elapsing between inoculation and the appearance of the first clinical symptoms, each erythrocytic cycle leads to a roughly logarithmic expansion of the parasite biomass. The incubation period varies between species and is dependent on immunity and antimalarial medication. The incubation period for *P. falciparum* is generally 9 to 14 days, *P. vivax* 12 to 17 days (although primary attack may occur up to 6 to 12 months after inoculation), *P. ovale* 16 to 18 days, and *P. malariae* 18 to 40 days.

Pathogenesis of Severe Malaria

The pathophysiology of severe malaria remains incompletely understood, but a number of processes have been proposed. First, the etiology may involve mechanical obstruction of the microvasculature mediated by a number of factors including cytoadherence of parasitized red blood cells (pRBCs) to endothelial cells within the small vessels of many tissues (10). This phenomenon is called sequestration, and is likely to be important by contributing to high total body parasitemia and focusing pathology in specific sites, for example the brain. Several postmortem studies have demonstrated greater pRBC sequestration in the brain compared with other organs (11–13). In addition to adhering to endothelial cells, mature-stage pRBC can also adhere to noninfected RBCs, forming rosettes, and to other pRBCs, forming clumps (with platelets) or autoagglutinates, which have been also been implicated in contributing to disease severity (14). Infection is also associated with a decrease in red cell deformability in both pRBCs and non-pRBCs (15). Studies have show that there is a stage-dependent decrease in the deformability of red cells as *P. falciparum* matures, and that mature parasites require correspondingly larger pressures (four- to sixfold, compared with controls) to allow entry of parasitized red cells into small (3-μm capillaries). These changes may result in reduced blood flow in the downstream (postcapillary) venules, and create a climate favorable to other pathophysiologically important processes such as cytoadherence (reviewed in ref. 16). Taken together these processes may result in reduced microvascular perfusion and lead to tissue hypoxia and acidosis. Second, the release of a variety of toxins and other soluble mediators including tumor necrosis factor-α (TNF-α) and interleukin-1 (IL-1), reactive oxygen species and neurotransmitters appears to be important (reviewed in refs. 17 and 18). In cerebral malaria (CM), since the parasites are confined to the intravascular space, the toxins produced must cross the blood–brain barrier (BBB) to affect the central nervous system (CNS). Moreover, a breakdown of the BBB leading to increased vascular permeability has been invoked to explain the features of CM (19,20).

What has become apparent is that severe malaria encompasses a complex syndrome affecting many organs, resulting in biochemical and hematologic derangements, which have many features in common with the pathophysiologic derangement seen in children with the sepsis syndrome. Among these, metabolic acidosis (manifesting as respiratory distress) has emerged as a central feature of severe malaria, and is widely recognized as the best independent predictor of a fatal outcome in adults and children (reviewed in refs. 17,21,22), mortality being greatest in the children in whom acidosis and impaired consciousness coexist. Thus, in severe malaria, impaired organ perfusion (including perfusion of the brain) appears to be an important component of the acidosis, as well as contributing to the neurologic dysfunction of CM.

Clinical Presentation

Malaria should be considered in any patient presenting with a fever who has traveled to or come from an endemic area. Although most patients present within a few weeks or months of their return, presentation may be delayed particularly in the semi-immune, those who have taken prophylaxis, and in *P. vivax, P. ovale,* and *P. malariae* infections. Ninety percent of travelers who contract malaria do not become ill until after they return home. Imported malaria is easily treated if diagnosed promptly, but follows a serious course in 12% of people, mainly due to delays in diagnosis and inappropriate treatment (23). The usual presentation is with fever within 2 weeks of exposure, but in children the presentation can sometimes be with nonspecific symptoms including cough, headache, malaise, vomiting, and diarrhea. Common supportive findings in malaria include splenomegaly, mild thrombocytopenia, and anemia. Mild jaundice is the more usual presentation in adults but is unusual in children. However, malaria should be considered in any child with fever and mild jaundice (24). While the clinical symptoms and signs do not help distinguish the infecting *Plasmodium* species, the travel history is extremely helpful (especially travel to Africa where *P. falciparum* is the most frequent infecting species) in imported malaria cases and in guiding drug selection. Noninfectious disease specialists are more likely to make errors in therapy than are infectious diseases specialists, so prompt referral is recommended. Specialist advice is recommended for children infected with *P. falciparum* returning from Southeast Asia, where multidrug resistant malaria is endemic.

Definition of Severe Malaria in Children

A precise definition of severe malaria in nonimmune children is problematic, since little information is available on the clinical spectrum of severe malaria in children outside of Africa. Furthermore, the suitability of the clinical definition of severe malaria in non- or semi-immune adults is questionable since a number of features are rarely reported in African children with severe malaria, specifically jaundice, pulmonary edema, and renal failure (24). A working definition has been proposed to guide initial assessment and emergency treatment, which draws mainly from the experience of working with critically ill African children. The definition aims to identify those at greatest risk in whom appropriate emergency management is required, but also to identify groups at risk of complications and who require close monitoring or parental medication (Table 13.1).

TABLE 13.1. Recognition of severe malaria

High: immediate risk of dying and urgent need of supportive treatment
Depressed conscious state (any level)
Status epilepticus
Irregular respirations or obstructed airway
Tachypnea or increased work of breathing (Kussmaul breathing)
Hypoxia (oxygen saturations <95%)
Hypotension (systolic blood pressure <2 SD)
Evidence of compensated shock (tachycardia, increased work of breathing, cool peripheries, capillary refilling time ≥2 seconds)
Dehydration
Severe hyperkalemia (potassium >5.5 mmol/L)
Intermediate: need for close monitoring
Hemoglobin <10 g/DL
History of convulsions in this illness
Hyperparasitemia >5%
P. falciparum in a child with sickle cell disease (due to high risk of complicated disease)
Low risk: need admission for parental medication
Vomiting or unable to take or comply with oral medication

SD, standard deviation.

Diagnosis and Laboratory Investigations

Parasitology

For those arriving back from a malarious area, three *thick* blood films taken 12 hours apart will exclude most malaria infections in any patient exposed to malaria. If clinical suspicion is high, further films are warranted. Thick films are necessary to diagnose malaria (especially when the parasite density is low), and a thin film is required to speciate the malaria. The microscopist should examine 100 thick-film high-magnification fields. Failure to prepare and rigorously examine a thick film may lead to a false-negative malaria film especially in nonimmune patients who often present with scant parasitemias. Despite this, some scanty infections may escape detection. There are now a number of other tests that are used to detect parasitemia. The *Para*Sight-F antigen-capture test uses a monoclonal antibody to histidine-rich protein 2 of *P. falciparum*. It is used on urine, requires limited expertise, and has a sensitivity and specificity of >90%. However, it is expensive, nonquantitative, and only detects the presence of *P. falciparum* but, as it is antibody dependant, it remains positive for 28 to 35 days, even when the parasite has been cleared. Newer tests such as the Optimal-IT® test (Diamed) that depend upon parasite lactate dehydrogenase and can differentiate falciparum from other species. Therefore it is less vulnerable to false positive tests once parasitemia has been cleared. The quantitative buffy coat (QBC™) technique involves centrifugation of the patient's blood in commercially supplied collection tubes that are then examined under a microscope fitted with a Paralens™ (Becton Dickson) using ultraviolet drop (UV light. The method has been reported to be easier and more sensitive than traditional thick-film analysis. However, potential drawbacks include difficulties in quantification of the parasite density, species differentiation, and wide variation between operators. Polymerase chain reaction (PCR) is useful, especially for low-level parasitemia, but it is time-consuming, expensive, and requires considerable experience.

Once the diagnosis is made, repeat blood films for parasite counts may be useful in following the progress of the disease. However, the pediatrician should be aware that, as quinine acts on the later stages (schizonts), which are the generally sequestered in the microcirculation and thus not generally visible to the microscopist examining the blood film (which generally examines the circulating younger ring stages), peripheral parasitemia might continue to increase over the first 24 hours of effective treatment. In cases presenting from Africa (where quinine resistance is rarely encountered), this rarely indicates quinine resistance and should not cause undue alarm.

Other Laboratory Investigations

To determine the range of biochemical and hematologic derangements we suggest the following basic investigations: full blood count, electrolytes (including potassium magnesium, phosphate, and calcium), urea (BUN) or creatinine, blood glucose, lactate, and a blood gas. These should be measured serially, at least 12 hourly, if the child remains critically ill. Additional blood should be obtained for blood cultures and for blood grouping, in case a transfusion is required subsequently.

Management of Malaria

Uncomplicated Malaria

For this review we focus on the management of severe malaria. For those children not fulfilling the criteria for severe disease, prompt diagnosis and specialist referral is recommended. A number of new mediations are available for those with uncomplicated falciparum malaria, including mefloquine (Lariam), atovaquone-proguanil (Malarone), or lumefantrine-artemether (Riamet or Coartem); the latter is currently the only fixed-ratio artemether combination therapy that has been developed up to international standards (Table 13.2). Due to worldwide problems with chloroquine resistance, we suggest that falciparum malaria should not be treated with chloroquine, unless the child has visited a zone without any prior reports of resistance. Similarly, for those infected in Africa, Fansidar (sulfadoxine-pyrimethamine) should also not be prescribed due to widespread resistance. Furthermore, owing to its bitter taste, compliance with an oral course of quinine is difficult for most children.

Severe Falciparum Malaria

In an analogous manner to the triage of any critically ill child, the hierarchy of the clinical assessment in severe malaria should focus on the early recognition of impending respiratory failure initially, followed by shock and then neurologic dysfunction, thus guiding early management toward the complications that are

Table 13.2. Antimalarial medication recommended for children with uncomplicated and severe malaria

Drug	Uncomplicated malaria (oral medication)	Complicated malaria (parenteral medication)
Mefloquine (Lariam)	15 mg base/kg followed by a second dose of 10 mg/kg 8–24 hours later	Quinine hydrochloride[a]: Loading dose 20 mg salt/kg IV over 4 hours then 10 mg/kg IV 8 hourly (with ECG monitoring).
Proguanil with atovaquone (Malarone)	Daily dose for 3 days: 11–20 kg: 1 tablet, 21–30 kg: 2 tablets 31–40 kg: 3 tablets >40 kg: 4 tablets (adult dose)	Quinine should be given for 7 days but in practice oral medication can be prescribed once children is able to take medication[b]
Artemether with lumefantrin (Riamet)	Given at 0, 8, 24, 36, 48, and 60 hours[c] 5–15 kg: 1 tablet 15–25 kg: 2 tablets 25–35 kg 3 tablets ≥5 kg: 4 tablets (adult dose)	Avoid oral quinine in children as the bitter taste may affect compliance

[a]In the U.S. where quinine is not routinely available, quinidine gluconate is used instead. A loading dose of 10 mg/kg is infused over 1 hour followed by a 0.02 mg/kg/min continuous infusion until parasites cleared (ECG monitoring recommended). This should be followed by a course of oral antimalarial medication (see below).
[b]Complete treatment with Malarone, Mefloquine (12 hours after preceding quinine dose), or Riamet. The *full* oral course of these follow on medications must be taken.
[c]Treatment course shown is the intensive 3-day course designed for nonimmune children and treatment where multidrug resistance is present or suspected, i.e., 8 hourly treatment on the first day, 12 hourly thereafter.

the most life-threatening (Fig. 13.1) (25). Assessment and immediate management should not be delayed while awaiting laboratory confirmation of malaria, since immediate management in suspected cases is the management of respiratory failure or shock. Within endemic areas most deaths from severe malaria occur within hours of admission (26). These generally arise from the failure to recognize impending circulatory collapse similar to that seen in septic shock, or compromised airway and respiratory failure in children with prolonged or complex seizures. Deaths arising after the first 12 hours include a small number of cases with features of raised intracranial pressure (ICP) (27). Although raised ICP is an uncommon complication, the potential to develop this complication has major implications for the initial management in those presenting in deep coma (inability to localize a painful stimulus) complicated by features of hypovolemic shock, and warrants a cautious approach to volume resuscitation in such cases. The chapter gives a detailed outline of management guideline proposed for the United Kingdom which has been previously summarized (28).

Initial Assessment and Emergency Treatments

Characteristic Respiratory Patterns of Severe Malaria

Irregular Breathing/Hypoventilation. The presence of respiratory depression or irregular breathing should alert the clinician to the presence of complex seizures, iatrogenic respiratory depression (due to multiple anticonvulsant

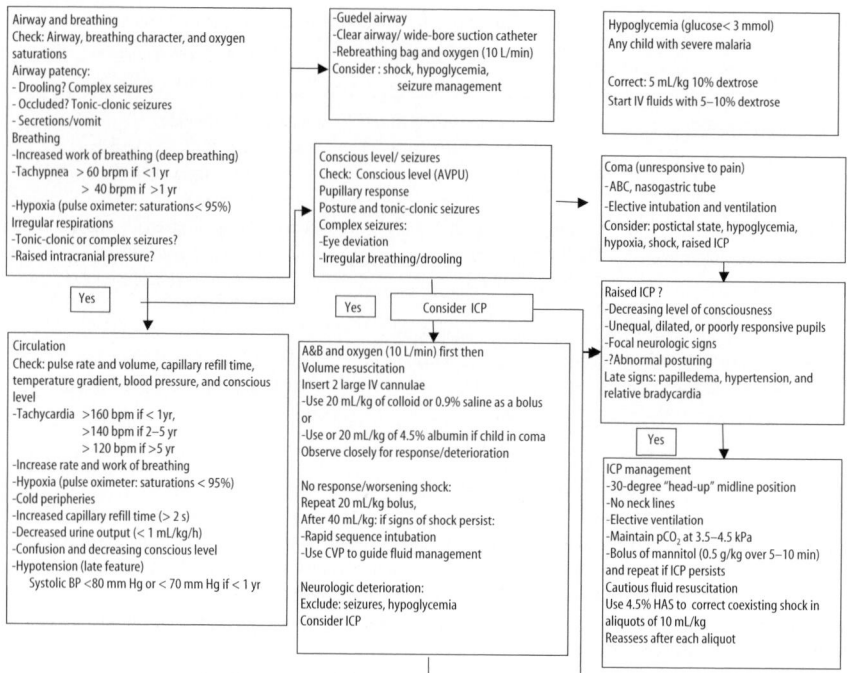

Airway and breathing
Check: Airway, breathing character, and oxygen saturations
Airway patency:
- Drooling? Complex seizures
- Occluded? Tonic-clonic seizures
- Secretions/vomit
Breathing
-Increased work of breathing (deep breathing)
-Tachypnea > 60 brpm if <1 yr
                    > 40 brpm if >1 yr
-Hypoxia (pulse oximeter: saturations< 95%)
Irregular respirations
-Tonic-clonic or complex seizures?
-Raised intracranial pressure?

-Guedel airway
-Clear airway/ wide-bore suction catheter
-Rebreathing bag and oxygen (10 L/min)
Consider : shock, hypoglycemia,
                  seizure management

Hypoglycemia (glucose< 3 mmol)
Any child with severe malaria

Correct: 5 mL/kg 10% dextrose
Start IV fluids with 5–10% dextrose

Conscious level/ seizures
Check: Conscious level (AVPU)
Pupillary response
Posture and tonic-clonic seizures
Complex seizures:
-Eye deviation
-Irregular breathing/drooling

Coma (unresponsive to pain)
-ABC, nasogastric tube
-Elective intubation and ventilation
Consider: postictal state, hypoglycemia,
hypoxia, shock, raised ICP

Yes

Yes   Consider ICP

Raised ICP ?
-Decreasing level of consciousness
-Unequal, dilated, or poorly responsive pupils
-Focal neurologic signs
-?Abnormal posturing
Late signs: papilledema, hypertension, and
relative bradycardia

Circulation
Check: pulse rate and volume, capillary refill time,
temperature gradient, blood pressure, and conscious
level
-Tachycardia >160 bpm if < 1yr,
                     >140 bpm if 2–5 yr
                     > 120 bpm if >5 yr
-Increase rate and work of breathing
-Hypoxia (pulse oximeter: saturations < 95%)
-Cold peripheries
-Increased capillary refill time (> 2 s)
-Decreased urine output (< 1 mL/kg/h)
-Confusion and decreasing conscious level
-Hypotension (late feature)
          Systolic BP <80 mm Hg or < 70 mm Hg if < 1 yr

A&B and oxygen (10 L/min) first then
Volume resuscitation
Insert 2 large IV cannulae
-Use 20 mL/kg of colloid or 0.9% saline as a bolus
or
-Use or 20 mL/kg of 4.5% albumin if child in coma
Observe closely for response/deterioration

No response/worsening shock:
Repeat 20 mL/kg bolus,
After 40 mL/kg: if signs of shock persist:
-Rapid sequence intubation
-Use CVP to guide fluid management

Neurologic deterioration:
Exclude: seizures, hypoglycemia
Consider ICP

Yes

ICP management
-30-degree "head-up" midline position
-No neck lines
-Elective ventilation
-Maintain pCO₂ at 3.5–4.5 kPa
-Bolus of mannitol (0.5 g/kg over 5–10 min)
and repeat if ICP persists
Cautious fluid resuscitation
Use 4.5% HAS to correct coexisting shock in
aliquots of 10 mL/kg
Reassess after each aliquot

FIGURE 13.1. Emergency triage assessment and management of children with severe malaria. A&B, airway and breathing; AVPU, alert, responds to voice, responds to pain, unconscious; bpm, beats per minute; brpm, breaths per minute; HAs, human albumin solution; ICP, intracranial pressure.

medications), or the possibility of raised ICP. In children with severe malaria, around 25% of seizures are subtle or subclinical (only demonstrated by electroencephalogram [EEG]) (29), frequently manifesting as eye deviation, an irregular respiratory pattern or drooling. High-flow oxygen and appropriate airway management are as important as the administration of anticonvulsants. Hypoglycemia (blood sugar <3 mmol/L) may precipitate seizures or abnormal posturing and should be considered in such cases (30).

Respiratory Distress. Children with severe malaria frequently present with respiratory distress (31). Formerly this was thought to indicate the presence of pulmonary edema, biventricular heart failure, or lower respiratory tract infection. However, studies from Kilifi, Kenya, have shown that the vast majority of cases of malaria with respiratory distress (about 95%) have a metabolic acidosis (base deficit ≥10 mmol/L) (32). This hyperventilation is typically the deep breathing of Kussmaul respiration with minimal features of intercostal indrawing. Deep breathing is typically associated with other features of shock and multiorgan impairment including cold peripheries, prolonged capillary refill time (>2 seconds), hypoxia (oxygen saturations <95%), convulsions, impaired consciousness, and hypoglycemia.

Circulation

Recognition of Shock in Severe Malaria. Many children with severe malaria have features of compensated shock. These include an increased work of breathing, tachycardia with bounding peripheral pulses or cool peripheries, prolonged capillary refill time ($\geq$2 seconds), low central venous pressure, and some alteration of consciousness (33). The question of whether any of the perturbation of conscious level in this situation is primarily a neurologic manifestation of cerebral malaria (secondary to sequestered red cells in postcapillary vascular beds within the brain), or whether they are part of a multisystem disorder akin to the severe inflammatory response syndrome is unclear. Nevertheless, since metabolic acidosis (base deficit >5 mmol/L) commonly accompanies these features of shock, including cases with impaired consciousness, we suggest that these features are due to hypovolemia and should be treated with volume expansion (33,34). Moreover, in children with severe malaria, prolonged capillary refill time ($\geq$2 seconds) has been shown to have good prognostic value, and is associated with other features of circulatory failure, such as shock and metabolic acidosis (35).

Recommendations for Volume Resuscitation. Several resuscitation fluids are available for the treatment of severe dehydration or shock in children. Simple electrolyte solutions are of proven benefit in most situations where excess water and electrolyte depletion has resulted from severe diarrhea or vomiting. In conditions such as septic shock or severe malaria there is still debate over the optimum fluid and the safety of volume resuscitation. As in sepsis, some advocate the use of colloidal solutions, which will replete water, electrolytes, and plasma oncotic pressure, thus theoretically reducing the risk of exacerbating raised ICP. There is undoubtedly some risk that aggressive volume expansion would accentuate ICP. Noncolloidal solutions, such as 0.9% saline, move rapidly from the intravascular compartment into the tissues with the potential risk of exacerbating raised ICP and pulmonary edema. It has been shown recently that volume resuscitation with 20 to 40 mL/kg of either 0.9% saline or 4.5% human albumin solution (HAS) leads to correction of the hemodynamic features of shock and improved renal function (36). Volume expansion with either 0.9% saline or HAS in children *without coma* appeared to be safe and led to a reduced case fatality of one in 72 patients (1.4%) compared to a historic controls (15% to 20%), indicating the potential value and safety of volume expansion in this high-risk group. Nevertheless, we advise caution when treating children with coma (inability to localize pain). In the same trial, children presenting in coma together with features of shock, 11 of 24 (46%) receiving 0.9% saline died, compared to only one of 21 (5%) of those receiving 4.5% HAS (relative risk, 9.6; 95% confidence interval [CI] 1.4–68; p = .002 (36). Until further data become available from larger trials, we recommend that 4.5% HAS should be considered the resuscitation fluid of choice in the subgroup of children with severe malaria who present with coma and shock. The relative benefit of albumin over other resuscitation fluids including saline and gelatin-based colloids has been recently

established in a small phase II trail (volume expansion with albumin compared to gelofusine in children with severe malaria: results of a controlled trial. Plos Clinical Trials [36a]).

Volume resuscitation should proceed cautiously and be terminated once there is a satisfactory cardiovascular response to the volume challenge. In these children urinary output should be monitored from the outset, as it is a good indicator of renal perfusion. A reduction in urine output to <1 mL/kg/h is likely to indicate, in the absence of urinary retention, impaired renal perfusion secondary to hypovolemia. Reevaluation of the respiratory and circulatory status after each intervention is important. For any child with persisting features of shock after 40 mL/kg of fluid resuscitation, elective tracheal intubation and ventilation, and placement of a central venous line to guide further fluid management is recommended. Pulmonary edema is a rare complication of volume expansion (<0.5%) (36).

The Child with Impaired Consciousness

The presentation of an acute neurologic syndrome characterized by impaired consciousness, convulsions, abnormal neurologic signs, and opisthotonic posturing indicates the features of (CM) (37,38). However, in a small number of children, these features may also suggest raised ICP (27). Intracranial pressure monitoring and postmortem studies in a two different series of patients with a prolonged and complicated course have demonstrated that brain swelling is a major feature in fatal cases (13,27). Nevertheless, in most cases, signs suggestive of raised ICP developed in the later stages of the illness, along with features compatible with transtentorial herniation in the agonal stages. The pathogenesis of the intracranial hypertension in cerebral malaria is unclear (39). Cranial computed tomography (CT) studies in adults and children with CM have failed to demonstrate hydrocephalus (39,40), and there is a lack of gross cerebral edema at postmortem (13). It has been suggested that the raised ICP stems from an increase cerebral blood volume (CBV) (41). Increases in the CBV may result from the red cell sequestration in the cerebral venules, leading to impaired venous return, or increased cerebral blood flow caused by seizure activity and anemia.

Management of the Unconscious Child. The initial management should include maintenance of the airway, support of breathing, and immediate correction of hypoglycemia and volume deficits. This will correct hypoxia, hypoglycemia, and shock, which are potential contributors to the depressed conscious level. Rapid assessment of neurologic function should include an assessment of the conscious level, pupillary size, and reaction to light, in addition to observing the child's posture and convulsive movements, if present. Finally, meningitis should be considered as an alternative diagnosis in a child with neck stiffness or a full fontanel.

A child who is unresponsive to pain (coma) or a child with impaired consciousness and features suggestive of raised ICP warrants elective tracheal intubation and ventilation. For those with seizures, the decision to ventilate could be delayed if they are in a postictal state, as long as the airway is patent.

Repeated seizures and a whole range of posturing movements are commonly seen in severe malaria, making the diagnosis of raised ICP difficult. Nevertheless, owing to the potential risk of raised ICP, artificial ventilation should aim to optimize the pCO_2 in the normal range (38). Other supportive treatments and standard management should continue as recommended. Patients with severe acidosis may self-ventilate their pCO_2 to very low levels as compensation for the metabolic acidosis. Great care should be taken when initiating ventilation to avoid a sudden rise of pCO_2, even to normal levels, before the metabolic acidosis has been partially corrected. If the patient is still shocked or if the shocked state returns, then treatment of shock should take priority, since brain perfusion depends on adequate cardiac output. The therapeutic dilemma in this group of children is reminiscent of the similar predicament in the treatment of meningitis, in which it was customary in the past to volume restrict. Recent studies in meningitis have shown that, when compared to volume expansion, modest fluid restriction is detrimental to outcome (42,43). We suggest cautious volume expansion with 4.5% HAS and careful close monitoring.

Raised Intracranial Pressure

From personal experience, this complication is uncommon in nonimmune children with imported malaria. However, it should be suspected in those with signs of raised ICP, which include a declining level of consciousness; focal neurologic signs, such as unequal, dilated, or poorly responsive pupils; abnormal posturing; hypertension; and relative bradycardia (27,38). Papilledema is a late finding in acutely raised ICP. In a series of children who developed raised ICP in severe malaria, the only sign that was associated with the development of intermediate or severe intracranial hypertension was sluggish or absent pupillary response (39). Other signs (such as absent or extensor motor response, pupillary dilatation, decerebrate posturing, or absent oculocephalic reflexes) were not predictive. Caution is advocated for the diagnosis of raised ICP in children in the peri- or postictal state, where the pupillary signs and conscious level may be difficult to interpret.

The development of features suggestive of raised ICP in children is an emergency and should be treated by urgent tracheal intubation, with CO_2 monitoring by capnography (44). To optimize and stabilize cerebral blood flow, the pCO_2 should be kept within the normal range. Mannitol (0.5 g/kg infused over 5 to 10 minutes) may be effective in lowering the ICP, but previous studies conducted with ICP monitoring showed that its short-lived effect meant that repeated doses were often necessary. The use of steroids to control brain swelling in severe malaria is not recommended, as their effect on raised ICP remains unclear, and their use has been show to lead to adverse outcome in adults with severe malaria (24).

Seizure Control

Seizures are very common in childhood malaria. Most present as tonic-clonic convulsions. However, complex seizures are also common and may manifest as bizarre posturing, eye deviation, an irregular respiratory pattern, or drooling (45,46). After ensuring adequate airway and respiratory support, specific management should follow local protocols or evidence-based guidelines, such as the one recommended by the Advanced Paediatric Life Support Group, in the United Kingdom (47) (Fig. 13.2). The routine use of phenobarbitone or phenytoin for seizure prophylaxis is not recommended (24). Both phenytoin and phenobarbitone appear to be safe in children with severe malaria, but a previous trial has shown an increased risk of death in those receiving a 20-mg/kg phenobarbitone loading dose, particularly if administered to children receiving two or more doses of diazepam over the following 24 hours (48). Phenobarbitone (18 mg/kg) has been used to treat status epilepticus in these children (49),

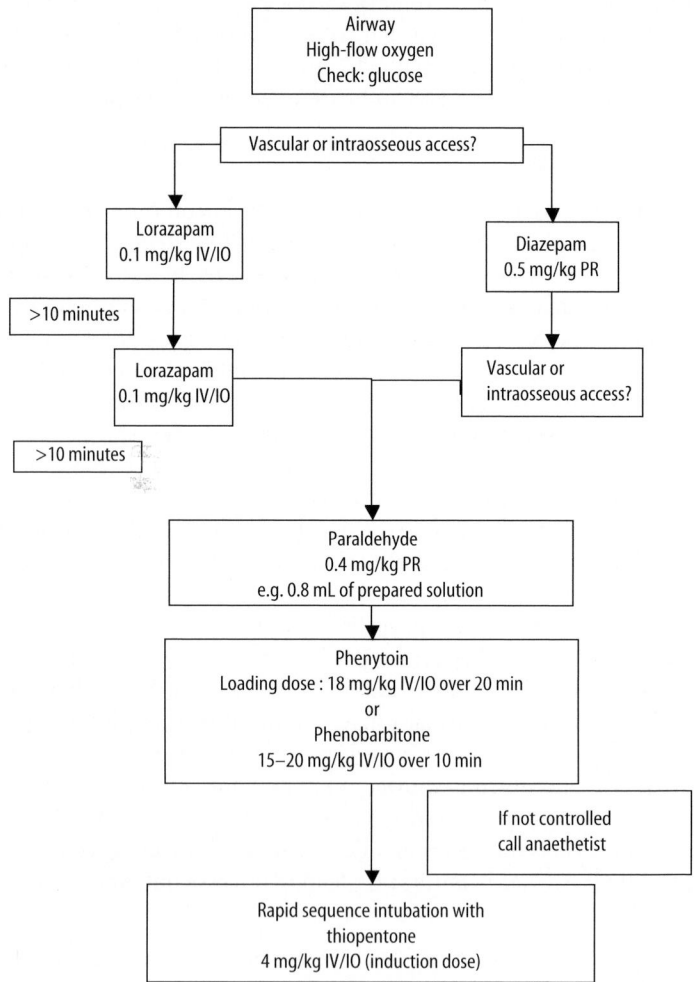

FIGURE 13.2. Suggested algorithm for management of seizures. IO, intraocular; PR, per rectum.

but phenytoin may be a better alternative (50). The safe use of anticonvulsants in a modern PICU setting is likely to differ greatly from that in African centers, where ventilatory support is not available. Control of convulsions should therefore follow the standard algorithm shown in Figure 13.2.

General Management and Complications

Antimalarial Medications. Parenteral quinine, prescribed as quinine dihydrochloride (122 mg salt contains 100 mg quinine base), remains the first-line treatment of severe falciparum malaria. An initial loading dose of 20 mg quinine salt/kg should be infused over 4 hours, followed by 10-mg/kg infusions every 8 hours thereafter. Intravenous quinine should also be prescribed to any child with *P. falciparum* malaria who is unable to take oral medication or is vomiting. Caution is recommended for those who have taken mefloquine (Lariam) prophylaxis in the previous 24 hours. Mefloquine is a synthetic analogue of quinine, and the quinine-loading dose should be omitted if the patient has taken mefloquine prophylaxis in the previous 24 hours or received a treatment dose within the previous 3 days. Quinine should be prescribed for 7 days; however, once the child can take oral medication, follow-up treatment with another antimalarial is recommended (since quinine's bitter taste precludes its oral prescription to children as it substantially increase the likelihood of poor compliance and therefore effective parasitological cure). Mefloquine (Lariam), atovaquone-proguanil (Malarone), and lumefantrine-artemether (Coartem; currently the only fixed ratio artemether combination therapy that has been developed up to international standards), are potential choices for completion of treatment. The dosing schedule is outline in Table 13.2. For travelers returning from Southeast Asia where quinine resistance is problematic, advice regarding the use of intravenous artesunate should be sought from specialist tropical medicine centers.

Metabolic Derangement. Children with severe malaria often have profound derangements in acid–base balance (metabolic acidosis and respiratory compensation) (51,52), glucose metabolism (hypoglycemia) (30), and electrolyte perturbations (53). Acidosis generally resolves with the correction of hypovolemia by adequate fluid resuscitation or blood transfusion in children developing anemia. The management of severe acidosis, which is refractory to volume expansion, is a difficult problem. Severe acidosis may depress myocardial function and increase the risk of cardiac arrest. However, correction with sodium bicarbonate carries the risk of paradoxical worsening of intracranial acidosis, as the resultant reduction in respiratory drive and increase in carbon dioxide (CO_2) production may increase blood pCO_2. As CO_2 rapidly diffuses across the BBB, it may paradoxically worsen intracranial acidosis. This dilemma in the use of bicarbonate is reminiscent of the situation in diabetic ketoacidosis. A pragmatic solution is to administer bicarbonate only to patients with profound acidosis resistant to resuscitation and only with careful control of ventilation to maintain pCO_2 in the normal range. Hypoglycemia (blood glucose <3 mmol/L) is a common finding, and usually correlates with severity of illness. It should be corrected (Fig. 13.1) and the provision of maintenance fluids containing 5% to 10% glucose should be started once resuscitation is complete, to prevent recurrence. Although quinine may cause hypoglycemia secondary to insulin release, its occurrence in African children has been less frequently observed than in Thai adults (54).

Fluids and Electrolytes. Once fluid deficits have been corrected, patients should be on maintenance intravenous fluid until they are able to take oral fluids. Electrolyte derangements are common in children with severe malaria, especially cases complicated by acidosis. Hypercalcemia (corrected total calcium >2.62 mmol/L) and hyperkalemia (potassium >5.5 mmol/L) may be present at admission, the latter being associated with a poor prognosis. Hyperkalemia probably results from the lysis of potassium-rich red blood cells, an inevitable consequence of malaria infection. Mild, asymptomatic deficiencies of magnesium (25% to 30%) and phosphate (about 30%) develop after admission. In areas where point-of-care monitoring is not possible, the deficiencies of magnesium and phosphate were left uncorrected and were not associated with an adverse outcome (53). Hypocalcemia appears to be an infrequent complication. Conversely, hypokalemia (potassium <3.0 mmol/L) is a common complication of severe malaria; however, it is often not apparent on admission. On correction of the acidosis, plasma potassium may fall precipitously due to transcellular shifts and increased fractional excretion of potassium and the transtubular gradient of potassium indicating abnormal renal potassium loss (55). Careful, serial monitoring of serum potassium is suggested, and potassium supplementation should be considered for most children within 24 hours of admission, but only prescribed after correction of volume deficits (>8 hours).

Other Supportive Treatment. Secondary bacterial infection may occur and empiric broad-spectrum antibiotics are warranted, for example ceftriaxone 100 mg/kg/day. In cases complicated by impaired consciousness, lumbar puncture to exclude meningoencephalitis should be deferred until after the acute phase of cerebral malaria, especially in the presence of focal (in particular brainstem) neurologic signs and until the possibility of raised ICP has been excluded. Hyperpyrexia is common and increases the risk of convulsions in children, so it should be treated with antipyretics and sponging with tepid water. Acetaminophen and ibuprofen may be used, but the latter should be used cautiously in children with evidence of renal impairment and thrombocytopenia (platelet count $<50 \times 10^9$/L). All patients with malaria have some reduction of hemoglobin concentration. Most remain stable and do not require transfusion. The decision to transfuse may be influenced by the parasitemia level and clinical condition of the patient. The presence of anemia and respiratory distress may indicate the presence of lactic acidosis, and generally responds to whole blood transfusion, since these children are frequently both anemic and hypovolemic. In many hospitals in Africa, up to 50% of children admitted with severe malaria receive a blood transfusion (56), so in order to make blood available for the most needy, blood transfusion is generally only recommended for those with a hemoglobin concentration of less than 5 g/dL (24). In areas where there is provision of a safe, readily available supply of blood for transfusion, we suggest transfusion if the hemoglobin concentration falls below an absolute value of 7 g/dL, but transfusion should be considered at a higher level of hemoglobin, for example, <10 g/dL in children with sustained features of severity or hyperparasitemia (>5%). The platelet count is invariably low and the degree of thrombocytopenia is related to the severity of the disease, but bleeding is rare (57). In severe falciparum malaria, adhesion molecule upregulation has been demonstrated (58,59) and thrombomodulin levels have been reported to be high (59,60), suggesting that any coagulation activation seen might be due to endothelial dysfunction. Few detailed studies exist of coagulation abnormalities in severe malaria. Frank disseminated intravascular coagulation (DIC) is rare (57,61) despite frequent thrombocytopenia, and purpura fulminans has been reported in isolated case reports. In children, coagulopathy is a rare occurrence but should be corrected with fresh frozen plasma.

Role of Exchange Transfusion

Exchange transfusion (ET) was first reported as an adjunct to the treatment of severe malaria in 1974 (62). Since then, numerous accounts based on small case series have been published reporting its successful use in the treatment of severe malaria. The role of red cell exchange transfusion has also been advocated in the same condition (63). Although there have been no randomized trials of exchange transfusion in either adults or children (62), the World Health Organization (WHO) advocates its use in cases with hyperparasitemia (>10%) in adult intensive care unit (ICU) settings, despite evidence to suggest that it may not confer a better outcome (64). In the vast number of reports, poor study design including the use of historic control groups, groups from different centers, or even different malaria endemicities (hence differences in immunity between the subjects) make interpretation difficult. In addition, comparing data between reports is further complicated by a lack of uniformity in the definitions of severe malaria, in the criteria dictating the use of ET, in the protocols for the procedure itself, and in the outcome measures.

The vast majority of children, even those with high degree parasitemia (up to 25%), respond rapidly to the support outlined above. Nevertheless, there are a number of theoretical advantages of exchange transfusion including the provision of new red cells, thus improving the rheologic properties of circulating red cell mass. We suggest that ET should be considered as an adjunctive therapy in children with persistent acidosis and multiorgan impairment who are not responsive to the resuscitation outlined above. Exchange transfusion may be considered as a means of rapidly reducing the level of abnormal red cells, or parasite toxins. One group that may derive substantial benefit from ET or red cell ET are children with sickle cell disease, due to the inherent propensity of the red cell to become rigid under stress, and a group in whom the prognosis is much more guarded. Nevertheless, the value of ET or red cell ET should be regarded as experimental until further data become available.

Further Management and Prognosis

Coma is often of 2 to 3 days' duration even in the absence of raised ICP. Unlike sepsis, refractory shock rarely complicates severe malaria, perhaps owing to the lack of gross capillary leak syndrome. Nevertheless, complications of fluid overload, including pulmonary edema or raised ICP, should be closely monitored. Raised ICP may complicate cases, especially in children presenting in coma. Frequent reassessment and close monitoring of critically ill children identify most complications, which have been covered above. The outlook for those surviving malaria is good. However, data from African children suggest that approximately 10% of children with CM (defined by coma) will have a severe neurologic deficit at discharge (4). An even greater number have learning and language disorders. Nevertheless, most experience has been drawn from a population for which there are often significant delays in presentation to hospital, and access to modern intensive care facilities is not possible.

Dengue

Transmission and Epidemiology

The dengue virus is a small single-stranded, positive-sense RNA virus. Four closely related but antigenically distinct viral serotypes (DENV-1, -2, -3, and -4) exist, and together constitute one subgroup of the genus *Flavivirus*, family Flaviviridae (65). Humans are the primary vertebrate hosts, and Aedes mosquitoes of the subgenus *Stegomyia* are the primary mosquito vectors for all four serotypes. The major vector, *Ae. aegypti,* is a day-biting highly domesticated mosquito that is well adapted to urban environments.

Dengue is estimated to affect 50 to 100 million people each year, and some 2.5 billion people live in areas of risk (66,67). Intermittent outbreaks of what is thought to have been dengue have been known for more than 200 years. However, during the latter half of the 20th century a dramatic and progressive increase in the number and severity of reported cases occurred, particularly in the heavily populated urban centers of Southeast Asia. Dengue is now endemic in many Asian cities, with major epidemics occurring at 3- to 5-year intervals. In addition, the geographic distribution of the dengue viruses and their mosquito vectors has gradually expanded, and dengue has emerged as a significant public health problem in the Pacific region and the Americas, as well as throughout Asia (68). Cases have also been reported from some African countries and from parts of Australia. A map showing the world distribution of dengue in the year 2000 is shown in Figure 13.3. The diagnosis must be considered in all patients presenting with a febrile illness within 2 weeks of travel to any of these areas.

Infection with any of the four serotypes can cause a wide variety of clinical disease manifestations in infected individuals, ranging from asymptomatic infection to life-threatening hypovolemic shock and hemorrhage (Fig. 13.4) (69). The classic view has been that two distinct disease entities exist: dengue

World Distribution of Dengue–2000

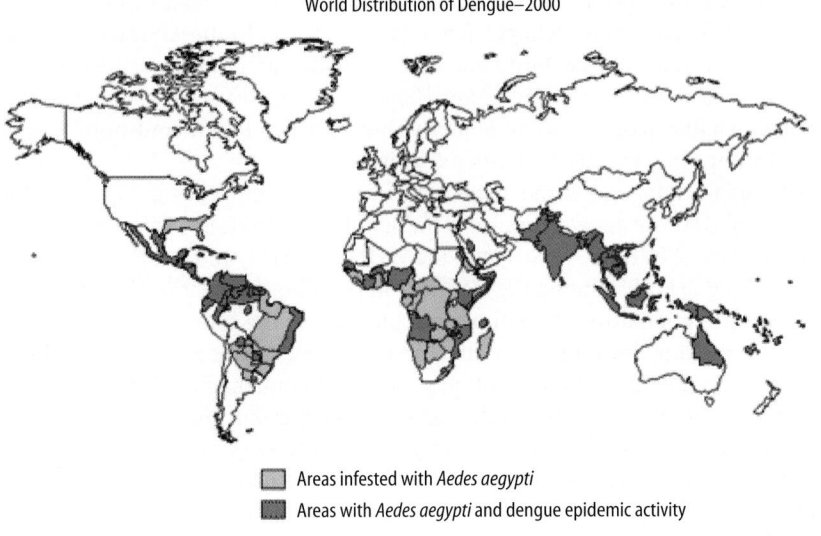

☐ Areas infested with *Aedes aegypti*
■ Areas with *Aedes aegypti* and dengue epidemic activity

CDC

Figure 13.3. Map showing areas of the world reporting epidemic dengue activity in the year 2000, together with the distribution of the major mosquito vector for the dengue virus. (From cdc.gov/ncidod/dvbid/dengue/)

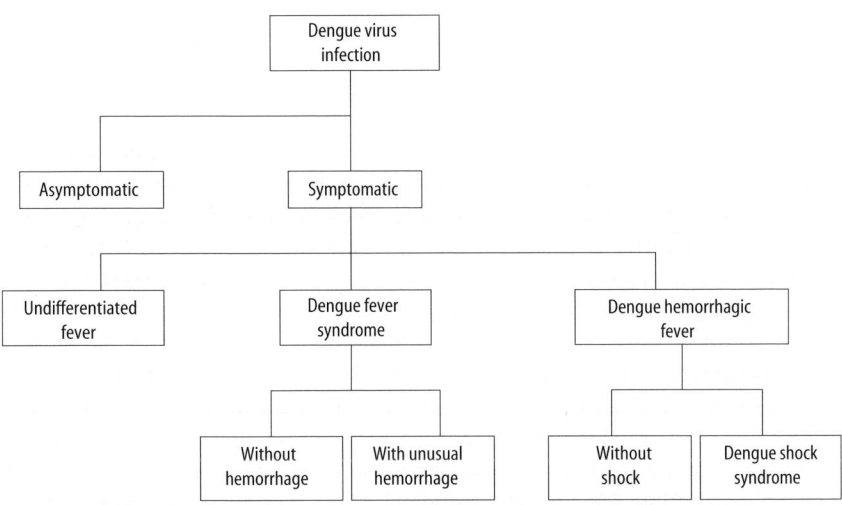

Figure 13.4. Schematic diagram illustrating the common clinical manifestations of dengue infection. (From Reference 67.)

fever (DF), a nonspecific febrile illness with prominent constitutional symptoms; and dengue hemorrhagic fever (DHF), a syndrome characterized by increased vascular permeability and altered hemostasis, resulting respectively in capillary leak syndrome and hemorrhage. In recent years, however, this view has been challenged, and there is increasing evidence that a continuous, or at least overlapping, spectrum of disease exists (70–72).

Although adults sometimes experience serious complications, globally the burden of DHF or severe disease falls mainly on children. Some 250,000 to 500,000 cases of DHF are reported to the WHO each year, and in many countries in Asia dengue ranks among the leading causes of hospitalization and death for the pediatric population. Infection with any one of the four dengue serotypes provides lifelong immunity to that serotype, but without cross-protective immunity to the other three serotypes. Dengue hemorrhagic fever occurs predominantly in older children and young adults experiencing a second (or subsequent) infection with a dengue virus serotype different from that encountered during any prior infection (73,74). However, only a small proportion of second infections result in DHF. By adulthood, most people living in endemic areas have already been exposed to all the local serotypes and are immune to subsequent infection unless a new serotype is introduced.

Among patients who do develop DHF, shock is less frequent and less severe in older age groups (75), probably reflecting maturation in intrinsic vascular permeability control mechanisms with increasing age (76). Unfortunately, however, infants with residual transmitted maternal antibody experiencing their first dengue infection are also at risk of DHF and may develop profound shock.

Pathogenesis

The pathogenesis of dengue is poorly understood. The theory of antibody-dependent enhancement (ADE) was the first to be invoked to explain the observation that more severe disease was associated with secondary infections. The ADE hypothesis suggests that heterotypic nonneutralizing antibodies elicited in response to the first infection bind to the virus introduced in the second infection, and form antibody-virus complexes that bind to Fc receptors of monocytes and macrophages, increasing uptake and productive infection in these cells, and setting in train a cascade of inflammatory events (77,78). Rapid mobilization of serotype cross-reactive memory T cells, the phenomenon of "original antigenic sin," has been suggested as an alternative mechanism to trigger the inflammatory cascade, release vasoactive molecules, and precipitate DHF (79). Cross-reactive memory cells may be less effective at clearing the infecting serotype, leading to higher viral loads and increased immunopathology. Other possible mechanisms for which there is some supportive evidence include molecular mimicry (80,81), immune complex mediated disease (82–84), and complement activation (85–87). However, although a range of markers of immune activation have been found in association with severe disease in secondary dengue infections (88–90), these responses do not differ significantly from those occurring in other viral infections, most of which do not progress to a hemorrhagic shock syndrome.

Although most cases of DHF occur in patients experiencing a second dengue virus infection, or in very young children with residual maternal antibodies, it is also occasionally seen in primary infections, indicating that viral virulence factors may play a role (91–92). Epidemics associated with significant DHF occurrence have been recorded for all four serotypes, but it has been suggested that the sequence of acquisition of the serotypes may be relevant (74). In addition, considerable genetic variation exists within serotypes, and there is epidemiologic evidence to indicate that certain strains, for example the Southeast Asian DENV-2 strain, are more virulent than others (93). Various human genetic markers have also been examined, and a variety of human leukocyte antigen (HLA) alleles and polymorphic non-HLA host genetic factors associated with both susceptibility and resistance to severe disease have been identified (94–96).

A complex interaction between host and virus is likely to determine disease severity, and it is probable that many of the factors mentioned above do play an important role in pathogenesis. However, the two characteristic features of severe dengue infection, increased vascular permeability and disordered hemostasis, suggest involvement of the endothelium in the disease process, but as yet no clear link between any of these factors and vascular endothelial dysfunction has been demonstrated. Although in vitro dengue virus has been shown to infect a wide range of cells of endothelial and epithelial derivation, the major sites of dengue virus replication in the human host remain uncertain (97). Infection of peripheral blood mononuclear cells definitely occurs, but there is currently no evidence to support infection of endothelial cells during acute disease. However, current theories on the control of microvascular permeability suggest that it is regulated at the level of the endothelial surface glycocalyx rather than by endothelial cells per se (98,99). Preliminary evidence from children with shock indicates that one of the important glycosaminoglycan constituents of the glycocalyx layer is altered during dengue infections, suggesting that structural or functional changes in the glycocalyx layer may be important in pathogenesis (100). Research efforts to try to link aspects of the inflammatory response to effector mechanisms at the vascular endothelial level continue.

Clinical Manifestations

Conventionally, clinical dengue disease is considered to consist of two separate entities, DF and DHF, although the idea of a continuous spectrum of disease is gaining credence. The important features differentiating DHF or severe dengue from uncomplicated infections are discussed below and summarized in Table 13.3.

TABLE 13.3. Recognition of severe dengue

High risk: need for immediate resuscitation/supportive care (ITU/HDU)
    Signs of cardiovascular compromise
        Pulse pressure ≤20 mm Hg
        Hypotension for age
        Weak pulse and poor peripheral perfusion (tachycardia often absent)
    Signs of respiratory compromise (usually only apparent after fluid resuscitation)
        Tachypnea/recession
        Pleural effusions or ascites
    Signs of cerebrovascular compromise
        Drowsiness, confusion, lethargy (late signs)
        Convulsions (rare)
    Significant mucosal bleeding, usually gastrointestinal
    Obvious jaundice

Intermediate risk: need for close observation and regular hematologic monitoring (HDU)
    High (>50%) or rapidly rising hematocrit
    Any spontaneous mucosal bleeding, or severe skin bleeding such as large hematomas at injection sites
    Marked thrombocytopenia (<20,000–30,000 platelets/mm^3)
    Increasing abdominal pain or marked hepatic tenderness

Low risk: admission required for symptom control (pediatric ward)
    Persistent vomiting

HDU, hemodialysis unit; ITU, intensive therapy unit.

Dengue Fever/Mild Dengue

Five to seven days on average following an infected mosquito bite, DF begins suddenly with high fever and nonspecific constitutional symptoms. Anorexia, nausea, and vomiting are common. Headache, retro-orbital pain, myalgia, and arthralgia are also often reported, but adults appear to be more symptomatic in this respect than children. On examination, a faint and evanescent macular rash may be seen, and the face may appear flushed, with conjunctival suffusion. Mild generalized lymphadenopathy and hepatomegaly are usual, but splenomegaly is rare. Minor skin bleeding and a positive tourniquet test are quite common, and occasionally major gastrointestinal bleeding occurs, usually in teenagers or young adults. The high fever persists for 5 to 7 days, sometimes with a saddleback pattern, and usually terminates abruptly. A maculopapular rash may appear on the face and limbs around this time, especially in older children and adults. Sometimes this convalescent rash is extremely florid, with an intensely erythematous appearance interspersed with islands of normal skin. The rash fades after a few days but desquamation and pruritus may occur subsequently. Adults often complain of extreme tiredness for weeks after recovery, and convalescence may be complicated by depression.

The differential diagnosis of classic DF includes other arboviral infections (such as chikungunya), as well as measles, rubella, enterovirus infections, adenovirus infections, and influenza. Other differential diagnoses that should be considered, depending on local disease prevalence, include typhoid, malaria, leptospirosis, hepatitis A, rickettsial diseases, and bacterial sepsis.

Dengue Hemorrhagic Fever/Severe Dengue

Shock is the most important manifestation of severe dengue in children. During the initial febrile phase DHF is indistinguishable from DF, except that vomiting, abdominal pain, and increasingly tender hepatomegaly are more prominent among patients with DHF. Increased vascular permeability is probably present from the early stages, but does not usually become apparent until 4 to 5 days into the illness, often around the time the fever settles. Although plasma proteins and fluid leak gradually from the intravascular compartment to the interstitium, initially plasma volume is maintained probably by a compensatory increase in lymphatic return to the circulation. However, after several days of ongoing protein loss, plasma volume becomes compromised, hematocrit starts to rise, and additional compensatory cardiovascular, renal, and adrenal mechanisms come into play. Eventually peripheral vasoconstriction occurs, and the diastolic blood pressure begins to rise and the pulse pressure to narrow. Paradoxically, many children do not develop a tachycardia despite profound hypovolemia, and during the later stages of the illness minor degrees of heart block may even be noted. Once the pulse pressure narrows to less than an arbitrary level of 20 mm Hg, the patient is considered to have dengue shock syndrome (DSS) (69), but may appear disconcertingly well and complain only of vague abdominal pain and tiredness. Narrowing of the pulse pressure is unique to DSS, and a fall in the systolic pressure is a late phenomenon; sequential blood pressure recordings of 100/70, 100/80, and 100/90 suggest that cardiovascular collapse is imminent. If fluid resuscitation is not instituted promptly, the ongoing depletion of plasma volume becomes critical, the systolic blood pressure falls rapidly, and irreversible shock and death may follow.

Clinical identification of increased vascular permeability is difficult until or unless cardiovascular decompensation develops. Diagnosis relies on serial hematocrit determinations during the febrile phase, with demonstration of a progressive rise over time. Accumulation of leaked fluid in the pleural and peritoneal cavities or the interstitium rarely becomes apparent until shock is established or considerable volumes of parenteral fluid therapy have been administered. Early presentation with shock (day 3 of fever) or very narrow pulse pressure (≤10 mm Hg) indicates very severe leakage (72). The increase in permeability is transient and usually resolves within 48 to 72 hours of becoming clinically apparent. Spontaneous reabsorption of the excess interstitial fluid begins around the sixth to eighth day of illness and progresses rapidly. With appropriate management the outcome is generally good and convalescence is usually short and uneventful, although a rash similar to that seen with DF may be apparent in older children and adolescents.

The term *dengue hemorrhagic fever* was coined to reflect the fact that some form of hemorrhagic manifestation was thought always to accompany the increase in vascular permeability. However, it is clear that patients with DF (i.e., without obvious vascular leakage) may also experience bleeding (101,102), and that many children with shock due to vascular leakage have no or only minor bleeding (72,103). Bleeding manifestations are more frequently encountered in adults infected with dengue. In most children bleeding is limited to the presence of skin petechiae, a positive tourniquet test, or bruising at venepuncture sites. Epistaxis, gum and gastrointestinal bleeding are less common but may occasionally be severe. Rarely, massive gastrointestinal bleeding has been reported to cause hemorrhagic shock, as distinct from shock due to vascular leak. However, significant gastrointestinal bleeding is usually seen only as a late phenomenon in children with very severe or protracted shock who are profoundly compromised (103). Intracranial hemorrhage is rare.

In addition to the major clinical categories discussed above, children with dengue may sometimes present with hepatic or neurologic problems. Although mild to moderate hepatomegaly is common in both DF and DHF, fulminant liver failure is unusual; if it occurs, mortality tends to be high (104,105). A possible association with aspirin or consumption of traditional medicine or herbal remedies has led some clinicians to suspect a Reye's-like syndrome, and occasionally ammonia levels have been found to be elevated. Dengue encephalopathy is a relatively rare occurrence usually seen in those with prolonged shock, hypoxia, and acidosis, or very rarely following an intracranial hemorrhage. However, there is now increasing awareness that a true encephalitis with direct viral invasion of the CNS does sometimes occur (106–108). Febrile convulsions are an infrequent occurrence in young children with dengue.

In the early stages of DHF the differential diagnosis encompasses the same range of disorders as DF, and familiarity with local disease patterns determines which specific diagnoses need to be considered. However, the occurrence of shock around the fourth or fifth day of a febrile illness in a child from a dengue endemic area is virtually pathognomonic for DSS.

Diagnosis

The World Health Organization Case Definitions for Dengue

The WHO has proposed clinical case definitions for DF, DHF, and DSS to assist with diagnosis and management, and to facilitate collection of epidemiologic data (69,109). Laboratory confirmation is required to support a diagnosis of DF, as the symptoms resemble those of many other viral infections common in childhood.

It is suggested that in endemic areas, DHF can be diagnosed provided the following four features are present: fever, a hemorrhagic tendency, thrombocytopenia with a platelet nadir of $\leq100,000/mm^3$, and evidence of plasma leakage. A diagnosis of DSS is made if all four criteria are present together with signs of circulatory failure. Unfortunately, some patients with confirmed dengue and vascular leakage of sufficient severity to result in shock are not identified as having DHF or DSS using these case definitions (71,72). In addition, differentiation between DF and DHF without shock is not always straightforward. Possible revisions to make the classification scheme more workable in clinical situations are under discussion.

Laboratory Diagnosis

During the febrile stage of the illness the optimal method for laboratory diagnosis is virus isolation by inoculation of plasma into *Toxorhynchites splendens* mosquitoes (110). Circulating virus remains readily detectable up to about 5 days after the onset of symptoms (111). Viral RNA can also be detected by reverse-transcription PCR, and this method is usually positive until later in the course of the illness. Several different protocols are available, including methods suitable to identify the infecting virus serotype (112–114).

Serologic diagnosis is complicated by the existence of cross-reactive antigenic determinants shared by dengue and other members of the flavivirus family. Capture enzyme-linked immunosorbent assay (ELISA) techniques are now the most commonly employed method for serologic diagnosis, but in view of this cross-reactivity it is necessary to include tests for other locally prevalent flaviviruses in parallel with dengue virus serology (115). In regions where JEV co-circulates with dengue, quantitative techniques that measure the relative levels of antidengue and anti-JEV immunoglobulin M (IgM) and IgG can differentiate between the two infections. The antibody response to a secondary infection is markedly different from that elicited by a primary infection. In primary infections virtually all patients will develop detectable levels of IgM within 2 days of defervescence, peaking within 2 weeks, and then decaying to become undetectable 2 to 3 months after infection. In secondary infections, IgG is detectable even in the acute phase, and the level rises quickly over the first 2 weeks, whereas IgM is absent or low, rises little in comparison to IgG, and declines quickly. Thus, the antidengue IgM and IgG capture ELISA responses can be used to discriminate primary from secondary infections.

Laboratory Investigations

Dengue Fever

Patients with DF are usually leukopenic for the first few days, but may go on to develop a lymphocytosis, often including many atypical lymphocytes (116). Thrombocytopenia is often noted, but the hematocrit and coagulation screening tests are said to be normal (117). However, very few patients with classic DF have been closely followed with respect to these indices. Hepatic transaminases are often mildly elevated.

Dengue Hemorrhagic Fever/Severe Dengue

In children with DHF, basic laboratory findings are usually more deranged, though similar to the findings in DF. Changes in hematocrit can be helpful in assessing the severity of the vascular leakage. An increase in hematocrit to ≥20% of the baseline value or the expected mean for the population is accepted as evidence of plasma leakage in the WHO dengue classification scheme (69). Unfortunately, many children do not present until hemoconcentration is well established, and baseline population data are rarely available. However, serial hematocrit measurements are very valuable for directing fluid therapy, particularly in those with shock.

Moderate to severe thrombocytopenia is very common in patients with DHF. A drop in the platelet count to ≤100,000/mm^3 forms one of the WHO diagnostic criteria for DHF (69), although in reality some patients do not reach this cutoff point even when shocked. Platelet nadirs of ≤20,000/mm^3 are not infrequent however, usually around the fifth or sixth day of illness. Function of the remaining platelets is also impaired (118,119). An increase in activated partial thromboplastin time with a reduction in the fibrinogen level is common, with a general trend toward increasing derangement of these parameters with increasing severity of dengue disease (103,120,121). In patients with shock, concentrations of procoagulant markers tend to be increased but not markedly so, and although anticoagulant protein concentrations are reduced, this appears to be due to vascular leak rather than consumption (103). It seems probable that dengue infection results in a specific coagulopathy with increased fibrinolysis, possibly due to the presence of a circulating anticoagulant, but the exact nature of this remains to be elucidated. The evidence for classic DIC is not convincing, except in those patients with profound shock who develop severe mucosal bleeding in the context of hypoxia, acidosis, and multisystem failure.

Moderate to severe hyponatremia is common. A marked reduction in plasma proteins, particularly albumin and the smaller proteins is seen, and the severity of the hypoproteinemia correlates with the severity of the vascular leak (100). However, it is important to take into account the vascular leak process when interpreting plasma concentrations of proteins and other factors. Not only are small molecules more likely to leak, but if the patient is hemoconcentrated at the time of sampling, measured plasma concentrations will be artificially increased. After administration of intravenous fluids, plasma protein concentrations drop further, but during the recovery phase re-equilibration occurs rapidly and protein concentrations return to normal.

Management

The only treatment currently available for symptomatic dengue infections is supportive. No specific drug treatments have been shown to be beneficial. Steroid therapy, employed regularly for the treatment of DHF during the 1970s and 1980s, demonstrated no convincing benefit in several randomized controlled trials and is no longer recommended (122,123).

For most patients, hospital admission is unnecessary during the first 2 to 3 days of illness. Oral rehydration should be encouraged with oral rehydration solutions or similar preparations, together with a light diet. Paracetamol (10 to 15 mg/kg, every 4 to 6 hours) is the preferred antipyretic agent, and aspirin and nonsteroidal antiinflammatory drugs are contraindicated. The child should be reviewed daily until the fever has settled, with the hematocrit and platelet count checked at each visit. Children unable to tolerate oral fluids require hospital admission and judicious use of parenteral fluids. Persistent vomiting or severe abdominal pain, mucosal bleeding or severe skin bleeding/bruising, a rapidly rising hematocrit, or a marked drop in the platelet count indicates the need for close observation on a well-staffed ward where vital signs and hematocrit can be checked frequently. Children who develop shock require admission to intensive care, as do those with major gastrointestinal bleeding. Management of shock and bleeding are described in detail below. Hepatic and neurologic dysfunction are rare except as consequences of hypovolemia. Supportive management of these complications is similar to that of any acute severe hepatitis or encephalopathy and will not be discussed further here.

Fluid Therapy for Children Without Shock

In the absence of cardiovascular compromise, intravenous fluid therapy is indicated for those with repeated vomiting or a very high or rapidly rising hematocrit early in the course of the illness. Parenterally administered fluids distribute between the intravascular, interstitial, and intracellular fluid compartments according to specific physicochemical properties of the individual solutions (124). In essence, the sodium content determines the efficacy of crystalloid solutions for intravascular volume replacement. Only isotonic crystalloid solutions such as 0.9% saline or Hartmann's or Ringer's lactate preparations, which distribute primarily between the intravascular and interstitial compartments, should be used. Hypotonic electrolyte solutions, which distribute across all three fluid compartments, provide less effective intravascular support and contribute to the development of fluid overload. Hypoglycemia is unusual in these children; if dextrose is considered necessary, it must be administered in an isotonic electrolyte preparation. The minimum volume of fluid possible to maintain cardiovascular stability and good urine output should be prescribed. In practice, a volume of 5 to 6 mL/kg/h is usually given for the first 1 to 2 hours, after which the infusion rate is reduced to maintenance levels of 2 to 3 mL/kg/h provided the cardiovascular parameters remain stable. Changes in the hematocrit are helpful in guiding fluid therapy, but it is important to recognize that if the patient is warm and well perfused with stable vital signs, then a relatively high but stable hematocrit (even 50% to 55%) is acceptable. It is likely that the hematocrit will start to fall rapidly once the reabsorptive phase of the disease begins, and fluid overload secondary to excess parenteral fluid administration is a major contributor to morbidity and mortality. Thrombotic events do not occur, probably because of the mild intrinsic dengue coagulopathy.

Fluid Therapy for Children with Shock (Fig. 13.5)

Shock is diagnosed if the pulse pressure is ≤20 mm Hg or the child is hypotensive for age. Treatment of established shock is a medical emergency. Resuscitation should be started with an isotonic crystalloid solution at a rate of 15 mL/kg over 1 hour. If the patient's clinical condition has stabilized after this time (wider pulse pressure, warm peripheries), the rate of fluid administration may be reduced to 10 mL/kg/h, and then gradually reduced to maintenance levels

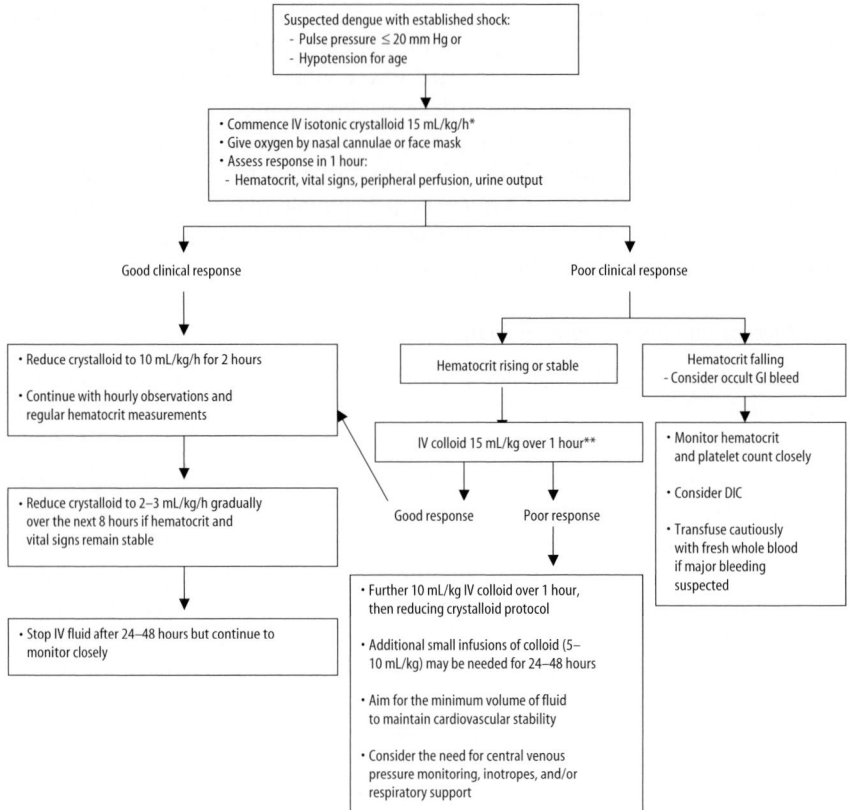

Figure 13.5. Volume replacement flow chart for patients with dengue shock syndrome. *Use only isotonic crystalloid solutions such as Ringer's lactate or normal saline. **Use a medium molecular weight iso-oncotic colloid preparation, e.g., 6% dextran 70 or 6% hydroxyethyl starch.

over the next 6 to 8 hours. Older children/teenagers and children who are overweight require proportionately less fluid per kilogram body weight, and the volumes given after the initial resuscitation should be adjusted downward. If there are signs of ongoing cardiovascular compromise after the first hour of treatment (no improvement in pulse pressure, persisting peripheral shutdown, a rising hematocrit), a colloid solution should be substituted for the crystalloid solution, at an initial rate of 10 to 15 mL/kg over 1 hour.

Immediate distribution of colloid solutions is primarily within the intravascular compartment limited by the permeability of the capillary wall to the particular colloid molecules. The molecules also increase plasma oncotic pressure, thereby altering the balance of fluid flux across the endothelium and providing volume expansion in excess of the actual volume of fluid infused. In general, small colloid molecules exert a relatively greater osmotic effect than larger molecules at the same concentration, but large molecules remain within the circulation longer as the small molecules are rapidly excreted by the kidneys or lost from the circulation by leakage into the interstitium. Since there is preferential leak of small molecules in children with DSS, larger molecular weight preparations may offer theoretical advantages (100). At present, however, there is no conclusive evidence as to which colloid solution is most effective for resuscitation of DSS, but isotonic preparations such as 6% dextran 70 or 6% hydroxyethyl starch (HES, molecular weight [MW] 200,000) have been used with equal success (124a).

After 1 hour of colloid infusion, treatment should revert to the reducing schedule of isotonic crystalloid as described above, provided the patient's condition has improved. If not, a further infusion of colloid at a rate of 10 mL/kg may be given over 1 hour. It is preferable to limit the use of any colloid preparation to the minimum necessary to support the circulation at any one time, since further supplementary treatment with small infusions of 5 to 10 mL/kg of colloid may be required in the ensuing 24 to 48 hours if the capillary leak persists. In most cases intravenous fluid therapy can be stopped after this time. A small proportion of patients develop mild transient hypertension immediately after the initial resuscitation, probably reflecting the adaptive cardiovascular/adrenal responses that have developed over the preceding days to offset the chronic plasma leakage. The rate of fluid administration should be reduced and the hypertension usually resolves over about 4 to 6 hours.

Management of Hemorrhagic Complications

Mucosal bleeding in the form of epistaxis, gum bleeding, or gastrointestinal or vaginal bleeding may occur in any patient, but is usually minor. For most children, routine inpatient observation with regular monitoring of the platelet count is all that is indicated. Intramuscular injections should be avoided. Platelet concentrates are of no value for the treatment of thrombocytopenia in the absence of major bleeding, since the thrombocytopenia improves rapidly during the second week of illness. Children with profound thrombocytopenia (<20,000 platelets/mm^3) should be managed expectantly with bed rest and protection from trauma. Transfusion is very rarely necessary, but if so fresh blood with or without platelet concentrates must be used.

In children with shock, major bleeding is almost always associated with very severe or prolonged cardiovascular compromise, and is usually from the gastrointestinal tract. Contributing factors include profound thrombocytopenia and DIC exacerbated by tissue hypoxia and acidosis superimposed on the underlying dengue coagulopathy. In addition, all colloid preparations can affect hemostatic competence adversely, and children with profound shock are likely to require repeated colloid infusions. Internal bleeding may not become apparent for many hours until the first melena stool is passed. Occult bleeding should be considered in all those who fail to improve clinically after appropriate fluid resuscitation, particularly if the hematocrit is stable or falling and the abdomen is distended and tender. Transfusion should be undertaken with extreme care because of the problem of fluid overload. In the event that major internal bleeding is suspected in a child with shock, a small volume of fresh whole blood (5 to 10 mL/kg) should be given very slowly and the response observed. Further small transfusions of blood, platelets, and fresh frozen plasma may be given subsequently if there is a good clinical response and significant bleeding is confirmed.

Fluid Overload

Clinically significant fluid overload develops in several situations. Most commonly it follows administration of inappropriate intravenous fluid in excessive amounts or too rapidly to patients with moderate capillary leak, or else continuation of parenteral fluid therapy once the reabsorptive phase of the disease has commenced. Rarely, it may be seen in patients with catastrophic leak for whom support of the circulation is not possible without administration of large volumes of fluid.

If shock has resolved and the cardiovascular indices are stable, children with mild to moderate overload should be observed on bed rest for 24 to 48 hours and all intravenous fluid therapy should be stopped. In most cases spontaneous reabsorption of fluid will occur with a concomitant diuresis and no further treatment is necessary. Symptomatic patients with tachypnea or breathlessness and large pleural/pericardial or other effusions should receive a diuretic (e.g., furosemide 1 mg/kg/dose oral or IV) once or twice daily for 24 hours, together with facial oxygen and strict bed rest. Temporary support with an inotropic agent may be considered for a brief period during the early reabsorptive phase until the diuretics take effect.

The rare patients, usually those with catastrophic capillary leak, who remain profoundly hypovolemic when fluid overload becomes apparent are extremely difficult to manage and have a high mortality. Central venous pressure monitoring is helpful, but lines should only be inserted by experienced staff in view of the marked thrombocytopenia and severe coagulopathy that are usually present by this stage. Repeated small boluses of colloid are frequently necessary to support the circulation, combined with inotropic agents often in high doses. Maintenance crystalloid therapy should be reduced to a minimum. Diuretics are contraindicated since their effect will be to deplete the intravascular compartment further. Aspiration of large pleural effusions or drainage of ascites is helpful in relieving respiratory symptoms, and early intervention with positive pressure ventilation, preferably before the development of frank pulmonary edema, may be lifesaving. Once pulmonary edema is established, the technical difficulties of mechanical ventilation become increasingly complex and the outlook is grave. Metabolic derangements, DIC, and multiorgan failure are common complications and contribute to the high mortality.

Outcome

Reliable outcome data for the different clinical disease presentations are lacking, in part due to the difficulties in diagnosis and classification mentioned above.

However, in experienced hands and with meticulous attention to detail, mortality rates of <1% are achievable for patients with established DSS, even in endemic areas without access to sophisticated intensive care (125). Mortality rates of >10% are still sometimes reported, and in many of these cases iatrogenic volume overload is likely to have contributed significantly to the adverse outcome. Death rates are proportionately higher in very young children, the elderly, and those with secondary as opposed to primary infections (75). In general, however, for the majority of hospitalized patients, full recovery is usual.

Japanese Encephalitis

Japanese encephalitis (JEV) is also a small single-stranded RNA virus, another member of the genus *Flavivirus*, family Flaviviridae. The virus exists naturally in an enzootic cycle involving pigs, birds, and *Culex* mosquitoes. Pigs act as an amplification host, developing high and prolonged viremia, but are not generally affected by the virus. They are the most important hosts for transmission to humans. The major vector is *Culex tritaeniorhynchus*, a mosquito that breeds in rice paddy fields and bites preferentially during the evenings or at night. People closely exposed to the enzootic life cycle become infected incidentally but are considered dead-end hosts, as the viremia is usually brief and onward transmission does not occur. Following the bite of an infected mosquito, only a small proportion of people (estimated at 1:25 to 1:1000) develop clinical disease (126,127), ranging from a mild flu-like illness to a fatal meningoencephalitis.

Epidemiology

Epidemics of encephalitis were initially reported in Japan from the 1870s onward, and became more frequent and widespread in the region during the 20th century. Japanese encephalitis is now endemic throughout most of Southeast Asia and is reported sporadically as far west as Pakistan and Nepal, and as far east as the islands of the Pacific Rim and northern Australia (128). Serologic surveys have shown that in rural Asia the majority of the population is infected during childhood or early adulthood and clinical disease is most often seen in these age groups. The incidence of infection is lower in infants and young children, probably reflecting limited exposure to the vector. In some countries such as Japan and Thailand, the number of reported cases has fallen in recent years, probably due to a combination of mass vaccination of children, changes in agricultural practices, and increasing industrialization (129). However, JEV remains one of the most important causes of viral encephalitis worldwide, with an estimated 50,000 cases and 15,000 deaths occurring annually (130). Vaccination is recommended for travelers staying in rural areas in endemic countries for more than 1 month, but in recent years several cases of severe meningoencephalitis have been reported in tourists spending less than 2 weeks in holiday resorts in Asia (131,132). The disease, therefore, must be considered in the differential diagnosis of all unvaccinated children presenting with acute neurologic disorders after travel to or from endemic areas.

Related neurotropic arboviruses such as Murray Valley encephalitis virus in Australia, St. Louis encephalitis virus in the U.S., and West Nile virus, previously endemic in large parts of Africa and now spreading rapidly across the U.S., exhibit many epidemiologic and clinical features similar to JEV but are much less common.

Pathogenesis

The factors determining which persons infected with JEV develop disease are unknown, but probably include viral factors, such as the titer and neurovirulence of the infecting virus, and host factors, such as age, genetic predisposition, preexisting immunity, and the acute response to the infection. Infection with JEV elicits lifelong immunity, but prior infection with related flaviviruses such as dengue may influence the clinical phenotype. After inoculation, JEV appears to amplify peripherally before invading the CNS. The mechanism by which it crosses the blood brain barrier (BBB) is unknown, but limited data available from pathologic studies indicate that once within the nervous system, the virus has a predilection for the thalamus, basal ganglia, and midbrain (133,134).

Clinical Manifestations

In the small proportion of infected patients who develop symptoms, the disease begins suddenly after an incubation period of 1 to 2 weeks, in the form of a nonspecific febrile illness in which headache and vomiting are conspicuous features. Neuropsychiatric manifestations are quite common during the early stages, especially in older children and adults, sometimes leading to an initial diagnosis of mental illness. After 3 to 4 days, confusion and drowsiness develop and the child may lapse into coma. One or two grand mal seizures often occur around this time. A number of children develop only aseptic meningitis or very mild encephalitis, but since a diagnosis of JEV infection is rarely considered, the proportion with this mild presentation remains unknown.

Among those with obvious encephalitis, approximately 20% deteriorate rapidly within the first 7 to 10 days. Signs of severe brainstem involvement (posturing, rigidity spasms, ocular abnormalities, loss of brainstem reflexes, etc.) are prominent in this group. Mortality is high, even with full intensive care support, and profound neurologic sequelae are common in survivors. Multiple, sometimes prolonged, or complex seizures may occur and are a poor prognostic sign (135,136).

Among the remaining 80%, most children remain deeply comatose for several days before regaining consciousness gradually during the second or third week of illness. Bizarre dystonic posturing and rigidity spasms in response to stimulation are common during this period and may reflect localized basal ganglia or brainstem involvement. A profound parkinsonian-like state often becomes apparent as the child recovers and initially it can be difficult to differentiate between this "locked-in" state and persisting coma. Tremor, cogwheel rigidity, and marked bradykinesia with a typical mask-like facies develop as the patient improves. Bilateral, symmetrical long tract signs may also be present, particularly in the lower limbs, with extremely brisk reflexes, marked clonus, and up-going plantar responses, but often little weakness of the limbs. Both the extrapyramidal signs and the long tract signs tend to improve gradually over a period of several weeks. It may be that acute swelling of lesions in the thalami, basal ganglia, and brainstem results in temporary compression of the corticospinal tracts, and as the edema regresses pressure on the tracts is released.

In a small number of children, unilateral upper motor neuron limb weakness is seen from an early stage, often involving the arm more than the leg. These signs are usually associated with significant lesions in the contralateral thalamus on magnetic resonance imaging (MRI), and probably indicate involvement of motor fibers in the internal capsule. Some recovery is usual, but if the initial weakness is profound, long-term sequelae can be expected. Another feature sometimes noted during the acute phase of the illness is a poliomyelitis like paralysis (137,138). Rapid onset of flaccid paralysis is noted in one or more limbs, usually but not exclusively in patients with some degree of impairment of consciousness. Weakness appears to be more frequent in the lower than the upper limbs and is usually asymmetrical. Rare cases present with respiratory paralysis similar to patients with severe bulbar poliomyelitis. Unfortunately, there is little recovery, and at followup, persistent weakness and marked wasting of the affected limbs is usual. Nerve conduction studies and electromyography indicate permanent anterior horn cell damage.

Neurologic progress during the recovery period is characterized by the development of several different but characteristic syndromes. Patients may exhibit any or all of the following problems. After about 4 to 6 weeks some children develop very severe choreoathetoid movement disorders or profound dystonic posturing, both of which may persist for weeks to months, although eventual recovery is the rule. Others develop severe difficulties with speech and swallowing, although involuntary facial movements and the gag reflex are preserved. Sometimes these problems are accompanied by major neuropsychiatric disturbance suggestive of a pseudobulbar palsy. Again, full recovery is the rule, although some children may remain mute for many weeks while able to comprehend speech and cooperate with examination.

The differential diagnosis of JEV infection is broad, and includes other viral encephalitides (e.g., neurotropic arboviruses, herpes viruses, enteroviruses, postinfectious and postvaccination encephalomyelitis), other CNS infections (bacterial and fungal meningitis, tuberculosis, cerebral malaria, leptospirosis, tetanus), other infectious diseases with CNS manifestations (typhoid encephalopathy), and noninfectious diseases (tumors, cerebrovascular accidents, Reye's syndrome, toxic encephalopathies, epilepsy). Distinguishing JEV from all these possibilities may be difficult during the early stages but the characteristic clinical features that develop over several weeks, together with the typical MRI findings are very helpful.

Diagnosis

Attempts to isolate JEV from clinical specimens are usually unsuccessful since the viremia is generally brief and of low magnitude. Diagnosis is routinely based on serology, using capture ELISA techniques to measure anti-JEV IgM and IgG. However, as with dengue, serologic diagnosis is complicated by the existence of cross-reactive antigenic determinants, and it is necessary to run the tests in parallel with tests for other locally prevalent flaviviruses. The presence of anti-JEV IgM in the cerebrospinal fluid (CSF) confirms the diagnosis, but may not develop until the second week of the illness. The presence of anti-JEV IgM in plasma alone is considered to be strongly supportive rather than diagnostic, however, since a coincidental asymptomatic JEV infection in a patient with another neurologic disease cannot be ruled out. Different antibody response patterns are seen when JEV is the first, as compared to a second, or later flavivirus encountered by the patient, but the relevance of this to disease severity is unclear at present.

Laboratory Investigations

A moderate lymphocytosis (10 to 100 cells/mm^3) is usually seen in the CSF during the first 1 to 2 weeks. Occasionally polymorphonuclear cells predominate early in the disease, with counts up to 1000 cells/mm^3 if the specimen is obtained during the first 1 to 2 days of fever. Red cells are not present except as a consequence of trauma. The CSF protein may be mildly increased (50 to 200 mg/dL), but the CSF/blood glucose ratio is normal. The CSF opening pressure is often mildly elevated; very high pressures are unusual, but if present the prognosis is poor.

Examination of the blood reveals a peripheral neutrophil leukocytosis in most patients. Hyponatremia is also fairly common; possible contributing factors include inappropriate parenteral fluid therapy, use of osmotic agents such as mannitol, and inappropriate secretion of antidiuretic hormone. Slight increases in hepatic enzymes may be noted, but most other blood parameters remain normal.

Imaging of the CNS reveals characteristic features and may be helpful for diagnosis (139–141). Magnetic resonance imaging is more sensitive than CT. Data from early scans are limited, but during the second week of illness, non-enhancing thalamic lesions are seen in most symptomatic children. These are often multiple and sometimes encroach on the internal capsule. A pattern of low signal on T1 and high signal on T2 images is typical. Small gliotic scars may remain visible on scans taken several months later. Similar lesions are often present in the basal ganglia and brainstem of children with moderate to severe disease, but involvement of the cerebral hemispheres and cerebellum is less common. Mild to moderate cerebral edema is seen in some cases, but the most severely affected patients often die before scanning is possible. Single photon emission tomography in a few patients has shown hypoperfusion of the thalamic nuclei in particular, confirming that the virus appears to have a predilection for this area of the brain (142,143).

Electroencephalographic abnormalities are consistent with the severity of the encephalitis (135,143). Diffuse slowing is apparent in most patients, but in those with severe neurologic involvement, more complex patterns are seen often together with epileptiform activity. In the latter group, subtle seizures and status epilepticus may occur and can be difficult to identify without electroencephalographic monitoring.

Management

No specific therapy is available and treatment remains supportive. During the acute stage, careful attention to fluid balance and nutrition, scrupulous nursing care to prevent pressure sores and aspiration pneumonia, physiotherapy, and antibiotic therapy for secondary infections are all important. Repeated seizures and obvious raised ICP occur in a minority of children and warrant appropriate therapy (136). However, in the majority of patients the role of raised ICP and tentorial herniation versus acute brainstem involvement remains uncertain; ICP monitoring may be helpful in centers with appropriate facilities.

For many years corticosteroids were used during the acute illness, but a formal trial in Thailand in the 1980s showed no benefit from dexamethasone, and corticosteroids are no longer recommended (144). Recently, treatment with interferon-α has been investigated. It is produced naturally in the CSF in response to infection with JEV and has in vitro activity against the virus. However, in a randomized double-blind placebo-controlled trial, daily injections of recombinant interferon-α failed to reduce mortality or influence the severity of neurologic sequelae (145).

The recovery phase may be very prolonged, and nutritional support is critical during this period, particularly in those children with severe movement disorders (who are often in ceaseless motion while awake and thus have a very high metabolic requirement), and in those with swallowing difficulties. Involvement of the family in physiotherapy and rehabilitation helps to reassure them that although progress may be slow, the eventual outcome is usually reasonable among those who survive the acute illness.

Outcome

Between 20% and 30% of patients diagnosed with JEV die, usually within a couple of weeks of the onset of symptoms. However, children with mild encephalitis or aseptic meningitis who recover quickly may not be identified as having JEV, so the overall mortality of symptomatic infections is likely to be lower. Recovery is long and complicated, but almost all the late manifestations improve over time. Unfortunately, the poliomyelitis-like flaccid paralysis does not improve, and affected children are often left with wasted limbs with little or no function. Most patients with upper motor neuron paralysis show some improvement and are able to function remarkably well despite residual abnormalities detectable on examination. By 1 year, the majority of survivors are back at school, although the presence of minor learning or behavioral difficulties is unknown.

Vaccine-Preventable Diseases

In the developed world, routine immunization has made many of the previously common serious infections of childhood into rarities. Major efforts by the WHO and other global bodies to establish and implement fully the Expanded Program of Immunization (EPI) have also resulted in improved control of these diseases in the world's poorest nations. However, despite these improvements, vaccine-preventable diseases are still responsible for the deaths of some 2 million children each year in the developing world. Many factors contribute to the difficulties in disease eradication: use of cheap vaccines of uncertain quality; incomplete vaccine deployment; and lack of basic infrastructure, limiting access to at-risk populations and compromising the cold chain. In addition, the disruptive effects of social unrest, wars, or natural disasters may both disrupt immunization programs and increase exposure to disease. Furthermore, unfounded anxieties about vaccine safety may have serious consequences. Recently, vaccine refusal in Nigeria resulted in a large epidemic of paralytic poliomyelitis spread across several countries, indicating how tenuous control of the disease, generally regarded as one of the WHO's major successes, remains.

Global immunization coverage for three doses of diphtheria, tetanus, and pertussis in infancy remains at less than 80% worldwide, with the lowest rates in sub-Saharan Africa and South Asia (Fig. 13.6). Inadequately vaccinated persons traveling to regions where such diseases remain common may either become ill themselves or may act as carriers returning home with the potential to infect others. It is important for physicians practicing in the industrialized world to be aware of the clinical manifestations and treatment of these rare diseases, since early diagnosis improves outcome and helps to limit spread. In this section, three of the vaccine-preventable diseases that are rarely seen in the developed world, diphtheria, tetanus and polio, are discussed. Although other diseases covered in routine infant immunization programs, such as pertussis and measles, remain major killers worldwide, they are likely to be more familiar to practitioners in the developed world. The focus of this section is on recognition and management of the diseases.

Immunization schedules differ slightly according to local policy and disease prevalence and are not discussed here. All these diseases are notifiable, and suspected cases should be reported immediately to the relevant public health authority so that antitoxin can be obtained without delay where necessary, and so that measures can be taken to minimize the likelihood of spread.

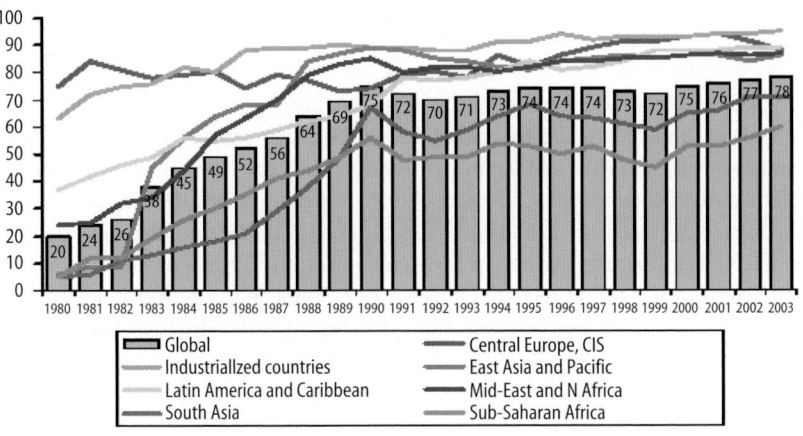

FIGURE 13.6. Global immunization coverage for three doses of diphtheria, tetanus, and pertussis vaccine in infancy. (From World Health Organization/UNICEF, 2004.)

Diphtheria

Diphtheria is an acute severe disease caused by exotoxin producing *Corynebacterium diphtheriae*. The organism is a nonmotile, unencapsulated nonsporulating gram-positive bacillus. Conventionally, three biotypes, gravis, intermedius, and mitis, are recognized, but toxin production depends on the presence of a lysogenic phage carrying the *tox* structural gene and is not related to biotype. The organism usually infects the respiratory tract, and humans are the only known reservoir. Cutaneous diphtheria is also common in many tropical countries but may be seen among alcoholics, the indigent, and the homeless in developed countries (146,147). The principal modes of spread are by respiratory droplets from acute cases or asymptomatic carriers, or by direct contact with infected skin lesions.

In the developed world, immunization against diphtheria became widespread during the 1940s and 1950s, and by the 1980s the disease had been virtually eliminated in many countries. However, it remains endemic in many parts of the world, particularly in Asian countries. During the 1990s a major resurgence of diphtheria occurred in the countries of the former Soviet Union, with rapid spread to neighboring states (148). Although this epidemic has now been successfully brought under control, the potential for rapid reemergence of the disease remains (149). Worldwide more than 5000 deaths from diphtheria were reported in 2002 (150). Imported cases continue to occur in Europe, particularly among inadequately vaccinated travelers to or from the Indian subcontinent, and deaths are not unknown (151,152).

Pathogenesis

The organism itself is not particularly invasive, but the exotoxin enters susceptible mammalian cells and blocks protein synthesis, resulting in cell death (153). At the site of infection, local toxin production induces tissue necrosis and the formation of a dense mass of fibrin, leukocytes, dead epithelial cells, and organisms, closely adherent to the underlying mucosa. The term *diphtheria* derives from the Greek root for leather or hide, reflecting the similarity in appearance of this pseudomembrane to a piece of leather. The pseudomembrane is found typically on the tonsils or posterior pharynx, but may develop anywhere in the respiratory tract. Marked cervical lymphadenitis may occur together with woody hard induration of local soft tissues, resulting in the typical "bull-neck" appearance and contributing to the severity of respiratory distress.

Local disease at the primary site of infection may be severe, but often the most serious clinical manifestations are those resulting from systemic absorption and dissemination of the extremely potent exotoxin. The toxin can affect all organs in the body, but the major clinical consequences generally involve the heart, kidneys, and nervous tissue after a variable latent period.

Non–toxin-producing *C. diphtheriae* usually induce only a mild inflammatory reaction in the superficial layers of the respiratory mucosa. Rarely however, nontoxigenic strains have been associated with significant invasive disease, suggesting that other virulence factors may exist (154,155). A closely related microorganism, *Corynebacterium ulcerans*, is also able to produce diphtheria toxin and has been associated with classic diphtheria as well as with milder symptoms.

Clinical Manifestations

Acute Disease

The incubation period is typically between 2 and 5 days. The initial disease is conveniently classified into several clinical types, according to the site of primary infection.

In pure nasal diphtheria, infection is limited to the anterior nares and a serosanguinous or seropurulent nasal discharge is seen, sometimes associated with a subtle membrane visible inside the nostril. Absorption of toxin is limited and systemic complications rare.

Faucial diphtheria, involving the tonsils or posterior pharyngeal structures, is more severe. Relatively mild upper respiratory tract symptoms are followed after 1 or 2 days by the development of membrane on one or both tonsils, sometimes extending upward to the uvula and soft palate or downward to the larynx and trachea. The extent of the membrane correlates with the severity of the bull-neck, the degree of airway obstruction, and the signs of acute systemic toxicity. In very severe cases massive toxin absorption results in cardiac and respiratory collapse, renal failure, and death within a few days. In most patients, however, after 5 to 7 days the membrane sloughs off and the patient recovers from the local infection, but remains at risk of the delayed cardiac and neurologic problems.

Laryngeal diphtheria generally represents downward extension of membrane from the pharynx and is correspondingly severe. Sometimes the membrane forms a cast of the whole of the tracheobronchial tree and in such cases death is virtually inevitable. Occasionally, however, the membrane is limited to the larynx alone; symptoms include hoarseness, a brassy cough, and rapidly progressive stridor and respiratory distress. Emergency tracheostomy often provides dramatic relief and, as absorption of toxin is limited in isolated laryngeal diphtheria, late complications are unusual.

Cutaneous, ocular, aural, and genital diphtheria are all reported but are rarely associated with significant toxin-mediated disease. Indolent nonhealing ulcers of cutaneous diphtheria are common in the tropics and may serve as a reservoir for the organism, while at the same time inducing good immunity in the host.

Late Complications

Characteristically, cardiac complications become evident during the second week of illness, and may be insidious in onset. Subtle electrocardiogram (ECG) abnormalities, such as minor ST-T wave changes, increased rates of ectopy, and first-degree heart block, are frequently detectable, but clinical cardiac dysfunction becomes apparent only in a subgroup of these patients (156–158). In this group, the minor ECG abnormalities progress rapidly to more complex conduction abnormalities, including atrioventricular dissociation and complete heart block, and myocardial dysfunction becomes apparent. Clinical signs may include profound bradycardia, diminished heart sounds, a gallop rhythm, and varying degrees of congestive failure. A hypotensive low-output state is a very poor prognostic sign, usually associated with major conduction disturbances, and suggests extensive myocardial damage. Ventricular and supraventricular tachyarrhythmias may also occur and are often fatal.

Neurologic complications occur in around 10% to 20% of patients, usually arising between the third and eighth weeks of illness. Signs are typically bilateral, and motor rather than sensory. Difficulty in swallowing with nasal regurgitation due to palatal paralysis is often the first manifestation. Ocular and other cranial nerve palsies indicating bulbar involvement may follow, in which case the course is often severe (159). Later still a peripheral polyneuropathy similar to Guillain-Barré syndrome may develop.

Diagnosis

The diagnosis of diphtheria should be made on the basis of clinical findings without waiting for laboratory confirmation, since any delay in treatment may have serious consequences. In developed countries where diphtheria is a rarity, it may easily be missed. A high index of suspicion is required, particularly in children without adequate immunization cover and in those who have recently visited an area endemic for diphtheria (160). Differential diagnoses include infectious mononucleosis, herpetic tonsillitis, Vincent's angina, streptococcal pharyngitis, and blood dyscrasias. Definitive diagnosis relies upon isolation of the organism using specific culture media. Elek's test or PCR are used to demonstrate toxigenicity of individual strains.

Management

Neutralization of free toxin with diphtheria antitoxin is the most important aspect of management. The antitoxin is only effective before the toxin enters cells, so prompt administration of adequate doses is critical. Empirical dosage recommendations are based on the site, extent, and duration of disease and are shown in Table 13.4 (161). The antitoxin is still raised in horses, so preliminary sensitivity testing should be performed, and facilities for resuscitation must be available even in the absence of a reaction to the test dose.

Antibiotic therapy should also be given to eliminate the organism and prevent spread. The organism is susceptible to a wide range of antibiotics, but penicillin and erythromycin are currently the antibiotics of choice. However, some erythromycin-resistant isolates have been identified (162). Treatment should be continued for 14 days, and the patient should be barrier nursed until eradication of the organism has been confirmed by culture of appropriate swabs. Clinical infection may not induce adequate levels of antitoxin for long-term protection, so patients should be formally immunized during convalescence.

Good supportive care is critical. Emergency tracheostomy may be lifesaving in children with severe airway obstruction in the initial stages of the illness. Ventilatory support is not usually required and manipulation of the upper airway should be avoided in case part of the membrane is dislodged and obstructs the lower airways. Secondary bacterial pneumonia may occur and should be treated with broad-spectrum antibiotics.

Careful clinical examination and regular ECG and echocardiographic monitoring allow early detection of conduction disturbances and heart failure. Cardiac pacing may be helpful in those with predominant involvement of con-

TABLE 13.4. Dosage of antitoxin recommended for various types of diphtheria

Type of diphtheria	Dosage (units)	Route
Nasal	10,000–20,000	Intramuscular
Tonsillar	15,000–25,000	Intramuscular or intravenous
Pharyngeal or laryngeal	20,000–40,000	Intramuscular or intravenous
Combined types or delayed diagnosis	40,000–60,000	Intravenous
Severe diphtheria, e.g., with extensive membrane or severe edema (bull-neck diphtheria)	40,000–100,000	Intravenous or part intravenous/ part intramuscular

ducting tissue rather than heart muscle, but in general severe conduction disturbances are associated with major myocardial involvement (163,164). If hypotension and renal compromise develop, the response to inotropic agents is poor and the outlook is bleak. Patients with mild to moderate cardiac failure can usually be managed successfully with bed rest, oxygen, diuretics, and angiotensin-converting enzyme inhibitors. However, recovery may take many weeks, and occasional patients are left with permanent conduction abnormalities. Steroids are of no benefit in the treatment or prevention of myocarditis (165). Ventilatory and nutritional support may be required for long periods in those patients who go on to develop severe neurologic complications, but eventual neurologic recovery is usual.

Outcome

Before the introduction of antitoxin, antibiotics, and routine immunization, the prognosis was grave. Currently mortality rates of around 5% to 10% are usual, with the majority of deaths occurring in those with overwhelming disease at presentation or those who develop severe myocarditis. If antitoxin is administered within 72 hours of onset of symptoms, severe disease and death are rare (166).

Tetanus

Clostridium tetani, the causative organism of tetanus, is an obligate anaerobic spore-forming bacillus. The spores are widely dispersed in the environment, particularly in soil, and are present in the intestinal flora of humans and many other animal species. They are extremely stable and remain viable for many years. The disease is caused by a potent exotoxin that is produced by the bacterium and has a very high affinity for nervous tissue. Despite the availability of an effective vaccine, tetanus remains common in the developing world, and is still occasionally encountered in developed countries. Approximately half a million deaths are attributed to tetanus each year, many of them neonates. In 2002, the WHO estimated that 200,000 deaths occurred worldwide due to neonatal tetanus (150).

Contamination of the umbilical stump in neonates, or of penetrating wounds or a chronically discharging ear in older children, are common routes of infection. Intramuscular injections, ear piercing, and minor trauma can also lead to disease, and in some patients no portal of entry is apparent.

Pathogenesis

Conditions that favor germination of tetanus spores into the vegetative toxin-producing form include low oxygen tension, tissue necrosis, hemorrhage, and sepsis. The toxin attaches to gangliosides on peripheral nerves close to the site of production. After internalization it moves to the CNS by retrograde axonal flow and interferes with mechanisms controlling release of the inhibitory neurotransmitter γ-aminobutyric acid. Sustained excitatory discharge of the α motor neurons causes the characteristic motor spasms. The toxin exerts its effects at many sites including the brainstem, spinal cord, peripheral nerves, and neuromuscular junctions. Involvement of the autonomic nervous system also occurs and may result in profound hemodynamic disturbances.

Clinical Manifestations

The incubation period varies from 24 hours to several months after inoculation, and reflects the distance the toxin must travel within the nervous system. In neonates the average incubation period is about 7 days following delivery. The period of onset is the time between the first symptom and the start of spasms. In general, the shorter these periods are, the more severe the disease is likely to be.

Muscle rigidity and spasms are the most typical features of generalized disease. The masseter muscles are among the first to be affected, resulting in trismus. Difficulty in sucking is often the presenting feature in neonates. Rigidity of the abdominal and spinal muscles also tends to develop early, with later progression to opisthotonus. Muscle spasms affecting the whole body occur at intervals, superimposed on the background rigidity; the frequency and duration of the spasms reflects the severity of the disease. The spasms may be induced by even very minor stimuli, are extremely painful, and can lead to laryngeal obstruction, respiratory arrest, and death. Localized tetanus results in pain and muscle rigidity at the site of an injury but without generalized spasms, and is much less severe than generalized tetanus.

Cardiac arrhythmias and extremely labile blood pressure due to autonomic dysfunction are seen in some patients with severe disease (167), but these complications appear to be less frequent in children than adults. Marked sweating and hyperpyrexia are also noted. Acute renal failure appears to be primarily due to hemodynamic dysfunction, although rhabdomyolysis and myoglobinuria may also contribute.

Diagnosis

The diagnosis is made on the clinical signs. Culture of the organism is difficult and frequently negative. Generalized tetanus is usually obvious, but early or localized disease may present difficulty, especially in developed countries where tetanus is rarely encountered. Differential diagnoses include tetany, drug-induced dystonic reactions, rabies, and oropharyngeal pathology. In neonates, sepsis, seizures, and kernicterus must also be considered.

Management

High-dose penicillin for 7 to 10 days remains the standard antimicrobial therapy in most parts of the world. Metronidazole is a safe and effective alternative. Careful wound debridement and removal of any foreign material are essential.

Administration of tetanus immunoglobulin neutralizes circulating toxin, but has no effect on toxin that is already bound to nerve cells. Human antitoxin has a much lower incidence of side effects than equine antitoxin, but is expensive and rarely available in countries where tetanus is common. Where possible, patients should receive 5000 to 8000 IU (neonates 500 IU) of human antitoxin intramuscularly, or 500 to 1000 IU/kg (neonates 5000 IU) of equine antitoxin, administered with full resuscitation facilities available in case of anaphylaxis. As yet there is no evidence that additional intrathecal therapy improves outcome (168). However, active vaccination with tetanus toxoid should be given to all patients, as this appears to boost the effect of the passive immunization, as well as stimulating the long-term protective response.

The mainstay of effective management is adequate sedation and muscle relaxation, together with appropriate ventilatory support. In patients with generalized tetanus, early tracheostomy allows maintenance of the airway during laryngeal spasms and facilitates removal of secretions. Benzodiazepines are the most commonly used sedative agents, but very high doses are often required which may lead to respiratory depression and coma, and necessitate mechanical ventilation. Neuromuscular blocking agents can be used in addition to sedation for control of very severe spasms in ventilated patients. Where mechanical ventilation is not an option, a cocktail of benzodiazepines, chlorpromazine, and paraldehyde or phenobarbitone can be used to control spasms (169). General supportive measures include avoidance of extraneous stimuli as far as possible, careful attention to fluid balance and nutrition, and good general nursing care to avoid aspiration and pressure sores.

Drugs such as beta-blockers, magnesium sulfate, clonidine, and labetalol have been used to treat autonomic dysfunction with mixed success. Skeletal muscle relaxants, such as baclofen, have been used in small numbers of patients and are reported to reduce the need for sedation and paralysis (170). Magnesium sulfate has also been used as adjunctive therapy to control spasms, and is currently undergoing formal evaluation in adults to see whether it has a role in the routine management of severe tetanus (171,172). If renal dysfunction develops, support with either hemofiltration or dialysis should be instituted early to prevent additional complications due to metabolic and electrolyte imbalances. Concomitant septicemia is common in neonates, most likely acquired by contamination of the umbilical stump with other bacteria as well as tetanus; the neonates should automatically receive cover with broad-spectrum antibiotics. Nosocomial infections, particularly with gram-negative organisms, are a frequent complication in all severely affected patients, and should be aggressively investigated and treated.

Outcome

The course of the disease is usually long and complicated, and outcome depends largely on the availability of mechanical ventilation and the standard of nursing care. Overall mortality rates of 10% to 30% are seen in older children and adults

(173). Respiratory failure, hemodynamic disturbance, and septicemia are the commonest causes of death. In those who survive, sequelae include contractures, chest deformities, seizures, myoclonus, and the consequences of hypoxia.

Neonatal tetanus occurs in very poor communities with limited access to health care and globally carries a mortality of approximately 60%, with many babies dying before they ever reach a hospital. It is entirely preventable by active immunization of women during pregnancy and improvements in education regarding care of the umbilical stump.

Poliomyelitis

Polioviruses are small RNA viruses within the genus *Enterovirus*, family Picornaviridae. Three serotypes exist, of which type 1 is the most frequent cause of epidemics. Humans are the main reservoir of the viruses in nature. The virus is highly infectious and transmission is primarily by the fecal-oral route.

The WHO commenced a major polio-eradication initiative in 1998, resulting in a decrease of more than 99% in the incidence of paralytic poliomyelitis in children by 2003. Less than 1000 deaths from poliomyelitis were reported from only six countries in the world in that year, suggesting that the WHO's goal of global eradication might be achievable. However, rumors of contaminated polio vaccine led to a suspension of immunization activities in northern Nigeria in mid-2003, resulting in a large polio epidemic that spread rapidly to at least 11 countries and reestablished transmission in several countries previously declared polio free (174,175). It is apparent that continuing commitment will be needed worldwide for many years to come to prevent resurgence of the disease (176).

Pathogenesis

After entry by the oral route, the virus multiplies at sites of implantation in the pharynx and gastrointestinal tract. It then invades local lymphoid tissue and enters the bloodstream, and may go on to infect cells of the CNS. Viral replication in motor neurons in the spinal cord and brainstem causes paralytic and bulbar poliomyelitis, respectively. Early changes are reversible, but destruction of the nerve cells leads to permanent paralysis.

Clinical Manifestations

The incubation period is commonly between 1 and 3 weeks, and the majority of infections are subclinical. Some children do experience a minor nonspecific illness, but very few develop clinical or laboratory evidence of CNS invasion. Nonparalytic aseptic meningitis develops in only 1% to 2% of all poliovirus infections, and true paralytic poliomyelitis is even rarer, with estimates of the ratio of inapparent to paralytic infections varying from 50:1 to 1000:1. Most paralytic cases involve unimmunized infants or young children, since adults living in a community where the virus still circulates are likely to have already acquired natural immunity.

The initial prodromal illness, consisting of fever, anorexia, lassitude, and gastrointestinal symptoms lasting a few days, may be followed immediately by headache, vomiting, and pain and stiffness in the neck, back, and legs. Alternatively, the illness may be biphasic with a brief symptom-free period before onset of these symptoms. Asymmetrical flaccid paralysis with absent reflexes then develops over several days, eventually reaching a plateau. Further extension is unlikely once the fever settles. Paralysis affects the lower limbs more frequently than the arms and characteristically involves large rather than small muscles. Sometimes spasms in the limbs and back occur, associated with severe myalgia. Sensory pathways remain intact. Infection of the brainstem results in bulbar poliomyelitis characterized by dysphagia, pooling of oral secretions, nasal speech, and sometimes respiratory and cardiovascular failure if the critical control areas in the medulla are affected. The majority of cases (approximately 80%) manifest pure spinal polio, with isolated bulbar polio only accounting for 2% to 5% of cases and the remainder with a mixed bulbospinal picture. Eventually, after a plateau period of days to weeks, there is gradual recovery of neurologic function and strength begins to return to the affected muscle groups.

Diagnosis

Recovery of a poliovirus from stool or a throat swab, or a significant rise in the titer of neutralizing antibody supports a diagnosis of poliomyelitis in patients with clinical disease, but since asymptomatic individuals may shed virus for several weeks concurrent with another neurologic disorder, only virus isolation from the CSF is considered definitive. This is rarely successful however.

The differential diagnosis of paralytic polio covers a variety of neurologic disorders, including Guillain-Barré syndrome, botulism, myasthenia gravis, tetanus, and paralytic rabies. In addition, a true poliomyelitis-like illness can follow infection with many of the other nonpolio enterovirus groups, and there is increasing awareness that very similar spinal cord involvement may occur in several of the arboviral encephalitides, in particular Japanese encephalitis and West Nile virus infections (177–179). Vaccine-associated paralytic poliomyelitis is a rare adverse event that may follow administration of live attenuated oral polio vaccine, probably as a result of reversion of the vaccine virus to a more neurotropic form. The clinical manifestations are identical to those caused by wild-type virus infection.

Examination of the CSF typically reveals a mild to moderate lymphocytic pleocytosis with slight elevation of the CSF protein, but a normal glucose. Spinal MRI may be helpful in confirming spinal cord involvement and excluding other local pathology.

Management

No specific treatment is available. The antiviral agent pleconaril has broad-spectrum activity against enteroviruses (180) and has been used occasionally in the treatment of poliomyelitis, but formal studies of efficacy have not been carried out.

Strict bed rest in the early paralytic phase may limit further deterioration. The extent and severity of paralysis must be documented frequently at this stage to allow early identification of respiratory involvement. Paralyzed muscles should be placed in the position of rest, and splints and supports used to try to maintain a normal posture and thus prevent development of contractures and deformities in the future. Analgesics may be required to relieve muscle pain, but sedatives should be avoided while there is a risk of developing respiratory paralysis. Active physiotherapy may begin once the fever has abated for a few days.

Early recognition of spinal respiratory paralysis is important to reduce the risk of secondary hypoxic damage. Intermittent positive pressure ventilation via a tracheostomy is required if there is significant respiratory dysfunction, and may be necessary for many weeks. The course may be complicated by secondary pneumonia, hypertension, urinary retention, and constipation. Patients with mild isolated bulbar polio, where the major problem is difficulty in swallowing, can be managed with nasogastric feeding and regular suction of secretions. More severe cases require tracheostomy, particularly if the cough is too weak to clear secretions, or stridor due to laryngeal paralysis occurs. Involvement of the cardiorespiratory center results in irregular and inefficient respiration, hyperpyrexia, arrhythmias, and fluctuations in blood pressure, and ultimately leads to cardiorespiratory arrest. Assisted ventilation and appropriate therapeutic measures to support cardiac function should be instituted but the prognosis is poor.

Outcome

The mortality for paralytic polio is usually less than 5% in children, although it may be up to 75% in those with bulbar involvement. In survivors, moderate recovery is often seen in the first couple of months, although permanent paralysis with rapid wasting occurs in muscle groups supplied by very severely affected nerves. Rehabilitation is a lengthy process, and improvements may still be seen up to 12 to 18 months from the onset of paralysis. Physiotherapy is very important. In severe cases children may require support from braces or calipers to become ambulant, and occasionally complex orthopedic procedures are necessary to correct severe contractures and deformities, although such options are rarely available to children in the developing world. Up to 40% of children go on to develop a postpolio syndrome after an interval of 30 to 40 years. Muscle pain recurs and new weakness or paralysis may develop together with exacerbation of any existing weakness. The syndrome is not an infectious process. The mechanism is thought to involve failure of oversized motor units created during the recovery process from the initial paralytic illness.

Emerging Viral Infections of Global Importance

A series of new and devastating viral infections has emerged in Asia over the last 10 years. The occurrence of highly pathogenic H5N1 avian flu in Hong-Kong (1997), Nipah virus encephalitis in Malaysia (1998), and, most dramatically, the advent of severe acute respiratory syndrome (SARS) in southern China (2002) have all posed significant threats to international health. Southeast Asia is particularly vulnerable to emerging zoonotic infections. It is densely populated with small family-run farms, and live animal/poultry markets are an integral part of the way of life even in urban centers. Many people live in very close proximity to animals and birds, increasing the risk of transmission between species. Alongside this traditional way of life, rapid industrial and economic developments have taken place in recent years and there has been a corresponding increase in communication with Western countries. Hong Kong in particular lies at the crossroads between the East and the West and experiences a heavy volume of international travel. The rapid worldwide spread of SARS from Hong Kong in 2003 drew attention to the importance of travel in the global epidemiology of disease, and underlines the necessity for physicians to maintain up-to-date knowledge of all serious infectious diseases, even those reported from apparently remote areas of the world.

At the present time, the recrudescence of H5N1 avian flu in Southeast Asia and more widely is of major concern, particularly with respect to the development of transmission potential between humans. If effective human-to-human transmission does develop, a worldwide influenza pandemic can be expected, and, given the severe pulmonary involvement seen in the human cases to date, global mortality in excess of that seen during the 1918 Spanish flu pandemic may occur. This final section of the chapter provides an overview of avian flu and SARS, the two most important emerging zoonoses of recent years.

Highly Pathogenic Avian Influenza A (H5N1)

Influenza viruses are single-stranded, negative-sense RNA viruses, with segmented genomes and great antigenic diversity. Both influenza A and B are responsible for widespread outbreaks of human disease. Although only one subtype of influenza B is recognized, influenza A viruses are classified into many subtypes according to the characteristics of two surface glycoproteins, hemagglutinin (H1-15) and neuraminidase (N1-9). Hemagglutinin attaches to sialic acid receptors on respiratory epithelial cells facilitating cellular entry, while neuraminidase is required for enzymatic cleavage of glycosidic linkages to sialic acid, so that viral progeny can leave infected cells. Hemagglutinin is the major antigenic determinant against which neutralizing antibodies are directed and is a crucial element in vaccine design. Neuraminidase is an important target for antiviral agents.

Influenza viruses have the ability to evolve rapidly, and are thus able to evade immune detection and cause repeated outbreaks of infection. Viral evolution occurs by two main mechanisms. Antigenic drift refers to the process by which point mutations occur in the surface glycopeptides of a viral subtype; emerging strains are antigenic variants that are closely related to strains circulating during previous outbreaks. In contrast, antigenic shift occurs when two influenza A viruses with different subtype characteristics infect a common host and reassortment of genomic segments takes place. Viruses with novel hemagglutinin or neuraminidase characteristics emerge that are antigenically quite distinct from previous viruses. Such viruses have the potential to cause global pandemics if transmission between people proves to be efficient. Aquatic birds are the natural reservoir for influenza viruses, and all subtypes have been recovered from them. However, only subtypes carrying the H1, H2, and H3, and N1 and N2 determinants have so far established stable lineages in the human population. Pigs are thought to be potential mixing vessels in which avian and human flu viruses might combine into new strains. The highly concentrated poultry and pig farming that is frequently seen in Asia, in conjunction with the traditional live animal markets, provide optimal conditions for such events to occur.

Epidemiology

During the 20th century three global influenza pandemics occurred on a background of substantial interpandemic disease activity. The "Spanish flu" (H1N1) epidemic of 1918 is thought to have been responsible for up to 50 million deaths worldwide. Following this epidemic, H1 viruses continued to cause intermittent outbreaks over many years. Then, in 1957, "Asian flu" (H2N2) emerged, to be followed in 1968 by "Hong Kong flu" (H3N2); both caused approximately one million deaths, but fortunately did not achieve the devastation of the 1918 epidemic.

In recent years several subtypes of highly pathogenic avian influenza A have crossed the species barrier and have caused serious human disease. Although H9 and H7 virus subtypes were implicated in causing human disease in China and the Netherlands in 1998 and 2003 respectively (181–183), it is the outbreaks of highly pathogenic H5N1 disease in Asia that are of major concern. In 1997 in Hong Kong 18 people, of whom 6 died, were infected with the avian H5N1 subtype during an outbreak affecting poultry (184). Formidable public health measures involving the rapid slaughter of more than a million chickens were required to control the outbreak, and no further human cases occurred until February 2003, when two members of a Hong Kong family were confirmed to have H5N1 infection following a visit to mainland China. Again, the isolates were of purely avian origin, although with evidence of significant antigenic drift in the hemagglutinin genes (185). From the end of 2003, large outbreaks of H5N1 infection were noted among poultry in many countries in Asia (Cambodia, China, Indonesia, Japan, Laos, South Korea, Thailand, and Vietnam), followed by an outbreak of lethal human H5N1 infection in Thailand and Vietnam in December 2003. By February 2004 more than 100 million birds had either died from the disease or been culled, the number of new human cases had slowed to a halt, and the outbreak appeared to have been controlled. Then in late June 2004, new outbreaks of H5N1 among poultry were again reported from several Asian countries followed by recrudescence of human disease. Subsequently, avian cases have been reported throughout Africa, the Middle East, and Europe. Between August 2004 and February 2006 over 100 human cases and about 60 deaths have been reported.

It seems that the disease is now endemic among bird populations worldwide, and that human cases are likely to continue to occur. Molecular characterization of viruses isolated over the last few years indicates that the precursor virus responsible for the initial H5N1 outbreak in Hong Kong in 1997 has evolved into a dominant pathogenic genotype, with an expanded host range that includes both terrestrial poultry and wild and migratory birds (185,186). Other studies suggest that the virus may have acquired the ability to infect and replicate in mammals. There are preliminary reports of H5N1 infection in pigs in southern China, and both domestic cats and tigers, previously considered to be resistant to influenza, have experienced serious disease (187,188). No conclusive evidence of sustained human-to-human transmission has emerged, although a single case of probable transmission within a family has been reported from Thailand (189). Similarly, no evidence for genetic reassortment between human and avian influenza virus genes has been found as yet. However, if H5N1 viruses do develop the capability for efficient human-to-human transmission, there is little preexisting natural immunity to H5N1 in the human population, and an influenza pandemic could result, with high rates of illness and death.

Pathogenesis

Human influenza viruses are predominantly transmitted from person to person via small particle aerosols released from the airway during coughing or sneezing. Once virus is deposited on the respiratory tract epithelium, it can attach to and penetrate columnar epithelial cells after which viral replication begins and cell death occurs. Viral shedding from the respiratory tract is usually first detected just before the onset of symptoms, rises promptly to a peak, and remains elevated for 24 to 48 hours before decreasing rapidly. Prolonged shedding of virus may occur in young children. Influenza in healthy children usually manifests as a tracheobronchitis, and pneumonia or other serious complications such as myocarditis or rhabdomyolysis are rare. Despite the occurrence of fever and systemic symptoms, infectious virus is rarely detected in the blood.

The exact method of transmission for avian viruses causing human disease remains uncertain, but a history of close contact with sick poultry or of visiting poultry markets is common among human cases infected with the H5N1 virus

(190,191). Infected birds shed virus in saliva, nasal secretions, and feces, and it is presumed that people become infected when they come into contact with infected secretions. There is also little information on the pathogenesis of avian influenza viruses in humans, although the major determinants of disease in avian species have been well defined. Cleavage of the viral hemagglutinin glycoprotein is required to activate virus infectivity, and the distribution of activating proteases in the host is one of the determinants of tissue tropism and pathogenicity (192). The hemagglutinins of highly pathogenic avian viruses are cleaved intracellularly by ubiquitously occurring proteases, and therefore have the capacity to infect various cell types and cause disseminated infections, whereas mammalian viruses are cleaved extracellularly, limiting their spread to tissues where the appropriate proteases are encountered. The high proportion of patients with gastrointestinal manifestations, liver dysfunction, renal dysfunction, and hematologic disorders in addition to respiratory involvement (see below) may reflect the wider tissue tropism of the H5N1 virus and explain the unusual severity of disease in human beings. Patients from both the 1997 and 2003 series have also been demonstrated to have markedly raised cytokine levels, and it is postulated that the increased severity of human H5N1 disease reflects a combination of increased viral replication and excess induction of cytokines leading to tissue damage (193,194).

Clinical Manifestations

Few case series have been reported (184,191). In the Hong Kong series from the 1997 outbreak, both children and adults up to 60 years old were affected, with children under 5 years of age generally experiencing only mild disease, predominantly short-lived upper respiratory tract symptoms. In contrast, in the more recent series from Vietnam, only older children and young adults were affected, and all had serious illness. This is in line with the finding that the dominant H5N1 genotype has become more virulent over the intervening years, although it is possible that milder cases were not identified in Vietnam, as facilities for virologic diagnosis are limited. The observed age distribution probably reflects the fact that children and young adults are more likely to be involved in the care of poultry in family farms or small holdings.

The illness usually begins abruptly fever with high fever, cough, and shortness of breath, commonly 3 to 4 days after exposure to sick or dying poultry. Sputum production, hemoptysis, and pleuritic pain are common features from early in the course of the illness, with tachypnea, respiratory distress, and focal respiratory signs apparent on examination. Thus, presentation tends to be with an acute severe pneumonia rather than with the upper respiratory tract symptoms, myalgia, and conjunctivitis that are more typically associated with normal human influenza virus infections. Diarrhea frequently coexists with the respiratory symptoms and is occasionally the primary presenting complaint (195). In addition, a recent case report identified H5N1 infection in a young child presenting with diarrhea and an acute neurologic syndrome, who did not develop pneumonia until later in the course of the disease (196). The virus was identified in both serum and CSF, suggesting that it has the ability to invade the CNS. Viable virus was also demonstrated in the feces of this patient, a finding that may have important implications for transmission potential and infection control. The case also raises the possibility that the spectrum of clinical disease may be broader than currently appreciated. In the future it will be important to establish whether the virus is also responsible for milder respiratory illnesses or other clinical presentations in regions where disease among poultry is common.

Even with aggressive intensive care support, the course of the illness is usually one of progressive deterioration. The acute respiratory distress syndrome (ARDS) develops rapidly, often accompanied by hepatic and renal dysfunction, and eventually multiorgan failure leads to death. Bleeding manifestations are sometimes seen, together with laboratory evidence of a coagulopathy. Secondary bacterial infection was not found at presentation in either of the case series, but obviously remains a concern in patients requiring prolonged intensive care.

Diagnosis

Reverse-transcription PCR (RT-PCR) using specific primers for H5 and N1 on respiratory specimens is used for laboratory confirmation of infection, although formal evaluation of sensitivity and specificity has not yet been carried out, and repeat analysis of specimens examined at the peak of the outbreak suggests that some cases may have been incorrectly categorized as negative. In the Vietnam series, rapid commercial tests using influenza A antigens were less sensitive than RT-PCR (191). Comprehensive tests for other respiratory pathogens should also be carried out to exclude other causes of pneumonia.

Laboratory Investigations

Profound leukopenia is seen in most patients at admission, with a marked reduction in the total lymphocyte count to less than 1000/mm^3 apparent by day 5 to 6 of illness. This is usually accompanied by moderate to severe thrombocytopenia. Bone marrow examination in two children with panyctopenia in the Hong Kong series showed reactive histiocytosis with hemophagocytosis. Biochemical evidence of liver dysfunction is common, and renal failure unrelated to rhabdomyolysis (often a feature if renal failure occurs in human influenza infections) may develop.

The chest x-ray is usually abnormal at first presentation, often showing extensive bilateral infiltrates, focal consolidation, air bronchograms, or lobar collapse. The radiologic abnormalities progress rapidly as the patient deteriorates. Air trapping or pneumothoraces may be seen in ventilated patients.

Management

Hypoxia develops rapidly and most patients require prompt intervention with mechanical ventilation and full intensive care support at an early stage. In common with all cases of severe ARDS, whatever the underlying etiology, ventilatory support tends to be very difficult, and iatrogenic complications are frequent and contribute to the overall severity of the illness. All patients should receive broad-spectrum antibiotics on admission, even though bacterial superinfection is rare at this stage. Inotropic support for hypotension, careful attention to fluid balance and biochemical indices, and vigilant detection and treatment of secondary infections, renal compromise, and coagulation abnormalities are important, but unfortunately overall outcome remains poor. Although no hospital staff member appears to have contracted symptomatic avian flu from patients, a study carried out in Hong Kong following the 1997 outbreak presented serologic evidence of transmission to a small number of health care workers (197). Thus it is important to remember that the potential for human-to-human transmission exists, and appropriate infection control measures must be adhered to strictly.

In terms of specific treatment, two major classes of antiviral drugs are active against influenza viruses (198). Amantadine and rimantadine bind to the M2 membrane protein of influenza A viruses, interfering with its ion channel function and inhibiting viral replication. However, genetic sequencing of H5N1 virus samples from recent human cases in Vietnam and Thailand has demonstrated resistance to this class of drugs, leaving only the neuraminidase inhibitors (oseltamivir and zanamivir) for use against the currently circulating strains (199). Neuraminidase normally cleaves terminal sialic acid from specific glycoproteins that serve as host cell receptors for attachment of influenza viruses. Destruction of these receptors is critical in allowing newly formed viruses to leave the cell. If neuraminidase is inhibited, viral progeny remain attached to the host cell and cannot spread to other cells (200). Zanamivir must be delivered locally into the lungs using an inhaler, while oseltamivir has good oral bioavailability and can be given parenterally, and is therefore the preferred drug. Oseltamivir was used in a number of patients in Southeast Asia during the 2003 and 2004 outbreaks but mortality remained high; at this stage, it is not possible to say whether there is in any benefit in using the drug once severe pneumonia has developed, but since adverse effects are infrequent most physicians elect to use it. Prophylaxis should be offered to family members who have experienced the same exposure as the index case. Recent research demonstrating that oseltamivir resistance developed rapidly in children infected with H3N2 influenza viruses who received oseltamivir treatment is a cause for concern (201). Both ribavirin and steroids have been used in some patients, sometimes in combination with oseltamivir, but again there is insufficient evidence to say whether these drugs conferred any benefit.

No vaccine that is effective against the H5N1 virus is available at present, but efforts to produce one are ongoing. Production of vaccine reference strains for pilot human clinical trials is under way, but mass production and availability of such a vaccine remain distant prospects.

Outcome

Approximately 60% to 70% of patients diagnosed to have H5N1 infection die, usually during the second or third week of illness. Those who survive remain ventilator dependent for long periods, and ongoing follow-up studies in the few existing survivors indicate that there is considerable destructive damage to the lungs that is likely to be long lasting. These outcome statistics bode ill for global mortality and morbidity should a worldwide pandemic develop, particularly given that the disease often attacks young previously healthy persons, many of them children.

The Severe Acute Respiratory Syndrome

In November 2002 increasing numbers of patients with an acute severe atypical pneumonia with a high mortality were noted in southern China. By February 2003 the disease had spread to Hong Kong, and from there it disseminated rapidly around the world. More than 8000 patients on five continents were infected and 774 deaths occurred before the epidemic was successfully brought under control in June 2003, following a major global public health effort. The new disease was named the severe acute respiratory syndrome (SARS), and within a remarkably short time a novel coronavirus (SARS-CoV) had been identified as the causative agent. Coronaviruses are a family of enveloped single-stranded RNA viruses that can infect both humans and animals. However, prior to the advent of SARS this group of viruses had only been responsible for mild respiratory symptoms in humans.

Epidemiology

The genome of SARS-CoV has been sequenced and does not match those of any of the previously known human or animal coronaviruses (202,203). It seems probable that SARS-CoV evolved as an animal virus and adapted to human-to-human transmission in the recent past. In support of this, many of the original Chinese patients were found to have links to the live animal market trade (204), and closely related viruses have been isolated from Himalayan palm civets and other animals found in live animal markets in China (205). However, the primary reservoir of the virus in nature remains uncertain. Detailed molecular epidemiology studies indicate that the earliest genotypes isolated from patients during the outbreak were similar to the animal SARS-like coronaviruses, but that over time one lineage of the virus became dominant, presumably as it adapted to human-to-human transmission (205,206).

One of the remarkable features of the outbreak was the speed with which it spread around the world, suggesting that the new virus is highly transmissible. This is no longer thought to be the case, but rather that a few infected individuals (so-called superspreaders) were responsible for several large case clusters and that, in general, the transmissibility of the virus is low (207,208). During the epidemic, transmission occurred primarily in hospital settings, after at least 5 days of illness and from patients who were severely ill; health care staff and close family members were prominent among secondary cases. The primary mode of transmission appears to have been through contact with infectious respiratory droplets or fomites, although fecal-oral transmission may also have played a role. In addition, airborne transmission was implicated in one large community outbreak in a single apartment complex (209). Aerosol-generating procedures such as endotracheal intubation were associated with large secondary clusters in several hospitals (210,211). Transmission to casual contacts was unusual but did occur in enclosed spaces such as taxis, trains, and aircraft (212). There have been no reported cases of transmission prior to the onset of symptoms.

Once exposed, the incubation period appears to be between 2 and 10 days, with exceptional reports of up to 20 days. During the outbreak, quarantine measures based on a maximal incubation period of 10 days were successful in interrupting transmission. Mild or asymptomatic human infections were rare and appeared to play no part in onward transmission (213,214). In general, children experienced less severe disease than adults and were thought to contribute little to transmission (215,216).

Pathogenesis

The mechanisms by which the virus causes disease are not clear at present. There are preliminary indications that higher initial viral load is associated with poor outcome (217,218), and that viral replication at different sites is important in determining the clinical manifestations (219). Virus has been detected in respiratory samples, feces, urine, blood, and cerebrospinal fluid, supporting the view that the infection is widely disseminated rather than confined to the respiratory tract. Similarly at postmortem, fatal SARS cases were found to have viral dissemination to multiple organs (220). Quantitative assays performed on respiratory specimens obtained during the course of the illness indicate that, unlike other respiratory viral infections in which viral shedding is greatest around the time symptoms develop, viral loads increase progressively to peak around 10 days from the onset of the illness, later decreasing as antibody levels rise. Virus culture is only positive during the first 3 weeks of infection (221), although viral RNA may be detected many weeks later (222). These features probably explain the epidemiologic finding that disease transmission is minimal in the early days of infection but tends to occur from the end of the first week. It is possible that viral replication continues beyond 3 weeks, but that the virus is complexed with antibody after this time and therefore not a viable means of transmission.

Postmortem studies have shown varying degrees of exudative and proliferative acute lung injury, with edema, inflammatory infiltrates, pneumocyte hyperplasia, fibrinous exudates, and later, organization and fibrosis (223,224). No specific features have been identified. It has been suggested that some of the lung damage may be immunopathologic in nature, particularly in patients who deteriorate after the second week when the viral load is decreasing.

Clinical Manifestations

Although SARS has affected people of all ages, pediatric cases have been infrequent and the disease is generally milder in children (225–227). However, children's exposure to live animal markets or seriously ill hospitalized patients is likely to have been limited. Presentation is typically acute, with high fever, myalgias, malaise, headache, and rigors. Cough is common, but upper respiratory symptoms such as coryza or sore throat are infrequent. During the second week of illness, shortness of breath, tachypnea, and pleuritic chest pain may develop, sometimes accompanied by focal respiratory signs. Watery diarrhea frequently occurs around this time. The majority of children start to improve after a few days with defervescence and improvement in clinical signs and radiologic abnormalities. In contrast, in about two thirds of adults the fever persists and the patient becomes breathless and hypoxic with increasingly severe respiratory compromise. Some 20% to 30% progress to respiratory failure and require admission to an intensive care unit for mechanical ventilation (228). Mortality in this group is high, particularly among the elderly, due to a combination of multiorgan failure, bacterial superinfection and intercurrent medical problems.

Diagnosis

The occurrence of lower respiratory disease in epidemiologically linked clusters is not unique to SARS, and no specific clinical or laboratory findings can distinguish SARS from other respiratory illnesses rapidly enough to inform critical management decisions at the time of presentation. The differential diagnosis includes a range of common respiratory pathogens, including influenza, parainfluenza and respiratory syncytial viruses, *Haemophilus influenzae*, *Mycoplasma pneumoniae*, *Legionella* species, and other atypical organisms. In March 2003, the WHO established preliminary case definitions to facilitate early diagnosis, based on a combination of clinical and epidemiologic features. These have been revised over time (229). Laboratory confirmation is required to confirm the diagnosis using either RT-PCR or serologic tests.

Although specimens from the lower respiratory tract are most useful for viral diagnosis, few patients have a productive cough early in the course of the illness. However, nasopharyngeal aspirates, nose and throat swabs, and plasma, urine and fecal specimens are all suitable for diagnosis using RT-PCR. The timing of specimen collection is important, and negative samples obtained within the first 5 days of illness should be repeated since the viral load is known to be low at this time. However, in view of the possibility of laboratory error and the serious consequences for global public health of a positive result, it is equally important that positive samples are confirmed by checking a second clinical sample and using techniques that target different parts of the genome. Serologic diagnosis is used for retrospective confirmation of SARS-CoV infection, as antibody is only detectable after the first week of illness. Late seroconversion has been seen in a few patients, so the second sample should be collected a minimum of 21 days from the onset of symptoms in order to rule out SARS conclusively.

Laboratory Investigations

Lymphopenia is common at presentation and progresses during the course of the illness (228). Thrombocytopenia and a prolonged activated partial thromboplastin time (APTT) may also be observed. Elevations of lactate dehydrogenase, liver enzymes, and creatine kinase have been noted, sometimes with electrolyte abnormalities, but there is no specific pattern to the derangements seen.

Abnormalities are noted on chest radiographs or CT scans in the majority of patients at first presentation, even within the first 3 to 4 days of illness. Typically patchy consolidation or ground-glass shadowing is seen in peripheral, subpleural, and lower zones of the lungs (230–232). At this time there may be little in the way of respiratory signs, often with a marked discrepancy noted between the clinical and radiologic findings. Serial radiologic examinations reveal progression to multifocal airspace consolidation or an ARDS picture as the patient deteriorates. Cyst formation and pneumothoraces may be seen, but mediastinal lymphadenopathy and pleural effusions are rare. Pneumomediastinum was noted in a series of patients without tracheal intubation or mechanical ventilation (233); it has been suggested that the subpleural pneumonic process has a pleurodesis-like effect so that air leaking from alveolar damage can only track along the bronchovascular bundles into the mediastinal space. Persisting radiologic abnormalities are common in survivors, even up to 6 months later (234).

Management

A number of different strategies were used to treat SARS patients around the world, but evidence documenting the efficacy of any of these therapies is lacking. Broad-spectrum antibacterial drugs were used to cover for typical and atypical community acquired pneumonias, while investigations were carried out to determine the underlying etiology of the disease. Intravenous ribavirin and high-dose intravenous corticosteroids were used in combination in many cases with severe pulmonary involvement. Oseltamivir was also used empirically in some hospitals. In vitro work is in progress looking at the effectiveness of various drugs including ribavirin, corticosteroids, and interferons-α and -β against the SARS-CoV.

The most important factor in bringing the epidemic under control was careful adherence to basic public health and infection control measures. Isolation and cohorting of patients, contact investigation and quarantine, strict infection control at health care facilities, and, in some cases, isolation of whole hospitals or communities were all employed. The effort involved was huge, and the financial costs considerable. In addition, commerce and travel were severely curtailed, resulting in major financial losses for the cities that bore the brunt of the outbreak.

Outcome

Worldwide the overall mortality rate associated with SARS was about 10%, but with considerable variation depending on age, geographical location, and comorbidity (235). In patients older than 65 years of age, particularly those with diabetes or heart disease, the death rate exceeded 50%. However, no deaths occurred in children, and relatively few required mechanical ventilation or intensive care support (227). Teenagers tended to resemble adults in their clinical presentation and disease progression, while most children younger than 12 years remained remarkably well, rarely even requiring supplemental oxygen.

Many adult survivors were left residual limitations in respiratory function as well as demonstrable radiologic abnormalities consistent with pulmonary fibrosis. Lung function testing up to 6 months after hospital discharge showed a restrictive pattern, but preliminary evidence suggests that these lung function abnormalities may improve in time (234,236). The sequelae of SARS are still largely unknown and it will be important to follow survivors to detect and manage any long-term sequelae appropriately.

Conclusion

The SARS epidemic was unprecedented in recent history for the rapidity and extent of its spread, as well as for the magnitude of its impact on the health systems and economies of the countries affected. However, the epidemic also demonstrated the effectiveness of basic infection control measures when rigorously applied, and established that international cooperation among clinicians, scientists, and health care agencies can work well when the stakes are high. Since the summer of 2003 a handful of additional cases have occurred in China, the majority following escape of the virus from laboratories working on the live virus, but fortunately onward transmission was limited in these incidents. It remains possible that further major epidemics of SARS may occur. In any event the experience with SARS serves as a reminder that new infectious diseases will undoubtedly continue to emerge and that a powerful, effective, and integrated international public health response is essential if such challenges to global health are to be contained.

References

1. Nothdurft H, Caumes E. Epidemiology of health risks and travel. In: Zuckerman J, ed. Principles and Practice of Travel Medicine. Chichester: Wiley, 2001.

2. Travel HSS. Illness in England, Wales, and Northern Ireland Associated with Foreign Travel: A Baseline Report to 2002. London: Health Protection Agency, 2003.

3. Guerin PJ, Olliaro P, Nosten F, et al. Malaria: current status of control, diagnosis, treatment, and a proposed agenda for research and development. Lancet Infect Dis 2002;2(9):564–573.

4. Snow R, Craig H, Newton C, Steketee R. The public health burden of Plasmodium falciparum malaria in Africa: Deriving the numbers. Working Paper No. 11, Bethesda, MD: Fogarty International Center, National Institutes of Health, 2003: 1–75.

5. Muentener P, Schlagenhauf P, Steffen R. Imported malaria (1985–95): trends and perspectives. Bull WHO 1999;77(7):560–566.

6. Jelinek T, Schulte C, Behrens R, et al. Imported Falciparum malaria in Europe: sentinel surveillance data from the European network on surveillance of imported infectious diseases. Clin Infect Dis 2002;34(5):572–576.

7. Robinson P, Jenney AW, Tachado M, et al. Imported malaria treated in Melbourne, Australia: epidemiology and clinical features in 246 patients. J Travel Med 2001; 8(2):76–81.

8. Amin NM. Malaria—a red alert. Am Fam Physician 1979;20(2):76–81.

9. Mouchet J. Airport malaria: a rare disease still poorly understood. Euro Surveill 2000;5(7):75–76.

10. Beeson JG, Brown GV. Pathogenesis of Plasmodium falciparum malaria: the roles of parasite adhesion and antigenic variation. Cell Mol Life Sci 2002;59:258–271.

11. Turner GD, Morrison H, Jones M, et al. An immunohistochemical study of the pathology of fatal malaria. Evidence for widespread endothelial activation and a potential role for intercellular adhesion molecule-1 in cerebral sequestration. Am J Pathol 1994;145(5):1057–1069.

12. Pongponratn E, Turner GD, Day NP, et al. An ultrastructural study of the brain in fatal Plasmodium falciparum malaria. Am J Trop Med Hyg 2003;69(4):345–359.

13. Taylor TE, Fu WJ, Carr RA, et al. Differentiating the pathologies of cerebral malaria by postmortem parasite counts. Nat Med 2004;10(2):143–145.

14. Roberts DJ, Pain A, Kai O, Kortok M, Marsh K. Autoagglutination of malaria-infected red blood cells and malaria severity. Lancet 2000;355(9213):1427–1428.

15. Dondorp AM, Angus BJ, Hardeman MR, et al. Prognostic significance of reduced red blood cell deformability in severe falciparum malaria. Am J Trop Med Hyg 1997;57(5):507–511.

16. Dondorp AM, Pongponratn E, White NJ. Reduced microcirculatory flow in severe falciparum malaria: pathophysiology and electron-microscopic pathology. Acta Trop 2004;89(3):309–317.

17. Maitland K, Newton CR. Acidosis of severe falciparum malaria: heading for a shock? Trends Parasitol 2005;21:111–116.

18. Clark IA, Cowden WB. The pathophysiology of falciparum malaria. Pharmacol Ther 2003;99(2):221–260.

19. Brown H, Hien TT, Day N, et al. Evidence of blood-brain barrier dysfunction in human cerebral malaria. Neuropathol Appl Neurobiol 1999;25(4):331–340.

20. Brown H, Rogerson S, Taylor T, et al. Blood-brain barrier function in cerebral malaria in Malawian children. Trans R Soc Trop Med Hyg 2001;64(3–4):207–213.

21. Mackintosh CL, Beeson JG, Marsh K. Clinical features and pathogenesis of severe malaria. Trends Parasitol 2004;20(12):597–603.

22. Maitland K. Severe malaria: lessons learned from the management of critical illness in children. Trends Parasitol 2006;22:457–462.
23. Croft A. Extracts from "Clinical Evidence." Malaria: prevention in travellers. BMJ 2000;321(7254):154–160.
24. Severe falciparum malaria. World Health Organization, Communicable Diseases Cluster. Trans R Soc Trop Med Hyg 2000;94(suppl 1):S1–90.
25. Group ALS. Advanced Paediatric Life Support: The Practical Approach, 3rd ed. London: BMJ Publishing Group, 2001.
26. Newton CR, Taylor TE, Whitten RO. Pathophysiology of fatal falciparum malaria in African children. Am J Trop Med Hyg 1998;58(5):673–683.
27. Newton CR, Kirkham FJ, Winstanley PA, et al. Intracranial pressure in African children with cerebral malaria. Lancet 1991;337(8741):573–576.
28. Maitland K, Nadel S, Pollard AJ, Williams TN, Newton CR, Levin M. Management of severe malaria in children: proposed guidelines for the United Kingdom. BMJ 2005;331:337–343
29. Crawley J, Smith S, Kirkham F, Muthinji P, Waruiru C, Marsh K. Seizures and status epilepticus in childhood cerebral malaria. Q J Med 1996;89(8):591–597.
30. White NJ, Miller KD, Marsh K, et al. Hypoglycaemia in African children with severe malaria. Lancet 1987;1(8535):708–711.
31. English M, Murphy S, Mwangi I, Crawley J, Peshu N, Marsh K. Interobserver variation in respiratory signs of severe malaria. Arch Dis Child 1995;72(4): 334–336.
32. English M, Waruiru C, Amukoye E, et al. Deep breathing in children with severe malaria: indicator of metabolic acidosis and poor outcome. Am J Trop Med Hyg 1996;55(5):521–524.
33. Maitland K, Levin M, English M, et al. Severe P. falciparum malaria in Kenyan children: evidence for hypovolaemia. Q J Med 2003;96(6):427–434.
34. Maitland K, Pamba A, Newton CR, Levin M. Response to volume resuscitation in children with severe malaria. Pediatr Crit Care Med 2003;4(4):426–431.
35. Pamba A, Maitland K. Capillary refill: prognostic value in Kenyan children. Arch Dis Child 2004;89:950–955.
36. Maitland K, Pamba A, English M, et al. Randomized trial of volume expansion with albumin or saline in children with severe malaria: preliminary evidence of albumin benefit. Clin Infect Dis 2005;40:538–545.
36a. Akech S, Gwer S, Idro R, et al. Volume Expansion with Albumin Compared to Gelofusine in Children with Severe Malaria: Results of a Controlled Trial. PLoS Clin Trials 2006;1:e21.
37. Newton CR, Hien TT, White N. Cerebral malaria. J Neurol Neurosurg Psychiatry 2000;69(4):433–441.
38. Group ALS. The Child with a Decreased Conscious Level, 3rd ed. London: BMJ Publishing Group, 2001.
39. Newton CR, Crawley J, Sowumni A, et al. Intracranial hypertension in Africans with cerebral malaria. Arch Dis Child 1997;76(3):219–226.
40. Looareesuwan S, Warrell DA, White NJ, et al. Do patients with cerebral malaria have cerebral oedema? A computed tomography study. Lancet 1983;1(8322):434–437.
41. Newton CR, Marsh K, Peshu N, Kirkham FJ. Perturbations of cerebral hemodynamics in Kenyans with cerebral malaria. Pediatr Neurol 1996;15(1):41–49.
42. Herson VC, Todd JK. Prediction of morbidity in Haemophilus influenzae meningitis. Pediatrics 1977;59(1):35–39.

43. Powell KR, Sugarman LI, Eskenazi AE, et al. Normalization of plasma arginine vasopressin concentrations when children with meningitis are given maintenance plus replacement fluid therapy. J Pediatr 1990;117(4):515–522.

44. The Artemeter-Quinine Meta-analysis Group. A meta-analysis using individual patient data of trials comparing artemether with quinine in the treatment of severe falciparum malaria. Trans R Soc Trop Med Hyg 2001;95(6):637–650.

45. Crawley J, English M, Waruiru C, Mwangi I, Marsh K. Abnormal respiratory patterns in childhood cerebral malaria. Trans R Soc Trop Med Hyg 1998;92(3): 305–308.

46. Ogutu BR, Newton CR. Management of seizures in children with falciparum malaria. Trop Doct 2004;34(2):71–75.

47. Group ALS. The Convulsing Child, 3rd ed. London: BMJ Publishing Group, 2001.

48. Crawley J, Waruiru C, Mithwani S, et al. Effect of phenobarbital on seizure frequency and mortality in childhood cerebral malaria: a randomised, controlled intervention study. Lancet 2000;355(9205):701–706.

49. Kokwaro GO, Ogutu BR, Muchohi SN, Otieno GO, Newton CR. Pharmacokinetics and clinical effect of phenobarbital in children with severe falciparum malaria and convulsions. Br J Clin Pharmacol 2003;56(4):453–457.

50. Ogutu BR, Newton CR, Muchohi SN, et al. Pharmacokinetics and clinical effects of phenytoin and fosphenytoin in children with severe falciparum malaria and status epilepticus. Br J Clin Pharmacol 2003;56:112–119.

51. Dondorp AM, Chau TT, Phu NH, et al. Unidentified acids of strong prognostic significance in severe malaria. Crit Care Med 2004;32(8):1683–1688.

52. English M, Sauerwein R, Waruiru C, et al. Acidosis in severe childhood malaria. Q J Med 1997;90(4):263–270.

53. Maitland K, Pamba A, Fegan G, et al. Perturbations in electrolyte levels in Kenyan children with severe malaria complicated by acidosis. Clin Infect Dis 2005; 40(1):9–16.

54. Taylor TE, Molyneux ME, Wirima JJ, Fletcher KA, Morris K. Blood glucose levels in Malawian children before and during the administration of intravenous quinine for severe falciparum malaria. N Engl J Med 1988;319(16):1040–1047.

55. Maitland K, Pamba A, Newton CR, Lowe B, Levin M. Hypokalemia in children with severe falciparum malaria. Pediatr Crit Care Med 2004;5(1):81–85.

56. Fleming AF. HIV and blood transfusion in sub-Saharan Africa. Transfus Sci 1997;18(2):167–179.

57. Ladhani S, Lowe B, Cole AO, Kowuondo K, Newton CR. Changes in white blood cells and platelets in children with falciparum malaria: relationship to disease outcome. Br J Haematol 2002;119(3):839–847.

58. Turner GD, Ly VC, Nguyen TH, et al. Systemic endothelial activation occurs in both mild and severe malaria. Correlating dermal microvascular endothelial cell phenotype and soluble cell adhesion molecules with disease severity. Am J Pathol 1998;152(6):1477–1487.

59. Boehme MW, Werle E, Kommerell B, Raeth U. Serum levels of adhesion molecules and thrombomodulin as indicators of vascular injury in severe Plasmodium falciparum malaria. Clin Invest 1994;72(8):598–603.

60. Hemmer CJ, Bierhaus A, von Riedesel J, et al. Elevated thrombomodulin plasma levels as a result of endothelial involvement in Plasmodium falciparum malaria. Thromb Haemost 1994;72(3):457–464.

61. Gerardin P, Rogier C, Ka AS, Jouvencel P, Brousse V, Imbert P. Prognostic value of thrombocytopenia in African children with falciparum malaria. Am J Trop Med Hyg 2002;66(6):686–691.

62. Gyr K, Speck B, Ritz R, Cornu P, Buckner CD. Cerebral tropical malaria with blackwater fever. A current diagnostic and therapeutic problem). Schweiz Med Wochenschr 1974;104(45):1628–1630.

63. Macallan DC, Pocock M, Robinson GT, Parker-Williams J, Bevan DH. Red cell exchange, erythrocytapheresis, in the treatment of malaria with high parasitaemia in returning travellers. Trans R Soc Trop Med Hyg 2000;94(4):353–356.

64. Riddle MS, Jackson JL, Sanders JW, Blazes DL. Exchange transfusion as an adjunct therapy in severe Plasmodium falciparum malaria: a meta-analysis. Clin Infect Dis 2002;34(9):1192–1198.

65. Lindenbach B, Rice C. Flaviviridae: The viruses and their replication. In: Knipe D, Howley P, eds. Fields Virology, 4th ed. Philadelphia: Lippincott Williams & Wilkins, 2001:991–1004.

66. Monath TP. Dengue: the risk to developed and developing countries. Proc Natl Acad Sci U S A 1994;91(7):2395–2400.

67. Hales S, de Wet N, Maindonald J, Woodward A. Potential effect of population and climate changes on global distribution of dengue fever: an empirical model. Lancet 2002;360(9336):830–834.

68. Gubler DJ. Dengue and dengue haemorrhagic fever: its history and resurgence as a global health problem. In: Gubler DJ, Kuno G, eds. Dengue and Dengue Haemorrhagic Fever. Wallingford: CAB International, 1997:1–23.

69. WHO. Dengue Haemorrhagic Fever: Diagnosis, Treatment, Prevention and Control. Geneva: World Health Organization, 1997.

70. Rigau-Perez JG, Bonilla GL. An evaluation of modified case definitions for the detection of dengue hemorrhagic fever. Puerto Rico Association of Epidemiologists. P R Health Sci J 1999;18(4):347–352.

71. Harris E, Videa E, Perez L, et al. Clinical, epidemiologic, and virologic features of dengue in the 1998 epidemic in Nicaragua. Am J Trop Med Hyg 2000;63(1–2):5–11.

72. Phuong CX, Nhan NT, Kneen R, et al. Clinical diagnosis and assessment of severity of confirmed dengue infections in Vietnamese children: is the world health organization classification system helpful? Am J Trop Med Hyg 2004;70(2):172–179.

73. Halstead SB, Nimmannitya S, Cohen SN. Observations related to pathogenesis of dengue hemorrhagic fever. IV. Relation of disease severity to antibody response and virus recovered. Yale J Biol Med 1970;42(5):311–328.

74. Sangkawibha N, Rojanasuphot S, Ahandrik S, et al. Risk factors in dengue shock syndrome: a prospective epidemiologic study in Rayong, Thailand. I. The 1980 outbreak. Am J Epidemiol 1984;120(5):653–669.

75. Guzman MG, Kouri G, Bravo J, Valdes L, Vazquez S, Halstead SB. Effect of age on outcome of secondary dengue 2 infections. Int J Infect Dis 2002;6(2):118–124.

76. Gamble J, Bethell D, Day NP, et al. Age-related changes in microvascular permeability: a significant factor in the susceptibility of children to shock? Clin Sci (Lond) 2000;98(2):211–216.

77. Halstead SB, O'Rourke EJ. Antibody-enhanced dengue virus infection in primate leukocytes. Nature 1977;265(5596):739–741.

78. Halstead SB. In vivo enhancement of dengue virus infection in rhesus monkeys by passively transferred antibody. J Infect Dis 1979;140(4):527–533.

79. Mongkolsapaya J, Dejnirattisai W, Xu XN, et al. Original antigenic sin and apoptosis in the pathogenesis of dengue hemorrhagic fever. Nat Med 2003;9(7): 921–927.

80. Markoff LJ, Innis BL, Houghten R, Henchal LS. Development of cross-reactive antibodies to plasminogen during the immune response to dengue virus infection. J Infect Dis 1991;164(2):294–301.

81. Lin CF, Chiu SC, Hsiao YL, et al. Expression of cytokine, chemokine, and adhesion molecules during endothelial cell activation induced by antibodies against dengue virus nonstructural protein 1. J Immunol 2005;174(1):395–403.

82. Petchclai B, Saelim P. Circulating immune complexes in dengue haemorrhagic fever. Lancet 1978;2(8090):638–639.

83. Ruangjirachuporn W, Boonpucknavig S, Nimmanitya S. Circulating immune complexes in serum from patients with dengue haemorrhagic fever. Clin Exp Immunol 1979;36(1):46–53.

84. Wang W, Chao D, Kao CL, et al. High levels of plasma dengue viral load during defervescence in patients with dengue hemorrhagic fever: implications for pathogenesis. Virology 2003;305(2):330–338.

85. Bokisch VA, Top FH Jr, Russell PK, Dixon FJ, Muller-Eberhard HJ. The potential pathogenic role of complement in dengue hemorrhagic shock syndrome. N Engl J Med 1973;289(19):996–1000.

86. Malasit P. Complement and dengue haemorrhagic fever/shock syndrome. Southeast Asian J Trop Med Public Health 1987;18(3):316–320.

87. Shaio MF, Chang FY, Hou SC. Complement pathway activity in serum from patients with classical dengue fever. Trans R Soc Trop Med Hyg 1992;86(6):672–675.

88. Bethell DB, Flobbe K, Cao XT, et al. Pathophysiologic and prognostic role of cytokines in dengue hemorrhagic fever. J Infect Dis 1998;177(3):778–782.

89. Green S, Vaughn DW, Kalayanarooj S, et al. Early immune activation in acute dengue illness is related to development of plasma leakage and disease severity. J Infect Dis 1999;179(4):755–762.

90. Green S, Vaughn DW, Kalayanarooj S, et al. Elevated plasma interleukin-10 levels in acute dengue correlate with disease severity. J Med Virol 1999;59(3):329–334.

91. Barnes WJ, Rosen L. Fatal hemorrhagic disease and shock associated with primary dengue infection on a Pacific island. Am J Trop Med Hyg 1974;23(3):495–506.

92. Scott RM, Nimmannitya S, Bancroft WH, Mansuwan P. Shock syndrome in primary dengue infections. Am J Trop Med Hyg 1976;25(6):866–874.

93. Rico-Hesse R, Harrison LM, Salas RA, et al. Origins of dengue type 2 viruses associated with increased pathogenicity in the Americas. Virology 1997;230(2):244–251.

94. Loke H, Bethell DB, Phuong CX, et al. Strong HLA class I–restricted T cell responses in dengue hemorrhagic fever: a double-edged sword? J Infect Dis 2001;184(11): 1369–1373.

95. Loke H, Bethell D, Phuong CX, et al. Susceptibility to dengue hemorrhagic fever in Vietnam: evidence of an association with variation in the vitamin d receptor and Fc gamma receptor IIa genes. Am J Trop Med Hyg 2002;67(1):102–106.

96. Stephens HA, Klaythong R, Sirikong M, et al. HLA-A and -B allele associations with secondary dengue virus infections correlate with disease severity and the infecting viral serotype in ethnic Thais. Tissue Antigens 2002;60(4):309–318.

97. Bhamarapravati N. Pathology of Infection. In: Gubler DJ, Kuno G, eds. Dengue and Dengue Hemorrhagic Fever. Wallingford, CT: CAB International, 1997: 115–132.

98. Hu X, Weinbaum S. A new view of Starling's hypothesis at the microstructural level. Microvasc Res 1999;58(3):281–304.

99. Michel CC, Curry FE. Microvascular permeability. Physiol Rev 1999;79(3): 703–761.

100. Wills BA, Oragui EE, Dung NM, et al. Size and charge characteristics of the protein leak in dengue shock syndrome. J Infect Dis 2004;190(4):810–818.

101. Hayes CG, Manaloto CR, Gonzales A, Ranoa CP. Dengue infections in the Philippines: clinical and virological findings in 517 hospitalized patients. Am J Trop Med Hyg 1988;39(1):110–116.

102. Kabra SK, Jain Y, Pandey RM, et al. Dengue haemorrhagic fever in children in the 1996 Delhi epidemic. Trans R Soc Trop Med Hyg 1999;93(3):294–298.

103. Wills BA, Oragui EE, Stephens AC, et al. Coagulation abnormalities in dengue hemorrhagic fever: serial investigations in 167 Vietnamese children with Dengue shock syndrome. Clin Infect Dis 2002;35(3):277–285.

104. Nimmannitya S, Thisyakorn U, Hemsrichart V. Dengue haemorrhagic fever with unusual manifestations. Southeast Asian J Trop Med Public Health 1987;18(3): 398–406.

105. Murgue B, Deparis X, Chungue E, Cassar O, Roche C. Dengue: an evaluation of dengue severity in French Polynesia based on an analysis of 403 laboratory-confirmed cases. Trop Med Int Health 1999;4(11):765–773.

106. Lum LC, Lam SK, Choy YS, George R, Harun F. Dengue encephalitis: a true entity? Am J Trop Med Hyg 1996;54(3):256–259.

107. Solomon T, Dung NM, Vaughn DW, et al. Neurological manifestations of dengue infection. Lancet 2000;355(9209):1053–1059.

108. Cam BV, Fonsmark L, Hue NB, Phuong NT, Poulsen A, Heegaard ED. Prospective case-control study of encephalopathy in children with dengue hemorrhagic fever. Am J Trop Med Hyg 2001;65(6):848–851.

109. WHO. Technical guides for diagnosis, treatment, surveillance, prevention and control of dengue haemorrhagic fever. Geneva: World Health Organization, 1975.

110. Rosen L, Gubler D. The use of mosquitoes to detect and propagate dengue viruses. Am J Trop Med Hyg 1974;23(6):1153–1160.

111. Gubler DJ, Suharyono W, Tan R, Abidin M, Sie A. Viraemia in patients with naturally acquired dengue infection. Bull WHO 1981;59(4):623–630.

112. Henchal EA, Polo SL, Vorndam V, Yaemsiri C, Innis BL, Hoke CH. Sensitivity and specificity of a universal primer set for the rapid diagnosis of dengue virus infections by polymerase chain reaction and nucleic acid hybridization. Am J Trop Med Hyg 1991;45(4):418–428.

113. Morita K, Tanaka M, Igarashi A. Rapid identification of dengue virus serotypes by using polymerase chain reaction. J Clin Microbiol 1991;29(10):2107–2110.

114. Lanciotti RS, Calisher CH, Gubler DJ, Chang GJ, Vorndam AV. Rapid detection and typing of dengue viruses from clinical samples by using reverse transcriptase-polymerase chain reaction. J Clin Microbiol 1992;30(3):545–551.

115. Innis BL, Nisalak A, Nimmannitya S, et al. An enzyme-linked immunosorbent assay to characterize dengue infections where dengue and Japanese encephalitis co-circulate. Am J Trop Med Hyg 1989;40(4):418–427.

116. Nimmannitya S, Halstead SB, Cohen SN, Margiotta MR. Dengue and chikungunya virus infection in man in Thailand, 1962–1964. I. Observations on hospitalized patients with hemorrhagic fever. Am J Trop Med Hyg 1969;18(6):954–971.

117. Dietz V, Gubler DJ, Ortiz S. The 1986 dengue fever outbreak in Puerto Rico. Dengue Surveill Summ 1987;40:1–2.
118. Mitrakul C, Poshyachinda M, Futrakul P, Sangkawibha N, Ahandrik S. Hemostatic and platelet kinetic studies in dengue hemorrhagic fever. Am J Trop Med Hyg 1977;26(5 Pt 1):975–984.
119. Srichaikul T. Pathogenesis of bleeding in DHF: role of platelet and coagulation abnormalities. J Med Assoc Thai 1989;72(4):239–242.
120. Krishnamurti C, Kalayanarooj S, Cutting MA, et al. Mechanisms of hemorrhage in dengue without circulatory collapse. Am J Trop Med Hyg 2001;65(6):840–847.
121. Huang YH, Liu CC, Wang ST, et al. Activation of coagulation and fibrinolysis during dengue virus infection. J Med Virol 2001;63(3):247–251.
122. Sumarmo, Talogo W, Asrin A, Isnuhandojo B, Sahudi A. Failure of hydrocortisone to affect outcome in dengue shock syndrome. Pediatrics 1982; 69(1):45–49.
123. Tassniyom S, Vasanawathana S, Chirawatkul A, Rojanasuphot S. Failure of high-dose methylprednisolone in established dengue shock syndrome: a placebo-controlled, double-blind study. Pediatrics 1993;92(1):111–115.
124. Griffel MI, Kaufman BS. Pharmacology of colloids and crystalloids. Crit Care Clin 1992;8(2):235–253.
124a. Wills BA, Nguyen MD, Ha TL, et al. Comparison of three fluid solutions for resuscitation in dengue shock syndrome. N Engl J Med 2005;353(9):877–889.
125. Halstead SB. Is there an inapparent dengue explosion? Lancet 1999;353(9158): 1100–1101.
126. Halstead SB, Grosz CR. Subclinical Japanese encephalitis. I. Infection of Americans with limited residence in Korea. Am J Hyg 1962;75:190–201.
127. Huang CH. Studies of Japanese encephalitis in China. Adv Virus Res 1982;27: 71–101.
128. Tsai TF. Factors in the changing epidemiology of Japanese encephalitis and West Nile fever. In: Saluzzo JF, Dodet B, eds. Factors in the Emergence of Arbovirus Disease. Paris: Elsevier, 1997:179–189.
129. Wu YC, Huang YS, Chien LJ, et al. The epidemiology of Japanese encephalitis on Taiwan during 1966–1997. Am J Trop Med Hyg 1999;61(1):78–84.
130. Solomon T, Dung NM, Kneen R, Gainsborough M, Vaughn DW, Khanh VT. Japanese encephalitis. J Neurol Neurosurg Psychiatry 2000;68(4):405–415.
131. Macdonald WB, Tink AR, Ouvrier RA, et al. Japanese encephalitis after a two-week holiday in Bali. Med J Aust 1989;150(6):334–336, 339.
132. Wittesjo B, Eitrem R, Niklasson B, Vene S, Mangiafico JA. Japanese encephalitis after a 10-day holiday in Bali. Lancet 1995;345(8953):856–857.
133. Desai A, Shankar SK, Ravi V, Chandramuki A, Gourie-Devi M. Japanese encephalitis virus antigen in the human brain and its topographic distribution. Acta Neuropathol (Berl) 1995;89(4):368–373.
134. Johnson RT, Burke DS, Elwell M, et al. Japanese encephalitis: immunocytochemical studies of viral antigen and inflammatory cells in fatal cases. Ann Neurol 1985; 18(5):567–573.
135. Misra UK, Kalita J. Seizures in Japanese encephalitis. J Neurol Sci 2001;190(1–2): 57–60.
136. Solomon T, Dung NM, Kneen R, et al. Seizures and raised intracranial pressure in Vietnamese patients with Japanese encephalitis. Brain 2002;125(pt 5):1084–1093.

137. Misra UK, Kalita J. Anterior horn cells are also involved in Japanese encephalitis. Acta Neurol Scand 1997;96(2):114–117.

138. Solomon T, Kneen R, Dung NM, et al. Poliomyelitis-like illness due to Japanese encephalitis virus. Lancet 1998;351(9109):1094–1097.

139. Kalita J, Misra UK. Comparison of CT scan and MRI findings in the diagnosis of Japanese encephalitis. J Neurol Sci 2000;174(1):3–8.

140. Kalita J, Misra UK, Pandey S, Dhole TN. A comparison of clinical and radiological findings in adults and children with Japanese encephalitis. Arch Neurol 2003;60(12): 1760–1764.

141. Prakash M, Kumar S, Gupta RK. Diffusion-weighted MR imaging in Japanese encephalitis. J Comput Assist Tomogr 2004;28(6):756–761.

142. Kalita J, Das BK, Misra UK. SPECT studies of regional cerebral blood flow in 8 patients with Japanese encephalitis in subacute and chronic stage. Acta Neurol Scand 1999;99(4):213–218.

143. Kalita J, Misra UK. EEG in Japanese encephalitis: a clinico-radiological correlation. Electroencephalogr Clin Neurophysiol 1998;106(3):238–243.

144. Hoke CH Jr, Vaughn DW, Nisalak A, et al. Effect of high-dose dexamethasone on the outcome of acute encephalitis due to Japanese encephalitis virus. J Infect Dis 1992;165(4):631–637.

145. Solomon T, Dung NM, Wills B, et al. Interferon alfa-2a in Japanese encephalitis: a randomised double-blind placebo-controlled trial. Lancet 2003;361(9360):821–826.

146. de Benoist AC, White JM, Efstratiou A, et al. Imported cutaneous diphtheria, United Kingdom. Emerg Infect Dis 2004;10(3):511–513.

147. Harnisch JP, Tronca E, Nolan CM, Turck M, Holmes KK. Diphtheria among alcoholic urban adults. A decade of experience in Seattle. Ann Intern Med 1989;111(1):71–82.

148. Galazka AM, Robertson SE, Oblapenko GP. Resurgence of diphtheria. Eur J Epidemiol 1995;11(1):95–105.

149. Dittmann S, Wharton M, Vitek C, et al. Successful control of epidemic diphtheria in the states of the Former Union of Soviet Socialist Republics: lessons learned. J Infect Dis 2000;181(suppl 1):S10–22.

150. WHO. The World Health Report 2004—Changing History. Geneva: World Health Organization, 2004:120–126.

151. Public Health Laboratory Services. A case of diphtheria from Pakistan. CDR Weekly 1994;4(37):173.

152. Nuorti P. Fatal case of diphtheria in an unvaccinated infant, Finland 2001. Eurosurveill Wkly 2002;6:4.

153. Pappenheimer AM Jr. Diphtheria toxin. Annu Rev Biochem 1977;46:69–94.

154. Zuber PL, Gruner E, Altwegg M, von Graevenitz A. Invasive infection with nontoxigenic Corynebacterium diphtheriae among drug users. Lancet 1992;339(8805): 1359.

155. Tiley SM, Kociuba KR, Heron LG, Munro R. Infective endocarditis due to nontoxigenic Corynebacterium diphtheriae: report of seven cases and review. Clin Infect Dis 1993;16(2):271–275.

156. Bethell DB, Nguyen Minh D, Ha Thi L, et al. Prognostic value of electrocardiographic monitoring of patients with severe diphtheria. Clin Infect Dis 1995;20(5): 1259–1265.

157. Loukoushkina EF, Bobko PV, Kolbasova EV, et al. The clinical picture and diagnosis of diphtheritic carditis in children. Eur J Pediatr 1998;157(7):528–533.

158. Lumio JT, Groundstroem KW, Melnick OB, Huhtala H, Rakhmanova AG. Electro-cardiographic abnormalities in patients with diphtheria: a prospective study. Am J Med 2004;116(2):78–83.

159. Logina I, Donaghy M. Diphtheritic polyneuropathy: a clinical study and comparison with Guillain-Barre syndrome. J Neurol Neurosurg Psychiatry 1999;67(4):433–438.

160. Bowler IC, Mandal BK, Schlecht B, Riordan T. Diphtheria—the continuing hazard. Arch Dis Child 1988;63(2):194–195.

161. Bonnet JM, Begg NT. Control of diphtheria: guidance for consultants in communicable disease control. World Health Organization. Commun Dis Public Health 1999;2(4):242–249.

162. Kneen R, Pham NG, Solomon T, et al. Penicillin vs. erythromycin in the treatment of diphtheria. Clin Infect Dis 1998;27(4):845–850.

163. Stockins BA, Lanas FT, Saavedra JG, Opazo JA. Prognosis in patients with diphtheric myocarditis and bradyarrhythmias: assessment of results of ventricular pacing. Br Heart J 1994;72(2):190–191.

164. Dung NM, Kneen R, Kiem N, et al. Treatment of severe diphtheritic myocarditis by temporary insertion of a cardiac pacemaker. Clin Infect Dis 2002;35(11):1425–1429.

165. Thisyakorn U, Wongvanich J, Kumpeng V. Failure of corticosteroid therapy to prevent diphtheritic myocarditis or neuritis. Pediatr Infect Dis 1984;3(2):126–128.

166. Quick ML, Sutter RW, Kobaidze K, et al. Epidemic diphtheria in the Republic of Georgia, 1993–1996: risk factors for fatal outcome among hospitalized patients. J Infect Dis 2000;181(suppl 1):S130–137.

167. Udwadia FE, Sunavala JD, Jain MC, et al. Haemodynamic studies during the management of severe tetanus. Q J Med 1992;83(302):449–460.

168. Neequaye J, Nkrumah FK. Failure of intrathecal antitetanus serum to improve survival in neonatal tetanus. Arch Dis Child 1983;58(4):276–278.

169. Okoromah CN, Lesi FE. Diazepam for treating tetanus. Cochrane Database Syst Rev 2004(1):CD003954.

170. Boots RJ, Lipman J, O'Callaghan J, Scott P, Fraser J. The treatment of tetanus with intrathecal baclofen. Anaesth Intensive Care 2000;28(4):438–442.

171. Attygalle D, Rodrigo N. Magnesium as first line therapy in the management of tetanus: a prospective study of 40 patients. Anaesthesia 2002;57(8):811–817.

172. Attygalle D, Rodrigo N. New trends in the management of tetanus. Expert Rev Anti Infect Ther 2004;2(1):73–84.

173. Brauner JS, Vieira SR, Bleck TP. Changes in severe accidental tetanus mortality in the ICU during two decades in Brazil. Intensive Care Med 2002;28(7):930–935.

174. Heymann DL, Aylward RB. Eradicating polio. N Engl J Med 2004;351(13):1275–1277.

175. Progress toward poliomyelitis eradication—poliomyelitis outbreak in Sudan, 2004. MMWR Morb Mortal Wkly Rep 2005;54(4):97–99.

176. Fine PE, Oblapenko G, Sutter RW. Polio control after certification: major issues outstanding. Bull WHO 2004;82(1):47–52.

177. Nash D, Mostashari F, Fine A, et al. The outbreak of West Nile virus infection in the New York City area in 1999. N Engl J Med 2001;344(24):1807–1814.

178. Solomon T, Willison H. Infectious causes of acute flaccid paralysis. Curr Opin Infect Dis 2003;16(5):375–381.

179. Sejvar JJ. West Nile virus and "poliomyelitis." Neurology 2004;63(2):206–207.
180. Romero JR. Pleconaril: a novel antipicornaviral drug. Expert Opin Invest Drugs 2001;10(2):369–379.
181. Peiris M, Yuen KY, Leung CW, et al. Human infection with influenza H9N2. Lancet 1999;354(9182):916–917.
182. Koopmans M, Wilbrink B, Conyn M, et al. Transmission of H7N7 avian influenza A virus to human beings during a large outbreak in commercial poultry farms in the Netherlands. Lancet 2004;363(9409):587–593.
183. Fouchier RA, Schneeberger PM, Rozendaal FW, et al. Avian influenza A virus (H7N7) associated with human conjunctivitis and a fatal case of acute respiratory distress syndrome. Proc Natl Acad Sci U S A 2004;101(5):1356–1361.
184. Yuen KY, Chan PK, Peiris M, et al. Clinical features and rapid viral diagnosis of human disease associated with avian influenza A H5N1 virus. Lancet 1998;351(9101): 467–471.
185. Guan Y, Poon LL, Cheung CY, et al. H5N1 influenza: a protean pandemic threat. Proc Natl Acad Sci U S A 2004;101(21):8156–8161.
186. Li KS, Guan Y, Wang J, et al. Genesis of a highly pathogenic and potentially pandemic H5N1 influenza virus in eastern Asia. Nature 2004;430(6996):209–213.
187. Kuiken T, Rimmelzwaan G, van Riel D, et al. Avian H5N1 influenza in cats. Science 2004;306(5694):241. Epub 2004 Sept 2.
188. Keawcharoen J, Oraveerakul K, Kuiken T, et al. Avian influenza H5N1 in tigers and leopards. Emerg Infect Dis 2004;10(12):2189–2191.
189. Ungchusak K, Auewarakul P, Dowell SF, et al. Probable person-to-person transmission of avian influenza A (H5N1). N Engl J Med 2005;352(4):333–340. Epub 2005 Jan 24.
190. Mounts AW, Kwong H, Izurieta HS, et al. Case-control study of risk factors for avian influenza A (H5N1) disease, Hong Kong, 1997. J Infect Dis 1999;180(2): 505–508.
191. Tran TH, Nguyen TL, Nguyen TD, et al. Avian influenza A (H5N1) in 10 patients in Vietnam. N Engl J Med 2004;350(12):1179–1188.
192. Steinhauer DA. Role of hemagglutinin cleavage for the pathogenicity of influenza virus. Virology 1999;258(1):1–20.
193. To KF, Chan PK, Chan KF, et al. Pathology of fatal human infection associated with avian influenza A H5N1 virus. J Med Virol 2001;63(3):242–246.
194. Peiris JS, Yu WC, Leung CW, et al. Re-emergence of fatal human influenza A subtype H5N1 disease. Lancet 2004;363(9409):617–619.
195. Apisarnthanarak A, Kitphati R, Thongphubeth K, et al. Atypical avian influenza (H5N1). Emerg Infect Dis 2004;10(7):1321–1324.
196. de Jong MD, Bach VC, Phan TQ, et al. Fatal avian influenza A (H5N1) in a child presenting with diarrhea followed by coma. N Engl J Med 2005;352(7):686–691.
197. Buxton Bridges C, Katz JM, Seto WH, et al. Risk of influenza A (H5N1) infection among health care workers exposed to patients with influenza A (H5N1), Hong Kong. J Infect Dis 2000;181(1):344–348.
198. Brooks MJ, Sasadeusz JJ, Tannock GA. Antiviral chemotherapeutic agents against respiratory viruses: where are we now and what's in the pipeline? Curr Opin Pulmon Med 2004;10(3):197–203.
199. Puthavathana P, Auewarakul P, Charoenying PC, et al. Molecular characterization of the complete genome of human influenza H5N1 virus isolates from Thailand. J Gen Virol 2005;86(Pt 2):423–433.

200. Matrosovich MN, Matrosovich TY, Gray T, Roberts NA, Klenk HD. Neuraminidase is important for the initiation of influenza virus infection in human airway epithelium. J Virol 2004;78(22):12665-12667.

201. Kiso M, Mitamura K, Sakai-Tagawa Y, et al. Resistant influenza A viruses in children treated with oseltamivir: descriptive study. Lancet 2004;364(9436): 759-765.

202. Marra MA, Jones SJ, Astell CR, et al. The Genome sequence of the SARS-associated coronavirus. Science 2003;300(5624):1399-1404. Epub 2003 May 1.

203. Rota PA, Oberste MS, Monroe SS, et al. Characterization of a novel coronavirus associated with severe acute respiratory syndrome. Science 2003;300(5624):1394-1399. Epub 2003 May 1.

204. Wang M, Xu HF, Zhang ZB, et al. [Analysis on the risk factors of severe acute respiratory syndromes coronavirus infection in workers from animal markets.] Zhonghua Liu Xing Bing Xue Za Zhi 2004;25(6):503-505.

205. Guan Y, Zheng BJ, He YQ, et al. Isolation and characterization of viruses related to the SARS coronavirus from animals in southern China. Science 2003;302(5643): 276-278. Epub 2003 Sep 4.

206. Consortium CSME. Molecular evolution of the SARS coronavirus during the course of the SARS epidemic in China. Science 2004;303(5664):1666-1669. Epub 2004 Jan 29.

207. Riley S, Fraser C, Donnelly CA, et al. Transmission dynamics of the etiological agent of SARS in Hong Kong: impact of public health interventions. Science 2003;300(5627):1961-1966. Epub 2003 May 23.

208. Anderson RM, Fraser C, Ghani AC, et al. Epidemiology, transmission dynamics and control of SARS: the 2002-2003 epidemic. Philos Trans R Soc Lond B Biol Sci 2004;359(1447):1091-1105.

209. Yu IT, Li Y, Wong TW, et al. Evidence of airborne transmission of the severe acute respiratory syndrome virus. N Engl J Med 2004;350(17):1731-1739.

210. Varia M, Wilson S, Sarwal S, et al. Investigation of a nosocomial outbreak of severe acute respiratory syndrome (SARS) in Toronto, Canada. Can Med Assoc J 2003; 169(4):285-292.

211. Scales DC, Green K, Chan AK, et al. Illness in intensive care staff after brief exposure to severe acute respiratory syndrome. Emerg Infect Dis 2003;9(10): 1205-1210.

212. Olsen SJ, Chang HL, Cheung TY, et al. Transmission of the severe acute respiratory syndrome on aircraft. N Engl J Med 2003;349(25):2416-2422.

213. Chan PK, Ip M, Ng KC, et al. Severe acute respiratory syndrome-associated coronavirus infection. Emerg Infect Dis 2003;9(11):1453-1454.

214. Lee HK, Tso EY, Chau TN, Tsang OT, Choi KW, Lai TS. Asymptomatic severe acute respiratory syndrome-associated coronavirus infection. Emerg Infect Dis 2003; 9(11):1491-1492.

215. Bitnun A, Allen U, Heurter H, et al. Children hospitalized with severe acute respiratory syndrome-related illness in Toronto. Pediatrics 2003;112(4):e261.

216. Chang LY, Huang FY, Wu YC, et al. Childhood severe acute respiratory syndrome in Taiwan and how to differentiate it from childhood influenza infection. Arch Pediatr Adolesc Med 2004;158(11):1037-1042.

217. Chu CM, Poon LL, Cheng VC, et al. Initial viral load and the outcomes of SARS. Can Med Assoc J 2004;171(11):1349-1352.

218. Cheng VC, Hung IF, Tang BS, et al. Viral replication in the nasopharynx is associated with diarrhea in patients with severe acute respiratory syndrome. Clin Infect Dis 2004;38(4):467–475. Epub 2004 Jan 29.

219. Hung IF, Cheng VC, Wu AK, et al. Viral loads in clinical specimens and SARS manifestations. Emerg Infect Dis 2004;10(9):1550–1557.

220. Farcas GA, Poutanen SM, Mazzulli T, et al. Fatal severe acute respiratory syndrome is associated with multiorgan involvement by coronavirus. J Infect Dis 2005; 191(2):193–197.

221. Chan KH, Poon LL, Cheng VC, et al. Detection of SARS coronavirus in patients with suspected SARS. Emerg Infect Dis 2004;10(2):294–299.

222. Chu CM, Leung WS, Cheng VC, et al. Duration of RT-PCR positivity in severe acute respiratory syndrome. Eur Respir J 2005;25(1):12–14.

223. Nicholls JM, Poon LL, Lee KC, et al. Lung pathology of fatal severe acute respiratory syndrome. Lancet 2003;361(9371):1773–1778.

224. Hwang DM, Chamberlain DW, Poutanen SM, Low DE, Asa SL, Butany J. Pulmonary pathology of severe acute respiratory syndrome in Toronto. Mod Pathol 2005;18(1): 1–10.

225. Hon KL, Leung CW, Cheng WT, et al. Clinical presentations and outcome of severe acute respiratory syndrome in children. Lancet 2003;361(9370):1701–1703.

226. Wong GW, Li AM, Ng PC, Fok TF. Severe acute respiratory syndrome in children. Pediatr Pulmonol 2003;36(4):261–266.

227. Leung CW, Chiu WK. Clinical picture, diagnosis, treatment and outcome of severe acute respiratory syndrome (SARS) in children. Paediatr Respir Rev 2004;5(4): 275–288.

228. Lee N, Hui D, Wu A, et al. A major outbreak of severe acute respiratory syndrome in Hong Kong. N Engl J Med 2003;348(20):1986–1994.

229. WHO. WHO Guidelines for the Surveillance of Severe Acute Respiratory Syndrome (SARS)—Updated Recommendations, October 2004. Geneva: World Health Organization, 2004.

230. Muller NL, Ooi GC, Khong PL, Nicolaou S. Severe acute respiratory syndrome: radiographic and CT findings. AJR Am J Roentgenol 2003;181(1):3–8.

231. Babyn PS, Chu WC, Tsou IY, et al. Severe acute respiratory syndrome (SARS): chest radiographic features in children. Pediatr Radiol 2004;34(1):47–58.

232. Muller NL, Ooi GC, Khong PL, Zhou LJ, Tsang KW, Nicolaou S. High-resolution CT findings of severe acute respiratory syndrome at presentation and after admission. AJR Am J Roentgenol 2004;182(1):39–44.

233. Peiris JS, Chu CM, Cheng VC, et al. Clinical progression and viral load in a community outbreak of coronavirus-associated SARS pneumonia: a prospective study. Lancet 2003;361(9371):1767–1772.

234. Ng CK, Chan JW, Kwan TL, et al. Six month radiological and physiological outcomes in severe acute respiratory syndrome (SARS) survivors. Thorax 2004;59(10): 889–891.

235. Wang JT, Chang SC. Severe acute respiratory syndrome. Curr Opin Infect Dis 2004;17(2):143–148.

236. Chan KS, Zheng JP, Mok YW, et al. SARS: prognosis, outcome and sequelae. Respirology 2003;8(suppl):S36–40.

14
Cardiac Infections in the Pediatric Intensive Care Unit

Laura M. Ibsen and Irving Shen

In a general pediatric intensive care unit that includes cardiac surgical patients, the most common cardiac infections encountered are postsurgical complications. Patients who are acutely ill with endocarditis, myocarditis, or pericarditis may also require intensive care. After immediate stabilization, the general principles of taking a thorough history and considering patient exposures remains paramount. An integrated team approach, involving critical care specialists, infectious disease specialists, cardiologists, and surgeons, is vital to providing excellent care for these patients.

Mediastinitis and Sternal Wound Infections in Cardiac Surgical Patients

Mediastinitis and sternal wound infection are uncommon but important infectious complications of cardiac surgery that may be associated with significant morbidity and mortality.

Epidemiology of Sternal Wound Infections

Surgical wound infections after pediatric cardiac surgery can be broadly categorized as superficial or deep (1). Superficial wound infections are limited to the soft tissue above the sternum, whereas deep mediastinal infections or mediastinitis either originates from or extends below the sternum and involves the mediastinal structures. The incidence of wound infections after pediatric cardiac surgery is uncommon, occurring in approximately 0.1% to 5% of surgical patients (2–8). Many factors have been implicated to increase the risk of postoperative wound infections, including active infection at the time of surgery (9), active infection during the convalescent period, low birth weight or prematurity at the time of operation, extended length of operation, long cardiopulmonary bypass time, improper wound closure leading to sternal nonunion, nasal swab positive for *Staphylococcus aureus* (10), large volume transfusion of blood or blood products, open sternum after surgical repair (11), reexploration for postoperative bleeding, prolonged intensive care unit (ICU) stay, prolonged indwelling central venous catheter, and failure to use prophylactic antibiotics at the time of skin incision. None of these factors has been consistently found to increase the risk of postoperative wound infection, although some are perceived to have an association.

The most common organisms associated with sternal wound infections are *Staphylococcus epidermidis, S. aureus, Enterococcus* species, and *Candida* species. Both enteric and nonenteric gram-negative organisms are also reported but are much less common (11–13).

Diagnosis and Treatment of Sternal Wound Infections

Postoperative wound infection can occur up to 6 to 8 weeks after the initial surgery. Initial presentation may be subtle, including nonspecific symptoms such as irritability, low-grade fever, lethargy, and poor feeding. These symptoms are usually accompanied by wound erythema with or without purulent discharge. Timely diagnosis usually relies on a high index of suspicion. Computed tomography of the chest is usually not helpful because pockets of fluid collections in the mediastinum may be normal postoperative findings after cardiac surgery. Likewise echocardiography is not helpful except to look for evidence of intracardiac vegetations to rule out endocarditis.

Cursory visual inspection of the wound is usually not adequate to judge how deep the infection extends. This often requires thorough exploration of the wound and debridement, usually under general anesthesia. This is necessary because at the time of exploration, the surgeon must be prepared to reopen the sternum to determine whether the infection extends into the pericardial and mediastinal space. Broad-spectrum antibiotics should be instituted as soon as blood and wound cultures are obtained. Antibiotic selection can be changed to target the specific offending organism once the culture and sensitivity results are available.

The most common superficial wound complication after pediatric cardiac surgery is a sterile suture abscess. This is due to an immunologic reaction to the suture material used to close the incision. In the case of suture abscess, draining the abscess and removing the offending suture is curative. A prolonged course of antibiotic therapy is not necessary.

Superficial bacterial cellulitis of the wound may be treated with a course of antibiotics targeted specifically toward the responsible organism. If the cellulitis is accompanied with drainage and abscess formation, operative drainage and debridement along with a course of antibiotic will be necessary. The incision is usually left open and allowed to heal by secondary intention (Fig. 14.1).

The treatment of deep mediastinal infection in children after cardiac surgery historically has mirrored the treatment used for adults. This entails aggressive operative drainage and debridement, including partial or complete sternectomy and muscle or omental flap coverage. However, recent experience suggests that such an aggressive approach may not be necessary in the pediatric

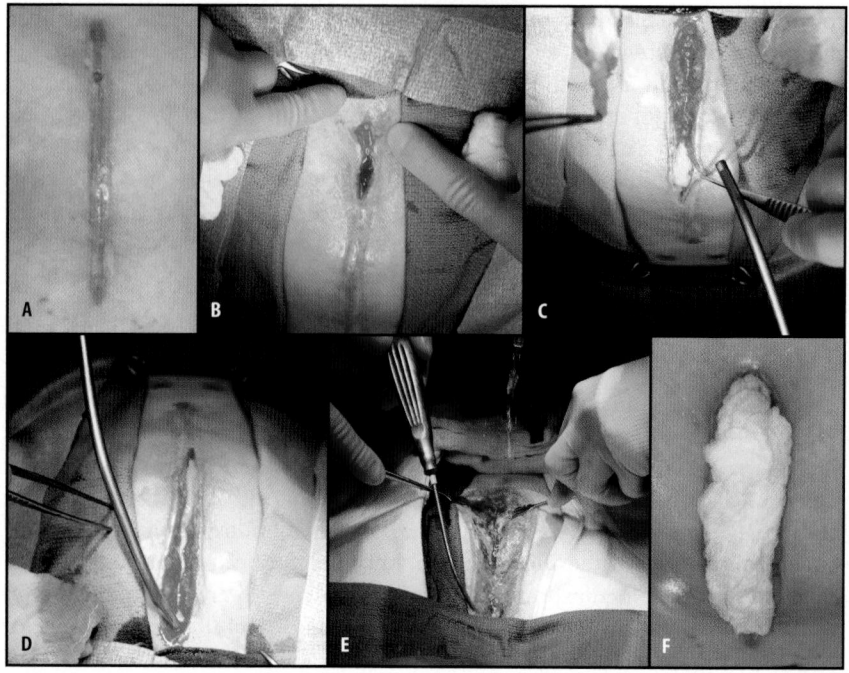

FIGURE **14.1.** A 10-year-old girl with deep sternal wound infection 2 weeks after a Ross procedure. (A) Erythematous incision with beginning of dehiscence. (B–D) In the operating room, the wound is opened. (E) The wound is copiously irrigated. (F) The wound is left open and packed.

population (14). Most pediatric patients, even ones with purulent mediastinitis, can be successfully treated with aggressive drainage and debridement followed by primary sternal closure and antibiotics. The reason why children react to mediastinal infection so differently than adults do is unclear. It may be because the internal thoracic artery, which provides the majority of the blood supply to the sternum, is often harvested for coronary bypass grafting in adults (15). The sternum in children may have better collateral blood supply, allowing for better penetration of systemic antibiotics to the site of sternal infection.

Antibiotic treatment should begin as soon as sternal wound infection is suspected and appropriate cultures have been obtained. The initial antibiotic regimen should consist of broad-spectrum gram-positive coverage, with the addition of gram-negative coverage if deep sternal wound infection or mediastinitis is suspected. Superficial wound infections are frequently managed with gram-positive coverage alone. Factors to be considered when deciding whether or not to use vancomycin empirically include prevalence of methicillin-resistant *S. aureus* (MRSA) in the community, MRSA colonization of the patients, and severity of the infection. For those who are known to be colonized with *Pseudomonas, Enterobacter,* or *Serratia species*, additional aminoglycoside coverage should be considered. Antibiotics are then tailored when culture results are known. Superficial wound infections should be treated for 2 weeks (intravenous plus oral), and mediastinitis should be treated for 4 to 8 weeks with intravenous antibiotics. If cultures from the sternum are positive, antibiotics should be continued for a minimum of 6 weeks for presumed osteomyelitis. If blood cultures are positive and the patient has indwelling foreign material (e.g., mechanical or tissue valve), endocarditis should be assumed and antibiotics continued for a minimum of 6 weeks.

Endocarditis

Infective endocarditis (IE) is rare in the pediatric population. Over the past several decades, as the incidence of rheumatic heart disease in developed countries has declined and the survival of children with congenital heart disease (CHD) has increased, CHD has become an increasingly important underlying condition in children with IE in developed countries. Gram-positive cocci are the most common offending organisms, but gram-negative organisms and fungal species are increasingly seen in critically ill patients who have been hospitalized for a prolonged period of time. Most episodes of IE can be treated successfully with a prolonged course of intravenous antibiotics. Surgical intervention is usually reserved for complications resulting from the infection or for lack of response to medical therapy.

Epidemiology

Infective endocarditis occurs less frequently in children than in adults, but the frequency appears to be increasing in children both with and without cardiac defects (16,17). The increased incidence in children with cardiac defects is in part due to recent improvement in survival after undergoing operative repair of their lesions. Correcting the underlying cardiac defect should theoretically decrease the risk of developing endocarditis; however, some patients continue to have abnormal anatomic blood flow after repair and therefore are still at increased risk of developing IE. Furthermore, multiple episodes of bacteremia can occur during the operative repair or during the convalescent period in the ICU that may predispose them to postoperative endocarditis. Finally, prosthetic material used in the repair of congenital cardiac defects in the forms of patches, grafts, or valves also can provide a potential nidus of infection. The increased incidence in children without cardiac defects can be attributed to two groups. The first group is the increasing number of survivors after treatment of childhood malignancy or organ transplantation. This group of patients, along with the increasing number of critically ill premature newborns who are surviving due to improvement in neonatal critical care, often requires long-term indwelling central venous catheter use, and this may predispose them to IE even in the absence of structural heart defects. Congenital or acquired immunodeficiency does not appear to increase the risk of IE in children (18).

The published guidelines by the American Heart Association stratify patients into different risk categories for the development of IE (19). In the pediatric population, the high-risk group includes patients with prosthetic heart valves (including bioprosthetic valves and homograft valves), complex cyanotic congenital heart defects (single ventricle, transposition of great arteries, tetralogy of Fallot), surgically constructed systemic to pulmonary shunts, and a previous history of endocarditis. The moderate-risk group includes patients with uncorrected congenital cardiac defects other than the ones in the high-risk category (patent ductus arteriosus [PDA], ventricular septal defect [VSD], primum atrial septal defect [ASD], coarctation of the aorta, bicuspid aortic valve), acquired valvular dysfunction, and hypertrophic cardiomyopathy. The negligible risk category includes patients who have isolated uncorrected secundum ASD or who had surgical repair of their cardiac lesion more than 6 months ago without any residual defect. These patients have the same risk of developing IE as the general population without any cardiac defects. The need for prophylaxis in the presence of mitral valve prolapse is controversial, but in general it is considered a moderate risk if there is valvar regurgitation or thickened valve leaflets.

Dental procedures, oral surgery, and certain respiratory, gastrointestinal, and genitourinary tract procedures are associated with bacteremia, and antibiotic prophylaxis is therefore recommended in the above groups. Routine ICU procedures such as endotracheal intubation and central line placement through antiseptically cleaned skin, as well as cardiac catheterization, do not require antibiotic prophylaxis. Prophylactic antibiotics are recommended for patients who undergo cardiac surgery (19). Patients who undergo invasive procedures performed in the ICU, such as opening or closing the sternum, should probably receive prophylactic antibiotics, though there is little evidence to support a given regimen.

Pathogenesis

Injury to the lining of the heart, from turbulent blood flow as a result of a structural cardiac defect, from intravenous catheters, or from other direct trauma such as surgery, stimulates fibrin and platelet deposition to form a sterile thrombus on the area of damaged endothelium. Subsequent episodes of bacteremia or fungemia allow circulating organisms to seed this sterile thrombus, and the thrombus shields these organisms from detection and eradication by the host defense mechanism. The organisms start to proliferate in this protected environment, and the thrombus grows. Transient bacteremia associated with oral hygiene, skin care in neonates, and medical procedures involving the oral, respiratory, gastrointestinal, and genitourinary tract is thought to be responsible for most cases of IE, although the inciting event cannot always be determined.

Microbiology

Gram-positive cocci, including *Streptococcus* and *Staphylococcus* species, are the most common causative organisms of IE in children (20–22). *S. aureus*, coagulase-negative staphylococci, and *Candida* species are the most common organisms causing IE in neonates (23,24). Less common organisms that can cause IE, such as gram-negative bacilli or fungi, may be identified in patients who are immunosuppressed, those who are hospitalized for a prolonged period of time, and in neonates. Infections of prosthetic patches or valves in the heart early after implantation (less than 3 months) are most likely due to contamination at the time of surgery. The most common organism found in early postoperative endocarditis is *S. epidermidis*, although *S. aureus*, diphtheroids, gram-negative bacilli, and fungi are also relatively more common than in community-acquired IE (25). Late postoperative endocarditis is caused by a similar spectrum of organisms to that of the general population.

In up to 10% of cases of IE, a causative organism can never be isolated in culture even though there is strong clinical or echocardiographic evidence to support the diagnosis (18,26). This condition is termed culture-negative IE. The reasons organisms cannot be identified in culture-negative IE are either due to antibiotic therapy at the time of blood sampling, which will suppress the growth of the organism in culture, or to infection with one of the fastidious organisms that grows very slowly or poorly in vitro. These include *Chlamydia*, fungi, and the HACEK organisms (*Haemophilus, Actinobacillus, Cardiobacterium, Eikenella corrodens,* and *Kingella* spp.).

Clinical Manifestations

The clinical presentation of IE in children can be very diverse, ranging from vague and nonspecific symptoms like weight loss, myalgias, arthralgias, chest pain, night sweat, malaise, anorexia, or fever, to fulminant overwhelming sepsis, heart failure, multiorgan system failure, and death (Table 14.1). The physical examination of the child with IE is highly variable. Splenomegaly is common, but the classic peripheral manifestations of IE, like petechiae, Osler's nodes, Janeway lesions, Roth spots, and subungual splinter hemorrhage, are rare. The cardiac examination depends on the underlying heart defect(s) and whether there are any cardiac complications associated with the infection. Damage to valve leaflets results in regurgitation murmurs, whereas infection in a systemic to pulmonary shunt may not result in a new or changed murmur but in decreased systemic oxygen saturations due to obstruction to pulmonary blood flow. Intracardiac abscess formation can lead to fistulas between cardiac chambers, which may manifest as a new murmur, or to conduction delay or block. Severe valvular damage, large septal defects, or high degree heart block may lead to heart failure.

Infected vegetations on the right side of the heart can embolize to the lungs and result in pulmonary infection, abscesses, or infarcts. Embolization of

TABLE **14.1.** Clinical features of infective endocarditis

Presenting symptoms
    Fever
    Malaise
    Weight loss, anorexia
    Congestive heart failure
    Arthralgias
    Gastrointestinal symptoms
    Chest pain
    Neurologic symptoms
Physical examination findings
    Fever
    Congestive heart failure
    Splenomegaly
    Petechiae
    Embolic phenomenon (pulmonary or systemic)
    New or altered cardiac murmur
    Decreased oxygen saturations in patient with systemic to pulmonary artery shunt
    Osler nodes, Janeway lesions, Roth spots

left-sided vegetations can cause infection or infarction of systemic end organs. Up to 20% of the children with IE have some form of neurologic symptoms, including altered sensorium, seizure, ataxia, aphasia, hemiplegia, or coma. These neurologic symptoms may be due to embolization to the brain or to the systemic sequelae of overwhelming sepsis.

Neonates with IE may present with variable and nonspecific findings that are consistent with sepsis or congestive heart failure from any cause. Septic emboli leading to osteomyelitis, meningitis, pneumonia, or neurologic abnormalities are common. Immunologic phenomenon such as Osler nodes, Roth's spots, and Janeway lesions are not described in neonates (18,24,27,28).

Diagnosis

Because of the highly variable and sometimes indolent clinical manifestations of IE, a number of diagnostic criteria have been developed and modified. The first was proposed by Pelletier and Petersdorf (29) in 1977, who categorized cases as definite, probable, or possible. Definite cases required histologic evidence of infected tissue from surgery or autopsy. The criteria were fairly specific but not sensitive enough for routine clinical use.

In 1981, von Reyn and colleagues (30) modified the Pelletier and Petersdorf criteria, improving their specificity and clinical utility. Cases were categorized as definite, probable, possible, and rejected. Definite cases still required histologic evidence of disease, and because many patients do not require surgery and do not die, many cases were classified as probable or possible.

In 1994, Durack and colleagues (31) proposed new diagnostic criteria, now known as the Duke criteria, that featured echocardiographic data prominently.

The Duke criteria rely on major and minor criteria (Table 14.2) and uses both clinical and pathologic findings to classify cases as definite, possible, or rejected (Table 14.3). The Duke criteria have been validated in several studies in adults (31–35) and in children (23). Modifications to the criteria include considering *S. aureus* bacteremia and positive Q-fever serology as major criteria (36).

A complete blood count may demonstrate some degree of leukocytosis with predominantly mature and immature neutrophils. Other nonspecific laboratory findings include elevated erythrocyte sedimentation rate, rheumatoid factors, or C-reactive protein; hemolytic anemia or anemia of chronic disease; immature forms on peripheral blood smear; hematuria; proteinuria; and renal insufficiency. The ability to grow the offending organism in culture from peripheral blood samples is crucial in establishing the diagnosis and guiding the antibiotics choice for therapy. In IE, bacteremia is usually continuous so it is not necessary to obtain cultures during a particular phase of the fever cycle. Three to six blood cultures obtained over a 48-hour period from separate venepunctures before starting empiric antibiotics will detect 97% of the cases of IE (37). For adult patients, 20 mL of blood should be obtained from each venipuncture. Recommendations for pediatric patients suggest that for neonates, 1 to 2 mL should be obtained from each venepuncture, for infants 2 to 3 mL, for older children 3 to 5 mL, and for adolescents 10 to 20 mL (38). Whenever possible, blood cultures should be obtained from fresh venepunctures rather than through indwelling catheters (38,39). If the patient is not acutely ill, antibiotics can be withheld while additional cultures are obtained. If IE is suspected and the patient is acutely ill, cultures can be obtained over a short time period and empiric antibiotic treatment started (18).

TABLE **14.2.** Duke clinical criteria for diagnosis of infective endocarditis (IE)

Definite IE
  Pathologic criteria
  Microorganisms: demonstrated by culture or histology in a vegetation, in a vegetation that has embolized, or in an intracardiac abscess, or
  Pathological lesions: vegetation or intracardiac abscess present, confirmed by histology showing active endocarditis
  Clinical criteria
  Using specific definitions listed in Table 14.3
  Two major criteria, or
  One major and three minor criteria, or
  Five minor criteria
Possible IE
  Findings consistent with IE that fall short of "definite" but not "rejected"
Rejected
  Firm alternate diagnosis for manifestations of endocarditis, or
  Resolution of manifestations of endocarditis with antibiotic therapy for <4 days, or
  No pathologic evidence of IE at surgery or autopsy, after antibiotic therapy for <4 days

Source: Durack et al. (31), with permission from Excerpta Medica Inc.

TABLE 14.3. Definitions of terms used in the Duke criteria for the diagnosis of infective endocarditis (IE)

Major criteria
1. Positive blood culture for IE
   A. Typical microorganism consistent with IE from two separate blood cultures as noted below:
      i.   Viridans streptococci,* *Streptococcus bovis*, or HACEK group, or
      ii. Community-acquired *Staphylococcus aureus* or enterococci, in the absence of a primary focus, or
   B. Microorganisms consistent with IE from persistently positive blood cultures defined as
      i.   ≥2 positive cultures of blood samples drawn >12 hours apart or
      ii. All of 3 or a majority of ≥4 separate cultures of blood (with first and last sample drawn ≥1 hour apart)
2. Evidence of endocardial involvement
   A. Positive echocardiogram for IE defined as
      i.   Oscillating intracardiac mass on valve or supporting structures, in the path of regurgitant jets, or on implanted material in the absence of an alternative anatomic explanation, or
      ii. Abscess, or
      iii. New partial dehiscence of prosthetic valve, or
   B. New valvular regurgitation (worsening or changing of preexisting murmur not sufficient)
Minor criteria
1. Predisposition: predisposing heart condition or intravenous drug use
2. Fever: temperature ≥38.0°C
3. Vascular phenomena: major arterial emboli, septic pulmonary infarcts, mycotic aneurysm, intracranial hemorrhage, conjunctival hemorrhages, and Janeway lesions
4. Immunologic phenomena: glomerulonephritis, Osler's nodes, Roth spots, and rheumatoid factor
5. Microbiological evidence: positive blood culture but does not meet a major criterion as noted above† or serologic evidence of active infection with organism consistent with IE
6. Echocardiographic findings: consistent with IE but do not meet a major criterion as noted above

*Includes nutritionally variant strains (*Abiotrophia* species).
†Excludes single positive cultures for coagulase-negative staphylococci and organisms that do not cause endocarditis.
Source: Durack et al. (31), with permission from Excerpta Medica Inc.

Echocardiography has become the primary modality to detect IE, follow its progression, and detect any cardiac complications that are associated with the infection. Serial examination can detect changes in vegetation size, valvular function, myocardial function, and abscess or fistula formation. Transthoracic echocardiography (TTE) has a sensitivity of about 80% in detecting vegetations in children (40,41), and is more useful in the pediatric population than in the adult population. Although lesions as small as 2 mm can be visualized if they contrast sufficiently with surrounding structures, the vegetation may not always be visible, particularly in the setting of complex congenital heart disease.

The routine use of transesophageal echocardiography (TEE) to investigate IE in children has not been evaluated, but it may be useful in the obese or very muscular adolescent, in the presence of pulmonary hyperinflation, or after cardiac surgery. It may be particularly important in the evaluation of aortic valvular endocarditis, as TEE is useful for assessing left ventricular outflow tract structures, particularly the development of aortic root abscess (42). The need to use cardiac catheterization in the diagnosis of IE is rare. In fact, it may be contraindicated due to the risk of precipitating embolization.

Clinical Course and Management

The treatment of IE should be an aggressive course of intravenous antibiotics that specifically target the organism identified in blood culture. The duration of antibiotic therapy is usually 4 to 8 weeks. Longer courses of antibiotic therapy may be necessary for some organisms that are particularly virulent, those that have a slow metabolic growth rate, or if cardiac prosthetic material is involved; 80% of IE cases are successfully treated with antibiotic therapy alone. Empiric antibiotics can be started if the clinical suspicion of IE is high while the blood culture results are pending. Empiric antibiotics should have a broad spectrum of coverage. Because a prolonged course of antibiotics is needed to treat IE, it is important to establish a firm diagnosis. Antibiotic therapy may be withheld for 48 hours or more if additional blood cultures are needed and if the patient is not acutely ill (18). Specific choice of antibiotic and the duration of treatment depend on both the organism cultured and whether prosthetic materials, such as valves, shunts, patches, or conduits, are present. Fungal endocarditis can be difficult to cure with medical therapy alone, and many have considered surgery necessary in combination with antifungal therapy (43,44), although there are several reports of candida endocarditis that was treated with medical therapy alone. In the absence of embolization of infected vegetations or hemodynamic instability, medical therapy alone may be successful (45–47). If the source of bacterial seeding, such as an infected long-term indwelling catheter or a tooth abscess, is still present, it should be removed. In culture-negative IE, antibiotics should be directed against the most common causative organisms including *Staphylococcus*, *Streptococcus*, and the HACEK organisms. These patients should be managed in consultation with an infectious disease specialist.

Complications of IE include congestive heart failure, periannular extension of an abscess, systemic or pulmonary embolic events, arrhythmia, valve dehiscence, shunt obstruction, mycotic aneurysms, glomerulonephritis or renal failure, and persistent bacteremia or fungemia (18,48) (Table 14.4). Factors that predispose children to the development of complications include the presence of prosthetic valves, left-sided IE, *S. aureus*, fungal IE, previous IE, the presence of symptoms for longer than 3 months, cyanotic congenital heart disease, and systemic-to-pulmonary shunts (48).

Embolic complications may occur in any patient with IE but are particularly common with large (>1 cm), left-sided lesions (49,50) and *Streptococcus viridans* infections (51). Emboli generally involve major arterial beds with high blood flow, including lungs, coronary arteries, spleen, bowel, extremities, and the middle cerebral artery of the brain. *S. aureus* and fungal infections have the highest risk of embolization regardless of vegetation size. Although embolism can occur at any time, most embolic events occur within the first 2 to 4 weeks of therapy (18,48). Although vegetation size does not predict embolization in the absence of large vegetations, increasing vegetation size during the fourth to eighth weeks of therapy is predictive of embolic complications (48).

TABLE 14.4. Complications of infective endocarditis

Congestive heart failure: gradual development
Gradual development of valve incompetence
Congestive heart failure: acute development
Perforation of a valve leaflet
Rupture of mitral valve cordae
Periannular leak or dehiscence of prosthetic valve
Periannular extension of infection
Valve dehiscence or rupture
Abscess or fistula formation
Systemic to pulmonary artery shunt obstruction
Embolic events
Middle cerebral artery
Coronary artery
Spleen
Bowel
Extremities and cutaneous
Lungs
Mycotic aneurysm (particularly intracerebral mycotic aneurysm)
Glomerulonephritis

Mycotic aneurysms result from embolization of infected vegetation material to the vasa vasorum of an artery or the intraluminal space, with spread of the infection through the vessel intima and vessel wall. They occur most commonly at arterial branching points. Although they are relatively uncommon, they most frequently occur in the intracranial arteries and carry a high morbidity and mortality. They may rupture, greatly increasing the risk of mortality. The clinical presentation of intracranial mycotic aneurysm is variable and may include focal neurologic signs, headache, altered mental status, or meningeal irritation (48).

Surgical treatment of IE is usually reserved for complications that are associated with the infection, or for lack of response to medical therapy. In the past, surgical treatment for IE was usually reserved as a last resort when all other options had failed. These patients usually were critically ill with systemic sepsis, multiorgan system failure, hemodynamic instability, and extensive cardiac tissue destruction. Consequently this approach resulted in very high operative mortality. The current trend is toward earlier surgical intervention in order to improve the outcome and to preserve the structure and function of native tissue and organs.

Lack of response to medical therapy in the treatment of IE is the most common indication for surgical intervention (52). Signs of failure of medical therapy include persistent fever, ongoing sepsis, bacteremia, increasing vegetation size, and recurrent embolization despite appropriate antibiotic choice and dosage. Another common indication for surgical intervention is the development of cardiac complications that are associated with the infection. These complications include invasion of cardiac tissues leading to conduction disturbances, abscesses, aneurysm, pseudoaneurysm, fistula formation, heart failure, hemodynamic deterioration due to valvular destruction, or cardiac outflow tract obstruction by large vegetation. In fact, any patient with IE who has hemodynamic or conduction disturbance should undergo surgical assessment. In some other special circumstances such as prosthetic valve endocarditis (53), infection with difficult-to-treat organisms such as fungus or *Pseudomonas*, infection of other intracardiac prosthetic materials such as patches and shunts, or rapid relapse following a full course of antibiotic therapy, may also benefit from surgical intervention. In adults with left-sided IE, vegetations that are greater than 10 mm in diameter are found to be at much greater risk of embolization, and therefore this is an indication for surgical debridement (54). However, there is less correlation with size of vegetation and risk of embolization in children, and therefore the absolute requirement for surgical debridement is less clear.

Myocarditis

Myocarditis is an inflammatory process that leads to myocardial necrosis and degeneration that is not caused by coronary artery stenosis or other diseases. While a viral etiology is most common, bacteria, fungi, and parasites, as well as autoimmune etiologies can also rarely lead to myocarditis. The clinical presentation of myocarditis may range from asymptomatic to fulminant, making it difficult to estimate the true incidence.

Epidemiology and Microbiology

Because of the variable presentation and difficulties with making an accurate diagnosis of myocarditis, it is difficult to determine accurately the prevalence in children. In developed countries, viruses are the most common cause of myocarditis, most frequently Coxsackie B and adenovirus (55,56). Bacteria and fungi infrequently cause myocarditis in nonneutropenic children. Among nonneutropenic children, *S. aureus* and *Neisseria meningitidis* are the most commonly identified bacterial causes of myocarditis (57,58). *Trypanosoma cruzi* (Chagas' disease) and *Corynebacterium diphtheriae* (diphtheria) are infrequent in the United States but are important causes of myocarditis in developing countries (Table 14.5). Various autoimmune diseases are associated with myocarditis, and there exists a rare and frequently fatal entity known as giant cell myocarditis that is often associated with systemic autoimmune diseases.

Pathology and Pathophysiology

Most of our understanding of the pathophysiology of myocarditis comes from animal models of Coxsackievirus B3–induced murine myocarditis. In the first 4 days of illness, virus can be detected in the myocardium itself, as well as the

TABLE 14.5. Infectious causes of myocarditis

Viral: Coxsackie B*, adenovirus*, cytomegalovirus, echovirus, Epstein-Barr virus, HIV, hepatitis C, measles, rubella, varicella, mumps, vaccinia, variola, parvovirus, influenza A and B, respiratory syncytial virus, herpesvirus, poliomyelitis, rabies, arbovirus, dengue, yellow fever
Bacterial: *Staphylococcus**, *Streptococcus*, *Pneumococcus*, *Neisseria meningitides**, *Salmonella*, *Borrelia burgdorferi*, *Corynebacterium diphtheriae**, *Haemophilus influenzae*, *Mycoplasma pneumoniae*, *Brucella*, *Chlamydia psittaci*, *Coxiella brunetti*
Fungal: aspergillus*
Parasitic: *Trypanosoma cruzi**, *Toxoplasma gondii*, *Trichinella spiralis*

*Most commonly identified etiologies.

interstitium where macrophages are activated. The secondary phase involves altered immune regulation in which CD4$^+$ T-helper cells and CD8$^+$ cytotoxic T cells are stimulated along with proinflammatory cytokines. Nitric oxide is produced by the myocytes and appears to play an important role in the damage to myocardial tissue (59,60). Persistence of viral RNA may play a role in the development of dilated cardiomyopathy (61). A specific myocardial receptor for adenovirus and Coxsackie B virus, the Coxsackie-adenovirus receptor (CAR), has been identified (62) and may provide an explanation for the propensity of these organisms to cause myocarditis.

There is emerging evidence that viral persistence is related to the development and severity of dilated cardiomyopathy in some patients. The role of autoantibodies in the pathophysiology of myocarditis and dilated cardiomyopathy is an area of ongoing investigation (56,63).

Diagnosis

The clinical presentation of myocarditis is extremely variable, ranging from indolent disease with only subtle findings on electrocardiogram (ECG) or echocardiogram to fulminant heart failure and death. Typical initial symptoms in acute viral myocarditis include a flu-like prodrome with fatigue, chest pain, dyspnea, and tachypnea. Signs of heart failure such as pulmonary rales, a third heart sound, and hepatomegaly, along with weak pulses and poor perfusion if the progression is rapid, may be present. Infants and young children may present with feeding difficulties or lethargy and clinical suspicion must be high. Myocarditis can also present with sudden unexplained death in previously asymptomatic children or adults (64–66).

Electrocardiography findings that are suggestive of myocarditis include generalized low-voltage QRS complex along with tachycardia, flattened T wave, or T-wave inversion in the left chest leads, and dysrhythmias. Atrial and ventricular dysrhythmias, heart block, and ECG patterns suggestive of infarct are sometimes seen.

Echocardiography usually demonstrates globally reduced ventricular function, usually left greater than right, although segmental wall motion abnormalities are not uncommon. There may also be atrioventricular (AV) valve regurgitation and pericardial effusion present.

Cardiac troponin T appears to be an accurate indicator for myocarditis in patients whose clinical presentation is suggestive (67). Viral antibody titers as well as blood polymerase chain reaction (PCR) testing may provide evidence of a specific infectious agent but generally do not help to establish the diagnosis of myocarditis. If bacteria or fungal myocarditis is suspected, blood cultures should be obtained.

Cardiac magnetic resonance imaging (MRI) can characterize inflammation in the setting of viral myocarditis, and serial MRI scans can demonstrate the progression from focal to generalized myocardial inflammation (68). Magnetic resonance imaging may also be a valuable tool in guiding the location from which biopsies are taken in order to increase the sensitivity of biopsy (69).

Endomyocardial biopsy has for many years been the "gold standard" for diagnosing myocarditis. In 1984 a working standard for the U.S. Myocarditis Treatment Trial was developed, known as the Dallas criteria, and is now used by most investigators to define the disease (70) (Table 14.6). Biopsies are typically taken from the right ventricular septum. Because the inflammation in myocarditis may be patchy, the sensitivity of biopsy is variable (71,72). Repeat biopsy may be useful if the initial biopsy is borderline (73). Biopsies from patients presenting late in the course of their disease may be less helpful as they may demonstrate only fibrosis.

Molecular biologic techniques have enhanced the diagnostic sensitivity of myocardial biopsy. Biopsy specimens can be processed and evaluated by various PCR techniques in order to detect the presence of viral genomes in the myocardium. Typically specimens are investigated for the presence of Coxsackie B virus and adenovirus, along with cytomegalovirus (CMV), Epstein-Barr virus (EBV), parvovirus b19, hepatitis C virus, influenza virus A and B, and respiratory syncytial virus in selected laboratories (74,75). The precise etiologic definition of myocarditis may provide important prognostic information and help guide treatment decisions (56,74).

TABLE 14.6. Dallas criteria: histopathologic definition and classification

First biopsy
    Myocarditis with/without fibrosis
    Borderline myocarditis
    No myocarditis
Subsequent biopsies
    Ongoing (persistent) myocarditis with/without fibrosis
    Resolving (healing) myocarditis with/without fibrosis
    Resolved (healed) myocarditis with/without fibrosis

Note: The inflammatory infiltrate should be classified by type (lymphocytic, eosinophilic, neutrophilic, giant cell, granulomatous, or mixed), amount (mild, moderate, or severe), and location (focal, confluent, or diffuse). The fibrosis should be characterized as endocardial, replacement, or interstitial.

Clinical Course and Management

In adults, myocarditis has been classified according to clinical and histologic features as fulminant, acute, chronic active, and chronic persistent myocarditis (76) (Table 14.7). Adults with fulminant myocarditis have a better prognosis compared to those with active myocarditis (77). The prognosis of children with myocarditis remains unclear, as most reports involve small numbers of children and do not precisely define the population under review. In general, children with myocarditis usually survive but some percentage of them will continue to have ventricular dysfunction and some will develop dilated cardiomyopathy (DCM), although reliable estimates of prognosis are not available. Of children who are diagnosed with DCM, approximately 30% to 40% have evidence of prior myocarditis (78), although it is not known how many children with myocarditis will go on to develop DCM.

Heart failure and dysrhythmias are the most frequent indications for intensive care monitoring or therapy for patients with myocarditis. Supportive therapy for heart failure associated with myocarditis ranges from diuretic therapy and afterload reduction to addition of inotropic support, to placing the patient on an extracorporeal membrane oxygenator (ECMO) or ventricular assist device (VAD).

Because digoxin increases the expression of proinflammatory cytokines and mortality in a murine model of myocarditis, it is not recommended in the acute phase of myocarditis (63), but if it is used for specific rhythm disturbances, lower doses without a loading regimen should be given (79). In mild heart failure, angiotensin-converting enzyme (ACE) inhibitors such as captopril provide afterload reduction. In murine models of viral endocarditis, captopril decreases the amount of inflammation and necrosis when administered within the first 30 days of infection (79).

In more severe heart failure, intravenous inotropic support may be needed. Dopamine and dobutamine increase contractility but also increase heart rate and myocardial oxygen demand. The phosphodiesterase inhibitor milrinone improves contractility while also reducing afterload. In most patients, milrinone, with dopamine added if needed to treat hypotension, is well tolerated.

Raised intrathoracic pressure reduces left ventricular afterload and may improve cardiac output in the setting of heart failure. Continuous positive

TABLE 14.7. Clinicopathologic classification of myocarditis

Fulminant myocarditis: There is an acute illness after a distinct viral prodrome, and patients have severe hemodynamic compromise. There are multiple foci of inflammation on biopsy specimens. Ventricular function either resolves spontaneously or results in death.
Acute myocarditis: There is a less distinct onset of illness and ventricular dysfunction is established and may progress to dilated cardiomyopathy.
Chronic active myocarditis: There is a less distinct onset of illness and there may be clinical and histologic relapses despite apparent initial response to immunosuppressive therapy.
Chronic persistent myocarditis: There is a less distinct onset of illness and a persistent histologic infiltrate but without ventricular dysfunction.

airway pressure (CPAP) is generally well tolerated and beneficial and avoids the necessity of sedation and endotracheal intubation, which may precipitate sudden decompensation. If mask CPAP is not tolerated or the patient's hemodynamic status worsens substantially, endotracheal intubation should proceed with caution, and medications needed for resuscitation should be available. Removing the work of breathing and the beneficial effects of positive intrathoracic pressure usually improve the hemodynamics in the patient with heart failure, although the initial sedation and the procedure of endotracheal intubation may lead to some initial instability. Although most patients with heart failure are volume overloaded, care must be taken to ensure that the patient is not hypovolemic, as positive intrathoracic pressure will reduce central venous return and lead to hypotension in the setting of hypovolemia.

Extracorporeal membrane oxygenator or VAD support is generally indicated in the setting of fulminant myocarditis with severe hemodynamic instability despite conventional supportive therapy, as it may successfully bridge the patient to heart transplant or to recovery (80–82). Dysrhythmias may be severe, and heart block may necessitate transvenous pacing, and occasionally rhythm disturbances may be so severe as to require mechanical support. Because the prognosis for fulminant myocarditis is relatively good if the patient survives the acute period, aggressive mechanical support is indicated.

Some specific causes of acute myocarditis may be treated with antimicrobial agents. Diphtheritic myocarditis should be treated with antitoxin and antibiotics, known bacterial or fungal pathogens should be treated with appropriate antibacterial or antifungal agents, and parasitic infections should be treated with appropriate antiparasitic medications. Although treatment of viral myocarditis with medications such as ganciclovir, acyclovir, amantadine, neuroaminidase inhibitors, pleconaril, interferon-α, and ribavirin has been suggested, and a number of case reports published, the efficacy of antiviral medications in improving the outcome of myocarditis has not been well established. Nevertheless, if a specific viral etiology is found and there is viral persistence in the myocardium, antiviral therapy should be strongly considered.

Because the sequelae of myocarditis appears to be related to activation of cellular and humoral immunity, immunosuppressive therapy has been the subject of several studies in children and adults with myocarditis and recent onset of dilated cardiomyopathy, yet its use and application remains controversial. The heterogeneity of the infecting agents, the heterogeneity of the host response in myocarditis and dilated cardiomyopathy, and the variability in the timing of intervention in the disease course between different case series and controlled trials compounds the controversy. Nevertheless, it is possible that there is a subset of patients who would particularly benefit from immunosuppressive therapy (83,84).

In a retrospective review of children with acute myocarditis, those treated with intravenous immunoglobulin (IVIG) had improved recovery of ventricular function compared with historical controls (85). The use of IVIG in adult patients with recent onset (<6 months) of dilated cardiomyopathy did not show a similar benefit, but the population did not consist entirely of patients with acute myocarditis (86). There has not been a large randomized, placebo-controlled trial of IVIG in children with acute myocarditis.

The use of prednisone in adults with dilated cardiomyopathy was associated with marginal clinical benefit in those patients who had evidence of inflammation on biopsy (87). In 1995 the American Myocarditis Treatment Trial published the results of a large trial comparing the use of azathioprine and prednisone, cyclosporine and prednisone, and placebo in patients with evidence of myocarditis on biopsy, and onset of heart failure within the preceding 2 years. This study did not demonstrate any benefit of immunosuppressive therapy (88). Children with biopsy-proven acute myocarditis treated with prednisone and cyclosporine or prednisone and azathioprine appeared to have improved clinical outcome and survival (89–91).

The immune response of infants and children differs from that of adults, and trials of immunomodulatory therapy in adult populations cannot necessarily be extrapolated to the pediatric population. At the present time, there is not conclusive evidence that immunosuppressive therapy is beneficial in the setting of myocarditis, but there is some suggestion that immunosuppression in children with proven acute viral myocarditis may be effective, although optimal medication and dosing strategies remain unknown (92). Table 14.8 outlines one possible immunosuppressive regimen. Most therapeutic regimens investigated, including IVIG, corticosteroids, and azathioprine or cyclosporine, were well tolerated in published studies.

In the future, application of combined histologic and microbiologic diagnostic methods may improve our ability to target therapy more specifically. The European Study of Epidemiology and Treatment of Cardiac Inflammatory Diseases (ESETCID) is an ongoing investigation of the use of treatment specific

TABLE 14.8. Immunosuppressive treatment strategy for acute myocarditis

Solu-Medrol: weaning schedule can be adjusted as indicated and prednisone can substitute for methylprednisolone when lower doses reached and patient tolerating oral medications.	
Day 1	10 mg/kg/d
Day 2	10 mg/kg/d
Day 3	10 mg/kg/d
Day 4	5 mg/kg/d
Day 5	2.5 mg/kg/d
Day 6	1.75 mg/kg/d
Day 7	1 mg/kg/d
Day 8	0.5 mg/kg/d
Day 9	0.3 mg/kg/d
Day 10 to 3 months: much slower weans 1 week at a time	
Wean over the next 3 months to discontinuation based on suspicion of original diagnosis, subsequent biopsies, and development of side effects.	
Intravenous immunoglobulin (IVIG): 2 g/kg over 36 to 48 hours	

Source: Courtesy of Yuk Law, M.D.

to the etiology of myocarditis: enterovirus-positive patients (as found on PCR) are treated with interferon-α; CMV and adenovirus positive patients are treated with IVIG; and those with autoimmune myocarditis are treated with azathioprine and prednisolone (93).

Pericarditis

Pericarditis involves inflammation of the pericardium and may or may not present with pericardial effusion. Pericarditis may present as an acute, subacute, or chronic illness and may be associated with a wide variety of infectious and noninfectious conditions. The causes of pericarditis can be classified as infectious, immunoreactive, neoplastic, traumatic, metabolic, and idiopathic. Infectious causes of pericarditis include bacterial, viral, tuberculous, fungal, rickettsial, and parasitic. In developing countries, *Mycobacterium tuberculosis* is an important cause of pericarditis, but it is rare in developed countries. In at least 30% to 50% of cases, the underlying etiology is not found despite thorough investigation (94–97).

Pathology and Anatomy

The pericardium is a double-layered sac that envelops the heart and proximal great vessels, consisting of the inner serosal layer that adheres to the myocardium, and the outer fibrous parietal pericardium. The two layers are 1 to 2mm thick and normally contain 15 to 35mL of pericardial fluid in the adult.

The normal pericardium limits chamber dilation, particularly the right atrium and ventricle, and equalizes the compliance between the right and left ventricles, leading to ventricular interdependence. This is normally not physiologically important, but in the presence of increased intrapericardial pressure, as with effusion, or if the pericardial dimension is fixed, as with constriction, ventricular interdependence is exaggerated.

Epidemiology and Microbiology

The incidence and prevalence of pericarditis, particularly in children, is difficult to determine. In adults, it is estimated that it may account for 5% of the patients presenting the emergency departments for nonmyocardial infarction chest pain (98). Autopsy studies suggest that pericarditis may frequently be subclinical (99).

A wide variety of organisms may cause pericarditis, but viruses are the most frequently identified or probable cause. Organisms that cause myocarditis are commonly found, including enteroviruses, adenoviruses, and influenza. Bacterial causes of pericarditis include *S. aureus, Haemophilus influenzae, N. meningitidis,* and various others (100), and may result from contiguous extension of infection or from seeding during bacteremia. In patients with HIV and in developing countries, mycobacterial infections are important causes of pericarditis (95).

Pericarditis after cardiac surgery is relatively common, and is thought to be immunoreactive in etiology. In the typical pediatric intensive care unit setting, the most common cause of pericarditis is usually postpericardiotomy syndrome. This may occur quickly, or up to several months after surgery or trauma.

Diagnosis of Pericarditis

Acute pericarditis typically presents with progressive, sharp chest pain that is worse when lying supine and is relieved by sitting upright. The pain may radiate to the neck, arms, or left shoulder. A pericardial friction rub is best heard at end expiration with the patient leaning forward. An effusion may lessen the friction rub and heart sounds may become muffled. If an effusion is present and is impairing cardiac filling, there may be increasing tachycardia. Pulsus paradoxus (drop in systolic blood pressure of >10 mm Hg during inspiration) suggests decreased venous return to the heart due to the presence of a pericardial effusion.

Chest radiography is frequently normal in the setting of uncomplicated pericarditis or with small effusions, but an increased cardiac shadow may be seen if there is a large effusion. The pericardium can distend and accommodate the effusion if it accumulates slowly, whereas rapidly accumulating effusions are less well tolerated. For that reason, the size of the effusion may not correlate with clinical findings.

Electrocardiographic findings classically reveal widespread upwardly concave ST segment elevation and commonly PR segment depression. The ST segment changes are not regional as with ischemia and there are no Q waves. Classically the abnormalities are described as progressing through four phases: ST elevation and upright T waves (stage I), evolution over several days to normal (stage II), T-wave inversion (stage III), and finally evolution to normal (stage IV) (94). With early diagnosis and treatment, except in the setting of purulent pericarditis, generally stage I is the only ECG finding seen.

Echocardiography is useful to assess for complications of pericarditis, such as effusion, tamponade, or constriction, and to determine their physiologic significance. In assessing for the presence of tamponade it is important to consider the volume status of the patient as well as the underlying compliance of the ventricles (95). Newer echo modalities such as tissue Doppler imaging may be useful in distinguishing between constrictive pericarditis and restrictive cardiomyopathy.

Computed tomography (CT) and MRI may be useful adjuncts in the evaluation of suspected pericarditis. Computed tomography provides detailed anatomic resolution of the entire pericardium and can reveal calcifications as well as determine pericardial thickness; MRI provides better characterization of the effusion and does not require contrast. Computed tomography and MRI are particularly important in the evaluation of suspected constrictive pericarditis or neoplasm (101).

Laboratory investigations commonly reveal leukocytosis, elevated C-reactive protein, and elevated erythrocyte sedimentation rate. Troponin I may be elevated in pericarditis and does not carry an adverse prognosis (102). Acute and convalescent serology may be useful in identifying viral etiologies, *Rickettsia*, and *Mycoplasma*.

Pericardiocentesis is indicated if there is a pericardial effusion with evidence of tamponade or if there is a suspicion of purulent pericarditis or neoplasm. Pericardial fluid should be analyzed for glucose, protein, cell count, and differential. Gram, acid-fast, and silver stains and well as cytologic examination should be performed, and fluid should be cultured for bacteria, fungi, mycobacteria, and viruses. Polymerase chain reaction techniques may be indicated for viruses or *Mycobacterium tuberculosis*. In the case of pericarditis caused by *M. tuberculosis*, pericardial biopsy and culture is often necessary (103).

Complications of Pericarditis

Recurrent pericarditis is relatively common and may occur for several years after an initial episode of pericarditis, but the development of tamponade or constrictive pericarditis with recurrence is uncommon. As with acute pericarditis, treatment is usually supportive.

Pericardial effusion and tamponade can occur with pericarditis of any etiology. Small effusions are usually not significant unless they develop rapidly or when constriction is also present. Moderate or large effusions are more common with bacterial, tuberculous, or malignant pericarditis. If the effusion is large or accumulates quickly so that the pericardium cannot stretch to accommodate it, increased intrapericardial pressure and pericardial constraint increase ventricular interdependence and respiratory variation in filling. On echocardiography, there is substantial respiratory variation in transmitral and tricuspid Doppler inflow, diastolic collapse of the right atrium and ventricle, and an enlarged inferior vena cava (95).

Constrictive pericarditis occurs when there is chronic fibrous thickening or calcification of the pericardium and produces abnormal diastolic filling due to the rigid, noncompliant pericardium. In developing countries, tuberculosis has been a significant cause of constrictive pericarditis. It may be difficult to distinguish constrictive pericarditis from restrictive cardiomyopathy, but the distinction is important both prognostically and in terms of available treatment, as constrictive pericarditis is potentially treatable with pericardiectomy and carries a better prognosis.

Treatment

Appropriate treatment of pericarditis depends on the etiology and complications present at initial presentation. The natural history of acute pericarditis of viral, idiopathic, or postsurgical etiology is frequently benign and management is largely aimed at symptomatic pain relief. Nonsteroidal antiinflammatory drugs (NSAIDs) are usually effective for fever, pericardial, pain, and inflammation in uncomplicated cases (95,104). The most commonly used NSAID is ibuprofen (94). These patients should be followed carefully and repeat imaging performed if there is any evidence of pericardial effusion and to watch for the development of constriction.

Colchicine is frequently added in adults with recurrent pericarditis and may be used as monotherapy for patients who are intolerant to NSAIDs (94,97). There are limited data on its effectiveness in children with pericarditis, but it appears to be similarly efficacious (105,106).

Corticosteroid treatment is considered important in the treatment of tuberculous pericarditis (107–109), but its use in other settings is controversial. In nontuberculous pericarditis, corticosteroids are effective in controlling symptoms, but there is a theoretical risk of reactivating infection and an increased incidence of chronic relapsing pericarditis (94).

Broad-spectrum antibiotics should be initiated empirically if purulent pericarditis is suspected, and pericardiocentesis with drainage of the purulent effusion is considered mandatory (100,110). Antibiotics are generally continued for 3 to 4 weeks. Fungal pericarditis similarly generally requires surgical drainage along with medical therapy (111).

Tuberculous pericarditis is treated with antituberculous drugs and generally with corticosteroids to hasten the time to resolution of symptoms and decrease reaccumulation of pericardial fluid. The role of open surgical drainage remains controversial but does allow for pericardial biopsy which may be needed for diagnosis (103,108).

References

1. Garner JS, Jarvis WR, Emori TG, Horan TC, Hughes JM. CDC definitions for nosocomial infections, 1988. Am J Infect Control 1988;16:128–140.
2. Edwards MS, Backer CJ. Median sternotomy wound infections in children. Pediatr Infect Dis J 1982;2:105–109.
3. Jimenez-Martinez M, Arguero-Sanchez R, Rerez-Alvarez JJ, Mina-Castaneda P. Anterior mediastinitis as a complication of median sternotomy incisions: diagnostic and surgical considerations. Surgery 1970;67:929–934.
4. Stiegel RM, Beasley ME, Sink JD, et al. Management of postoperative mediastinitis in infants and children by muscle flap rotation. Ann Thorac Surg 1988;46:45–46.
5. Grant RT, Breitbart AS, Parnell V. Muscle flap reconstruction of pediatric poststernotomy wound infections. Ann Plast Surg 1997;38:365–370.
6. Erez E, Kaatz M, Sharoni E, et al. Pectoralis major muscle flap for deep sternal wound infection in neonates. Ann Thorac Surg 2000;60:572–577.
7. Pasaoglu I, Arsan S, Yorgancioglu AC, Yuksel BA. A simple management of mediastinitis. Int Surgery 1995;80:239–241.
8. Mehta PA, Cunningham CK, Colella CB, Alferis G, Weiner LB. Risk factors for sternal wound and other infections in pediatric cardiac surgery patients. Pediatr Infect Dis J 2000;19:1000–1004.

9. Huddleston CB. Mediastinal wound infections following pediatric cardiac surgery. Semin Thorac Cardiovasc Surg 2004:108–112.

10. Ruef C, Fanconi S, Nadal D. Sternal wound infection after heart operations in pediatric patients associated with nasal carriage of *Staphylococcus aureus*. J Thorac Cardiovasc Surg 1996;113:681–686.

11. Tabbutt S, Duncan BW, McLaughlin D, et al. Delayed sternal closure after cardiac operations in a pediatric population. J Thorac Cardiovasc Surg 1997;113: 886–893.

12. Tortoriello TA, Friedman JD, McKenzie ED, et al. Mediastinitis after pediatric cardiac surgery: a 15-year experience at a single institution. Ann Thorac Surg 2003;76:1655–1660.

13. Maher KO, VanDerElzen K, Bove EL, et al. A retrospective review of three antibiotic prophylaxis regimens for pediatric cardiac surgical patients. Ann Thorac Surg 2002;74:1195–2000.

14. Ohye RG, Maniker RB, Graves HL, Devaney EJ, Bove EL. Primary closure for postoperative mediastinitis in children. J Thorac Cardiovasc Surg 2004;128:480–486.

15. Combes A, Trouillet J, Baudot J, et al. Is it possible to cure mediastinitis in patients with major postcardiac surgery complications. Ann Thorac Surg 2001;72:1592–1597.

16. Van Hare GF, Ben-Shachar G, Liebman J, Boxerbaum B, Riemenschneider TA. Infective endocarditis in infants and children during the past 10 years: a decade of change. Am Heart J 1984;107:1235–1240.

17. Martin JM, Neches WH, Wald ER. Infective endocarditis: 35 years of experience at a children's hospital. Clin Infect Dis 1997;24:669–675.

18. Ferrieri P, Gewitz MH, Gerber MA, et al. Unique features of infective endocarditis in childhood. Pediatrics 2002;109:931–943.

19. Dajani AS, Taubert KA, Wilson W, et al. Prevention of bacterial endocarditis: recommendations by the American Heart Association. Clin Infect Dis 1997;25: 1448–1458.

20. Wells WJ. Surgical problems of endocarditis in children. J Card Surg 1989;4: 313–316.

21. Nomura F, Penny DJ, Menahem S, Pawade A, Karl TR. Surgical intervention for infective endocarditis in infancy and childhood. Ann Thorac Surg 1995;60:90–95.

22. Alexiou C, Langley SM, Monro JS. Surgery for infective valve endocarditis in children. Eur J Cardiothorac Surg 1999;16:653–659.

23. Stockheim JA, Chadwick EG, Kessler S, et al. Are the Duke criteria superior to the Beth Israel criteria for the diagnosis of infective endocarditis in children? Clin Infect Dis 1998;27:1451–1456.

24. Millard DD, Shulman ST. The changing spectrum of neonatal endocarditis. Clin Perinatol 1988;15:587–608.

25. Karl TR, Wensley D, Stark J, et al. Infective endocarditis in children with congenital heart disease: comparison of selected features in patients with surgical correction or palliation and those without. Br Heart J 1987;58:57–65.

26. Saiman L. Endocarditis and Intravascular Infections. In: Long SS, ed. Principles and Practice of Pediatric Infectious Diseases, 2nd ed. New York: Elsevier, 2003:250–256.

27. Oelberg DG, Fisher DJ, Gross DM, Denson SE, Adcock EW 3rd. Endocarditis in high-risk neonates. Pediatrics 1983;71:392–397.

28. Symchych PS, Crauss AN, Winchester P. Endocarditis following intracardiac placement of umbilical venous catheters in neonates. J Pediatr 1977;90:287–289.
29. Pelletier LL, Petersdorf RG. Infective endocarditis. Medicine 1977;56:287–313.
30. Von Reyn CF, Levy BS, Arbeit RD, Friedland G, Crumpacker CS. Infective endocarditis: utilization of specific echocardiographic findings. Ann Intern Med 1981;94:505–518.
31. Durack DT, Lukes AS, Bright DK. New criteria for diagnosis of infective endocarditis: utilization of specific echocardiographic findings. Am J Med 1994;96: 200–209.
32. Bayer AS, Ward JI, Ginzton LE, Shapiro SM. Evaluation of new clinical criteria for the diagnosis of infective endocarditis. Am J Med 1994;96.
33. Hoen B, Selton-Suty D, Danchin N, et al. Evaluation of the Duke criteria versus the Beth Israel criteria for the diagnosis of infective endocarditis. Clin Infect Dis 1995;21:905–909.
34. Dodds GA, Sexton DJ, Durack DT, et al. Negative predictive value of the Duke criteria for infective endocarditis. Am J Cardiol 1996;77:403–407.
35. Heiro M, Nikoskelainen J, Hartiala JJ, Saraste MK, Kotilainen PM. Diagnosis of infective endocarditis: sensitivity of the Duke vs von Reyn criteria. Arch Intern Med 1998;158:18–24.
36. Li J, Sexton DJ, Mick N, et al. Proposed modifications to the Duke criteria for the diagnosis of infective endocarditis. Clin Infect Dis 2000;30:633–638.
37. Washington JAN. The role of the microbiology laboratory in the diagnosis and antimicrobial treatment of infective endocarditis. Mayo Clin Proc 1982;57: 22–32.
38. Towns ML, Reller LB. Diagnostic methods: current best practices and guidelines for isolation of bacteria and fungi in infective endocarditis. Infect Dis Clin North Am 2002;16:363–376.
39. Everts RJ, Vinson EN, Adholla PO, Reller LB. Contamination of catheter-drawn blood cultures. J Clin Microbiol 2001;39:3393–3394.
40. Kavey RE, Frank DM, Byrum CJ, et al. Two-dimensional echocardiographic assessment of infective endocarditis in children. Am J Dis Child 1983;137:851–856.
41. Bricker JT, Latson LA, Huhta JC, Gutgesell JP. Echocardiographic evaluation of infective endocarditis in children. Clin Pediatr 1985;24:312–317.
42. Karalis DA, Bansal RC, Hauck AJ, et al. Transesophageal echocardiographic recognition of subaortic complications in aortic valve endocarditis. Clinical and surgical implications. Circulation 1992;86:353–362.
43. Pierrotti LC, Baddour LM. Fungal endocarditis, 1995–2000. Chest 2002;122: 302–310.
44. Rex JH, Walsh TJ, Sobel JD, et al. Practice guidelines for the treatment of candidiasis. Clin Infect Dis 2000;30.
45. Sanchez PJ, Seiegel JD, Fishbein J. Candida endocarditis: successful medical management in three preterm infants and review of the literature. Pediatr Infect Dis J 1991;10:239–243.
46. Aspesberro F, Beghetti M, Oberhansli I, Friedli B. Fungal endocarditis in critically ill children. Eur J Pediatr 1999;158:275–280.
47. Minette M, Ibsen LM. Survival of candida sepsis on extracorporeal membrane oxygenation. Pediatr Crit Care Med 2005;6:709–711.
48. Bayer AS, Bolger AF, Taubert KA, et al. Diagnosis and management of infective endocarditis and its complications. Circulation 1998;98:2936–2948.

49. Mugge A, Daniel WG, Frank G, Lichtlen PR. Echocardiography in infective endocarditis: reassessment of prognostic implications of vegetation size determined by the transthoracic and the transesophageal approach. J Am Coll Cardiol 1989;14:631–638.

50. Sanfilippo AJ, Picard MH, Newell JB, et al. Echocardiographic assessment of patients with infectious endocarditis: prediction of risk for complications. J Am Coll Cardiol 1991;18:1191–1199.

51. Steckelberg JM, Murphy JG, Ballar D, et al. Emboli in infective endocarditis: the prognostic value of echocardiography. Ann Intern Med 1991;114:635–640.

52. Tolan RWJ, Kleiman MB, Frank M, King H, Brown JW. Operative intervention in active endocarditis in children: report of a series of cases and review. Clin Infect Dis 1992;14:852–862.

53. John MD, Hibberd PL, Karchmer AW, Sleeper LA, Calderwood SB. *Staphylococcus aureus* prosthetic valve endocarditis: optimal management and risk factors for death. Clin Infect Dis 1998;26:1310–1311.

54. Jaffe WM, Morgan DE, Pearlman AS, Otto CM. Infective endocarditis, 1983–1988: echocardiographic findings and factors influencing morbidity and mortality. J Am Coll Cardiol 1990;15:1227–1233.

55. Martin AB, Webber S, Fricker FJ, et al. Congenital cardiovascular disease/diabetes: acute myocarditis: rapid diagnosis by PCR in children. Circulation 1994;90: 330–339.

56. Calabrese F, Rigo E, Milanesi O, et al. Molecular diagnosis of myocarditis and dilated cardiomyopathy in children: clinicopathologic features and prognostic implications. Diagn Mol Pathol 2002;11:212–221.

57. Garcia NS, Castelo JS, Ramos V, Rezende GS, Pereira FE. Frequency of myocarditis in cases of fatal meningococcal infection in children: observations on 31 cases studied at autopsy. Rev Soc Bras Med Trop 1999;32:517–522.

58. Wasi F, Shuter J. Primary bacterial infection of the myocardium. Front Biosci 2003;8:228–231.

59. Batra AS, Lewis AB. Acute myocarditis. Curr Opin Pediatr 2001;13:234–239.

60. Leonard EG. Viral myocarditis. Pediatr Infect Dis J 2004;23:665–666.

61. Fuse K, Kodama M, Okura Y, et al. Predictors of disease course in patients with acute myocarditis. Circulation 2000;102:2829–2835.

62. Bergelson JM. Receptors mediating adenovirus attachment and internalization. Biochem Pharmacol 1999;57:975–979.

63. Feldman AM, McNamara DM. Myocarditis. N Engl J Med 2000;343:1388–1398.

64. Cioc AM, Nuovo GJ. Histologic and In Situ viral findings in the myocardium in cases of sudden, unexpected death. Mod Pathol 2002;15:914–922.

65. Dettmeyer R, Baasner A, Schlamann M, Haag C, Madea B. Coxsackie B3 myocarditis in 4 cases of suspected sudden infant death syndrome: diagnosis by immunohistochemical and molecular-pathologic investigations. Pathol Res Pract 2002;198:689–696.

66. Baasner A, Dettmeyer R, Graebe M, Rissland J, Madea B. PCR-based diagnosis of enterovirus and parvovirus B19 in paraffin-embedded heart tissue of children with suspected sudden infant death syndrome. Lab Invest 2003;83: 1451–1455.

67. Lauer B, Niederau C, Kuhl U, et al. Cardiac troponin T in patients with clinically suspected myocarditis. J Am Coll Cardiol 1997;30:1354–1359.

68. Friedrich MG, Strohm O, Schulz-Menger J, et al. Contrast media-enhanced magnetic resonance imaging visualize myocardial changes in the course of viral myocarditis. Circulation 1998;97:1802–1809.
69. Mahrholdt H, Goedecke C, Wagner A, et al. Cardiovascular magnetic resonance assessment of human myocarditis: a comparison to histology and molecular biology. Circulation 2004;109:1250–1258.
70. Aretz HT, Billingham ME, Edwards WD, et al. Myocarditis: a histopathologic definition and classification. Am J Cardiovasc Pathol 1987;1:3–14.
71. Hauck AJ, Kearney DL, Edwards WD. Evaluation of postmortem endomyocardial biopsy specimens from 38 patients with lymphocytic myocarditis: implications for role of sampling error. Mayo Clin Proc 1989;64:1235–1245.
72. Wu LA, Lapeyre AC, Cooper LT. Current role of endomyocardial biopsy in the management of dilated cardiomyopathy and myocarditis. Mayo Clin Proc 2001;76:1030–1038.
73. Dec GW, Fallon JT, Southern JF, Palacios I. "Borderline" myocarditis: an indication for repeat endomyocardial biopsy. J Am Coll Cardiol 1990;15:283–289.
74. Calabrese F, Thiene G. Myocarditis and inflammatory cardiomyopathy: microbiological and molecular biological aspects. Cardiovasc Res 2003;60:11–25.
75. Bowles NE, Ni J, Kearney DL, et al. Detection of viruses in myocardial tissues by polymerase chain reaction: evidence of adenovirus as a common cause of myocarditis in children and adults. J Am Coll Cardiol 2003;42:466–472.
76. Lieberman EB, Hutchins GM, Hershkowitz A, Rose NR, Baughman KL. Clinicopathologic description of myocarditis. J Am Coll Cardiol 1991;18:1617–1626.
77. McCarthy R, Boehmer JP, Hruban RH, et al. Long-term outcome of fulminant myocarditis as compared with acute (nonfulminant) myocarditis. N Engl J Med 2000;342:690–695.
78. Nugent AW, Daubeney PE, Chondros P, et al. The epidemiology of childhood cardiomyopathy in Australia. N Engl J Med 2003;348:1639–1646.
79. Bohn D, Benson L. Diagnosis and management of pediatric myocarditis. Paediatr Drugs 2002;4:171–181.
80. Duncan BW, Bohn D, Atz AM, et al. Mechanical circulatory support for the treatment of children with acute fulminant myocarditis. J Thorac Cardiovasc Surg 2001;122:440–448.
81. Fiser WP, Yetman AT, Gunselman RJ, et al. Pediatric arteriovenous extracorporeal membrane oxygenation (ECMO) as a bridge to cardiac transplantation. J Heart Lung Transplant 2003;22:770–777.
82. Tabbutt S, Leonard M, Godinez RI, et al. Severe influenza B myocarditis and myositis. Pediatr Crit Care Med 2004;5:403–406.
83. Cunnion RE, Parrillo JE, Maisch B, et al. Immunosuppressive therapy for myocarditis. N Engl J Med 1995;333:1713–1714.
84. Frustaci A, Chimenti C, Calabrese F, et al. Immunosuppressive therapy for active lymphocytic myocarditis: virological and immunologic profile of responders versus nonresponders. Circulation 2003;107:857–863.
85. Drucker NA, Colan SD, Lewis AB, et al. Congenital heart disease: gamma-globulin treatment of acute myocarditis in the pediatric population. Circulation 1994;89:252–257.
86. McNamara DM, Holubkov R, Starling RC, et al. Controlled trial of intravenous immune globulin in recent-onset dilated cardiomyopathy. Circulation 2001; 103:2254–2259.

87. Parrillo JE, Cunnion RE, Epstein SE, et al. A prospective, randomized, controlled trial of prednisone for dilated cardiomyopathy. N Engl J Med 1989;321: 1061–1068.

88. Mason JW, O'Connell JB, Hershkowitz A, et al. A clinical trial of immunosuppressive therapy for myocarditis. N Engl J Med 1995;333:269–275.

89. Balaji S, Wiles HB, Sens MA, Gillette PC. Immunosuppressive treatment for myocarditis and borderline myocarditis in children with ventricular ectopic rhythm. Br Heart J 1994;72:354–359.

90. Camargo PR, Snitcowsky R, da Luz PL, et al. Favorable effects of immunosuppressive therapy in children with dilated cardiomyopathy and active myocarditis. Pediatr Cardiol 1995;16:61–68.

91. Gagliardi MG, Bevilacqua M, Bassano C, et al. Long-term follow-up of children with myocarditis treated by immunosuppression and of children with dilated cardiomyopathy. Heart 2004;90:1167–1171.

92. Hia CP, Yip WC, Tai BC, Quek SC. Immunosuppressive therapy in acute myocarditis: an 18 year systematic review. Arch Dis Child 2004;89:580–584.

93. Hufnagel G, Pankuweit S, Richter A, Schonian U, Maisch B. The European Study of Epidemiology and Treatment of Cardiac Inflammatory Diseases (ESETCID). First epidemiological results. Herz 2000;25:279–285.

94. Spodnick DH. Acute pericarditis: current concepts and practice. JAMA 2003;289: 1150–1153.

95. Troughton RW, Asher CR, Klein AL. Pericarditis. Lancet 2004;363:717–727.

96. Levy P, Corey R, Berger P, et al. Etiologic diagnosis of 204 pericardial effusions. Medicine 2003;82:385–391.

97. Permanyer-Miralda G, Sagrista-Sauleda J, Soler-Soler J. Primary acute pericardial disease: a prospective series of 231 consecutive patients. Am J Cardiol 1985;56: 623–630.

98. Launbjerg J, Fruergaard P, Hesse B, et al. Long-term risk of death, cardiac events and recurrent chest pain in patients with acute chest pain of different origin. Cardiology 1996;87:60–66.

99. Friman G, Fohlman J. The epidemiology of viral heart disease. Scand J Infect Dis Suppl 1993;88:7–10.

100. Feldman WE. Bacterial etiology and mortality of purulent pericarditis in pediatric patients: a review of 162 cases. Am J Dis Child 1979;133:641–644.

101. Breen JF. Imaging of the pericardium. J Thorac Imaging 2001;16:47–54.

102. Imazio M, Demichelis B, Cecchi E, et al. Cardiac troponin I in acute pericarditis. J Am Coll Cardiol 2003;42:2144–2148.

103. Trautner BW, Darouiche RO. Tuberculous pericarditis: optimal diagnosis and management. Clin Infect Dis 2001;33:954–961.

104. Schifferdecker B, Spodnick DH. Nonsteroidal anti-inflammatory drugs in the treatment of pericarditis: clinical review. Cardiology Rev 2003;11:211–217.

105. Adler Y, Guindo J, Finkelstein Y, et al. Colchicine for large pericardial effusion. Clin Cardiol 1998;21:143–144.

106. Yazigi A, Abou-Charaf LC. Colchicine for recurrent pericarditis in children. Acta Paediatr 1998;87:603–604.

107. Strang JI, Kakaza HH, Gibson DG, Girling DJ, Nunn AJ, Fox W. Controlled trial of prednisolone as adjuvant in treatment of tuberculous constrictive pericarditis in Transkei. Lancet 1987;2(8573):1418–1422.

108. Strang JI, Kakaza HH, Gibson DG, et al. Controlled clinical trial of complete open surgical drainage and of prednisolone in treatment of tuberculous pericardial effusion in Transkei. Lancet 1988;2(8614):759–764.
109. Mayosi BM, Ntsekhe M, Volmink JA, Commerford PJ. Interventions for treating tuberculous pericarditis. The Cochrane Database of Systematic Reviews 2004;4.
110. Finkelstein Y, Adler Y, Nussinovitch I, Varsano I. A new classification for pericarditis associated with meningococcal infection. Eur J Pediatr 1997;156:585–588.
111. Schrank JHJ, Dooley DP. Purulent pericarditis caused by *Candida* species: Case report and review. Clin Infect Dis 1995;21:182–187.

15
Pediatric Critical Care: Acute Central Nervous System Infection

Thomas Iolster and Robert C. Tasker

Clinical Syndromes of Central Nervous System Infection in the Pediatric Intensive Care Unit

A variety of infectious organisms affect the central nervous system (CNS). From the perspective of pediatric critical care, each organism has the potential for generating distinctive clinical syndromes (Table 15.1), and these are discussed in this chapter.

Purulent Meningitis

Purulent meningitis is characterized by the presence of more than 1000 neutrophils/mm^3 in the cerebrospinal fluid (CSF). It is always considered to be of bacterial origin, even though bacteria may not be cultured. In countries with effective immunization against *Haemophilus influenzae* type B (Hib), *Neisseria meningitidis* and *Streptococcus pneumoniae* cause most cases of purulent meningitis in infants and children (1,2). During the neonatal period, the likely causative pathogens are different, with the most frequent being group B streptococcus, *Escherichia coli, Streptococcus pneumoniae, Listeria monocytogenes, Neisseria meningitidis,* other gram-positive bacteria, and other gram-negative rods (3,4). Rare causes of neonatal meningitis may also include staphylococci, enterococci, and viridans streptococci (5). The discussion in this chapter focuses on the small infant and child and not the neonate managed on the neonatal intensive care unit.

Pathogenesis

In most cases bacteria gain access to the CSF via the nasopharynx, bloodstream, and leptomeninges. However, bacteria may also spread to the CSF from an extradural focus, penetrating trauma, fractures, neurosurgical procedures (e.g., CSF diversion shunts), cochlear implants, or rupture of an intracranial abscess. The local inflammatory response to bacteria multiplying in the CSF involves

TABLE 15.1. Clinical syndromes of central nervous system (CNS) infection

1. Purulent meningitis
2. Aseptic meningitis
3. Acute encephalitis
4. Paralysis and weakness syndromes
    4.1 Poliomyelitis
    4.2 Guillain-Barré syndrome
    4.3 Botulism
5. Acute disseminated encephalomyelitis
6. Tetanus-like illness
7. Neurosurgical conditions
    7.1 Ventriculitis and infected shunts
    7.2 Brain abscess
    7.3 Subdural effusion
    7.4 Spinal abscess

polymorphonuclear leukocytes, the endothelium, complement, and chemical mediators. The result is an alteration in the cerebral blood flow (CBF), vasculitis, and obstruction to CSF outflow and reabsorption.

Clinical Features

Purulent meningitis leading to intensive care admission is often associated with acute complications and severe outcome. The diagnosis is particularly difficult in young infants since fever, lethargy, irritability, apnea, crying when handled, and poor eye contact are nonspecific signs. In addition, a bulging anterior fontanel and neck stiffness may not be present. Convulsion that is associated with fever, especially when there is not a prompt recovery of the state of consciousness, may be another presentation. In the older child fever, headache, and vomiting at an early stage, and irritability, photophobia, altered mental state, and neck stiffness later on, is the usual clinical progression. Focal signs and seizures may also be present; Kernig and Brudzinski signs are often absent in children. Last, at any age, signs of systemic involvement and distress may be present (e.g., tachycardia, poor perfusion, hypotension, tachypnea, purpura, or petechiae).

Diagnosis

The diagnosis of purulent meningitis is confirmed by recovering bacteria from the CSF. However, invariably in the comatose intensive care patient, lumbar puncture (LP) has to be postponed due to the risks of tentorial herniation (Table 15.2). When there is an acute CSF sample, it typically has a cloudy or turbid appearance, and the cell count is more than 1000 neutrophils/mm^3. The CSF glucose concentration is usually low and the protein concentration is usually elevated. Measurement of inflammatory mediators in the serum, such as C-reactive protein (CRP), may be helpful for diagnosis. A normal CRP (i.e.,

≤10 mg/L) has a high negative predictive value for the diagnosis of bacterial meningitis (6).

Meningitis may be difficult to diagnose in patients receiving oral antibiotics. In these cases, likely diagnosis should be based on the history, clinical presentation, and characteristics of the CSF. Low glucose, high protein, and a few white blood cells in the CSF can be suggestive of bacterial meningitis. In these cases bacterial antigen testing in the CSF may help to confirm the diagnosis.

Acute Complications

Brain Swelling

Patients can progress from being alert and irritable to being profoundly comatose. It is normally at this stage that referral is made for intensive care. In this state, our major concern is the development of brain swelling and raised intracranial pressure (ICP). The worst consequence of brain swelling is cerebral tentorial herniation.

Seizures

Convulsions that occur in the earlier stages of meningitis are usually generalized, and have less prognostic significance than those occurring later. Brain swelling, diffuse ischemia, cerebral inflammation, hyponatremia, subdural effusion, or focal infarction may cause seizures in meningitis.

Syndrome of Inappropriate Secretion of Antidiuretic Hormone

The syndrome of inappropriate secretion of antidiuretic hormone secretion (SIADH) is characterized by the presence of hyponatremia and hypo-osmolarity without signs of hypovolemia. The urine is concentrated and there is continued urinary sodium excretion in the absence of renal disease.

TABLE 15.2. Contraindications to lumbar puncture

Presence of shock
Glasgow Coma Scale <13
Signs of increased intracranial pressure
Abnormal pupil size and reaction, absent doll's-eye movements
Abnormal tone, tonic posturing
Respiratory abnormalities
Papilledema, hypertension, and relative bradycardia
Seizures
Within 30 minutes of short seizure, or following prolonged seizure (>30 minutes) or ongoing focal or tonic seizures
Local superficial skin infection
Coagulation disorder

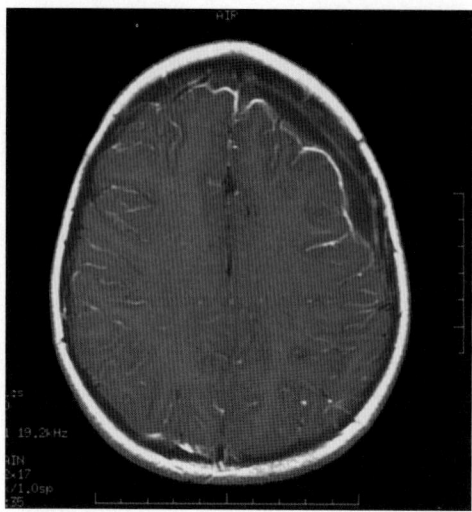

FIGURE 15.1. Magnetic resonance imaging (MRI) of a 9-year-old girl with left-sided sinusitis who developed large left-sided frontoparietal subdural empyema.

Subdural Effusion

The subdural space does not normally contain fluid. However, up to 50% of children with meningitis accumulate fluid in this space (Fig. 15.1). In these children, subdural effusions usually occur several days after the onset of illness, but they may be present from admission. The pathogenesis most likely involves increased permeability of cerebral blood vessels, increased ICP, and changes in local blood flow that favors the passage of proteins and fluid into the space. Subdural effusions often resolve spontaneously. However, if the effusion is large, if it is associated with seizures or focal signs, or if there is raised ICP, then surgical drainage should be considered.

When a fluid sample is collected, it is usually sterile. A positive bacterial culture indicates subdural empyema. In this instance, the fluid is purulent, contains more than 5000 leukocytes/mm^3, and there is an association with more severe neurologic outcome (7).

Obstructive Hydrocephalus

Obstructive hydrocephalus occurs when pus in the ventricles blocks the outflow of CSF, and is more frequent in small infants. Communicating hydrocephalus is caused by inadequate absorption of CSF, and it may develop 2 weeks after the onset of illness.

Medical Treatment

Antimicrobial Therapy

Early diagnosis and early parenteral antimicrobial therapy are essential. The specific choice of antibiotics depends on the likely cause and local epidemiology and antibiotic sensitivities. Before the cultures become available, the initial choice of treatment is based on the age of the patient. In small infants, 1 to 3 months old, a combination of ampicillin and cefotaxime or ceftriaxone is used. After age 3 months, treatment with ceftriaxone or cefotaxime is adequate (4). If there is suspicion of cephalosporin-resistant pneumococcus, or in cases where LP has been deferred, use vancomycin (8). The duration of antibiotic therapy depends on the infecting organism. Meningococcal meningitis is treated for 4 to 7 days, Hib meningitis for 7 to 10 days, and pneumococcal meningitis for 10 to 14 days. A repeat lumbar puncture at 24 to 48 hours of treatment should be done in cases of cephalosporin-resistant pneumococcus.

Steroids

Whether to use steroids as part of the acute treatment of bacterial meningitis in children is the subject of ongoing debate. Early use of dexamethasone has been shown to diminish hearing loss in children with Hib meningitis and to improve outcome in adults with pneumococcal meningitis (9). Its role, however, in the treatment of other types of meningitis in children is less clear (10). One concern is that steroids may interfere with the entry of cefotaxime and vancomycin into the CSF. There is also concern that steroids may worsen the outcome of viral meningitis.

If dexamethasone is used, it must be administered with or before the first dose of antibiotics, and therapy should be discontinued if the patient does not have bacterial meningitis. The recommended dose is 0.15 mg/kg, every 6 hours, for 4 days. Alternatively, 0.4 mg/kg, every 12 hours, for 2 days, is equally beneficial (11).

Chemoprophylaxis

Chemoprophylaxis is recommended for Hib and Meningococcal meningitis. In Hib meningitis, rifampin prophylaxis is recommended for all household contacts. This policy includes infants younger than 12 months who have not had complete primary immunization. The recommended dose of rifampin for Hib meningitis contacts is 20 mg/kg/d (maximum 600 mg/d) for 4 days.

In meningococcal meningitis, rifampin prophylaxis is recommended for all household (and "kissing") contacts as well as child care or nursery school contacts during the week before illness in the index case. The recommended dose of rifampin for meningococcal meningitis contacts is 10 mg/kg/d for 2 days. Alternatively, intramuscular ceftriaxone (125 mg in patients <15 years of age; 250 mg in patients >15 years) or ciprofloxacin 500 mg, one dose for people 18 years or older.

Aseptic Meningitis

Aseptic meningitis refers to meningitis that is not produced by bacteria. Aseptic meningitis can be serious but it is rarely fatal in children with normal immunity. The physical findings are similar to those in bacterial meningitis, but they are frequently less severe and the CSF usually shows fewer white cells than in bacterial meningitis (10 to 500 leukocytes/mm^3) and no bacteria on microscopy and culture.

Viruses cause most cases of aseptic meningitis. The term *viral meningitis* should not be used in these cases because there are other important causes to consider. Echovirus and Coxsackie virus, members of the enterovirus family, are the most frequent viral causes (12); these infections are more frequent in the summer and early autumn. Less frequent viral causes include adenovirus, measles, Epstein-Barr virus (EBV), and arbovirus. *Mycoplasma pneumoniae*, Lyme disease, cat-scratch disease, *Chlamydia psittaci,* and leptospirosis are rare nonviral causes. Other infectious causes, such as fungi, are often seen in immunosuppressed children, for example, *Cryptococcus, Candida albicans,* coccidioidomycosis, aspergillosis, histoplasmosis, and mucormycosis.

Noninfectious causes of aseptic meningitis include spinal anesthetics, chemicals injected into the subdural space for diagnosis or therapy, intracranial bleeding, vasculitides, and cerebral neoplasm. Kawasaki disease can also present with sterile CSF pleocytosis.

Pathogenesis

The pathogenesis of aseptic meningitis depends on its cause. When a virus is the cause, spread is usually via the fecal-oral or respiratory route. The virus replicates in the intestinal epithelial and lymphoid tissue, or in the respiratory epithelium, and then spreads to susceptible organs through the blood.

Clinical Features

Fever, headache, vomiting, neck stiffness, and photophobia are classic signs and symptoms of aseptic meningitis. Other symptoms may include arthralgia, myalgia, sore throat, and weakness. More specific signs, depending on the cause, are herpangina, papulovesicular lesions on the feet and hands, and a skin rash that blanches to pressure. The clinical picture in infants and children younger than 2 years old may be indistinguishable from bacterial meningitis or systemic sepsis. In this age group, fever, irritability, crying when handling, lethargy, and apneas should prompt consideration of CSF examination.

Diagnosis

A detailed history and study of the CSF are essential for a specific diagnosis of aseptic meningitis. The CSF usually shows 10 to 500 leukocyte/mm^3, although more than 1000 leukocytes may sometimes be present. Polymorphonuclear cell predominance may be present in the majority of the patients with enteroviral meningitis (13). The CSF protein concentration is usually normal, although in some cases it may be slightly raised. The CSF glucose concentration is usually low (i.e., 60% or less of the blood glucose) in aseptic meningitis, partially treated bacterial meningitis, tuberculosis, fungi, amoebae, toxoplasmosis, and some types of viral meningitis. Most of the viral meningitides, mycoplasma, and chlamydia meningitis have normal CSF glucose.

Medical Treatment

Antimicrobial Therapy

Children who need admission to the pediatric intensive care unit (PICU) are seriously ill. Antibiotics should always be started and the treatment modified when results from the LP are available (remembering that it may not be safe to perform an LP for a few days). Negative CSF cultures should prompt the clinician to search for other treatable causes (e.g., tuberculosis, *Mycoplasma*, Lyme disease), and a second lumbar puncture may be necessary. In cases where viral infection is confirmed, antibiotics can be stopped. In tuberculous meningitis the recommended treatment is a combination of isoniazid (10 to 20 mg/kg/d, up to 300 mg), rifampicin (10 to 20 mg/kg/d, up to 600 mg), and pyrazinamide (15 to 30 mg/kg/d, up to 2 g per day). Ethambutol or streptomycin may be added if initial response to treatment is poor (14). Steroids are effective in reducing ICP and may improve survival in patients over 14 years of age (15). Last, fungal meningitis is treated with amphotericin B.

Acute Encephalitis

Acute encephalitis, or meningoencephalitis, can be differentiated from aseptic meningitis by the presence of severe disturbances of consciousness. Acute encephalitis should also be differentiated from postinfectious encephalomyelitis, which usually follows a nonspecific viral infection, and noninfectious encephalopathies (e.g., metabolic, vascular, demyelinating disease, Reye's syndrome).

The most frequent causes of acute encephalitis in children include *Mycoplasma pneumoniae*, enterovirus, herpes simplex virus, varicella zoster, EBV, adenovirus, and influenza virus (16,17). Arboviruses are major causes of encephalitis in many areas of the world and should be routinely screened in endemic areas. Mumps, measles, and rubella infection are now infrequent. Other rare infectious causes include toxoplasmosis, lymphocytic choriomeningitis virus, rabies, adenovirus, hepatitis A virus, legionnaires' disease, and tuberculosis.

Clinical Findings

Fever and malaise usually precedes acute viral encephalitis. Then, the clinical findings that define encephalitis are severe, nontransient disturbance of consciousness and focal or generalized neurologic symptoms reflecting brain involvement. The neurologic signs include ataxia, disturbances of speech or vision, focal neurology, and focal or generalized seizures. Herpes simplex virus (HSV) encephalitis usually produces temporal lobe symptoms, focal paralysis, and lateralized seizures. *Mycoplasma pneumoniae* infection is often preceded by respiratory symptoms (18).

Diagnosis

The diagnosis of viral encephalitis can be difficult. As in aseptic meningitis a detailed history and CSF investigation are essential, but the latter may have to wait until it is safe. The CSF can be completely normal, but usually it contains more than 10 leukocytes/mm^3, mildly decreased glucose, and mildly increased protein. In children with HSV encephalitis, the CSF may contain red blood cells. Polymerase chain reaction (PCR) in CSF for enterovirus and HSV has shown high diagnostic sensitivity and specificity (19). It is also useful for the diagnosis of *Mycoplasma pneumoniae* and is being used for the detection of other organisms such as varicella zoster virus, cytomegalovirus, EBV, and *Mycobacterium tuberculosis*. Also, CSF or blood serology may be diagnostic, but unfortunately the results are not usually available during the acute illness.

Other investigations may help with the diagnosis. In HSV, cranial computed tomography (CT) shows edema and contrast enhancement in the temporal lobe after the third day of illness. Magnetic resonance imaging (MRI) may show abnormality in these regions earlier. The electroencephalogram may show periodic lateralized epileptiform discharges. Last, in some instances brain biopsy may be used. This investigation should be reserved for cases in whom the diagnosis is not clear, or in cases of HSV with progressive deterioration despite treatment with acyclovir (20). The main benefit of brain biopsy is that it excludes other diagnoses such as subdural empyema, brain tumour, toxoplasmosis, and other viruses.

Medical Treatment

Acyclovir has changed the previous, often fatal, course of HSV. There should be no delay in starting this treatment whenever HSV is suspected. The dose of acylovir is 30 mg/kg/day, given in three divided doses, for 10 days. The treatment should be repeated if there are signs of recurrence.

When *Mycoplasma pneumoniae* is suspected, antibiotics with good penetration into the brain (e.g., ciprofloxacin, doxycycline, chloramphenicol, or azithromycin) should be used (21).

Acute Paralysis and Weakness Syndromes

A wide variety of viruses can produce weakness and paralysis syndromes, including poliovirus, Coxsackie, rabies, HSV, influenza, EBV, and St. Louis encephalitis. *Clostridium botulinum* and *Campylobacter jejuni* are bacterial causes, and *M. pneumoniae* is another cause.

Poliomyelitis

Wild-type poliovirus infection is now eradicated with global immunization. However, poliomyelitis may result from the oral vaccine. It typically produces aseptic meningitis that may be associated with asymmetric flaccid paralysis. Severe forms with paralysis are caused by destruction of the anterior horn cells of the spinal cord. Sometimes compromise in bulbar and airway function may be present because of involvement of motor nuclei of cranial nerves. The CSF findings include elevated protein concentration and pleocytosis. The diagnosis is confirmed by isolation of poliovirus from the oropharynx and stools, or by serology.

Other pathogens that very rarely cause a poliomyelitis-like syndrome are Coxsackie, mumps, echovirus, HSV, St, Louis encephalitis, and *Mycoplasma*.

The course of severe forms of poliomyelitis may vary.

Guillain-Barré Syndrome

Guillain-Barré syndrome (GBS) is an immune-mediated polyneuropathy that typically presents after a viral or bacterial infection. It is the most frequent cause of acute paralysis in developed countries and is characterized by progressive, symmetrical motor weakness and areflexia, although sensory and autonomic disturbances may also be present. The pathogenesis involves immune response against an infective organism that cross-reacts with peripheral nerve components. Infections known to precede GBS are cytomegalovirus, EBV, varicella zoster virus, *C. jejuni*, and *M. pneumoniae*. Other infections that may precede GBS include HIV, Coxsackie virus, HSV-2 encephalitis, tuberculosis, psittacosis, malaria, tularemia, and toxoplasmosis.

Clinical Features

An acute infectious illness, most frequently upper respiratory tract infection or gastroenteritis, precedes the onset of neurologic symptoms by 1 to 3 weeks. The most frequent clinical presentation involves an acute inflammatory demyelinating polyradiculoneuropathy (AIDP) that produces ascending hypotonic paralysis and areflexia. Initially it affects the legs. Involvement of the arms and face is less frequent; so too are sensory loss in a glove-stocking distribution and autonomic disturbances. Other variants in clinical presentation include acute motor-sensory axonal neuropathy (AMSAN), acute motor-axonal neuropathy (AMAN), and the Miller-Fisher syndrome with ophthalmoplegia, ataxia, and areflexia. The symptoms of GBS may progress for up to 4 weeks, and recovery should begin 2 to 4 weeks after progression ceases.

Diagnosis

The diagnosis of GBS is clinical and can be aided by laboratory and electro-physiologic studies. The CSF shows high protein concentration with less than 10 leukocytes/mm³, typically during the second or third week after onset of symptoms. Electrophysiology studies show decreased conduction velocity in the peripheral nerves, and there may be other findings in the clinical variants of GBS.

Medical Treatment

Specific therapies that shorten the evolution of symptoms include plasma exchange and high-dose intravenous immunoglobulin (IVIG). Plasma exchange should be used as early as possible within the first 2 weeks of illness. Two courses for mild GBS and four to five courses for severe GBS. Intravenous immunoglobulin is as effective as plasma exchange and it has the added benefit that it is easier to administer; it is safe and it is more widely available than plasma exchange. The recommended dose of IVIG is 2 g/kg/d for 2 or 5 days, although the shorter course of treatment may be associated with early relapse (22). Steroids provide no added benefit and so should not be used (23).

Botulism

Botulism is caused by *Clostridium botulinum* toxin. Toxins enter the blood-stream either via the gastrointestinal tract or via an infected wound.

Clinical Features

Symptoms may start as early as 6 hours after exposure to toxin, or they may start some time later, up to 6 days. The cranial nerves are usually involved first, and swallowing is often affected as well as speech and eye movement. Other signs and symptoms include nausea, vomiting, dry mouth, and abdominal cramps. As the disease progresses it causes weakness or paralysis of the extrem-ities and the respiratory muscles. Patients must be monitored for signs of respiratory failure and autonomic dysfunction, and mechanical ventilation should be started whenever it is needed. In infants the disease can also be mild with hypotonia as the only sign.

Diagnosis

In the acute phase of illness the best way to diagnose botulism is with electro-myography using repetitive nerve stimulation. Recovery of *C. botulinum* toxin from stools or serum serology confirms the diagnosis, but these investigations usually take longer.

Medical Treatment

Specific therapy with antitoxin is useful to remove circulating toxin but it does not affect toxin already at the neuromuscular junction. In infant botulism, however, antitoxin is not recommended because the prognosis is good. Rather, antibiotics are used to eradicate the source of toxin production. Treatment with penicillin and metronidazole is effective in these cases. Aminoglycosides may worsen the neuromuscular transmission defect.

Acute Disseminated Encephalomyelitis

Acute disseminated encephalomyelitis (ADEM) is an inflammatory demyelinating disease of the CNS. It has a monophasic evolution and so can be differentiated from multiple sclerosis. It is considered a parainfectious disease, and the precipitants include infection with measles, mumps, rubella, chickenpox, EBV, influenza, group A streptococcus, and *Mycoplasma*. The most frequent precipitant in immunized populations is a nonspecific upper respiratory tract infection.

Clinical Features

The acute presentation of ADEM is usually with decreased level of consciousness or behavioral changes, combined with focal or multifocal neurologic deficits. Neurologic findings include pyramidal tract signs, ataxia, cranial neuropathy, optic neuritis, seizures, and sensory abnormalities. Other signs and symptoms include fever, headache, malaise, and meningism.

Diagnosis

In ADEM there should be evidence of demyelination on neuroimaging, and no evidence of direct infection of the CNS. MRI is preferred to CT scanning because the CT scan is usually normal (24). The MRI sequences (e.g., T2 and fluid-attenuated inversion recovery [FLAIR]) show multiple, disseminated asymmetrical lesions that affect the white matter throughout the CNS (Fig. 15.2). Lumbar puncture should be performed to exclude direct infection of the CNS. The CSF may show normal white cell count, or mild pleocytosis (100 to 200 cells/mm^3), and mild protein elevation. The CSF culture and virologic studies should be negative.

Medical Treatment

Usually, by the time of admission to the PICU, children with ADEM have already been started on antimicrobial therapy for meningitis and encephalitis. These drugs should be stopped once the diagnosis of ADEM is confirmed. In general, the prognosis for this condition is usually good, and many children may recover spontaneously in days to months. However, steroid therapy is currently used in most cases. One regimen that has been used is methylprednisolone 30 mg/kg/d (maximum 1 g), for 3 days, followed by oral prednisolone

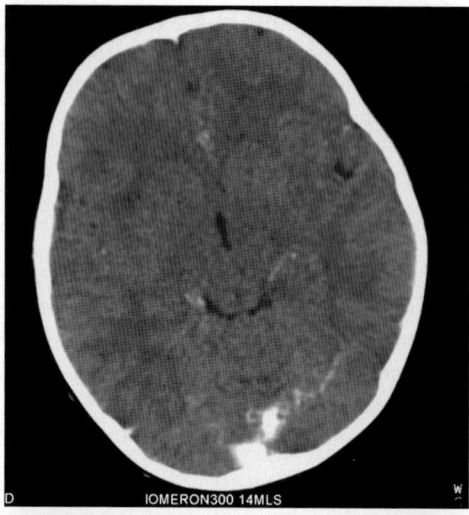

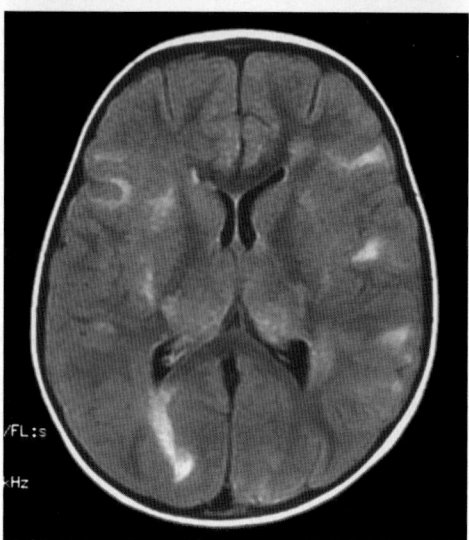

FIGURE 15.2. A 3-year-old boy with acute disseminated encephalomyelitis (ADEM). (A) Computed tomography (CT) scan. (B) Head MRI (T2 fluid-attenuated inversion recovery [FLAIR]). Note how the lesions (white patches on the T2 FLAIR) are more evident on the MRI.

2 mg/kg/d, for 2 weeks, followed by a 4-week weaning schedule (25). A non-tested treatment for relapsed, or refractory, ADEM may be plasma exchange or IVIG.

Tetanus-Like Illness

Tetanus is a neurologic syndrome caused by *Clostridium tetani* toxin. The toxin acts by disabling central inhibitory neurotransmission in the anterior horn cells of the spinal cord, causing lack of inhibition of excitatory impulses. The consequence is the characteristic muscle contractions: muscular rigidity, episodes of muscular spasm, and trismus. When the spasms are generalized there is a posture that resembles decorticate posturing. Generalized seizures may occur after such episodes. In many developing countries tetanus is endemic and still produces high mortality, especially in newborns of nonimmunized mothers. Most of the cases of tetanus in children and adults are secondary to trauma with dirty objects, or less frequently animal bites, burns, abscesses, or chronic ulcers.

Specific treatment for tetanus includes use of human tetanus immunoglobulin in a single dose of 3000 to 6000 units, given intramuscularly, to neutralize toxin still being released from the site of entry (26). Antibiotics are used to eradicate any *C. tetani*. The first choice antibiotic is metronidazole 30 mg/kg/d, in four divided doses (26,27). Alternatively, use penicillin 100,000 to 250,000 units/kg/d.

The Neurosurgical Patient

Ventriculitis and Shunt Infection

Inflammation of the ventricles is usually associated with ventricular shunt devices, but it may also be secondary to meningitis or rupture of a cerebral abscess into the ventricular system. The diagnosis is confirmed by the presence of more than 25 leukocytes/mm^3, or a positive culture from CSF obtained from the ventricles. Ventriculoperitoneal (VP) shunt malfunction predisposes to infection, but infection may also arise secondary to colonization of the shunt tubing with bacteria from the skin, which may happen during the first month after insertion. Premature birth, young age, previous shunt infection, and intra-operative use of neuroendoscopy have been described as risk factors for VP shunt infection (28). The common pathogens are coagulase-negative *Staphylococcus* species, *S. aureus*, and gram-negative rods (28,29).

Clinical Features

The diagnosis of VP shunt infection may be delayed because of the absence of specific signs of CNS infection. The symptoms of shunt infection include fever, seizures, headache, bulging fontanel, poor feeding, nausea, vomiting, lethargy, and exacerbation of strabismus. Fever is important and present in most instances, so, in any patient with a VP shunt, who develops fever, infection should be considered. However, other more frequent infections like otitis media, viral upper respiratory infection, or urinary infection should be excluded as they may also produce fever.

Diagnosis

Brain imaging may show worsened ventricular enlargement (which you can identify by reviewing all of the child's imaging) as evidence of VP shunt dysfunction. However, to rule out infection, CSF should be obtained from the shunt reservoir. More than 25 leucocytes/mm³, elevated protein, and normal or mildly decreased glucose are the usual CSF findings in infection. Elevated protein in the absence of pleocytosis may be the result of obstruction without infection.

Medical Treatment

Optimal management of VP shunt infections requires removal of the shunt and antibiotic treatment. Ideally, antibiotics should not be started until the diagnosis has been confirmed with CSF studies, or until two sets of cultures have been obtained. The dose of antibiotics should be as high as possible (because of poor penetration into the infected area) and long enough so that relapse is avoided. Initially, empiric treatment with vancomycin is used (especially in hospitals in which *S. aureus* and coagulase-negative staphylococci are methicillin-resistant) together with a third-generation cephalosporin to cover gram-negative infections. In proven staphylococcal infections, vancomycin can be used together with rifampicin, which better penetrates the blood–brain barrier. In cases where infection is caused by multidrug-resistant gram-negative rods, treatment with carbapenems or fluoroquinolones is needed (30). The duration of treatment is controversial and can range from 3 days for mild coagulase-negative infections to 10 days beyond CSF sterilization for other bacteria.

Brain Abscess

Brain abscesses are unusual, but they are the most common cause of focal CNS infection. Most cases occur in children with congenital heart disease, sinusitis, otitis, or mastoiditis. Other causes include trauma, local instrumentation, and rarely meningitis. Abscess in the temporal lobe is usually associated with otitis media or mastoiditis. Abscess in the frontal lobe is associated with frontal sinusitis or a fracture. Cyanotic congenital heart disease is usually associated with abscess in the distribution of the middle cerebral artery. In children, the most frequent bacterial causes—often mixed in nature—of brain abscess are streptococci, staphylococci, Enterobacteriaceae, and anaerobes. Fungal infections are very rare, but they may occur in immunocompromised children.

Clinical Features

The clinical presentation of cerebral abscess varies according to its size and location. Most children present with fever, evidence of increased ICP, and focal neurologic signs. Acutely, the neurologic examination may show any of the following signs: (1) focal deficits, (2) focal findings that progress rapidly to a diffuse alteration in sensorium, (3) diffuse depression of cerebral function, and (4) multiple deficits. In this context, the general alteration in cerebral function is often a sign of elevated ICP.

Diagnosis

Brain abscess is diagnosed using a CT scan. The typical lesion shows a hypodense area surrounded by a ring that enhances with contrast. An MRI allows earlier identification of the initial lesion (Fig. 15.3). In children with a space-occupying lesion such as cerebral abscess, an LP can be very dangerous because of the risk of tentorial herniation. When a CSF sample is collected, preferably at surgery, it usually shows nonspecific inflammatory findings. Other laboratory findings are equally inconclusive. For example, the peripheral white blood cell count can be normal or elevated, and the inflammatory markers, erythrocyte sedimentation rate (ESR) and CRP are usually elevated.

Medical Treatment

In most cases admitted to the PICU, surgical excision and drainage are needed. The initial choice of antibiotic therapy depends on the source of infection, and it is important to consider covering mixed infections (Table 15.3). Treatment can be modified once results of cultures and antibiotic sensitivities become available (31). The use of steroids is controversial, but may be used by neurosurgeons in instances where the mass is acting as a space-occupying tumor because of perilesional edema.

Subdural Empyema

Subdural empyema may be a complication of meningitis, especially when it occurs in infants or young children. However, subdural empyema can also be a distinct entity, usually related to local spread of infection from a site of

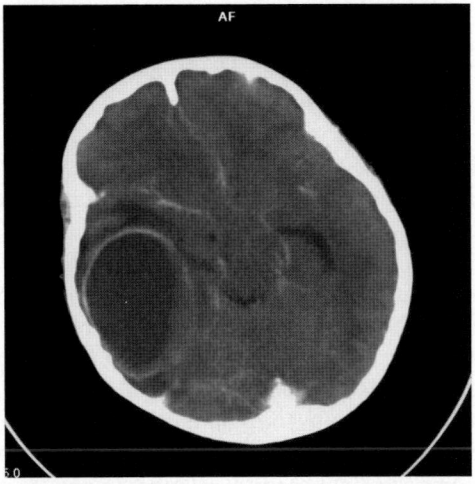

FIGURE 15.3. MRI of an 8-year-old boy with group A streptococcal brain abscess (right-sided temporoparietal region).

TABLE 15.3. Initial treatment with antibiotics based on source of infection

Sinusitis/teeth
Penicillin or cefotaxime/ceftriaxone + metronidazole + chloramphenicol/sulbactam

Chronic otitis/mastoiditis
Penicillin + metronidazole + ceftazidime

Postoperative
Vancomycin + ceftazidime

Penetrating head trauma
Oxacillin/vancomycin + cefotaxime/ceftriaxone

Metastatic spread
Oxacillin/vancomycin + cefotaxime/ceftriaxone + metronidazole

Congenital heart disease
Cefotaxime/ceftriaxone + metronidazole + chloramphenicol/sulbactam

trauma, sinusitis, otitis media, or cranial osteomyelitis. The type of infecting organisms depends on the source of the infection. The clinical findings include signs of increased ICP, nuchal rigidity, seizures, or focal neurology.

Antibiotic treatment depends on the source of infection and may include continuation of treatment for meningitis, or empirical treatment similar to that used in patients with brain abscess (see above). Surgical drainage is usually necessary, especially when collections are not related to bacterial meningitis.

This condition is still associated with high mortality and morbidity. High suspicion, rapid diagnosis, adequate antibiotic treatment, and prompt surgical intervention are essential.

Spinal Abscess

Spinal epidural abscess can lead to paraplegia. Early recognition and treatment is essential if severe consequences are to be avoided.

Spinal epidural abscesses occur more frequently in the posterior area and are usually located in the thoracic or lumbar region. They may occur after hematogenous dissemination, penetrating injuries, or local invasive procedures like an LP. In addition, they may arise from a contiguous infection (e.g., osteomyelitis, spondylodiscitis, perinephric abscess, psoas abscess, retropharyngeal abscess, and decubitus ulcers). Spinal abscess may produce problems such as direct compression of the spinal cord, mechanical compression of the blood vessels, or vasculitis with compromise of local blood flow. S. aureus is the most frequent cause of spinal abscess, followed by Streptococcus viridans, Streptococcus pneumoniae, Salmonella enteritidis, and other gram-negative bacilli. Rare causes include M. tuberculosis and fungi.

The clinical features of spinal abscess are initially nonspecific (e.g., fever or irritability). Localized pain or weakness and paralysis may follow later. In infants and small children the pain may be difficult to identify, and the diagnosis of a spinal lesion should be considered as part of the differential diagnosis of acute muscle weakness. The investigation of choice is an urgent spinal MRI. Once the diagnosis is confirmed, the patient should be referred for surgery; the treatment includes laminectomy, epidural drain, and antibiotics (32). Blood cultures and cultures of surgical material are essential for identification of the infecting organism. The initial empirical treatment should cover *S. aureus* and gram-negative organisms (33).

General Pediatric Intensive Care Unit Management of the Child with Central Nervous System Infection

Admission to the PICU should be considered in all patients with an altered level of consciousness, an inability to maintain their airway, respiratory distress, or circulatory instability. Even in stable patients, especially those who are likely to develop complications, high-dependency nursing care for monitoring is entirely appropriate. Overall, medical therapy should be aimed at, first, making the unstable child stable; second, diagnosing the underlying problem; and third, starting as fast as possible specific treatment, but when this is not possible, starting empirical therapy instead. The goal should be to limit the period from initial assessment and examination of the patient to initiation of antimicrobial therapy to less than 1 hour. In the following three subsections we discuss issues of general management pertinent to neurocritical care. General intensive care practice is covered elsewhere in this book.

Initial Survey

The assessment of the airway, breathing, and circulation should be undertaken during the first contact with the patient. Once the respiratory and circulatory states are safe, a thorough survey should continue with evaluation of the patient's neurology. This examination should focus on whether there are any signs of increased ICP. The findings from a detailed physical examination and history (Table 15.4) may help to guide the choice of diagnostic tests and initial treatments.

Airway and Breathing

Respiratory failure can be a major cause of morbidity and death in the acute phase of severe neurologic infectious disease. Patients can present with respiratory impairment secondary to loss of airway protective reflexes, muscular weakness, and alteration in the ventilatory drive or signs of pulmonary aspiration. Rapid assessment of airway patency and reflexes, respiratory effort, and gas exchange are needed. Supplemental oxygen must be given via face mask during the initial assessment. Cerebral anoxia or raised ICP can be avoided by preventing hypoxemia and hypercapnia.

TABLE 15.4. Summary of intracranial syndromes and presenting findings

Syndrome	Possible clinical findings
Purulent meningitis	Fever, headache, photophobia, vomiting, stiff neck
	Depressed consciousness
	Seizures
	Systemic involvement
	Purpuric rash
Aseptic meningitis	Fever, headache, photophobia, vomiting, stiff neck
	Systemic involvement
	Signs and symptoms are usually milder than in purulent meningitis
Encephalitis	Fever, headache, photophobia, vomiting, stiff neck
	Severe disturbance of consciousness
	Seizures
Space occupying infections	Fever, headache, vomiting, stiff neck
	Focal signs
	Seizures
Infected shunts	Fever, headache, vomiting
	Eye deviation
	Depressed consciousness
Acute disseminated encephalomyelitis (ADEM)	History of recent infection
	Fever
	Depressed consciousness, behavioral changes
	Focal or multifocal neurological deficits
	Seizures

In the child with an illness involving the CNS, the indications for endotracheal intubation are decreased level of consciousness (Glasgow Coma Scale <9), deteriorating level of consciousness, signs of increased ICP, inability to protect the airway, hypoxemia refractory to supplemental oxygen, hypoventilation, and shock. Airway management and intubation should be attempted by a skilled operator so as to avoid delays that could precipitate hypoxemia or acute elevations in ICP.

Circulation

Shock is usually secondary to sepsis, particularly meningococcal disease (34). Evaluation of mental state is essential in the assessment of cerebral perfusion. (Shock syndromes are considered elsewhere in this book. However, the reader should be aware that blood pressure support and hemodynamic monitoring are also central to brain-directed critical care.)

Raised Intracranial Pressure

Signs of raised ICP indicate the possibility of cerebral herniation (35) and low cerebral perfusion pressure, which together are associated with poor outcome in CNS infections (36,37). Raised ICP is more frequent in patients with severe bacterial meningitis, intracranial collections, encephalitis, and infected shunts, and it may be present in late phases (after 1 week) of herpetic encephalitis. The presence of raised ICP is less likely in postinfectious diseases.

Invasive monitoring of ICP in the comatose child with CNS infection has been reported by a number of clinical groups. However, there is no clear evidence about the benefits of such monitoring in children (or even adults) with CNS infections (38–40). Clinical signs of increased ICP in a child with CNS infection should prompt endotracheal intubation and mechanical ventilation. Normocapnic ventilation (P_aCO_2 4.5 to 5.0 kPa) should be used along with continuous monitoring of end-tidal CO_2 and serial arterial blood gases. Unnecessarily frequent endotracheal tube suction and painful procedures should be avoided as they lead to acute elevations in ICP. The child's head should be nursed in a midline position and the head of the bed can be elevated up to 30 degrees. Fever increases CBF and consequently ICP, so it should be treated aggressively with antipyretics and slow external cooling while trying to avoid shivering.

There is no evidence about the benefits of osmotherapy for children with CNS infections; however, mannitol (500 mg/kg/dose to 1g/kg/dose) is frequently used when there are signs of severely increased ICP. Close control of plasma osmolarity is essential when mannitol is used. Use of barbiturates and craniotomy are also controversial and are not to be used routinely in the treatment of these patients.

Seizures

Seizures are a frequent complication of CNS infections and they should be treated aggressively. It is important to consider the underlying cause that might require specific treatment; electrolyte surveillance, CT when indicated, and EEG may help determine this. Acute treatment with intravenous lorazepam (100 µg/kg/dose) followed by phenytoin (18 mg/kg loading dose) or phenobarbitone (20 mg/kg loading dose) is a standard anticonvulsant protocol. High-dose barbiturates can affect the level of consciousness and make evaluation of a comatose child more difficult.

Fluid Management

Excessive fluid administration, especially when hypotonic, exacerbates brain edema. However, fluid restriction has not been shown to improve outcome in CNS infection (41). One possible drawback of fluid is that the normal response aimed at maintaining intravascular volume—increased sympathetic activity—results in raising the lower limit of cerebral perfusion pressure. The consequence is that the child will be at risk of impaired CBF despite an apparently "normal" blood pressure. The type of fluid to be administered varies with age. In neonates glucose-containing salt solution is necessary, and in older children isotonic saline is usually a reasonable choice to avoid hyponatremia (42). Hyponatremia occurs frequently in patients with CNS infections and might exacerbate cerebral edema. It is usually secondary to excessive fluid administration, use of hypotonic fluids, or SIADH.

Glucose

Blood glucose concentration should be monitored closely in severely ill patients. Hypoglycemia may be present in the acute phase, especially in neonates. Hyperglycemia, on the other hand, may be present as part of the stress response. The question of whether to treat such children with insulin is unanswered. Normal saline or fluids with low glucose content should be administered in this situation.

Lumbar Puncture

Examination of CSF should be undertaken a soon as it is considered to be safe to do an LP (43). The contraindications to LP are listed in Table 15.2. Brain tissue herniation can occur if there is a space-occupying lesion, acute hydrocephalus, or brain swelling. Signs of raised ICP are nonspecific, and in the intubated, sedated child it is better to be cautious, unless one is sure that the neurologic examination is normal. Focal signs, abnormal extensor posturing, pupillary abnormalities, papilledema, and bradycardia with hypertension may all indicate increased ICP. A CT scan may be helpful in identifying a space-occupying lesion, but a normal scan does not rule out the possibility of herniation occurring after an LP (44,45). The problem is that CSF may continue to leak from the site of the LP. So, while a normal scan may indicate normality at the time of the LP, it does not guarantee against brain swelling developing in the hours after the LP. If there is a site of CSF leak below the brainstem (e.g., LP site), then the consequence will be downward herniation and central syndrome.

If an LP is performed, opening pressure should be measured. The normal opening CSF pressure is 180 mm H_2O in children and adults, and approximately 100 mm H_2O in neonates. If pressure is increased, the minimum amount of CSF should be obtained. Routine CSF investigations should include white cell count, glucose concentration, protein concentration, Gram stain, and bacterial culture. Polymerase chain reaction for enterovirus and other pathogens should be considered when the Gram stain is negative. Other tests may be indicated depending on the clinical findings and regional epidemiology.

References

1. Davison KL, Ramsay ME. The epidemiology of acute meningitis in England and Wales. Arch Dis Child 2003;88:662–664.
2. Dawson KG, Emerson JC, Burns JL. Fifteen years of experience with bacterial meningitis. Pediatr Infect Dis J 1999;18:816–822.
3. Holt DE, Halket S, de Louvois J, et al. Neonatal meningitis in England and Wales: 10 years on. Arch Dis Child (Fetal Neonatal Ed) 2001;84:F85–89.

4. Saez-Llorens X, McCracken GH Jr. Bacterial meningitis in children. Lancet 2003;361:2139–2148.

5. Chavez-Bueno S, McCracken GH Jr. Bacterial meningitis in children. Pediatr Clin North Am 2005;52:795–810.

6. Reefhuis J, Honein MA, Whitney CG, et al. Risk of bacterial meningitis in children with cochlear implants. N Engl J Med 2003;349:435–445.

7. Sormunen P, Kallio MJ, Kilpi T, et al. C-reactive protein is useful in distinguishing Gram stain-negative bacterial meningitis from viral meningitis in children. J Pediatr 1999;134:725–729.

8. McMaster P, McIntyre P, Gilmour G, et al. The emergence of resistant pneumococcal meningitis—implications for empiric therapy. Arch Dis Child 2002;87:207–210.

9. de Gans J, van de Beek D. Dexamethasone in adults with bacterial meningitis. N Engl J Med 2002;347:1549–1556.

10. Molyneux EM, Walsh AL, Forsyth H, et al. Dexamethasone treatment in childhood bacterial meningitis in Malawi: a randomised controlled trial. Lancet 2002;360: 211–217.

11. Schaad UB, Lips U, Gnehm HE, et al. Dexamethasone therapy for bacterial meningitis in children. Lancet 1993;342:457–461.

12. Atkinson PJ, Sharland M, Maguire H. Predominant enteroviral serotypes causing meningitis. Arch Dis Child 1998;78:373–374.

13. Negrini B, Kelleher KJ, Wald ER. Cerebrospinal fluid findings in aseptic versus bacterial meningitis. Pediatrics 2000;105:316–319.

14. Newton RW. Tuberculous meningitis. Arch Dis Child 1994;70:364.

15. Thwaites GE, Nguyen DB, Nguyen HB, et al. Dexamethasone for the treatment of tuberculous meningitis in adolescents and adults. N Engl J Med 2004;351: 1741–1751.

16. Kolski H, Ford-Jones EL, Richardson S, et al. Etiology of acute childhood encephalitis at the Hospital for Sick Children, Toronto, 1994–1995. Clin Infect Dis 1998;26:398–409.

17. Koskiniemi M, Korppi M, Mustonen K, et al. Epidemiology of encephalitis in children. A prospective multicentre study. Eur J Pediatr. 1997;156:541–545.

18. Lin WC, Lee PI, Lu CY, et al. Mycoplasma pneumoniae encephalitis in childhood. J Microbiol Immunol Infect 2002;35:173–178.

19. Huang C, Morse D, Slater B, et al. Multiple-year experience in the diagnosis of viral central nervous system infections with a panel of polymerase chain reaction assays for detection of 11 viruses. Clin Infect Dis 2004;39:630–635.

20. Whitley RJ, Lakeman F. Herpes simplex virus infections of the central nervous system: therapeutic and diagnostic considerations. Clin Infect Dis 1995;20:414–420.

21. Bitnun A, Ford-Jones E, Blaser S, et al. Mycoplasma pneumoniae encephalitis. Semin Pediatr Infect Dis 2003;14:96–107.

22. Korinthenberg R, Schessl J, Kirschner J, et al. Intravenously administered immunoglobulin in the treatment of childhood Guillain-Barre syndrome: a randomized trial. Pediatrics 2005;116:8–14.

23. van Koningsveld R, Schmitz PI, Meche FG, et al. Effect of methylprednisolone when added to standard treatment with intravenous immunoglobulin for Guillain-Barre syndrome: randomised trial. Lancet 2004;363:192–196.

24. Leake JA, Albani S, Kao AS. Acute disseminated encephalomyelitis in childhood: epidemiologic, clinical and laboratory features. Pediatr Infect Dis J 2004;23: 756–764.

25. Dale RC. Acute disseminated encephalomyelitis. Semin Pediatr Infect Dis 2003; 14:90–95.

26. American Academy of Pediatrics. Tetanus. In: Pickering LK, ed. 2000 Red Book: Report of the Committee on Infectious Diseases, 25th ed. Elk Grove Village, IL: American Academy of Pediatrics, 2000:563–568.

27. Ahmadsyah I, Salim A. Treatment of tetanus: an open study to compare the efficacy of procaine penicillin and metronidazole. Br Med J 1985;291:648–650.

28. McGirt MJ, Zaas A, Fuchs HE, et al. Risk factors for pediatric ventriculoperitoneal shunt infection and predictors of infectious pathogens. Clin Infect Dis 2003; 36:858–862.

29. Pople IK, Bayston R, Hayward RD. Infection of cerebrospinal fluid shunts in infants: a study of etiological factors. J Neurosurg 1992;77:29–36.

30. Anderson EJ, Yogev R. A rational approach to the management of ventricular shunt infections. Pediatr Infect Dis J 2005;24:557–558.

31. Saez-Llorens X. Brain abscess in children. Semin Pediatr Infect Dis. 2003; 14:108–114.

32. Bair-Merritt MH, Chung C, Collier A. Spinal epidural abscess in a young child. Pediatrics 2000;106:E39.

33. Rubin G, Michowiz SD, Ashkenasi A, et al. Spinal epidural abscess in the pediatric age group: case report and review of literature. Pediatr Infect Dis J 1993;12: 1007–1011.

34. Pollard AJ, Britto J, Nadel S, et al. Emergency management of meningococcal disease. Arch Dis Child 1999;80:290–296.

35. Horwitz SJ, Boxerbaum B, O'Bell J. Cerebral herniation in bacterial meningitis in childhood. Ann Neurol 1980;7:524–528.

36. Goitein KJ, Tamir I. Cerebral perfusion pressure in central nervous system infections of infancy and childhood. J Pediatr 1983;103:40–43.

37. Lindvall P, Ahlm C, Ericsson M, et al. Reducing intracranial pressure may increase survival among patients with bacterial meningitis. Clin Infect Dis 2004;38:384–390.

38. Oates-Whitehead R, Maconochie I, Baumer H, et al. Fluid therapy for acute bacterial meningitis. Cochrane Database Syst Rev 2005;3:CD004786.

39. Czosnyka M, Pickard JD. Monitoring and interpretation of intracranial pressure. J Neurol Neurosurg Psychiatry 2004;75:813–821.

40. van de Beek D, de Gans J, Tunkel AR. Community-acquired bacterial meningitis in adults. N Engl J Med 2006;354:44–53.

41. Arnal LE, Stein F. Pediatric septic shock: why has mortality decreased? The utility of goal-directed therapy. Semin Pediatr Infect Dis 2003;14:165–172.

42. Carcillo JA, Fields AI, American College of Critical Care Medicine Task Force Committee Members. Clinical practice parameters for hemodynamic support of pediatric and neonatal patients in septic shock. Crit Care Med 2002;30:1365–1378.

43. Kneen R, Solomon T, Appleton R. The role of lumbar puncture in children with suspected central nervous system infection. BMC Pediatr 2002;2:8.

44. Shetty AK, Desselle BC, Craver RD, et al. Fatal cerebral herniation after lumbar puncture in a patient with a normal computed tomography scan. Pediatrics 1999;103:1284–1287.

45. Tasker RC, Matthew DJ, Kendall B. Computed tomography in the assessment of raised intracranial pressure in non-traumatic coma. Neuropediatrics 1990;21: 91–94.

16
Respiratory Infection in Pediatric Intensive Care Unit

D.R. O'Donnell and R.G. Branco

The respiratory system is the most frequently affected system in pediatric intensive care unit (PICU) admissions. Lower respiratory reserve in infants and children than in adults, and the close interaction of the respiratory system with other systems contribute to the high incidence of respiratory dysfunction. Infectious diseases are the most common cause of acute illness in children, and, respiratory infections account for a large proportion of acute PICU admissions. Worldwide acute respiratory infections (ARIs) cause more deaths in children under 5 than do diarrhea, malaria, or HIV.

Respiratory Tract in Neonates and Children

There are significant differences in the airways in different stages of life. During the first months of life the infant has a predominantly nasal respiration, and up to 60% of term neonates are unable to convert to oral breathing in the case of nasal obstruction. The tongue is relatively large for the oral cavity and readily obstructs the airway. Situations associated with an increase in the size of the tongue (e.g., Beckwith's syndrome) or a decrease in the size of the midface (e.g., Down and Crouzon's syndrome) increase potential airway obstruction. The larynx is high (C4) and anterior, making laryngoscopy more difficult. The larynx has a funnel shape compared with cylindrical morphology in adults. During infancy, the larynx and carina descend, assuming the adult position at C6 and T4 (larynx and carina, respectively). The subglottic region is the narrowest part of the airway in children, and infection in this area (e.g., croup) can critically increase air-flow resistance.

In early infancy breathing is primarily diaphragmatic and the ribs more horizontal in position reducing the thoracic component of breathing. There are fewer type I diaphragmatic fibers, thus increasing the risk of fatigue. The chest wall is more elastic due to the soft rib cage, which allows deflation that is close to the lung closing volume even in the well infant. The lungs themselves are less compliant and elastic, increasing airway resistance. Alveoli at birth are bigger and less numerous, increasing greatly in number especially during the first 2 years, achieving a maximum at 8 years.

The size of the airways is important: resistance to flow in a cylinder is proportional to the fourth power of the radius of the lumen (Poiseuille's law), and small changes in airway lumen due to mucosal edema can cause critical obstruction either in the upper airway (e.g., croup) or in the lower airways (e.g., bronchiolitis).

Intact airway mucosa, normal mucus secretion, and ciliary activity are responsible for the mechanical defenses of the respiratory system. These activities are preserved in the newborn and young infant in the absence of specific diseases (e.g., cystic fibrosis, ciliary dyskinesia, pulmonary aspiration syndrome).

Indirect cigarette smoke in a child's environment is an important factor that reduces ciliary activity and damages airway epithelial cells. These functions are also impaired by several infections; for example, *Mycoplasma pneumoniae* attaches to ciliated epithelium, liberating hydrogen peroxide and other toxic products, and influenza A virus infects and destroys ciliated epithelial cells, resulting in desquamation.

In the newborn infant, immunologic defenses are relatively immature. Cellular immunity (T cell) is reduced at birth and only achieves normal function by 6 to 12 months of age. Immunoglobulin production probably reaches adult levels by about 5 years of age. Immunoglobulin G (IgG) levels are lower until the second year of life, which this contributes to the risk of infection with encapsulated organisms (e.g., *Haemophilus* spp., pneumococcus, coliforms). During the first few months, passive transfer of maternal immunoglobulin (IgG placental transfer during the last trimester of pregnancy, and secretory IgA in the breast milk) are helpful in infant immune defense. Immunoglobulin A protects the respiratory epithelium that is in continuous contact with the external environment. It helps to neutralize and prevent adhesion of bacterial and viral pathogens. Innate production of IgA is relatively slow during the first year of life.

Respiratory Tract Infections

Infections of the respiratory tract can be classified according to the anatomic localization of the infection. Although the same organism can cause infections in different sites, anatomic classifications help guide clinical treatment pending definitive microbiologic diagnosis, especially when children are very sick. This section describes specific infections in pediatric critical care, according to common clinical patterns.

Pneumonia

Worldwide, pneumonia is a leading cause of death in the pediatric population. Each year, an estimated 4 million children die from pneumonia, mainly in developing countries. In developed countries mortality due to pneumonia has been reduced by up to 97% over the last 50 years. The incidence of pneumonia, however, remains high in the U.S. and Europe, with rates of 4 per 100 child-years in those under 5, and 0.7 per 100 child-year in 12- to 15-year-olds. Only a small number of children with community-acquired pneumonia require intensive care. Children who require PICU admission present either the most severe infections, serious complications such as empyema or lung abscess, or more moderate infections in children with underlying conditions such as chronic lung disease of prematurity, cerebral palsy, or immunodeficiency. Table 16.1 summarizes the etiology and guidance for treatment of community acquired pneumonia.

TABLE 16.1. Community-acquired pneumonia

Age group	Usual pathogens	Empiric antibiotic therapy	Comments
Neonate (<1 month)	• Group B streptococci • *Listeria monocytogenes* • Gram-negative enteric bacilli • *Klebsiella* • *Staphylococcus aureus*	• Ampicillin (50 mg/kg/dose, IV, every 6–8 hours) + gentamicin (4.5 mg/kg/dose, IV, every 24 hours)	If meningitis is suspected or sepsis evident, use ampicillin 100 mg/kg/dose; gentamicin levels should be monitored
1 to 3 months	• *Chlamydia trachomatis* • Group A and B streptococci • Enterobacteriaceae • *Streptococcus pneumoniae* • *Haemophilus influenzae* • *Staphylococcus aureus* • *Listeria monocytogenes*	• Cefotaxime (50 mg/kg/dose, IV, every 12 hours) ± erythromycin (12.5 mg/kg/dose, IV/PO, every 6 hours)	For patients with associated meningitis or severe presentation of pneumonia, or patients with cystic fibrosis, frequency of cefotaxime should be increased to four times a day
3 months to 5 years	• *S. pneumoniae* • *H. influenzae* • *S. aureus* • Group A streptococci • *Mycoplasma pneumoniae* • *Chlamydia pneumoniae*	• Mild: floxacillin (25 mg/kg/dose, PO, every 6 hours) • Moderate–severe: cefotaxime (50 mg/kg/dose, IV, every 12 hours) + erythromycin (12.5 mg/kg/dose, IV/PO, every 6 hours)	
More than 5 years	• *M. pneumoniae* • *S. pneumoniae* • *H. influenzae* • *C. pneumoniae* • *S. aureus* • Group A streptococci	• Mild: erythromycin (12.5 mg/kg/dose, PO, every 6 hours) or azithromycin (10 mg/kg/day, PO) • Moderate–severe: cefotaxime (50 mg/kg/dose, IV, every 12 hours) + erythromycin (12.5 mg/kg/dose, IV/PO, every 6 hours)	

Definition

Pneumonia may be defined clinically as an infection of the lower respiratory tract that involves the airways and lung tissues. However, clinical definitions of pneumonia are heterogeneous, ranging from a broad diagnosis based only on signs and symptoms or on radiologic or microbiologic evidence of a responsible organism.

Etiology

Pneumonia is caused by a range of both viral and bacterial pathogens. Viral pneumonias are discussed more fully below.

Streptococcus pneumoniae is the single most commonly identified bacterial cause of pneumonia, but etiology of pneumonia varies according to age and geographical region. Vaccination against specific pathogens such as *Haemophilus influenza* type b or *S. pneumoniae* alters the relative frequency of these infections in different populations.

The First Year of Life

In the first 3 weeks of life pneumonia is uncommon, but when present the most common agents are those associated with perinatal infection. Group B *streptococcus, Listeria monocytogenes, Escherichia coli,* and *Klebsiella* spp. are common causes of bacterial infection in this age group, causing severe respiratory distress within a few days of life, and often as part of a widespread infection. Occasional agents also include *S. pneumoniae* and *Haemophilus influenzae* type b.

From 3 weeks to 3 months of age, the perinatal infections became gradually less common, but the incidence of other agents, such as *Chlamydia trachomatis* (the most frequent agent in this age group), *S. pneumoniae,* and *H. influenzae,* increases.

After 3 months, the incidence of *Chlamydia trachomatis* decreases while *S. pneumoniae* and *H. influenza* became more common pathogens.

After the First Year

After the first year of life, the most common causative agent of nonviral pneumonia is *S. pneumoniae* followed by *H. influenzae,* but the incidence of *Mycoplasma pneumoniae* steadily increases. After 5 years of age the most common causative agent of pneumonia is *M. pneumoniae,* followed by *S. pneumoniae, Chlamydia pneumoniae,* and *H. influenzae.* Older children without any underlying morbidity infrequently require intensive care treatment due to community-acquired pneumonia; therefore, a high index of suspicion is needed for more aggressive etiologic agents, such as *Staphylococcus aureus* or forms of invasive *S. pneumoniae.* In children with sickle cell anemia, *M. pneumoniae* is a common cause of severe pneumonia and acute chest syndrome, often requiring PICU admission.

Clinical Features

The hallmark signs of pneumonia are fever, tachypnea, and malaise. However, there is great variability in the presentation of the disease. Signs and symptoms of pneumonia vary with age, etiologic agent, severity of disease, and immunologic status of the child. Newborns can present with early severe respiratory distress, or signs of respiratory distress may be minimal or absent, with pneumonia presenting only with apnea, poor feeding, or with a clinical picture of sepsis. Out of the neonatal period, signs of respiratory distress are frequent, with respiratory rate being one of the most important signs. In infants, chest indrawing or respiratory rate over 50 breaths per minute have a positive predictive value of 45% and a negative predictive value of 83% of radiologic evidence of consolidation. In children less than 5 years of age, tachypnea had the best sensitivity (74%) and specificity (67%) of all clinical signs. In older children, a history of difficulty in breathing has a good association with pneumonia. In infants, fine crackles that are commonly heard in older children are often absent. Because of the relatively small size of the child's thorax and the thin chest, classic findings of consolidation can be masked by broad transmission of breath sounds.

High fever in infants or children is often considered an important sign of pneumonia, but infection with atypical organisms (such as *Mycoplasma* and *Chlamydia*) frequently present with little or no elevation in temperature. Wheeze occurs in 30% of *Mycoplasma* pneumonias and is more common in older children. Presence of wheeze is not associated with severity of disease. Signs of severe disease are oxygen desaturation to less than 92%, severe tachypnea, difficulty in breathing, grunting, nasal flaring, apneas, and failure to feed (in small children).

The British Thoracic Society suggests four criteria to consider PICU admission in children with pneumonia:

- Failure to maintain an oxygen saturation of >92% in $FiO_2 > 0.6$
- Evidence of shock
- Recurrent apnea or slow irregular breathing
- Rising respiratory rate and rising pulse rate with clinical evidence of severe respiratory distress and exhaustion, with or without a raised carbon dioxide tension (PCO_2)

Radiologic Investigations

Although not routinely recommended in children with mild uncomplicated lower respiratory infection, chest radiography can add significant information to the management of children with pneumonia associated with severe illness. Where they occur, radiologic changes from scattered infiltrates to dense lobar pneumonia or pleural effusion have a high diagnostic certainty. Radiographic findings are poorly predictive of the causative agent, but taken into consideration in the clinical context help to plan empiric therapy and perhaps further interventions. In the intensive care setting, there is debate about whether routine repeat imaging should be performed, and the ability of chest radiography to influence overall intensive care management. The little data available suggest that small children with active cardiopulmonary problems and two or more interventions, such as central venous catheter, endotracheal tube, or chest drain, are more likely to benefit from routine chest radiography.

Routine chest radiography may also be helpful with acute respiratory deterioration or in those patients not improving. The clinical diagnosis of complications of pneumonia (e.g., pleural effusion or lung abscess) can be difficult, and chest radiography can be helpful in this context. Because radiographic changes often lag significantly behind clinical improvement, chest radiography is rarely useful during recovery. Other radiologic investigations, such as chest ultrasound (US) or computerized tomography (CT), have restricted indications and are discussed later in this chapter (see Parapneumonic Effusions and Empyema).

Laboratory Investigations

Acute-phase reactants (peripheral white cell count and differential, erythrocyte sedimentation rate, and C-reactive protein [CRP] level) are widely used in pediatric practice. In critically ill children they are often used to monitor patient response to therapy. Acute-phase reactants are elevated in many stress situations. C-reactive protein is frequently elevated in children requiring PICU admission and may not be associated with bacterial infection. Interpretation of results should still take into account the overall clinical picture and may be more useful as a tool to evaluate improvements. Another acute-phase reactant, procalcitonin, has more recently been used to predict organ dysfunction and outcome of children admitted to PICU. However, further studies are necessary to define its role in PICU practice.

Electrolytes are checked routinely in children with pneumonia. Inappropriate secretion of antidiuretic hormone is well described, and adults with pneumonia have been shown to have a latent vasopressin-dependent impairment of renal water excretion. Therefore, electrolytes are often deranged in children with pneumonia, with hyponatremia present in 27% of hospital admissions.

The ideal diagnostic criterion for treatment in pneumonia is identification of the causative agent. Children younger than 18 months with signs of lower respiratory infection should have a nasopharyngeal aspirate (NPA) performed for viral antigen (with or without culture) detection. Indirect immunofluorescence is highly specific for detection of viral antigen and may be very useful when the diagnosis is uncertain.

Identification of a viral infection does not exclude the possibility of bacterial co-infection. Microbiologic evaluation of tracheal aspirate in children with tracheostomy or endotracheal intubation is often used to identify an etiologic agent.

The results of bacterial culture require experience and knowledge of local antibiotic sensitivities. There is a high incidence of contamination from colonizing organisms, and results may not reflect a pathogenic organism. Guided or nonguided bronchoalveolar lavage (BAL), discussed below, is also a useful test to identify possible etiologic agents. Blood culture has a good specificity but a very low sensitivity (10%). Due to the difficulty in obtaining adequate samples and the low sensitivity of blood cultures, often no etiologic diagnosis is made in children with pneumonia. Other investigations relevant to diagnosis and treatment of pneumonias in children are described later in this chapter.

Treatment

The cornerstone of treatment of bacterial pneumonia is antibiotic therapy. Since identification of the etiologic agent is uncommon in children with pneumonia, especially early during presentation, guidance to empiric antibiotic therapy should follow diagnostic algorithms that begin with the age of the child, consider clinical and epidemiologic factors, and take into account results of other investigations, such as chest radiography and serum acute phase reactants. A guide to antibiotic therapy for uncomplicated pneumonia according to age is described in Table 16.1.

Children presenting to intensive care should receive broad-spectrum antibiotics unless a clear etiologic diagnosis is available that enables targeted antimicrobial therapy. Infants should receive empiric cover with ampicillin and gentamicin, and all other ages should receive a second- or third-generation cephalosporin (some suggest adding an aminoglycoside if signs of systemic sepsis are present, until an organism is identified). In small infants with a history of cough and respiratory failure, macrolides are often added to cover *Bordetella pertussis,* and, in children over 3 years of age, to cover *Mycoplasma pneumoniae* infection. In children with a prolonged hospital stay or children with chronic lung disease such as cystic fibrosis, anti-*Pseudomonas* treatment may have to be considered if the patient is known to be colonized or if the infection is not responding to conventional antibiotic therapy. In immunocompromised patients, therapy should follow local guidelines. The risk of severe gram-negative infection bacterial, in particular, may require aminoglycoside or extended spectrum cephalosporins to be used. The risk of fungal infection may necessitate the use of newer triazole or echinocandin antimycotic agents to be considered. In view of the shift in epidemiology of infections associated with febrile neutropenia over the last few decades, most oncology guidelines recommend the use of a glycopeptide antibiotic such as vancomycin or teicoplanin to cover gram-positive organisms, including coagulase-negative staphylococci.

Fluid Management

Fluid management of critically ill patients, in particular patients with pneumonia or acute respiratory distress syndrome (ARDS), remains controversial.

Some argue that in stress situations, such as severe pneumonias, there is an increased secretion of antidiuretic hormone, and impairment of renal water excretion; therefore, fluids administration should be restricted (50–70% of expected maintenance) to avoid fluid overload and increment in pulmonary water/lung edema. Others argue that the amount of fluid administration has little or no effect on lung water content and that a more liberal fluid management helps to prevent hypovolemia, which is deleterious in the intensive care setting. The ARDS Network is currently performing a study to address this issue in adults. For now, we suggest a regimen using 70% of the expected fluid maintenance requirement, but remain alert to any signs of hypovolemia, which should be treated with normal saline boluses, and whenever the hemodynamic status allows, aim for a neutral fluid balance plus insensible losses, for example, 20 mL/kg/day.

Other Aspects of Care

Chest physiotherapy is a common practice in children ventilated to assist bronchial toilet. However, there is little clinical evidence of benefit of such therapy. Chest positioning has been shown to directly influence ventilation in children with unilateral pneumonia; positioning the affected side up helps to aerate the affected lung, but it is associated with higher risk of bacteremia and worsens ventilation. In animal models with unilateral pneumonia, a protective strategy of mechanical ventilation, (i.e., high peak end-expiratory pressure [PEEP] (>8 mm Hg) and low tidal volume), reduced the risk of ventilation-induced bacterial and inflammatory mediator dissemination.

General measures, such as analgesic and antipyretic medications, prevention of hypoxemia, and fractionated feeding. are also recommended.

Prevention

The use of vaccines has led to an important reduction in incidence of pneumonias. Introduction of the *Haemophilus influenzae* type b (Hib) vaccine led to a significant reduction in the incidence of pneumonia, despite Hib not having been recognized as a pathogen frequently associated with pneumonia. Vaccination against *Bordetella pertussis* has also reduced the incidence of severe pneumonic infection associated with this pathogen. However, recently an increasing number of younger children have been found to require PICU admission due to *B. pertussis* lower airway infection.

Recent introduction of the conjugated pneumococcal vaccines have reduced the incidence of invasive pneumococcal disease. There is some evidence of a reduction in the incidence of pneumococcal pneumonias in adults following widespread introduction of pneumococcal vaccination in infants and children. However, studies to evaluate population cost-effectiveness are still needed. In the intensive care setting, methods to prevent nosocomial pneumonia are mostly associated with measures to prevent ventilator-associated pneumonia.

Hospital-Acquired Pneumonia and Ventilator-Associated Pneumonia

Pneumonia is the second most frequent cause of hospital-acquired infection in children, accounting for 18% of cases. In the PICU this figure is similar, as pneumonia accounts for nearly 20% of PICU-acquired infections. Unlike adults, where hospital-acquired pneumonia is associated with 30% mortality, mortality in children due to hospital-acquired pneumonia is low, and closer to 8%. The etiology of PICU-acquired pneumonia may extensively differ among PICUs and according to the duration of PICU or hospital stay preceding infection. In children who develop PICU-acquired pneumonia during early hospitalization, the pathogens are likely to be similar to those associated with community-acquired pneumonias. After 3 days of hospitalization there is an increment in gram-negative infections (*P. aeruginosa* and *K. pneumoniae*). The most commonly identified pathogens are *P. aeruginosa* and *S. aureus* (around 20%) followed by *H. influenzae, Enterobacter* spp., and *K. pneumoniae*. The mechanisms involved in hospital-acquired pneumonia are mainly associated with upper airway or gastric mucosa colonization, although it can also occur via hematogenous spread or aerosolization. Other factors also likely to influence etiology include the use of H2 blockers and prior antibiotic treatment, which suppresses normal flora and facilitates gram-negative bacillary colonization.

Diagnosis of PICU-acquired pneumonia, except ventilator-associated pneumonia, is similar to that of community-acquired pneumonia, and includes radiographic evidence of pneumonia plus clinical signs. Children with hospital-acquired pneumonia are likely to require supportive therapy such as supplemental oxygen and mechanical ventilation. Broad antibiotic cover taking into account local resistance patterns is recommended until microbiologic evidence is available. In units with a low incidence of resistant pathogens, empiric therapy might include a third-generation cephalosporin and a macrolide. Where the incidence of resistant pathogens is high, the local protocol should be followed, and a glycopeptide antibiotic may need to be added to the previously suggested regimen.

Parapneumonic Effusions and Empyema

The accumulation of fluid in the potential space between the parietal and visceral pleurae of the thorax occurs in association with a range of clinical scenarios including infection, malignancy, autoimmune disease, and anatomic abnormality, or it may be due to iatrogenic causes.

Pleural effusions in association with pulmonary infection may also be referred to as either uncomplicated parapneumonic effusion or empyema. An uncomplicated parapneumonic effusion is associated with pneumonia and contains pleural fluid, which is usually sterile or contaminated with a low number of organisms. On the other hand, empyema represents an effusion with features of infection, evidenced by the presence of a large number of organisms or a large number of inflammatory cells and fibrin. Hippocrates wrote that a person "with empyemata . . . shall die on the fourteenth day, unless something favorable supervene[s]."

In the antibiotic era with early recognition and treatment, parapneumonic effusions in children carry a very low associated mortality. In reality, empyema and parapneumonic effusion represent parts of a spectrum of disease. Three stages of progression are described:

1. Exudative: accumulation of fluid within the pleural cavity, with few cells and without the presence of loculations (uncomplicated parapneumonic effusion)
2. Fibropurulent: an outpouring of inflammatory cells with thickening and fibrin deposition within the pleural space (empyema)
3. Organizing: fibroblast adhesion with pleural rind formation

Parapneumonic effusions and empyema have an incidence of around 3.3 per 100,000 children. Like community-acquired pneumonias, described above, the incidence and epidemiology of these effusions are influenced by time-dependent change in pathogens, local profiles, cluster infections with specific pathogens, and introduction of new vaccines.

The most commonly associated infections are *S. pneumoniae,* group A *Streptococcus, S. aureus,* and *H. influenzae.* Immunization for Hib has been associated with a drastic reduction in the frequency of this pathogen. In the 1990s the incidence of pleural effusions has risen sevenfold in the United Kingdom and fivefold in the United States. In both countries this has been attributed to a rise in detection of *S. pneumoniae* by polymerase chain reaction (PCR) and specifically the emergence of serotype 1. The reason for this is unknown, but *S. pneumoniae* may represent a virulent clone of pneumococcus. The introduction of new polyvalent pneumococcal conjugate vaccines changed the incidence of invasive pneumococcal disease (IPD), especially in the U.S. The seven-valent conjugated pneumococcal vaccine protects against serotypes 4, 6B, 9V, 14, 18C, 19F, and 23F, but not serotype 1. Serotype analysis of parapneumonic effusions pre- and postvaccination showed a rise in the incidence of *S. pneumoniae,* especially serotype 1. Approximately 50% of these children required intensive care admission. Data for 9- and 11-valent pneumococcal vaccine that protects against serotype 1 are not yet available.

Staphylococcus aureus is the most common causative agent of empyema in developing countries. In these populations *S. aureus* is present in up to 30% of empyemas, especially in children under 1 year of age. Resistance of *S. aureus* worldwide is an increasing problem, with methicillin-resistance *S. aureus* (MRSA) being reported in up to 80% of *S. aureus* isolates from empyema in some regions. Antibiotic resistance in *S. pneumoniae* is also increasing. However, in the U.S. the rate of penicillin-nonsusceptible *S. pneumoniae* isolates is decreasing following introduction of the conjugated polyvalent pneumococcal vaccine.

Gram-negatives including *Klebsiella* and *Pseudomonas aeruginosa* are infrequently associated with empyema, but their importance increases significantly in children with prolonged hospital stay and prolonged mechanical ventilation. *Candida* infections can occur in children with immunosuppression especially after prolonged antibiotic treatment for persistent effusion. In children, anaerobes are infrequently associated with empyema except in association with aspiration pneumonia.

Mycoplasma pneumoniae pneumonia is associated with a 20% incidence of pleural effusion; however, the overall incidence is low.

Mycobacterial and fungal pleural effusions are rare in children. Tuberculous empyema is unusual in the U.K. but may account for up to 6% of cases in developing countries, often in association with HIV infection. Histoplasmosis has been associated with pleural effusion in up to 6% of childhood histoplasmosis cases. Blastomycosis and other fungi (*Aspergillus*, *Coccidioides*) have also been described. Parasitic infections presenting with pleural effusions are uncommon but are found in patients with *Entamoeba histolytica* disease. Certain viruses, such as adenovirus and influenza, can cause effusion, but they are usually small, rarely requiring intervention.

Diagnosis

Clinical Presentation

Clinical presentation is mostly associated with symptoms and signs of pneumonia. There may be chest, abdominal, or shoulder pain in association. In children with pneumonia who remain pyrexial for more than 48 hours, further investigation for pleural effusion should be considered. Signs of respiratory distress and grunting respiration may be present. Clinical examination reveals a decrease in breath sounds, dullness to percussion, and bronchial breathing in the lung adjacent to the empyema.

Imaging

Radiographic examination of the chest can identify most pleural effusions. Posteroanterior or anteroposterior images are sufficient, with no necessity for lateral radiography in children. Obliteration of the costophrenic angle is the earliest sign of an effusion, followed by a rim of fluid ascending the chest wall (meniscus sign). Larger effusions appear as opacification covering the dependent positions of the lungs, generally above the diaphragm. In large effusions, compression of the lungs and shift of the trachea away from the effusion may occur. Repeat imaging or follow-up computed tomography (CT) is rarely helpful because radiographic improvement lags significantly behind clinical improvement.

Ultrasonography (US) is extremely useful in the diagnosis and management of pleural effusions. Portable US can easily be performed at the bedside to identify fluid in the pleural space, differentiate pleural thickening from fluid collection, estimate the size of effusion, and guide the optimal position for drainage.

Chest CT is not routinely recommended in children with pleural effusions. In complicated cases, however, CT can assist planning for surgery if considered.

Other Investigations

Blood cultures are indicative of the pathogens associated with empyema in 10% to 20% of cases. Serum acute phase reactants such as C-reactive protein (CRP), erythrocyte sedimentation rate (ESR), procalcitonin, and white cell count are nonspecific and do not add to the diagnosis or management of pleural effusion. There is no evidence to support the usefulness of serial measurements of CRP in assessing clinical progress, but they are widely used in clinical practice. Culture of tracheal secretions can also be helpful. Special consideration should be given to culture secretions for *M. pneumoniae* and immunofluorescence of respiratory viruses. Serologic tests can also be considered, especially when *Chlamydia* is suspected. Mantoux testing should be performed if tuberculosis is suspected.

Pleural Fluid

Many practitioners consider biochemical analysis of pleural fluid unnecessary in the management of parapneumonic effusions and empyema. However, protein, glucose, and lactate dehydrogenase (LDH) concentrations are often measured and are determined by the nature of the inflammatory process. This metabolic activity also leads to excretion of lactate and CO_2, resulting in a low pleural fluid pH. Lactate dehydrogenase, however, is increased due to its cellular origin (rather than a filtration from serum). The Light criteria have been widely used in adults to differentiate between transudates and exudates, but their usefulness in children is questionable.

Characteristics of exudates are a pleural/systemic protein ratio higher than 0.5, a pleural/systemic LDH ratio higher than 0.6, and a pleural LDH higher than two thirds of the upper limit of the normal serum LDH value.

In general, exudates have protein concentration higher than 3 g/dL or a specific gravity of greater than 1.016. Pleural glucose level usually is less than 3.3 mmol/L in exudates, or pleural/serum glucose ratio is less than 0.5. Exudative pH is usually less than 7.2, but production of ammonia by urea-splitting bacteria (e.g., *Proteus* species) may increase pleural fluid pH instead of diminishing it.

If tuberculosis is suspected, adenosine deaminase activity in the pleural fluid can be helpful. Other tests should be tailored according to the child's risks, including amylase (gastrointestinal disorders), triglycerides (chylothorax), cholesterol, rheumatoid factor, antinuclear antibodies, among others.

Cytology is mandatory in the analysis of pleural fluid. Gram stain is often positive in empyemas and can be used to direct empiric therapy. The differential cell count usually shows a white blood cell count >50,000/mm³ (>10,000/mm³ suggests exudate). A neutrophil predominance is present in bacterial infection and early tuberculosis. Eosinophilia may be seen in parasitic, fungal, and tuberculous infection, or in hypersensitivity. A large number of small lymphocytes suggest malignancy or tuberculosis. Evidence of erythrocytes in the fluid is nonspecific and can be associated with necrotizing infection, tuberculosis, and neoplasia. When tuberculosis is suspected, staining and culture for acid-fast bacilli should be performed. If available, PCR and tuberculostearic acid by mass spectroscopy can help in the diagnosis of tuberculosis.

Microbiology should always be performed, although culture results are often not positive in children admitted to the PICU who have usually already received antibiotics for some time before admission. Cultures are especially important in children who are immunocompromised and in children with ventilator-associated pneumonia (VAP). The PCR techniques are extremely useful, identifying a pathogen in up to 75% of culture negative cases.

Treatment

The principles of treatment are early drainage and adequate antibiotic treatment. In small clinically insignificant effusions, drainage may be avoided, but only in clinically stable children, with a known diagnosis.

Drainage

The principles of drainage are to use the least invasive method that will efficiently drain as much of the fluid as possible, causing the least amount of harm to the child. There are essentially three methods to choose from; in order of least to most invasive, they are simple pleural drainage, video assisted thoracoscopic surgery (VATS), and open thoracotomy.

Open thoracotomy is reserved for a very small minority of children in whom the presentation is late (organizing stage) and who continue to have life-threatening disease, and is usually carried out in a center where VATS is not available. VATS should be reserved for a small minority of cases where there is extensive loculation or organization with ongoing severe illness. Overwhelmingly, the vast majority of children should be treated by placement of a simple pleural drain or pigtail drain by an experienced specialist using appropriate analgesia, usually with the assistance of a pediatric anesthetist.

General anesthesia offers the advantage of minimizing the traumatic experience for the child and facilitating insertion of a peripherally inserted intravenous central catheter (PICC) at the same time to allow prolonged intravenous antibiotic therapy in the community, where available. Some PICUs offer an alternative to the operating theater for drainage and for intravenous access to be undertaken, having ventilation, sedation, analgesia, and full physiologic monitoring available.

Fibrinolytics such as urokinase are often recommended to be given via the pleural drain to maintain patency and optimize drainage.

Antibiotics

Most children can be successfully treated with intravenous antibiotics against *S. pneumoniae* and group A *streptococci*, such as benzylpenicillin or a cephalosporin. Antibiotics should be started as early as possible for all children with parapneumonic effusion. In cases where aspiration pneumonia is suspected, anaerobic cover should be considered. Antistaphylococcal cover is important if pneumatoceles are evident, and in areas with high incidence of MRSA, glycopeptide antibiotics such as vancomycin are recommended. Clindamycin is also often effective against MRSA and should also be considered. Children previously hospitalized or after surgical procedure should receive extended-spectrum coverage for gram-negative organisms such as *Pseudomonas* and *Klebsiella*. Empiric antibiotic therapy should be reviewed as soon as the results from the cultures are available.

There is no firm evidence regarding duration of antibiotic treatment, but it is usually prolonged, on average between 2 and 6 weeks. Clinical improvement, including resolution of fever, improved activity, and weight regain, is sometimes used to guide practice. Complete resolution of fever may be prolonged, taking up to 2 to 3 weeks. The use of prolonged courses of third-generation cephalosporins is associated with a significant incidence of skin rashes, often of dramatic appearance but rarely of clinical significance, that may require the antibiotics to be changed. Where community resources are in place, the use of intravenous antibiotics via PICC lines at home, such as daily ceftriaxone or teicoplanin, can very significantly reduce the hospital stay.

Follow-up investigation to rule out underlying immunodeficiency should be considered. Studies suggest that final resolution of radiologic abnormalities and lung function may take up to 12 months in some cases. Serious complications such as bronchopleural fistula, the need for lobectomy, trapped lung, and scoliosis are now uncommon with early effective management.

Ventilator-Associated Pneumonia

Ventilator-associated pneumonia (VAP) is defined as nosocomial pneumonia in mechanically ventilated patients that develops after 48 hours of initiation of mechanical ventilation. It is the most common hospital-acquired infection among patients requiring mechanical ventilation, resulting in excess mortality, prolonged length of hospitalization, and increased medical care costs.

Etiology

Pathogens responsible for VAP are similar to the ones responsible for PICU-acquired pneumonia. During the first days of ventilation, *S. pneumoniae, H. influenzae,* and anaerobes are most common. This profile changes with an increment in the incidence of *Pseudomonas aeruginosa, S. aureus,* and *Klebsiella* spp., with *P. aeruginosa* being the more frequent pathogen after 96 hours of mechanical ventilation. With prolonged ventilation there is an increment in the number of resistant pathogens, such as MRSA, extended-spectrum β-lactamase resistant (ESBR) *Klebsiella* species, and *Candida* species, especially in children receiving antibiotic therapy. Viruses are not frequently associated with VAP except in infants where nosocomial transmission of respiratory syncytial virus can be devastating.

Epidemiology

The prevalence of VAP in children admitted to the PICU ranges from 3% to 67%, and causes from 2 to 12 additional ventilator days/1000 ventilator days. The highest incidence of VAP is among children of age 2 months to 12 months. The most important risk factor for VAP, evidently, is the use and duration of mechanical ventilation. Mechanical ventilation potentially exposes the lungs to pathogens by eliminating several of the physiologic defense mechanisms. Colonization of the aerodigestive tract can happen within hours of tracheal intubation, creating a source for bacterial microaspiration. The endotracheal tube may allow a biofilm to be created that is a reservoir of pathogenic bacteria, resisting eradication by standard antimicrobial therapy. Direct delivery to the lower respiratory tract through mechanical suctioning or high-pressure airflow may occur. Elimination of the cough reflex and bypass of upper airway cleansing system also contribute to the risk of acquiring VAP. A few studies have evaluated the risk factors associated with VAP in children. The most recognized risk factors are need for reintubation, use of neuromuscular blockade, transport out of the PICU, genetic syndromes, and immunodeficiency (or use of immunosuppressants).

Diagnosis

Diagnosis of VAP remains a challenge in the PICU setting. Microbiologic evidence obtained from upper airway secretions does not necessarily reflect the lower respiratory tract, from where specimens are more difficult to collect, are easily contaminated, and have a low sensitivity. In mechanically ventilated children, a clinical diagnosis of pneumonia or the presence of radiographic changes has a poor predictive value for VAP. The National Nosocomial Infection Surveillance (NNIS) criteria to diagnose VAP requires development of new and persistent radiographic evidence of focal infiltrates 48 hours or more after the initiation of mechanical ventilation, plus two of the following criteria: temperature instability (defined as temperature >38.4°C or <37°C for children 1 to 12 years of age, and temperature >38°C for children 13 years of age or older), leukocytosis/leukopenia, and purulent sputum. It is believed, however, that such a definition (as with other clinical definitions) overestimates the incidence of VAP and may only be useful as a screening method.

A diagnostic algorithm for the diagnosis of VAP adapted from adult recommendations is provided in Figure 16.1. Ventilator-associated pneumonia should be suspected in mechanically ventilated children with clinical signs of

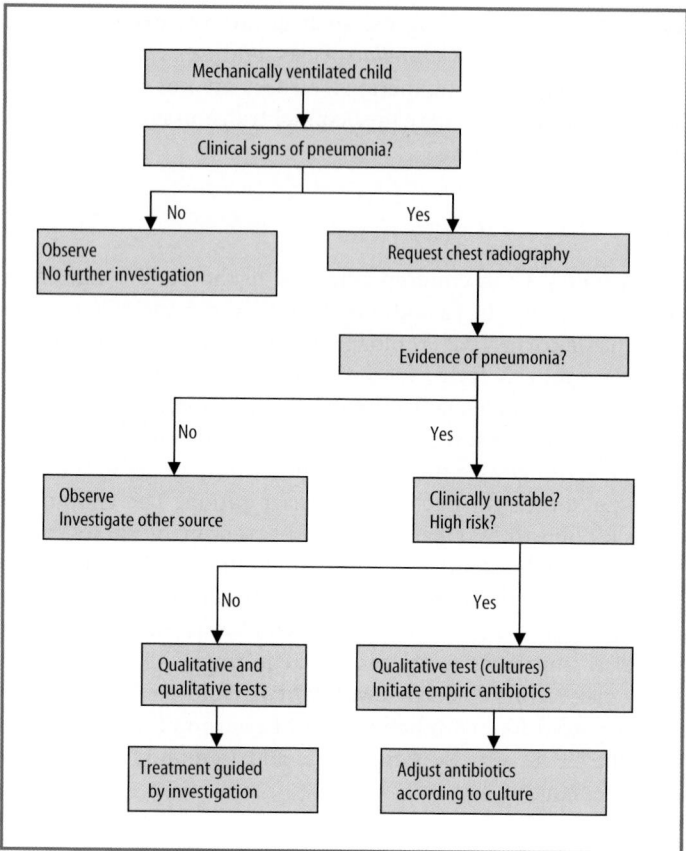

FIGURE 16.1. A decision tree that may be used in the investigation and treatment of ventilator associated pneumonia.

pneumonia: fever or hypothermia, leukocytosis (while blood count [WBC] >15,000) or leukopenia (WBC < 4000), purulent sputum, and decreased PaO_2/FiO_2 ratio. In the absence of these findings, a diagnosis of VAP is unlikely. If two or more of these abnormalities are present, however, a chest radiograph may be helpful. The choice of investigation depends on the clinical status of the children and on the availability of special techniques in the PICU. Endotracheal aspirate and blood culture should usually be performed. Use of more invasive procedures should be carefully considered, taking into account the clinical status of the child and the possible benefits of the procedure. Nonbronchoscopic BAL of the lower airway is easy to perform and well tolerated. Guided sampling is not always tolerated in severely ill children, and requires skilled personal with appropriate expertise in pediatric bronchoscopy. Qualitative tests such as culture and PCR can orientate the therapy of choice.

Acute Epiglottitis

Acute epiglottitis is a life-threatening illness with rapid onset and progression, and without treatment an upper airway obstruction and death frequently occur. The disease is characterized by cellulitis, with marked inflammation and edema of the supraglottic structures, which include the epiglottis, the aryepiglottic folds, and the arytenoid cartilages. It is possible that George Washington died of either epiglottitis or bacterial tracheitis in the winter of 1799 associated with an epidemic of influenza.

Etiology

Haemophilus influenzae type b is the most common causative agent, being isolated in most children with epiglottitis. Other causative organisms are rarely found but include group A *Streptococcus* and *S. pneumoniae*, *S. aureus*, *H. parainfluenzae*, and *H. influenzae* type a. Organisms are spread from person to person by secretions or large droplets.

The incidence of epiglottitis decreased dramatically after introduction of conjugated *H. influenzae* type b vaccine. The actual incidence in children is described to be around 1 per 100,000. Typically, children between 1 and 5 years old are the most commonly affected, with a predominance in boys. However, a few studies have described a change in the age group affected after vaccination from 3 to 6.5 years.

Clinical Presentation and Diagnosis

The typical presentation includes acute onset of cough and stridor, leading to respiratory distress, with no or minimal prodromal symptoms. A few hours of high fever, dysphasia, hoarseness, sore throat, and whispering stridor are typical. Children usually tend to sit up, in an attempt to keep airway open, since lying down often increases the degree of obstruction. Drooling is common because swallowing is painful. Typically the associated stridor is not severe, but suprasternal retraction and nasal flaring are often prominent. Septicemia is frequently present, and children commonly look "toxic."

When examining a child with suspected epiglottitis, direct visualization of the oropharyngeal cavity without preparation for immediate intubation is contraindicated. Any procedure that can potentially cause distress to the child (e.g., intravenous cannula insertion, blood sampling, forcing the child to lie down) should be avoided.

Diagnosis is usually clinical and confirmed by direct visualization of an inflamed and swollen epiglottis under general anesthesia before intubation. The causative agent can be isolated after a secure airway is obtained by blood culture (75% to 90%) or epiglottis swab (50%). Bacterial (e.g., Hib) antigens may also be detected in urine.

Treatment

The main treatment consists of maintaining a secure airway and controlling infection. Tracheal intubation should be performed in the operating room by an experienced pediatric anesthetist. Inhalational anesthetic agents are usually preferred to allow spontaneous ventilation during the procedure. An endotracheal tube 0.5 to 1.0 mm smaller than the expected for age is usually required. Humidified oxygen can be provided while waiting for intubation. In case of acute airway obstruction, bag-mask-valve ventilation is usually successful until tracheal intubation or tracheostomy is performed. In the catastrophic event of sudden acute obstruction, cricothyrotomy or tracheostomy may need to be performed. After the airway is secured, intravenous access should be obtained, blood cultures collected, and the child transferred to a PICU and antibiotics started. It is necessary to provide tube fixation and to restrict the child's movements to avoid accidental extubation. The duration of intubation is usually short (<2 days), and the criteria for extubation include the absence of fever, reduced swelling on direct laryngoscopy, and most importantly the presence of air leak around the endotracheal tube.

H. influenzae strains resistant to ampicillin have been isolated, with resistance mediated by a plasmid-transferred β-lactamase activity. Isolated *H. influenzae* strains, however, are sensitive to second- or third-generation cephalosporins. Thus, ceftriaxone (50 to 100 mg/kg/d), cefuroxime (50 to 200 mg/kg/d), or cefotaxime (100 to 200 mg/kg/d) have been used as the mainstay of antibiotic therapy. In previously vaccinated children, additional care should be taken, since other etiologic agents are more likely. Culture results should guide antibiotic therapy. In group A streptococcal infection, penicillin is the drug of choice, while in *S. aureus* infections, a semisynthetic penicillinase-resistant penicillin is preferred.

Complications can also occur, including pneumonia in up to 25% of affected children. Meningitis, arthritis, and cellulitis have been reported, but are rare. When Hib is the causative agent, all unvaccinated patients' contacts should receive antibiotic prophylaxis, usually with rifampicin.

Croup

Croup is a clinical syndrome characterized by cough, hoarseness, and stridor secondary to laryngeal obstruction. The term may derive from the Anglo-Saxon word *kropan,* which means "to cry aloud," or the Scottish term *roup,* which means "to cry out in a shrill voice." It has been used to describe several infections involving the larynx and the infraglottic region such as laryngitis, laryngotracheitis, laryngotracheobronchitis, laryngotracheobronchopneumonia, and bacterial croup. Epiglottitis and diphtheria have also been described historically as croup. Today the word *croup* is usually reserved for a viral illness associated with laryngotracheobronchitis that causes upper airway obstruction with stridor.

Croup usually starts with infection of the nasal and pharyngeal epithelia, with spread to the pharynx and trachea. Viral ability to impair ciliary function facilitates anatomic spread of the disease. When the disease spreads to the pharynx and trachea, edema and cellular infiltration of the lamina propria, submucosa, and adventitia occur. Inflammation of the trachea is seen on laryngoscopy, showing swelling and redness below the vocal cords, in the lateral walls of the trachea.

Croup affects 3% of children less than 6 years of age, with the highest incidence being at 18 months. It affects more boys than girls. Seasonal peaks of croup occur during late fall and winter and appear to mirror prevalence of parainfluenza virus type 1. Smaller peaks occur in late winter at a time when influenza virus types A and B or respiratory syncytial virus (RSV) infections are most commonly identified. Epidemic peaks usually reflect community parainfluenza type 1 and 2 or influenza A and B virus outbreaks. Close person-to-person contact is the main mechanism of spread, with large droplets containing viruses being transmitted by direct inoculation into the eye or nose, and airborne spread is much less common.

Laryngitis

Laryngitis is the mildest presentation of the croup syndrome, rarely leading to PICU admission. Etiology is most commonly viral, with influenza, adenovirus, rhinovirus, and RSV being the predominant agents. It occurs mainly in older children and adults. Prodromal symptoms of common cold and low-grade fever associated with barking cough and hoarseness are clinical signs of laryngitis. The disease is usually self-limited, requiring no specific treatment. Children with more severe presentation, requiring PICU admission, should raise suspicions about secondary infection or associated anatomic malformations (e.g., laryngo/tracheomalacia, tracheal stenosis).

Laryngotracheitis

Laryngotracheitis is a more severe presentation of laryngitis, with infection extending downward from the larynx to the trachea. It affects mainly children from 3 months to 3 years of age. Etiology is mainly viral, with parainfluenza type 1 and 2 being responsible for up to 75% of the infections. Influenza viruses, RSV, adenoviruses, enteroviruses, and coxsackieviruses are other potential causative agents. A prodromal period of coryza, followed by fever, barking cough, hoarseness, and later stridor, with mild to moderate signs of respiratory distress, are clinical symptoms of laryngotracheitis. Increasing tachypnea, tachycardia, sternal and chest retractions, and deepening cyanosis signal life-threatening airway obstruction.

Management of children with laryngotracheitis depends on the severity of the disease. Isolated clinical signs such as intercostal retractions or tachypnea are difficult to correlate with severity of disease; however, suprasternal retraction has been reported to be associated with imminent respiratory failure. A number of scoring systems have been developed and validated, to help clinical decision making in children with croup.

Initial management of a child with laryngotracheitis includes oxygen therapy if hypoxia is present, and avoidance of stressful factors for the child and parents. The child should be kept with parents all the time and only absolutely necessary procedures should be performed. Parents should be informed about the importance of reducing anxiety and calming the child. The use of sedatives should usually be avoided. Inhalation therapy with racemic epinephrine has shown good results in reducing respiratory distress and reducing need for tracheal intubation. Epinephrine may produce mucosal vasoconstriction and reduction of airway edema. A rebound effect has been described 2 to 3 hours after administration of epinephrine. Therapy with steroids including dexamethasone (intramuscular, oral, or intravenous) and budesonide (inhaled) have been shown to improve outcome. Use of inhaled Heliox may reduce airway resistance and improve work of breathing, and there are anecdotal reports of its use in self-limited upper airway obstruction. Antiviral therapy has not showed benefit in children with laryngotracheitis.

Children with severe forms of the disease, signs of critical airway obstruction, or signs of fatigue in the face of moderate obstruction should be closely monitored. In these two situations, endotracheal intubation is advised, in a controlled environment. The procedure should be preferably be performed by an experienced practitioner, for example a pediatric anesthetist. Usually tracheal intubation is performed under gas induction. The duration of illness is usually short in the mildly affected children, ranging from 3 to 5 days, although in severely affected children the duration ranges from 7 to 14 days.

Bacterial Croup

Laryngotracheobronchitis and Laryngotracheobronchopneumonia

Laryngotracheobronchitis and laryngotracheobronchopneumonia have been reported as variations of acute laryngotracheitis and occur less commonly. The initial presentation is similar to that of laryngotracheitis, but the child may deteriorate with increasing stridor and respiratory distress. The deterioration in the clinical status may be associated with secondary bacterial infection. Initial management is the same as for laryngotracheitis, and after deterioration treatment is the same as in bacterial tracheitis.

Bacterial Tracheitis

Bacterial tracheitis generally corresponds to a superinfection of the trachea, usually following a viral illness. Previous viral illness increases predisposition to colonization with potential bacterial pathogens by impairing ciliary activity and facilitating bacterial adherence to epithelial cells. The condition is uncommon (0.4 per 1000 pediatric admissions), with male predominance, and it may affect all ages until early adolescence. Children with Down syndrome, airway abnormalities, or those requiring endotracheal intubation or tracheostomy are at increased risk of developing bacterial tracheitis. The most common etiologic agents isolated are *S. aureus, H. influenzae,* and streptococcal infections. In immunosuppressed children, other organisms, including gram-negative bacteria, have been reported.

The clinical presentation is of upper respiratory infection progressing rapidly to severe respiratory dysfunction and systemic toxicity. The diagnosis is clinical and based on the finding of an exudative tracheitis. Guides to differentiation from epiglottitis are the presence of cough and marked prodromal symptoms, and the absence of drooling and neck hyperextension. White blood cell count is nonspecifically elevated, with an increase in polymorphonuclear cells. Upper airway radiographs, if performed, may show subglottic narrowing and cloudiness of the tracheal air column.

All children with presumed bacterial tracheitis should be observed in the PICU due to the risk of sudden respiratory failure. Early elective tracheal intubation is advisable in the presence of clinical deterioration. Recommendations for elective intubation are similar to those in epiglottitis. The use of inhaled epinephrine or steroids has been described in children with tracheitis, but there is usually poor response.

Blood cultures should be obtained when appropriate and antibiotics should be started as soon as possible. Empirical therapy should be direct against the most common pathogens. We recommend the use of a third-generation cephalosporin (cefotaxime or ceftriaxone) together with floxacillin or an aminoglycoside. In areas with a high incidence of MRSA, vancomycin should be considered as a primary treatment. Culture of tracheal secretions may be useful in identifying the causative agent and guiding antibiotic therapy. Bronchoscopy may help in guiding decision making about the timing of extubation, which may also be assessed by the onset of a marked decrease in the volume of tracheal secretions and the absence of fever.

Lemierre's Syndrome (Postanginal Sepsis)

Lemierre's syndrome, first described in the 1930s, is also known as postanginal sepsis. It is usually found as a complication of an oropharyngeal infection. The syndrome is due to infection by a gram-negative anaerobic bacillus, *Fusobacterium necrophorum. F. necrophorum* contains powerful cell wall–associated toxins and these are associated with clot formation and disseminated intravascular coagulation. The infection causes septicemia, septic thrombophlebitis of the internal jugular vein, and disseminated abscesses most commonly in the lung, leading to severe pneumonia or pneumonitis. The bacteria may be isolated from blood cultures. More common in the preantibiotic era, the infection is now very unusual but has a significant mortality. The illness may present with a very sore throat, rigors, and septicemia. There may be a history of oral or dental problems. Previously known to be sensitive to penicillin and clinda-mycin, there have been reports of resistance to β-lactam antibiotics. Anaerobic coverage with antibiotics such as metronidazole is usually indicated. Consideration should also be given to the concurrent use of low molecular weight heparin during treatment.

Pertussis Syndrome (Whooping Cough)

References in the medical literature to whooping cough date from 1540. Later the illness was named "pertussis," meaning violent cough. In the prevaccination era the annual incidence was approximately 100 to 200 cases per 100,000 population, and it is similar in some developing countries today. Routine immunization for pertussis started in the late 1940s in the U.S. and in late 1960s in the U.K., reducing incidences to less than 5 cases per 100,000 population. In the U.K., pertussis vaccination is given to children at 2, 3, and 4 months of age, using an acellular-pertussis–Hib combined vaccine (DTaP-Hib) [diphtheria/tetanus (DT)]. A preschool booster was added in 2001. The vaccination coverage is over 90%.

The vaccination program has proven very effective, markedly reducing the incidence in different countries. Periods of low adherence to vaccination, such as in the late 1970s when vaccination rates fell from 83% to less than 40%, was followed by a pertussis epidemic.

However, over the last decade the incidence of pertussis has increased in two populations, children under 6 months of age (who have not completed immunization) and adults (with waning immunity). Infants are at a high risk of complications and it is possible that the incidence of pertussis in the rest of the population is significantly underreported. In late 1990s, a study reported 58 patients with serologic or bacteriologic evidence of pertussis equivalent to an incidence rate of 330 cases per 100,000 per year. The official notification rate for the period under study was <4 per 100,000. The incidence in the PICU is also believed to be higher than reported; in a study of PICU admissions for severe respiratory infections, 25 of 126 infants (19.8%) had pertussis, only 28% (7/25) of whom had been suspected of having the disease.

Etiology

The main causative agent of pertussis syndrome is *B. pertussis*, being responsible for the most severe presentation of the disease. *B. parapertussis* is less frequent and often causes a milder illness. Other agents associated with pertussis syndrome are adenovirus, parainfluenza viruses, respiratory syncytial virus, and *Mycoplasma pneumoniae*.

Clinical Presentation

Classically the illness starts with a catarrhal stage, marked by nonspecific upper respiratory tract symptoms such as rhinorrhea, cough, and low-grade fever for 1 to 2 weeks. This is followed by a 2- to 4-week paroxysmal stage with the cardinal feature of pertussis syndrome: a paroxysmal cough followed by a characteristic whoop and sometimes vomiting. The paroxysms of coughing can be prolonged and may lead to cyanosis, bulging of the eyes, vomiting, and petechiae. In neonates and young infants the illness can present differently, with apnea as a first symptom, or minor respiratory symptoms followed by signs of overwhelming infection. Apneas or hypoxia are the leading causes for PICU admission. Eventually the convalescent stage refers to the slow decrease in severity and frequency of symptoms, and usually lasts for 1 to 2 weeks. The typical disease lasts from 6 to 8 weeks, with residual coughing persisting for months. Many present without the classic symptoms and at the times of the year when there is a high incidence of children with other respiratory infections, such as viral bronchiolitis, and this can make the diagnosis difficult.

Diagnosis

Diagnosis of pertussis syndrome is largely clinical, usually made on the basis of history and observations of coughing spasms. However, most children admitted to the PICU with pertussis are under 6 months of age (with a large percentage of children under 2 months of age) and do not present with the classic symptoms. A high index of suspicion should be maintained for children with respiratory failure of apparent infectious cause and apneas. A high leukocyte count associated with hyperlymphocytosis (absolute and relative) is frequently found in children with pertussis, but is nonspecific.

Laboratory methods to diagnose pertussis include PCR, culture, direct fluorescent antibody (DFA) testing, and serologic methods. Polymerase chain reaction is sensitive and specific; however, it is expensive, and differences in primer selection and detection systems sometimes lead to discrepancy in results. Culture has a poor sensitivity. Cotton swabs are not to be used to obtain cultures for pertussis since the cotton may inhibit *B. pertussis* growth. Small gramnegative bacilli such as *B. pertussis* and *B. parapertussis* do not easily grow in routine culture media; thus special culture media (i.e., Gengou agar) are used. Direct fluorescent antibody testing from nasopharyngeal smear can provide rapid diagnosis; however, its sensitivity is relatively low. Serologic tests measure antibodies to toxins (pertussis toxin, filamentous hemagglutinin, and agglutinins). Single measures are difficult to evaluate in immunized children since antibodies from vaccination may influence results. Paired samples are more specific. Combination of DFA and PCR may be the best strategies for laboratory diagnosis. When PCR in not available, DFA and culture provide a reasonable but less sensitive alternative. Chest x-rays in pertussis syndrome usually reveal perihilar infiltrate with focal collapses associated with plugs of secretions. More severe disease can present with multilobar pneumonia.

Treatment

Treatment for pertussis is mainly supportive. Antibiotics can reduce the length of disease if started in the catarrhal stage. Erythromycin (40 to 50 mg/kg/d for

7 to 14 days) is the treatment of choice; however, a high prevalence of intolerance may decrease adherence. Newer macrolides, such as clarithromycin and azithromycin, have been found to be as effective as erythromycin and have a lower prevalence of side effects.

Most complications of pertussis are associated with hypoxic episodes; thus, supplementary oxygen should be administered. In children with severe paroxysms or apneas, and children with diffuse pulmonary disease, ventilatory support should be provided.

There is no specific treatment for cough paroxysms; the use of β-adrenergic agents, steroids, and pertussis-specific immunoglobulin has been reported, with little evidence of efficacy.

Mechanical ventilation in children with pertussis can be difficult since children can continue to have cough paroxysms during ventilation, increasing risk of barotrauma, and air leak. Prolonged periods of muscle relaxation may be required to avoid complications of paroxysms. The mean duration of ventilation is 4 to 5 days. In refractory hypoxia, inhaled nitric oxide therapy has been described as an effective adjuvant therapy in anecdotal reports. The mortality associated with pertussis in the PICU is high (~10%), being associated with overwhelming pulmonary infection leading to severe hypoxemia and cardiovascular failure. Malignant pertussis is the most severe form of presentation, with mortality rates higher than 75%. It is characterized by very young age at onset, persistent tachycardia, dyspnea with early respiratory failure, neurologic involvement, severe hyperleukocytosis and hyperlymphocytosis, hyponatremia, and oliguria. There is no evidence of improved outcome using extracorporeal life support.

Other complications of pertussis include seizures and encephalopathy, subconjunctival hemorrhage, rectal prolapse, and hernias.

Prevention

Antibiotics (erythromycin) should be given to the index case, even in the late stages, to control transmission to other family members. Children admitted with pertussis should be placed on droplet precautions to prevent spread to hospital staff and should remain in such precautions until 5 days after initiation of antibiotics or 3 weeks after onset of paroxysms if no antibiotic is given. Close contacts should be also treated to prevent spread (40 to 50 mg/kg/d, up to 2 g/d, for 7 to 14 days) independently of age.

Bronchiolitis

Bronchiolitis is the most common cause of admission to hospital in infants under 1 year of age. Although intensive care support is needed in only a small minority of children, the number of admissions in the winter makes this illness important. The most common infectious agent is RSV, but other agents such as parainfluenza viruses, influenza viruses, adenoviruses, and human meta-pneumoviruses are also causes.

The peak age of admission with bronchiolitis is between 3 and 6 months. Younger infants, those born prematurely, or those with underlying cardiopulmonary disease including upper airway problems or with cell-mediated immunodeficiency are at special risk of severe disease. Children born prematurely remain at increased risk on average until about 44 weeks postconceptual age even without chronic lung disease. It is now known that adults, especially the very old, are also at high risk from RSV.

Respiratory syncytial virus is found in all populations and climates. In the U.S. the infection rate with RSV is 68.8% in the first year and 82.6% in the second year of life. Virtually all children have been infected at least once by 24 months of age, and half have been infected twice.

In the U.S. (with a population of 300 million), admission rates with RSV of about 100,000 per year were estimated to cost about $300 million. In Canada (with a population of 32 million), direct medical expenditure on admissions for hospitalized children with RSV was estimated to be about $18 million (in U.S. dollars). In Cambridge, U.K., of an estimated 4800 births 132 infants (2.75%) were admitted over a 2-year period, costing an estimated $332,000 (£215,000) in hospital costs. These figures suggest direct costs of about $0.50 to $1.50 per person per year for hospitalization for bronchiolitis.

Admission rates vary but are probably about 0.7% to 3.1%. Admissions due to bronchiolitis seem to have been rising perhaps by even 2.5-fold in the last 20 years. In some populations there appears to be a higher risk of hospitalization and ventilation; in populations of Native Americans, admission rates are reported as high as 9.1% to 15.6%. There is an increase in admission rates associated with crowded home conditions, and in areas of social deprivation admission rates may be twice as high as in more affluent areas. The local unemployment rate has been shown to be a predictor of the admission rate.

Admission rates vary not only internationally and by region, but by the route of admission. Children seen in general emergency rooms are about twice as likely to be admitted as those assessed in pediatric facilities. More male infants are admitted than females (1.5:1).

Diagnosis and Clinical Features

Bronchiolitis is essentially a clinical diagnosis consisting of respiratory distress in a child under 2 years of age caused by a viral infection with wheeze or crackles on auscultation. There is often a history of poor feeding, lethargy, and malaise. In some cases the infants have had a cough or the parents have noticed noisy breathing that is often described as "wheezing," although often the noises are transmitted from the upper airway. In very young infants, especially those less than 10 weeks old, the presentation may be with apneas. The infant is often coryzal, and may have recession, which may be intercostal, subcostal, suprasternal, or sternal. The oxygen saturation in air may be reduced (<95%), and signs of dehydration may be present. Admission to the hospital is usually based on the clinical presentation. The criteria for admission to the PICU vary with local policies, and in many centers nasal continuous positive airway pressure (CPAP) may be administered on general pediatric wards where children are nursed according to local high staffing protocols.

Virology

Identification of a causative virus is often reassuring, but co-infection can occur. The most commonly used method is direct immunofluorescence of nasopharyngeal aspirates, which is often accompanied by virus culture to improve sensitivity. Reverse-transcriptase PCR (RT-PCR) for viral genome is more sensitive but not widely available clinically. Methods of obtaining material for testing may also be by nasal brushings, nasal swabs, bronchial aspirates, and BAL. Once detected, repeated testing to establish clearance is not generally helpful because it is known that virus will be shed long after the child is likely to be discharged from hospital. Isolated, routinely available tests are not sensitive to rule out infection. In children with cell-mediated immunodeficiency, viral shedding can be extremely prolonged, even for many months.

There is conflicting evidence of whether the strain of RSV influences illness severity. Since nasopharyngeal aspirates are reported to have a sensitivity of 61% to 80%, repeated samples may be needed (up to three) to effectively rule out RSV infection.

Nosocomial infection is extremely important in the busy PICU environment. Nosocomial infection is most important in the care of vulnerable children in the PICU or elsewhere in the hospital.

Radiology

Chest radiography is often performed for bronchiolitis, for example as part of the confirmation of the correct endotracheal tube positioning. There are no studies from PICUs examining the impact of chest radiographs on management. Computed tomography scans are sometimes performed in RSV infections when the course is unusual; the patient is in a special group (such as the immunosuppressed) or when extubation has not been possible. Ko and colleagues studied the CT appearances in 10 lung transplant recipients. They reported that a ground-glass appearance (7/10), air-space opacities (5/10), and tree-in-bud opacities (4/10) were common and that acute bronchial dilatation (4/10) and wall thickening (4/10) were sometimes present. In their series some of the patients went on to develop bronchiolitis obliterans. In children where an alternative diagnosis is considered, or where there is an unusual course, chest CT scanning with or without angiographic reconstruction or magnetic resonance imaging can be helpful.

Predicting Severe Disease

Risk factors for more severe disease include a history of apnea or respiratory arrest during the acute illness before hospitalization, and pulmonary consolidation as shown on the chest radiograph if obtained at admission. Those with more severe RSV bronchiolitis are often relatively lymphopenic.

No reliable model to predict admission to intensive care with bronchiolitis has yet been developed. Severity indices including age at hospitalization, gestational age, the presence of an underlying condition, and RSV subtype predict outcome with a sensitivity of only 77% and a specificity of 76%. When the above model was modified by exclusion of viral subgroup, sensitivity increased to 94%, but specificity decreased to 46%. Once ventilated, Tasker et al. suggest that the time course can be predicted for many infants. In a retrospective group of 45 infants with RSV bronchiolitis, criteria were generated and then prospectively evaluated in 44 infants admitted later. In this work it was shown that four-quadrant consolidation on chest x-ray, the best alveolar arterial oxygen gradients (AaDO$_2$, torr) >400, and mean airway pressure >10 cm H$_2$O could distinguish a severe group (median duration of PICU stay 17 days) from a milder group (median stay 7 days).

Management

The mainstays of management are supportive, including maintaining adequate oxygenation, controlling fluid and electrolyte balance, maintaining normoglycemia, and treating associated shock. Specific antiviral therapy with ribavirin has now become much less common; its effective in vitro antiviral action has not translated to clinical benefit for the vast majority of children. There is one group of children in whom antiviral treatment is likely to be of benefit: those who are unfortunate enough to catch RSV around the time of bone marrow transplantation. In both adults and children in this group, the mortality of RSV if respiratory failure occurs approaches 100% without treatment. The combination of high-dose anti-RSV immunoglobulin or intravenous immunoglobulin with ribavirin appears to confer improved survival.

Antibiotics

In children admitted to the pediatric ward, there has been concern that antibiotics are overused. It is known that concurrent serious bacterial infections are rare in children admitted with RSV infection. For children admitted to the PICU where the severity of illness is greater, the judgment about antibiotics is influenced by the increased risk of failing to treat an undiagnosed bacterial illness. Many serious infectious diseases are more common during the winter, and either the diagnosis may be confused with bronchiolitis or there may be co-infection with more than one organism. For this reason in our experience, most children on the PICU receive antibiotics at some time during their admission if they are ventilated for bronchiolitis.

Bronchodilators

β_2-agonists and anticholinergics such as ipratropium have been used in bronchiolitis for more than 20 years. Initial studies with ipratropium bromide suggested a possible reduction in the work of breathing, but this was not supported by subsequent work. The most recent consensus suggests that bronchodilators offer no significant benefit in bronchiolitis and the risks of exacerbating the well-reported complication of cardiac dysrhythmias should be considered.

Epinephrine

Nebulized adrenaline has been used, and in the last 10 years there have been five published randomized controlled trials evaluating the effect of nebulized adrenaline in bronchiolitis; all have shown significant clinical improvement with adrenaline. It is probable that the α-adrenergic stimulation is the most useful in reducing bronchial mucosal edema and thickness.

DNAse

Nasr et al. described a randomized, double-blind, placebo-controlled trial of the use of recombinant human deoxyribonuclease I in children with bronchiolitis. Although they were able to show that chest radiographic appearances were significantly improved in the treatment group, no significant clinical benefit could be shown {Nasr SZ, Strouse PJ, Soskolne E 2001}.

Nitric Oxide

Inhaled nitric oxide has not been shown to be effective in infants with respiratory failure caused by RSV, although nitric oxide is widely used for ARDS and is likely to be tried in RSV infection.

Heliox

A few reports of the use of Heliox in RSV infection suggest it may have a role, but it is unlikely to be used widely until its efficacy in a wide variety of clinical scenarios has been proven.

Neuromuscular Blockade

Neuromuscular blockade (NMB) is widely used during ventilation of infants with RSV infection. One study that looked at all children with respiratory failure found that the subset of children with RSV infection receiving prolonged NMB had longer ventilator courses compared to those in whom NMB was not used, despite similar demographics, severity of illness, and oxygenation impairment. However, paralysis still has a use in the early stages of mechanical ventilation of children with respiratory failure.

Surfactant

Gene polymorphisms for surfactant proteins A and D have been associated with severe RSV infection. These studies suggest that surfactant may be important in the immune response to RSV. There is further evidence that surfactant protein A is involved in opsonization of RSV.

Surfactant production can be adversely affected by damage to the type 2 pneumocytes by viruses. Severe viral bronchiolitis is associated with an absence of surfactant activity. There is both a deficiency in surfactant levels and impaired functional activity. Two small studies have looked at surfactant therapy in severe bronchiolitis. Both suggested that treatment appeared to improve gas exchange, reduce airway pressures, and shorten duration of ventilation and ICU stay, but no measures of overall outcome were included. Larger trials are needed.

High-Frequency Oscillatory Ventilation

Many units including our own now use high-frequency oscillation ventilation (HFOV) for a proportion of infants with bronchiolitis. In the literature there are several case reports and short case series but no formal randomized controlled trials of HFOV specifically in this area. Larger studies of HFOV included data from infants with bronchiolitis, and it is now a familiar tool for ventilating infants and children.

Nasal Continuous Positive Airway Pressure Ventilation

Clinicians have extended the use of nasal CPAP (nCPAP) from its widespread application in neonatology to the management of infants with bronchiolitis. In some centers nCPAP by single nasal prong is preferred, but other centers have now introduced other devices such as the flow driver, which may by more effective in neonatal practice. Continuous positive airway pressure may reduce the work of breathing by improving functional residual capacity above the closing volume.

Extracorporeal Membrane Oxygenation

Extracorporeal membrane oxygenation (ECMO) now has an established role in children with severe respiratory failure that is unresponsive to conventional therapy. Extracorporeal membrane oxygenation in RSV bronchiolitis has a survival of up to 96%, with a very low rate of neurologic sequelae. When complications occur, they are often associated with cannula insertion and anticoagulation. The relatively prolonged therapeutic period and intensity of management have limited the use of ECMO to the very sickest children in whom conventional ventilation has failed.

Complications

Apnea

Apnea and bradycardia occur commonly in young infants with respiratory viral infections and may result in the need for admission to PICU and for mechanical ventilation. Respiratory syncytial virus infection causes apnea in 1.8% to 23.9% of cases depending on the criteria used for diagnosing apnea. Risk factors for RSV-related apnea include age below 2 months and premature birth. In one study, patients with apneas had a significantly lower temperature, higher pCO_2, and lower pH, and on chest radiography had more signs of atelectasis. Apnea associated with other viral infections is less common but has been reported in association with parainfluenza virus, influenza virus, adenovirus, and Epstein-Barr virus. The relative risk for mechanical ventilation increases with the number of episodes of apnea. The management of apnea associated with viral infections is generally supportive, using CPAP or intermittent mandatory ventilation. Caffeine has been tried but the results are as yet inconclusive.

Hypotension

Hypotension may occur during bronchiolitis, and fluid volume resuscitation using isotonic crystalloid solutions is usually the first-line therapy when this occurs. Where inotropic support is required, no clear evidence has been produced to direct treatment. Inotropes such as dopamine, dobutamine, and adrenaline have been reported in life-threatening infection. Myocarditis and pericardial effusion have been reported in association with RSV infection.

Central Nervous System

Case reports exist that have suggested that encephalopathy may occur with bronchiolitis. One study suggested an incidence of 1.8% and that seizures were the major presenting complication. Despite this, it has not been possible to detect RSV in cerebrospinal fluid, and the possible mechanisms remain unclear. Case reports of seizures during bronchiolitis have been reported.

Other Complications

Fluid and electrolyte balance dysregulation is often encountered in ventilated children with bronchiolitis. Hyponatremia is common even at presentation and may be severe. Caution should be exercised in the types and volumes of fluids given during intravenous fluid management. Excessive amounts of hypotonic solutions can exacerbate hyponatremia.

Special Children

Cerebral Palsy

A common problem seen in the PICU is the child with cerebral palsy with functional upper airway obstruction. Many children with these sorts of problems have bulbar dysfunction leading to poor hypopharyngeal tone and coordination. This often results in significant upper airway obstruction, which is exacerbated during viral infections. In addition, oropharyngeal secretions are handled poorly, and these children are at high risk of aspiration causing pulmonary collapse and consolidation. Poor muscular tone and a less effective cough can exacerbate the child's situation. Early gastrostomy and the treatment of gastroesophageal reflux has greatly improved the general nutrition of many children with cerebral palsy over recent years, but many of these children are still relatively less well nourished, leaving their immunity less able to withstand pulmonary illness.

Upper Airway Problems

Anatomic abnormalities may be unmasked during bronchiolitis. In particular, those with upper airway problems including tonsillar hypertrophy, vascular rings, vocal cord palsy, or papillomata, may have more severe or complicated disease.

Cyanotic Congenital Heart Disease

Those with cyanotic congenital heart disease and especially those with pulmonary hypertension are at greatly increased risk of severe disease with bronchiolitis. In the early years of pediatric intensive care, mortality in this group was reported to be as high as 44%. Today, although still associated with a significantly higher risk, the mortality is substantially better and probably under 9% in those who require ventilation.

Sequelae

The outcome for children admitted to PICU is improving with improvements in care. Shay et al. (16) reviewed deaths associated with bronchiolitis in the U.S. from 1979 to 1997 and suggested a death rate of 2.2 to 2.4 per 100,000 live births with a total of 1806 in the period studied.

Bibliography

1. Williams BG, Gouws E, Boschi-Pinto C, Bruce J, Dye C. Estimates of world-wide distribution of child deaths from acute respiratory infections. Lancet Infect Dis 2002; 2(1):25–32.
2. Kendig's Disorders of the Respiratory Tract in Children, 7th ed. 2006 Elsevier Victor Chernick, MD, FRCP (C), Thomas F. Boat, MD, Robert W, Wilmott, MD and Andrew Bush, MD, FRCP, FRCPCH.

Pneumonia

1. Graat ME, Stoker J, Vroom MB, Schultz MJ. Can we abandon daily routine chest radiography in intensive care patients? J Intensive Care Med 2005;20(4):238–246.
2. Tu CY, Hsu WH, Hsia TC, et al. Pleural effusions in febrile medical ICU patients: chest ultrasound study. Chest 2004;126:1274–1280.
3. Miller WT Jr, Tino G, Friedburg JS. Thoracic CT in the intensive care unit: assessment of clinical usefulness. Radiology 1998;209:491–498.

4. Boussekey N, Leroy O, Georges H, Devos P, d'Escrivan T, Guery B. Diagnostic and prognostic values of admission procalcitonin levels in community-acquired pneumonia in an intensive care unit. Infection 2005;33:257–263.
5. Luyt CE, Guerin V, Combes A, et al. Procalcitonin kinetics as a prognostic marker of ventilator-associated pneumonia. Am J Respir Crit Care Med 2005;171:48–53.
6. Light RW, Macgregor MI, Luchsinger PC, et al. Pleural effusions: the diagnostic separations of transudates and exudates. Ann Intern Med 1972;77(4):507–513.

Ventilator-Associated Pneumonia

1. Carvalho CE, Berezin EN, Pistelli IP, Mimica L, Cardoso MR. Sequential microbiological monitoring of tracheal aspirates in intubated patients admitted to a pediatric intensive care unit. J Pediatr (Rio J) 2005;81(1):29–33.
2. Chastre J, Fagon JY. Ventilator-associated pneumonia. Am J Respir Crit Care Med 2002;165(7):867–903.
3. Gauvin F, Dassa C, Chaibou M, Proulx F, Farrell CA, Lacroix J. Ventilator-associated pneumonia in intubated children: comparison of different diagnostic methods. Pediatr Crit Care Med 2003;4(4):437–443.
4. Burmester M, Mok Q. How safe is non-bronchoscopic bronchoalveolar lavage in critically ill mechanically ventilated children? Intensive Care Med 2001;27(4): 716–721.
5. Fagon JY, Chastre J, Wolff M, et al. Invasive and noninvasive strategies for management of suspected ventilator-associated pneumonia. A randomized trial. Ann Intern Med 2000;132(8):621–630.
6. Bush A. Bronchoscopy in paediatric intensive care. Paediatr Respir Rev 2003;4(1): 67–73.
7. Davies L, Dolgin S, Kattan M. Morbidity and mortality of open lung biopsy in children. Pediatrics 1997;99(5):660–664.
8. Luyt CE, Chastre J, Fagon JY. Value of the clinical pulmonary infection score for the identification and management of ventilator-associated pneumonia. Intensive Care Med 2004;30(5):844–852.
9. Singh N, Rogers P, Atwood CW, Wagener MM, Yu VL. Short-course empiric antibiotic therapy for patients with pulmonary infiltrates in the intensive care unit. A proposed solution for indiscriminate antibiotic prescription. Am J Respir Crit Care Med 2000;162:505–511.
10. Chastre J, Wolff M, Fagon JY, et al.; PneumA Trial Group. Comparison of 8 vs 15 days of antibiotic therapy for ventilator-associated pneumonia in adults: a randomized trial. JAMA 2003;290(19):2588–2598.

Empyema

1. Hippocrates. The book of Hippocrates. In: Adams F, ed. The Genuine Works of Hippocrates. London: C. and J. Adlard Printers, 1849.
2. Schultz KD, Fan LL, Pinsky J, et al. The changing face of pleural empyemas in children: epidemiology and management. Pediatrics 2004;113(6):1735–1740.
3. Henriques Normark B, Kalin M, Ortqvist A, et al. Dynamics of penicillin-susceptible clones in invasive pneumococcal disease. J Infect Dis 2001;184(7):861–869.
4. Alfaro C, Fergie J, Purcell K. Emergence of community-acquired methicillin-resistant Staphylococcus aureus in complicated parapneumonic effusions. Pediatr Infect Dis J 2005;24(3):274–276.

5. Buckingham SC, King MD, Miller ML. Incidence and etiologies of complicated parapneumonic effusions in children, 1996 to 2001. Pediatr Infect Dis J 2003;22(6):499–504.
6. Kyaw MH, Lynfield R, Schaffner W, et al.; Active Bacterial Core Surveillance of the Emerging Infections Program Network. Effect of introduction of the pneumococcal conjugate vaccine on drug-resistant Streptococcus pneumoniae. N Engl J Med 2006;354(14):1455–1463.
7. Ramirez S, Hild TG, Rudolph CN, et al. Increased diagnosis of Lemierre syndrome and other Fusobacterium necrophorum infections at a Children's Hospital. Pediatrics 2003;112(5):e380.
8. Byington CL, Korgenski K, Daly J, Ampofo K, Pavia A, Mason EO. Impact of the pneumococcal conjugate vaccine on pneumococcal parapneumonic empyema. Pediatr Infect Dis J 2006;25(3):250–254.
9. Balfour-Lynn IM, Abrahamson E, Cohen G, et al.; Paediatric Pleural Diseases Subcommittee of the BTS Standards of Care Committee. BTS guidelines for the management of pleural infection in children. Thorax 2005;60(suppl 1):i1–21.
10. Pierrepoint MJ, Evans A, Morris SJ, Harrison SK, Doull IJ. Pigtail catheter drain in the treatment of empyema thoracis. Arch Dis Child 2002;87(4):331–332.

Bronchiolitis

1. Arnold JH, Anas NG, Luckett P, et al. High-frequency oscillatory ventilation in pediatric respiratory failure: a multicenter experience. Crit Care Med 2000; 28:3913–3919.
2. Bont L, van Vught AJ, Kimpen JL. Prophylaxis against respiratory syncytial virus in premature infants. Lancet 1999;354:1003–1004.
3. Buck JJ, Debenham P, Tasker RC. Prophylaxis for respiratory syncytial virus infection: missing the target. Arch Dis Child 2001;84(4):375.
4. De PA, Davis PG, Faber B, Morley CJ. Devices and pressure sources for administration of nasal continuous positive airway pressure (NCPAP) in preterm neonates (Cochrane Review). Cochrane Database Syst Rev 2002;CD002977.
5. Green TP, Moler FW, Goodman DM. Probability of survival after prolonged extracorporeal membrane oxygenation in pediatric patients with acute respiratory failure. Extracorporeal Life Support Organization. Crit Care Med 1995;23: 1132–1139.
6. Hall CB. Respiratory syncytial virus and parainfluenza virus. N Engl J Med 2001;344:1917–1928.
7. Heilman CA, From the National Institute of Allergy and Infectious Diseases and the World Health Organization. Respiratory syncytial and parainfluenza viruses. J Infect Dis 1990;161:402–406.
8. Jansson L, Nilsson P, Olsson M. Socioeconomic environmental factors and hospitalization for acute bronchiolitis during infancy. Acta Paediatr 2002;91: 335–338.
9. Kellner JD, Ohlsson A, Gadomski AM, Wang EE. Bronchodilators for bronchiolitis. Cochrane Database Syst Rev 2000;CD001266.
10. Langley JM, Wang EE, Law BJ, et al. Economic evaluation of respiratory syncytial virus infection in Canadian children: a Pediatric Investigators Collaborative Network on Infections in Canada (PICNIC) study. J Pediatr 1997;131:113–117.

11. Mazzella M, Bellini C, Calevo MG, et al. A randomised control study comparing the Infant Flow Driver with nasal continuous positive airway pressure in preterm infants. Arch Dis Child Fetal Neonatal Ed 2001;85:F86–F90.

12. Medbo S, Finne PH, Hansen TW. Respiratory syncytial virus pneumonia ventilated with high-frequency oscillatory ventilation. Acta Paediatr 1997;86:766–768.

13. Meyer TA, Warner BW. Extracorporeal life support for the treatment of viral pneumonia: collective experience from the ELSO registry. Extracorporeal Life Support Organization. J Pediatr Surg 1997;32:232–236.

14. Muller-Pebody B, Edmunds WJ, Zambon MC, Gay NJ, Crowcroft NS. Contribution of RSV to bronchiolitis and pneumonia-associated hospitalizations in English children, April 1995–March 1998. Epidemiol Infect 2002;129:99–106.

15. Purcell K, Fergie J. Concurrent serious bacterial infections in 2396 infants and children hospitalized with respiratory syncytial virus lower respiratory tract infections. Arch Pediatr Adolesc Med 2002;156:322–324.

16. Shay DK, Holman RC, Newman RD, Liu LL, Stout JW, Anderson LJ. Bronchiolitis-associated hospitalizations among US children, 1980–1996. JAMA 1999;282:1440–1446.

17. Ko JP, Shepard JA, Sproule MW, et al. CT manifestations of respiratory syncytial virus infection in lung transplant recipients. J Comput Assist Tomogr 2000;24(2):235–241.

18. Trasker RC, Gordon I, Kiff K. Time course of severe respiratory syncytial virus infection in mechanically ventilated infants. Acta Paediatr 2000;89(8):938–941.

19. Nasr SZ, Strouse PJ, Soskolne E, et al. Efficacy of recombinant human deoxyribonuclease I in the hospital management of respiratory syncytial virus bronchiolitis. Chest 2001;120(1):203–208.

17
New Therapies for Sepsis

Liz Whittaker and Simon Nadel

There have been significant improvements in the outcome of sepsis in more recent years. The recently reported mortality rate of between 7% and 18% is a significant improvement from the more than 90% mortality reported in the 1960s (1–3). However, sepsis remains the second leading cause of death in children aged 1 to 14 years in the developed world, with an estimated financial burden of $1.97 billion per year in the United States (4).

The significant improvement in outcome over the last few decades is due in part to an increased understanding of the importance of rapid recognition of disease; early, aggressive fluid-resuscitation; and prompt, appropriate antibiotic therapy. In addition, improvements in organ-support technologies and intensive care techniques have dramatically widened therapeutic options. However, apart from antibiotics and supportive care, there are no approved adjunctive therapies for use in children.

The pathogenesis of the sepsis and septic shock is now becoming better understood. Greater understanding of the complex network of immune, inflammatory, and hematologic disturbances may enable the development of novel and rational therapies. Early recognition of sepsis and the systemic inflammatory response syndrome (SIRS) in the critically ill patient, and appropriate interventions to modify disease progression, may avoid the continuing morbidity, mortality, and financial burden associated with sepsis.

The clinical diagnosis of sepsis and SIRS in children may be very challenging. An international panel of experts in the fields of adult and pediatric severe sepsis and clinical research proposed a set of definitions for sepsis, with the aim of clarifying the diagnosis and treatment of these conditions and to aid interpretation of research in this field. These are more useful in the context of large, multicenter, international therapeutic trials rather than in a clinical setting, but can help in the understanding of the research and development occurring in this area currently (5). These definitions are described in Table 17.1.

Etiology

The causes of sepsis in the pediatric age group are influenced by age, host immune status, exposure to specific pathogens, and the presence of indwelling devices (Table 17.2) (see Chapter 1).

TABLE 17.1. Definitions of SIRS, infection, sepsis, severe sepsis, septic shock, and MODS

Systemic inflammatory response syndrome (SIRS)

The presence of at least two of the following four criteria, one of which must be abnormal temperature or leukocyte count:

- Core* temperature of >38.5°C or <36°C
- Tachycardia, defined as a mean heart rate >2 SD above normal for age in the absence of external stimulus, chronic drugs, or painful stimuli; or otherwise unexplained persistent elevation over a 0.5- to 4-hour time period or for children <1 year old: bradycardia, defined as a mean heart rate <10th percentile for age in the absence of external vagal stimulus, beta-blocker drugs, or congenital heart disease; or otherwise unexplained persistent depression over a 0.5-hour time period.
- Mean respiratory rate >2 SD above normal for age or mechanical ventilation for an acute process not related to underlying neuromuscular disease or the receipt of general anesthesia.
- Leukocyte count elevated or depressed for age (not secondary to chemotherapy-induced leukopenia) or >10% immature neutrophils.

Infection

A suspected or proven (by positive culture, tissue stain, or polymerase chain reaction test) infection caused by any pathogen or a clinical syndrome associated with a high probability of infection. Evidence of infection includes positive findings on clinical exam, imaging, or laboratory tests (e.g., white blood cells in a normally sterile body fluid; perforated viscus, chest x-ray consistent with pneumonia, petechial or purpuric rash, or purpura fulminans)

Sepsis

SIRS in the presence of or as a result of suspected or proven infection.

Severe sepsis

Sepsis plus the following: cardiovascular organ dysfunction, acute respiratory distress syndrome (ARDS), or two or more other organ dysfunctions.

Septic shock

Sepsis and cardiovascular organ dysfunction.

---

*Core temperature must be measured by rectal, oral, or central catheter probe.
Source: Goldstein et al. (5).

TABLE 17.2. Likely infecting pathogen causing systemic sepsis and age group and underlying disease

Patient group	Pathogen
Neonates	Group B streptococcus
	Enteric bacilli
	Listeria monocytogenes
	Haemophilus influenzae
	Streptococcus pneumoniae
	Chlamydia trachomatis
	Enterovirus
	Herpes simplex virus
Infant/child	*Streptococcus pneumoniae*
	Neisseria meningitidis
	Haemophilus influenzae type b
Underlying immunodeficiency, asplenia, neutropenia, T- and B-cell deficiency, chronic granulomatous disease, HIV, malnutrition, indwelling prosthetic device, nosocomial sepsis	*Streptococcus pneumoniae, Salmonella,* other encapsulated organisms, *Staphylococcus aureus, epidermidis* enterococci, *Pseudomonas aeruginosa,* other gram-negative bacilli α-hemolytic streptococci, clostridia and other anaerobes, fungi, *Enterovirus,* herpes simplex virus, other viruses, malaria

Vaccinations have dramatically altered the epidemiology of sepsis. In particular, the widespread introduction of Hib, meningococcal serogroup C, and heptavalent pneumococcal conjugate vaccines have significantly decreased the incidence of these invasive bacterial infections where they have been introduced into the routine vaccination schedules.

Pathophysiology

Septic shock and multiorgan dysfunction result from the activation of host defense mechanisms in response to a microbial invasion. The progression to SIRS is dependent on the host's immunocompetence, the virulence and quantity of the pathogen, and the therapeutic intervention attempted. Systemic inflammatory response syndrome may continue independently, regardless of eradication of the pathogen by antimicrobial agents, due to uncontrolled elaboration, release, and action of normal immune mediators. It is now understood that this pathophysiology is due to a complex cascade involving release of proinflammatory cytokines, vasoactive mediators, and reactive oxygen species.

Cytokines are soluble, low molecular weight glycoproteins that act to regulate both innate and specific immune responses and act as inflammatory mediators. Individual cytokines can be produced by multiple cells and have multiple, often overlapping functions, acting on various target cells in different ways depending on the timing of release and local concentration.

At low concentrations cytokines have a paracrine effect, whereas at increased concentrations, such as in sepsis, the cytokines have both paracrine and endocrine effects and may also act systemically. The sepsis syndrome commences with activation of the innate immune response by the pathogen in question. This triggers the secretion of pro- and antiinflammatory mediators, activates leukocytes and the coagulation cascade, and causes an increase in apoptosis (6). Thrombin created by coagulation activation contributes directly to inflammation as well as promoting fibrin deposition (7). Thus, the pathogenesis of tissue injury is complex and cannot be attributed to a single agent. Tissue injury occurs during inflammation and is a progressive process, which may eventually lead to organ dysfunction and failure, despite antibiotics and supportive care.

Clinically, the child presenting with septic shock has signs consistent with systemic inflammation. Fever, tachycardia, and tachypnea are the most common features present, but prolonged capillary refill time, abnormal temperature regulation, and decreased activity or poor feeding are frequently present. With the development of worsening disease, respiratory failure, circulatory and myocardial failure, coagulopathy, renal failure, hepatic failure, and decreased neurologic function become apparent.

At present, there is no straightforward, reliable investigation available for the diagnosis of sepsis. Markers of infection and inflammation have not to date proved themselves sensitive and specific enough to be used. Those currently used in clinical practice include C-reactive protein and total peripheral white blood cell count; however, there are many markers under review that may prove invaluable in future practice. These include procalcitonin, lipopolysaccharide-binding protein (LBP), specific rapid antigen assays, polymerase chain reaction (PCR), genomic testing, and proteomic testing. Measurements of cytokines (such as interleukin-6 [IL-6]) as markers for sepsis have not proven straight-forward, but used in combination with current techniques, these newer markers may prove beneficial for more rapid diagnosis in the future (8–11).

Therapies used in shock should encompass treatment of the cause, supportive management of the clinical state, and prevention/management of the inflammatory system driving the condition.

Antimicrobial Therapy

The only proven therapy for bacterial infection is appropriate antimicrobial therapy (Fig. 17.1). Empiric therapy for suspected sepsis should be targeted toward the likely causative pathogens (Table 17.2). If sepsis is suspected, anti-microbials should be administered promptly. Important considerations when selecting a suitable antimicrobial regimen include the patient's age, acquisition of infection (community or nosocomial), host immune status, and penetration

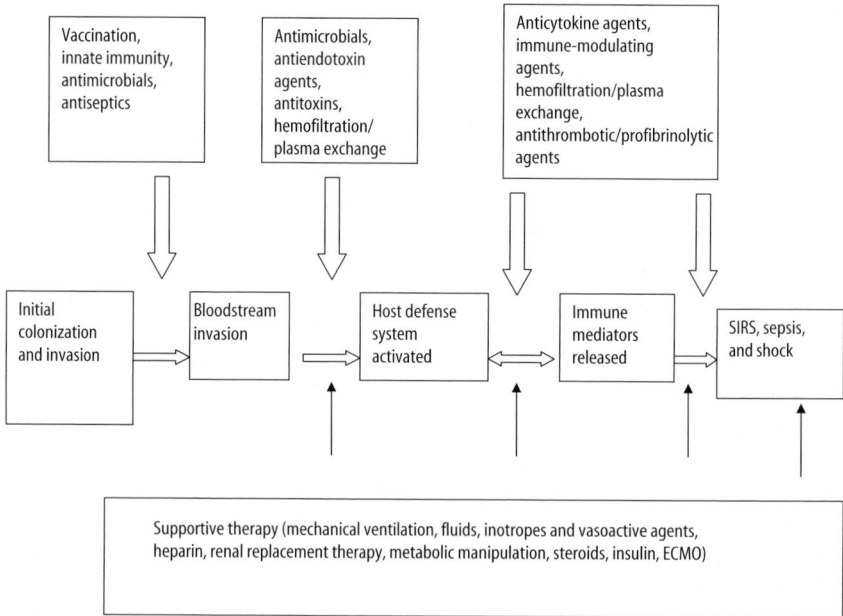

FIGURE 17.1. Potential areas for therapeutic intervention to interrupt disturbed physiology in sepsis and septic shock. SIRS, systemic inflammatory response syndrome; ECMO, extracorporeal membrane oxygenation.

into tissues and compartments (such as bone or central nervous system). Knowledge of organism susceptibility patterns is essential.

Once the causative organism is isolated and antibiotic susceptibilities available, then antimicrobial therapy can be tailored appropriately.

Supportive Care

Effective treatment of sepsis and septic shock is dependent on prompt recognition and initiation of supportive therapy, together with specific therapy.

The basic principles of immediate care include ensuring the ABCs: adequate airway patency, gas exchange (breathing), and circulation. The interventions required to achieve these goals depend on the specific physiologic state of the patient at the time of presentation.

Septic shock is the result of decreased intravascular volume, maldistribution of circulating volume, or impaired myocardial function, all of which may occur in various combinations at different times during the course of septic shock (12). Children with sepsis who receive early aggressive fluid resuscitation (>60 mL/kg in the first hour) demonstrate improved survival without increased risk of pulmonary edema, cerebral edema, or acute respiratory distress syndrome (ARDS) (13).

Clinical observation and careful monitoring determine the amount of circulatory support with fluid or vasoactive agents that is required. These factors include the patient's clinical state (e.g., capillary refill time, urine output, peripheral/core temperature gradient, neurologic state), and information obtained from monitoring devices (heart rate, blood pressure, central venous pressure, pulmonary artery pressure, cardiac output, stroke volume, and systemic vascular resistance). Septic shock causes multiple organ dysfunction, and it is important to evaluate and treat abnormalities in other organ systems including the respiratory, renal, and gastrointestinal systems.

Early recognition of sepsis allowing earlier initiation of organ support is essential in the effective management of the condition. The aim of initial resuscitation and supportive therapies is to maintain organ perfusion and oxygenation.

Hypoxemia should be treated with increased inspired oxygen concentrations and monitored with pulse oximetry and regular blood gas estimations. Mechanical ventilation is often required to support failing respiratory function and reduce the work of breathing due to noncompliant lungs. Cardiovascular support in the form of fluids, inotropes, or vasoconstrictors should be initiated. Increasing evidence suggests that those children who receive early aggressive fluid resuscitation have greater survival rates, with no increase in morbidity. Ongoing monitoring should continue and determine further management, taking into consideration the possible development of multiorgan failure (14).

Experimental Therapies for Sepsis

Understanding the pathophysiology of sepsis has allowed the development of multiple novel interventions in an attempt to interrupt the inflammatory process and reduce morbidity and mortality. Although none of these therapies has proven beneficial in the pediatric population, they remain important adjuncts in experimental sepsis, and several have been studied in both pediatric and adult populations. These are discussed below, and while most would not appear beneficial, it is likely that they will be the basis for future drug development and clinical trials in infants and children.

Antiendotoxin Therapies

Endotoxin is one of the most important bacterial components that contribute to the inflammatory process. Levels of endotoxin directly correlate with severity of meningococcal disease and other forms of sepsis, and with elaboration and release of inflammatory mediators, including the cytokines tumor necrosis factor-α (TNF-α) and IL-1 and -6, and the upregulation of the complement and coagulation pathways. Endotoxin has also been found in the presence of critical illness in children and adults, not related to documented gram-negative sepsis, where its presence appears to be related to severity of disease and outcome (15,16).

It is postulated that the presence of endotoxin in the blood in these circumstances is related to the altered gut permeability seen in critical illness or insult, allowing endotoxin to translocate into the systemic circulation, thus contributing to the inflammatory stimulus in these patients.

The assumption that the inflammatory process is related to the presence of endotoxemia is based on the finding that much of the pathophysiology of gram-negative sepsis can be reproduced by the administration of purified endotoxin or a variety of endotoxin-free inflammatory mediators, upregulated by endotoxin. In addition, many of these effects can be blocked, in vitro and in vivo, by agents that neutralize the effects of endotoxin or the elaborated downstream inflammatory mediators.

A variety of antiendotoxin strategies have been proposed, including agents that bind to and neutralize endotoxin, efforts to enhance endotoxin clearance, or agents that inhibit the interaction of endotoxin with its receptors.

Antiendotoxin Antibodies

For many years, investigators have attempted to produce neutralizing antibodies to the highly conserved elements in the core region of endotoxin (such as lipid A). This is a particularly attractive strategy as it would enable a single product, if effective, to be useful in all forms of gram-negative sepsis. Early studies indicated that passively administered antisera raised to rough mutant bacteria (such as *Escherichia coli* J5) protected against challenge from heterologous gram-negative bacteria (17,18). These rough mutant bacteria expose core elements of endotoxin on their surface. Based on the assumption that the antisera contained antibodies that bound to and neutralized endotoxin, researchers developed cross-protective monoclonal antibodies apparently directed against lipid A. Two particular antibodies were developed that were found to weakly bind, but not to neutralize endotoxin (19). Following encouraging results in initial studies, both antibodies went into larger studies in both adults and children.

A murine monoclonal IgM antibody, E5, was studied in a multicenter, placebo-controlled trial in adults with severe sepsis due to probable or confirmed gram-negative infection (20). The study was stopped after the second interim analysis; 1090 patients received study medication and 915 had gram-negative infection confirmed by culture. There were no significant differences in mortality between the E5 or placebo groups at day 14 (29.7% vs. 31.1%; $p = .67$) or day 28 (38.5% vs. 40.3%; $p = .56$). Patients presenting without shock had a slightly lower mortality when treated with E5, but this difference was not significant (28.9% vs. 33.0% for the E5 and placebo groups, respectively, at day 28; $p = .32$).

A humanized monoclonal IgG antibody against the lipid A moiety of endotoxin, HA-1A, was studied in two multicenter, randomized, double-blind, placebo-controlled trials in adults with sepsis and one trial in children with meningococcal septic shock. The two adult studies showed conflicting results, the first showing a significant benefit in patients with gram-negative septic shock (21). However, due to methodologic problems, this study was repeated in a larger number of patients. This study of 621 patients with presumed gram-negative infection and shock failed to repeat the positive results of the first study (22). Mortality rates in this study were as follows: placebo, 32% (95 of 293) and HA-1A, 33% (109 of 328) ($p = .864$). Mortality rates in the patients treated with HA-1A without gram-negative bacteremia were higher: placebo, 37% (292 of 793) vs. HA-1A, 41% (318 of 785) ($p = .073$). Following this study, HA-1A was abandoned as a potentially useful agent.

The study of HA-1A in children with meningococcal septic shock was completed before the second adult study reported. The pediatric study demonstrated a 33% absolute reduction in mortality in the treatment group (23). However, this did not reach statistical significance. The authors concluded that there may actually have been a genuine beneficial effect of HA-1A that was obscured by nonoptimal timing of intervention; that is, treatment with an effective antiendotoxin therapy is likely to be more effective if given earlier in the disease course. The median time from initiation of antibiotic therapy to administration of study medication in this study was 6.4 hours, with 25% of patients receiving study medication >9.7 hours following antibiotic therapy; thus the antiendotoxin therapy may have been given too late to have an effect.

However, another reason why this study was not positive may have been that the improvement in mortality may have been a chance finding. Since this study was reported, in vitro data have suggested that HA-1A has low affinity for endotoxin and no activity against some species of endotoxin (24).

Other Antiendotoxin Therapies

There are several other promising antiendotoxin therapies under development. These are derived from innate peptides and proteins in insects and animal species, which have evolved for the specific purpose of binding and neutralizing endotoxin.

Endotoxin, which is present in the circulation, forms complexes with circulating proteins and lipoproteins, such as the acute-phase reactant LBP, which facilitates the transfer of endotoxin to its receptors Toll-like receptor (TLR4), CD14, and lipoproteins (25). Endotoxin is also bound and neutralized by many neutrophil granule proteins, including the bactericidal/permeability-increasing protein (BPI) and the cationic antibacterial protein hCAP-18 (a cathelicidin) (26,27).

One compound derived from naturally occurring BPI has been the subject of controlled clinical trials. A recombinant form ($rBPI_{21}$) consisting of 21 amino acids of the N-terminal fragment of naturally occurring BPI has been shown to act synergistically with antimicrobials in the killing of many bacteria, and to bind and neutralize endotoxin. This recombinant protein has been the subject of an uncontrolled clinical study in children with severe meningococcal septicemia (28). This study evaluated 26 children (1 to 18 years of age) with meningococcal septicemia within 8 hours of receiving antibiotics. The study showed a significant reduction in mortality in the treated patients (only one death) compared with historical controls (expected four to eight deaths). The results of this study prompted a phase III randomized, double-blind, placebo-controlled study of $rBPI_{21}$ in meningococcal septic shock, which evaluated 393 children; 190 children received $rBPI_{21}$ and 203 received placebo. There was no significant difference in the mortality rate between the two groups, 14 (7.4%) in the $rBPI_{21}$ group and 20 (9.9%) in the placebo group ($p = .48$). However, fewer patients treated with $rBPI_{21}$ had multiple severe amputations (6 of 190 [3.2%] vs. 15 of 203 [7.4%]; odds ratio, 2.47 (0.94–6.51); $p = .067$), and more had a functional outcome at day 60 similar to that before illness (136 of 176 [77.3%] vs. 126 of 190 [66.3%]; $p = .019$) (29).

Any effective antiendotoxin agent is likely to be most beneficial if given early in the course of disease. This is particularly true in meningococcal sepsis, where disease progression is rapid. Mean time of delivery of the $rBPI_{21}$ in this study was 5.9 hours following initial antibiotic therapy (29).

It is possible that treatment with $rBPI_{21}$ would be more beneficial if it were given simultaneously with antibiotics. However, the study was confounded by the large number of children who died before starting or completing the infusion of $rBPI_{21}$. Analysis of the children who survived to complete study drug infusion showed a lower mortality in the $rBPI_{21}$ treated group (2.2%) compared with the placebo group (6.2%), but this was not statistically significant due to the small numbers involved ($p = .07$).

Despite the positive findings in the secondary end points, and the encouraging effects on the primary end point, there have been no further phase III studies of rBPI$_{21}$ in children with sepsis.

Statins

Endotoxin is known to bind to high-density lipoprotein (HDL), low-density lipoprotein (LDL), and very low density lipoprotein (VLDL). These particles appear to be involved in detoxification and clearance of circulating endotoxin through the reticuloendothelium (30). Preparations of HDL that are reconstituted from plasma are able to neutralize endotoxin more potently than are natural lipoproteins (31). The HDLs attenuate the proinflammatory response in animal models and humans by binding and neutralizing lipopolysaccharide (LPS), by inhibiting the expression of adhesion molecules and proinflammatory cytokines, by stimulating the release of nitric oxide, and by enhancing the activity and expression of antiinflammatory enzymes and proteins. These have shown promising results in adult volunteers challenged with endotoxin, where the volunteers showed reduction in symptoms, proinflammatory cytokines, and endotoxin-induced changes in leukocyte count (32). Although the mechanism of beneficial effects of HDLs are complex and will require further elucidation, there is a clear indication that HDLs, and some pharmacologic agents, such as fibrates, niacin, and statins, which have been shown to significantly elevate HDL levels, have the potential to become valuable therapeutic agents in the prevention and treatment of sepsis and septic shock (33).

Statins exert antiinflammatory effects by modifying leukocyte–endothelial cell interactions and by altering the responses of monocytes/macrophages and T cells. Statins also modulate inflammatory cell signaling and inflammatory gene expression, thereby reducing the release of inflammatory cytokines. Statins also have important antioxidant effects through a variety of mechanisms. Interesting data also demonstrate the antithrombotic properties of statins through effects on platelet function, coagulation, and fibrinolysis. They also appear to improve endothelial function by enhancing the expression of constitutive endothelial nitric oxide, and by inhibiting apoptosis. Lastly, statins directly inhibit major histocompatibility complex (MHC) class II expression induced by interferon-γ (IFN-γ), thereby modifying T-cell activity. These multiple antiinflammatory properties may be responsible for the beneficial effects of statins observed in clinical trials in other inflammatory, immune-mediated diseases such as multiple sclerosis and rheumatoid arthritis (34).

No data from randomized trials of statins in sepsis are yet available, but observational studies support a potentially important preventive, and possibly, a treatment effect.

The largest study to date is a population-based cohort study involving the linked administrative databases in Ontario, Canada, and included a matched cohort of 69,168 patients (35). The incidence of sepsis was substantially lower among patients receiving statins (hazard ratio [HR], 0.81; 95% confidence interval [CI], 0.72–0.91). The protective association between statins and sepsis persisted in high-risk subgroups, including patients with diabetes mellitus, malignancy, and those receiving oral steroids. Significant reductions in severe sepsis (HR, 0.83; 95% CI, 0.70–0.97) and fatal sepsis (HR, 0.75; 95% CI, 0.61–0.93) were also observed.

Retrospective cohort data from two U.S. teaching hospitals provided information on 787 patients with a discharge diagnosis of pneumonia (36). Patients were deemed to be on a statin if it was noted to be prescribed at admission. The 30-day and 90-day mortality rates were 9.2% and 13.6%, respectively. After adjusting for confounders, including using propensity analysis (a statistical technique to ensure that patients in both groups are equally likely to be prescribed a particular intervention, in this instance a statin), statin use at presentation was associated with an odds ratio for death at 30 days of 0.36 (95% CI, 0.14–0.92).

However, not all the data regarding statin use point toward a benefit. In a more recent study, investigators assessed effects of statin treatment before or during intensive care unit admission in 438 patients ventilated for more than 96 hours (37). Although there was a trend toward lower rates of infection and delayed onset of infection in statin-treated patients, these did not reach statistical significance. Hospital mortality was higher in statin-treated patients (61% vs. 42%, $p = .03$).

While due to their observational nature the studies presented above suffer from selection bias and other confounders, taken together, these early data suggest that statins may contribute toward preventing sepsis and potentially have a role in the treatment of sepsis. Future studies in children appear warranted.

Endotoxin Removal

Enhancement of clearance of endotoxin to reduce plasma levels is the basis for the anecdotal use of extracorporeal methods of endotoxin removal. These methods include plasmapheresis, exchange transfusion, hemofiltration, and hemadsorption. Despite many anecdotal reports of the use of these methods (particularly plasmapheresis or blood exchange) in patients with sepsis, there have been no well-controlled studies, and only a small number of patients have been recruited to these studies (38–41). Despite the impression of clinical improvement following initiation of therapy in many reports, properly conducted studies are required to prove clinical efficacy.

Despite these caveats, there does appear to be benefit from high-volume hemofiltration in critically ill adults. A large study comparing volumes of filtration per hour in acute renal failure patients treated with venovenous hemofiltration (only about 10% of whom had sepsis) demonstrated a significantly higher survival rate in those patients treated with at least 35 mL/kg/h of filtration (42). However, a study of 30 patients (including eight children) with septic shock, 14 of whom were randomized to treatment by plasma exchange, showed no difference between the two groups (43).

A study of plasma or whole-blood exchange in meningococcal septicemia showed transient reduction in soluble TNF-α receptors, which rebounded following exchange. There was no influence on mortality (44).

High-permeability hemofiltration (HP-HF) is a new mode of renal replacement therapy designed to facilitate the elimination of cytokines in sepsis. A study to investigate the effects of HP-HF in patients with septic shock in 16 patients with sepsis-induced multiple organ failure used intermittent high permeability hemofiltration (iHP-HF; nominal cutoff point: 60 kd) (45). Intermittent HP-HF was performed over 5 days for 12 hours per day and alternated with conventional hemofiltration. Intermittent HP-HF proved to be safe with regard to cardiovascular hemodynamics and its impact on the coagulation status. However, high transmembrane protein losses occurred, and cumulative 12-hour protein loss was 7.60 g (interquartile range: 6.2–12.0). The filtration capacity for IL-6 was exceptionally high. The IL-6 sieving coefficient approximated 1 throughout the study period. However, the TNF-α elimination capacity was poor. High permeability hemofiltration is a new approach that facilitates the elimination of cytokines.

Further studies are needed to analyze whether HP-HF is able to positively impact the course of sepsis.

Extracorporeal adsorption apheresis for elimination of endotoxin from plasma is under investigation. Use of polymyxin B or human albumin coated cartridges has been studied in humans, demonstrating significant reduction in circulating endotoxin levels (46,47). In addition, other adsorbents such as DEAE-cellulose mats have been subjected to clinical trials. In one such study of 15 critically ill patients with sepsis, a significant reduction in plasma endotoxin levels from a median of 0.61 to 0.39 EU/mL (EU, endotoxin units) (−35%) was achieved ($p < .001$) (48). Long-term comparison of the initial and posttreatment levels after a series of five to six individual apheresis treatments also showed a statistically significant decline in circulating endotoxin, IL-6, C-reactive protein (CRP), and fibrinogen levels, and an increase in cholesterol levels. Thus extracorporeal endotoxin removal may prove a promising therapeutic tool for patients suffering from bacterial sepsis and proven endotoxemia.

Antiinflammatory and Anticytokine Therapies

Cytokines play a central role in the pathogenesis of sepsis. They coordinate a wide variety of inflammatory reactions at tissue level. They interact in a complex network in which they influence each other's production and activity. The cytokine network can be roughly divided into those with proinflammatory activity and those with antiinflammatory activity. Prominent proinflammatory cytokines are TNF-α and IL-1. Antiinflammatory cytokines, of which IL-10 is probably the best studied example, inhibit the synthesis of proinflammatory cytokines and exert several direct antiinflammatory effects on different cell types. The action of proinflammatory cytokines can be inhibited further by naturally occurring soluble inhibitors, such as soluble TNF receptor type I and type II, which inhibit TNF activity, and soluble IL-1 receptor type II and IL-1-receptor antagonist (IL-1ra), which both inhibit IL-1 activity.

The plasma concentrations of cytokines vary greatly in patients with sepsis. In general, proinflammatory cytokines can be detected in only a subset of patients, whereas antiinflammatory cytokines and soluble inhibitors can be seen in virtually all patients with sepsis and even in healthy individuals. It has been argued that those patients who fulfill the clinical criteria for SIRS may not have detectable levels of proinflammatory cytokines in their circulation because they are studied late in the septic process (49). This may explain why the cytokines TNF-α, IL-1β, IL-12, and IFN-γ, which according to animal models play a central role in the pathogenesis of septic shock, are not consistently correlated with disease severity or outcome in patients with septic shock.

The kinetics of cytokine release have been studied in models of sepsis and systemic inflammation, induced by intravenous administration of either live bacteria or bacterial products such as endotoxin. In these models TNF-α is the first cytokine to be detected in the circulation. Infusion of either a relatively low dose of endotoxin in healthy people or a lethal dose of live *Escherichia coli* in baboons results in transient release of TNF-α, peaking after 90 minutes. There is a close positive correlation between the size of the bacterial challenge and the extent of TNF-α release. Other proinflammatory cytokines, including IL-1b, are released shortly after the release of TNF-α, in conjunction with several antiinflammatory mediators, in particular IL-10, IL-1ra, and soluble TNF receptors (50).

In 1985, it was first recognized that TNF-α production has a central role in systemic toxicity elicited by endotoxin. Pretreatment with antiserum to TNF-α was seen to protect mice against the lethal effect of endotoxin (51). Further studies showed that a monoclonal antibody to TNF protected baboons against lethal gram-negative bacteremia (52). Since that time anti-TNF strategies have proved to be protective in many experimental sepsis models.

Neutralization of IL-1 activity, by administration of recombinant IL-1ra, was also seen to reduce mortality induced by endotoxin or living bacteria in animal models. Importantly, administration of recombinant TNF-α or IL-1 to laboratory animals can reproduce most of the characteristics of the sepsis syndrome, and TNF-α and IL-1 have synergistic toxicity in experimental models (53). These landmark studies formed the basis of the design of clinical trials that use agents to neutralize the activity of TNF-α and IL-1.

The cytokine IL-10 mainly produced by antigen presenting and T-helper cells is engaged predominantly in antiinflammatory activities, decreasing the production of proinflammatory cytokines and endotoxin toxicity in vivo. Neutralization of endogenously produced IL-10 in endotoxemic mice is associated with increased production of several proinflammatory cytokines, including TNF-α, and was shown to be associated with increased mortality. Interleukin-10 gene-deficient mice showed increased mortality after endotoxin administration, together with high concentrations of TNF-α, IL-1, and other inflammatory mediators (54).

On the basis of these discoveries, it is believed that the sepsis syndrome and SIRS were likely to result from an infection triggering an excessive inflammatory response. Multiple clinical trials looking at the use of antiinflammatory agents have been performed based on this hypothesis.

One of the cytokines most extensively examined as a target for antiinflammatory strategies is TNF-α. In multiple studies of therapies designed to neutralize or block the functions of TNF-α, there have been no statistically significant improvements in survival in the experimental cohorts; indeed, in at least one study, of a recombinant TNF receptor construct, mortality was actually higher in the group receiving the experimental agent compared with placebo (55). A meta-analysis of these trials suggested a small but significant benefit for anti–TNF-α agents overall (56).

Tumor necrosis factor-α is known to trigger the release of multiple cytokines including IL-6. Increased IL-6 levels are associated with poor outcome in septic patients and are known to correlate with severity of illness. Hence, it was postulated that IL-6 levels might be a useful marker for sensitivity to anti–TNF-α therapies. One large multicenter, placebo-controlled trial of a murine monoclonal antibody to human TNF-α, Afelimomab, randomized 2634 patients with severe sepsis to either a 3-day course of Afelimomab or placebo (57). The authors found that mortality in those who received Afelimomab was lower than placebo in the patients with elevated IL-6 levels (43.6% vs. 47.6%, $p = .21$). Using logistic regression analysis, treatment with Afelimomab was associated with an adjusted reduction in the risk of death by 5.8% ($p = .041$) and a corresponding reduction of relative risk of death of 11.9%. Compared with placebo, this monoclonal antibody resulted in a more rapid resolution of organ failure and significant reductions in both TNF-α and IL-6 levels.

Interleukin-6 is the cytokine most closely correlated with severity of cardiovascular dysfunction in children with meningococcal disease (58). Although murine models have shown some reduction in the immune response following LPS stimulus by a combination of anti–IL-6 and anti–IL-6 receptor, there have been no clinical trials to date.

Efforts to inhibit IL-1 activity by the use of recombinant IL-1ra have not been proven to reduce mortality in several clinical trials. In one study of recombinant human IL-1 receptor antagonist (rhIL-1ra) in the treatment of 696 adults with severe sepsis and septic shock, the study was terminated after an interim analysis found that it was unlikely that the primary efficacy end points would be met (59). The 28-day, all-cause mortality rate was 33.1% (116/350) in the rhIL-1ra treatment group, and 36.4% (126/346) in the placebo group, yielding a 9% reduction in mortality ($p = .36$) (60). This study confirmed the findings of an earlier study of 893 patients with sepsis syndrome, which also failed to demonstrate any benefit of IL-1ra in this group of patients.

It is unclear why there is a discrepancy between the protective benefit of antiinflammatory therapies in preclinical studies compared with the effect on septic patients in clinical trials. While the effects of proinflammatory cytokines in models of systemic inflammation are clearly deleterious, these models do not accurately reflect clinical sepsis in humans. In human sepsis, the infection usually disseminates from a local infectious source, such as the lung, abdomen, or urinary tract, and this is the primary site of cytokine production. This focus is absent in the models of systemic inflammation. It has been shown that this localized proinflammatory cytokine production is essential for host defense. Increased morbidity and mortality has been recorded following neutralization of endogenous TNF-α in a model of murine pneumonia (61). Conversely, following the elimination of IL-10, an antiinflammatory cytokine, there was improved survival of murine pneumonia and decreased bacterial load within the lungs (62). This apparently paradoxical role of cytokines in bacterial infections has been recognized in other severe bacterial infections. Endogenous TNF-α has a protective role in the pathogenesis of gram-negative peritonitis, and IL-10 gene-deficient mice given intraperitoneal *E. coli* showed reduced dissemination of the infection to distant organs (63). However, systemic inflammation was increased and there was a higher lethality of the *E. coli.*

The role of cytokines in various models of sepsis (endotoxin administration, pneumonia, peritonitis) is clearly very different. Proinflammatory cytokines are vital for host defense at the site of infection, but appear to be detrimental in systemic inflammation, causing tissue damage and harm. Equally, antiinflammatory cytokines seem to weaken local antibacterial defense, while diminishing the systemic toxicity created by bacteria. The balance between proinflammatory actions and compensatory antiinflammatory mediator activity restricts inflammation to local sites of injury, prevents significant systemic inflammatory responses, and minimizes the potential adverse effects of proinflammatory mediators on host tissue

The concept of blocking a single elevated cytokine and expecting to block human sepsis is likely to be too simplistic. As patients move through different phases of the septic response, there may be intervals when it is appropriate to inhibit multiple cytokines while at other times it may be appropriate to augment the immune response.

Immunoparalysis

In most patients with sepsis, induction of antiinflammatory pathways to inhibit excessive proinflammatory activity can be demonstrated. This has led to the concept of compensatory antiinflammatory response (CARS), following SIRS in the time course. For example, the plasma levels of soluble TNF-α receptors and soluble IL-1 receptor II and IL-1 receptor antagonist increase substantially during the septic process, probably reflecting an attempt by the host to limit inflammation caused by TNF-α and IL-1. Similarly, severe sepsis is associated with detectable serum IL-10 levels in 80% to 100% of patients (64). In addition, shortly after the onset of sepsis, a "refractory state" develops that is characterized by a relative inability of host inflammatory cells to respond to proinflammatory stimuli (such as endotoxin challenge) (65). The mechanisms for this state remain unclear, but this is likely to be a purposeful adaptation of the host.

This adaptation or hyporesponsiveness of immune cells has also been referred to as "immunoparalysis" and anergy. It is likely that the antiinflammatory cytokines, particularly IL-10 and transforming growth factor-β (TGF-β) are involved. Plasma from patients with sepsis was shown to significantly diminish the capacity of normal monocytes to secrete TNF-α (65). Other mediators released during the initial hyperinflammatory phase of sepsis that could contribute to the subsequent underresponsiveness of blood leukocytes include catecholamines, glucocorticoids, and prostaglandins.

It has been suggested that immunoparalysis could contribute to the increased susceptibility to nosocomial infections and late mortality demonstrated in patients who survive the acute septic episode. As a result, strategies aimed at restoring immune function have been developed and partially evaluated in patients with sepsis. Cytokines able to reverse monocyte deactivation in experimental models are IFN-γ and granulocyte-macrophage colony-stimulating factor (GM-CSF). One pilot study with recombinant IFN-γ was performed in sepsis patients who had demonstrable immunoparalysis, defined as the presence of <30% human leukocyte antigen (HLA)-DR–positive monocytes for at least 2 days (66). Nine patients were treated with daily subcutaneous injection of IFN-γ until >50% of their monocytes were HLA-DR positive for 3 consecutive days. The IFN-γ treatment restored TNF-α production capacity of monocytes and was not associated with adverse effects. Although the efficacy of IFN-γ could not be established in this small uncontrolled study, eight patients recovered from sepsis shortly after treatment.

In a study of 60 infants with neutropenia and clinical signs of sepsis, daily subcutaneous injection of recombinant human GM-CSF for 7 consecutive days was associated with an increase in neutrophil count and a reduction in mortality (3/30 in the GM-CSF group vs. 9/30 in the control group) (67). Further studies are needed to assess the effects of immune stimulation in sepsis in general.

Intravenous Immunoglobulin

Intravenous immunoglobulin (IVIG) can be regarded as a treatment method that seeks to augment the host's immune responses. Intravenous immunoglobulin has sometimes been used in the treatment of severe sepsis. However, although plasma immunoglobulin concentration may be reduced in patients with sepsis, the use of IVIG as therapy is not supported by large randomized clinical trials. However, no individual well-designed trial has been undertaken in adults or children with sepsis. A small nonblinded study in 21 patients with streptococcal toxic-shock syndrome showed a reduced mortality (6% vs. 34%, p = .02) (68). Additionally, a meta-analysis has suggested that IVIG could be beneficial in sepsis, although even in this analysis patient numbers were low (69).

Corticosteroids

Since the 1960s there have been attempts to modulate the sepsis-induced inflammatory response with corticosteroids, given at pharmacologic doses. Numerous studies failed to show a beneficial effect of glucocorticoids in patients with sepsis, and this lack of efficacy was confirmed in several meta-analyses (70,71). However, recent investigations have indicated that glucocorticoids given in more physiologic doses could be beneficial to patients with septic shock.

Adrenal failure is common in critical illness and in particular in vasopressor-dependent septic shock. High baseline total serum cortisol together with a low response to a corticotropin-stimulation test (<9 µg/dL cortisol increase 60 minutes after 0.25 mg of corticotropin) is correlated with a poor outcome in sepsis (72).

Several studies in children and adults with septic shock have demonstrated abnormalities of control of adrenal corticosteroid secretion over the course of illness (73–75). Although it is rare to have severe adrenal insufficiency on presentation, a relative deficiency of adrenal steroid secretory function has been demonstrated in sepsis, often associated with resistance to high doses of inotropes, suggesting that replacement doses of corticosteroids may be beneficial in some patients with refractory shock.

Several studies have examined the effects of glucocorticoids given at physiologic doses that induce few or no immunosuppressive effects and have been limited to patients with septic shock requiring vasopressor. Especially promising was a study conducted by Annane et al. (76). This controlled study investigated the efficacy of stress-dose hydrocortisone (50 mg every 6 hours) plus 50 mg of fludrocortisone daily for 7 days in 299 adult patients who had septic shock for <8 hours. The target population included patients with an inadequate response in serum cortisol after adrenocorticotropic hormone stimulation. A 30% relative reduction in mortality was seen in patients treated with corticoids compared with placebo.

Various randomized controlled trials comparing hydrocortisone to placebo have been performed in septic shock. However, all these studies are not comparable, because despite using roughly similar inclusion criteria, they differ regarding the total daily dose, total duration, and weaning methods of hydrocortisone administration. However, there is general agreement that hydrocortisone supplementation improves the hemodynamic condition of vasopressor-dependent septic shock (77). Shock reversal is hastened, vasopressor needs are reduced more rapidly, and this benefit is observed whatever the duration of shock before hydrocortisone is instituted.

A strategy that would maximize benefit while minimizing potential toxicity or unnecessary treatment would include the use of low-dose corticosteroids (<1 mg/kg given every 6 to 8 hours) in children with septic shock. Corticosteroids should probably be given for 1 week from onset of shock, defined by the need of vasopressors. Corticosteroid administration should be preceded by an acute adrenocorticotropic hormone (ACTH) test. When the results of the test are available (preferably within a few hours), treatment should be continued only in patients with corticosteroid insufficiency defined by a random cortisol of 15 µg/dL or less, a peak cortisol of 20 µg/dL or less, or a cortisol increment of 9 µg/dL or less.

What remains more difficult to define is adrenal insufficiency, the optimal dose and timing of corticosteroid supplementation, whether this should then be tapered slowly, and the impact of corticosteroid supplementation on outcome. Several studies are ongoing in an attempt to answer these important questions in both adults and children.

Although no study has yet evaluated the efficacy of low-dose corticosteroids in children with sepsis, well-designed trials conducted in children with bacterial meningitis, many of whom had bacteremia when enrolled, have shown that early administration of *high-dose* dexamethasone is associated with significant reduction in hemodynamic instability in the 6 hours after initiation of steroid and antibiotic therapy (78).

Agents Affecting Arachidonic Acid Metabolism

Products of the cyclooxygenase and lipooxygenase pathways of arachidonic acid metabolism include leukotrienes, prostaglandins, and thromboxane. They appear to play a major role in causing vasodilatation and platelet aggregation, membrane lysis, and increased capillary permeability, which are the hallmarks of SIRS and shock. Agents that interfere with these pathways have been suggested as treatments for sepsis.

In a large randomized study using ibuprofen in 455 patients with sepsis, ibuprofen reduced prostacyclin and thromboxane levels and decreased fever, tachycardia, oxygen consumption, and lactic acidosis, but it did not prevent the development of shock or ARDS, or improve survival (79). A later study that examined the effects of ibuprofen on the physiology and survival of hypothermic patients with sepsis revealed a significant reduction in the 30-day mortality from 90% (18 of 20 placebo-treated patients) to 54% (13 of 24 ibuprofen-treated patients). Compared with febrile patients, the hypothermic group had exaggerated response of cytokines TNF-α and IL-6 and of the lipid mediators thromboxane and prostacyclin (80).

There is increasing evidence that cyclooxygenase (COX)-2 is involved in the endothelial dysregulation of sepsis. There is some recent evidence that COX inhibition may be beneficial in animal models of sepsis (81).

Pentoxifylline

Pentoxifylline, a xanthine derivative and a phosphodiesterase inhibitor, has been shown to have numerous potential beneficial effects in human and animal experimental models of sepsis. Pentoxifylline suppresses production of inflammatory mediators such as TNF-α. In adults and neonates it has been shown to decrease TNF-α, IL-1, and IL-10, but not IL-6 or IL-8 (82,83). Pentoxifylline delays the release of endothelin-1, abolishes TNF burst, and suppresses IL-6 and lactate, while improving survival from abdominal sepsis in rats. Pentoxifylline also augments hemodynamic performance during sepsis, and has been shown to prevent endothelial cell dysfunction; preserve endothelial thrombomodulin, protein C, and the protein S anticoagulant system; stimulate fibrinolysis associated with the increased release of tissue plasminogen activator; enhance prostacyclin release; and attenuate the release of thromboxane. These biologic and cellular effects of pentoxifylline have been attributed to the inhibition of cellular phosphodiesterase, with resultant increase in cyclic adenosine monophosphate (cAMP) concentration. Therefore, the numerous potential beneficial effects make pentoxifylline an interesting modality for the treatment of sepsis. No significant adverse effects have been reported.

There are few human controlled studies. A study in surgical patients with severe sepsis showed an improvement in organ dysfunction score in patients receiving pentoxifylline compared with placebo, but was too small to show any change in mortality (84). Two studies have been performed in neonates, which have included 107 infants (85,86). There was a significant reduction in all-cause mortality during hospital stay in neonates with sepsis who received pentoxifylline as an adjunct to antibiotics, compared to those who received placebo (relative risk [RR], 0.14; 95% CI, 0.03–0.76). The results from these two studies showed a statistically significant reduction in mortality and a trend toward earlier correction of metabolic and hemodynamic derangements in preterm neonates with confirmed late-onset sepsis. However, because of methodologic weaknesses of these studies, routine use of pentoxifylline cannot be recommended on the available data.

Anticoagulant Therapies

Abnormality in the regulation of coagulant pathways are almost universally demonstrated in patients with sepsis. These abnormalities can vary from subclinical alterations in clotting times to full-blown disseminated intravascular coagulation (DIC).

Tissue Factor Pathway Inhibitor

Tissue factor (thromboplastin) is a transmembrane cell surface receptor for plasma clotting factor VII, and exhibits homology with the cytokine-receptor family. It is a major initiator of coagulation. Tissue factor pathway inhibitor (TFPI) is an endogenous serine protease inhibitor, synthesized and secreted by endothelial cells, that inhibits factor Xa directly, and the factor VIIa/tissue factor catalytic complex in a Xa-dependent fashion. A significant portion of endogenous TFPI is bound to the microvasculature through low-affinity binding to glycosaminoglycans. This pool of TFPI is releasable into the circulation by exposure to heparin. A small pool of TFPI is stored in platelets and secreted on activation and degranulation. Most circulating TFPI is bound to lipoproteins. The circulating concentration of TFPI varies widely in healthy volunteers and in patients with sepsis. The functional properties of circulating TFPI are not well delineated.

Endothelial dysfunction is common, as shown by the presence of coagulation abnormalities in most septic patients. It has been suggested that TFPI may protect the endothelium from coagulation and sepsis-induced injury. This is supported by preclinical studies in which exogenous TFPI improved outcome in septic animals (87). Importantly, inhibition of tissue factor by either tissue-factor-antibody treatment or infusion of TFPI not only abrogated DIC in primates with bacteremia, but also prevented death. However, in the same sepsis model, intervention further downstream in the coagulation cascade by infusion of site-inactivated factor Xa did not alter survival despite complete protection against DIC (88). Thus, tissue factor may exert its effects on inflammatory mechanisms distinct from its effect on coagulation.

There have been several phase I and II studies that have examined recombinant TFPI in patients with sepsis. In the first study, a greater than expected effect on prothrombin time was seen in three patients receiving TFPI, which was associated with an increase in serious bleeding adverse events. Therefore, in subsequent studies, lower TFPI doses were given. A phase II study comparing placebo with 0.025 or 0.05 mg/kg/h TFPI in patients with severe sepsis showed no difference with respect to adverse effects between treatment arms, and a trend toward a reduced mortality in TFPI-treated patients (89).

In view of these data, a phase III randomized, double-blind, placebo-controlled, multicenter study evaluated the safety and efficacy of recombinant TFPI in 1754 adult patients with severe sepsis. The main outcome measure was all-cause 28-day mortality. There was no overall effect on 28-day mortality (rTFPI group, 34.2% vs. placebo group, 33.9%; $p = .88$) (90).

Antithrombin

Antithrombin is another anticoagulant protein that inhibits a number of clotting factors, including thrombin and factors IXa and Xa. Antithrombin also inhibits the activity of products of the contact system, such as factors XIa and XIIa, and kallikrein. Antithrombin also has antiinflammatory properties: it appears to modulate the inflammatory response by binding to the endothelium via cell-surface heparin-sulfate proteoglycans and may promote the release of prostacyclin. The antiinflammatory effects of antithrombin are only seen at supraphysiologic concentrations and in the absence of heparin. In animal models of sepsis, antithrombin therapy is protective against lethality and organ failure (91).

There have been several studies of the use of antithrombin in human sepsis that suggest that antithrombin therapy could be beneficial. In one study, continuous long-term antithrombin infusion was seen to attenuate SIRS, as indicated by reduction in the plasma concentrations of IL-6, soluble endothelial adhesion molecules, and diminished CRP response (92).

A randomized, prospective, placebo-controlled phase III multicenter clinical trial (KyberSept) was performed to test the efficacy of high-dose antithrombin therapy in patients with severe sepsis, and specifically examined patients concomitantly treated with heparin for deep venous thrombosis prophylaxis (93). From 2314 patients with severe sepsis (1157 placebo and 1157 antithrombin subjects each), 1616 patients (811 placebo and 805 antithrombin subjects) received heparin concomitantly with study drug (antithrombin 30,000 IU) over 4 days, whereas 698 patients (346 placebo and 352 antithrombin) did not. In patients who did not receive heparin, 28-day mortality was reduced in the antithrombin group compared with placebo (37.8% vs. 43.6%; absolute reduction: 5.8%; risk ratio: 0.860 [0.725–1.019]), which increased to day 90 (44.9% vs. 52.5%; absolute reduction: 7.6%; risk ratio: 0.851 [0.735–0.987]). In patients who did receive concomitant heparin, no effect of antithrombin on mortality was seen (28-day mortality: 39.4% vs. 36.6%; absolute increase: 2.8%; risk ratio: 1.08 [0.96–1.22]). The conclusions of this study were that treatment with high-dose antithrombin III may increase survival time up to 90 days in patients with severe sepsis and high risk of death. This benefit may even be stronger when concomitant heparin is avoided.

Despite this large study, which failed to show an overall beneficial effect of antithrombin treatment in septic patients, it is conceivable that antithrombin may be of benefit to subsets of patients with sepsis, in particular those who do not concurrently receive heparin, which appears to neutralize the effect of antithrombin.

Activated Protein C

Activated protein C (aPC) proteolytically inactivates clotting factors Va and VIIIa and thus is a natural anticoagulant. aPC is generated after an interaction of protein C with thrombin, when the thrombin/protein C complex binds to the endothelial cell-surface protein thrombomodulin (TM) and the endothelial protein C receptor (EPCR). aPC function is dependent on a circulating cofactor, protein S. aPC activity is impaired during sepsis as a result of increased consumption of protein S and protein C, decreased activation of protein C by downregulation of TM on endothelial cells and reduced expression of EPCR. Furthermore, protein S bioavailability is reduced by its binding to the acute-phase protein C4b-binding protein.

The hypothesis that aPC could be beneficial in sepsis is based on a number of preclinical observations. Infusion of aPC into septic baboons prevented hypercoagulability and death, whereas inhibition of endogenous protein C activation by a monoclonal antibody exacerbated the response to *E. coli* infusion, and converted a sublethal model into a severe-shock response associated with DIC and death (94). This monoclonal antibody prevented protein C from binding to the EPCR, thereby reducing protein C activation by the thrombin–TM complex (95). Hence, similar to the tissue factor–VIIa mediated pathway, the protein C pathway appears to have other effects on host response apart from its role in coagulation. The presence of EPCR is reduced in children with meningococcal sepsis, thus confirming that regulation of activation of the protein C pathway is disordered in acute sepsis in humans (96).

One mechanism that could contribute to the antiinflammatory properties of the protein C pathway system, is the capacity of protein C and protein S to inhibit endotoxin-induced production of TNF-α, IL-1, and IL-6 by monocytes in vitro, and the ability of aPC to reduce TNF-α release during endotoxemia in rats. Other antiinflammatory effects of aPC include inhibition of the interaction of monocytes and neutrophils with injured endothelium, and an increase in fibrinolysis by inhibiting the acute-phase protein inhibitor of plasmin generation, plasminogen-activator inhibitor type-1 (PAI-1) (97).

A large multicenter placebo-controlled trial on the efficacy of recombinant human aPC in 1690 patients with severe sepsis has been published (98). This was the first study of an adjunctive therapy for sepsis in more than 20 years to show a positive effect on 28-day all-cause mortality. The trial was designed to enroll 2280 patients but was stopped prematurely at the second planned interim analysis because the efficacy criteria were met. aPC was shown to significantly reduce mortality from 30.8% in the placebo group to 24.7% in the treatment group ($p = .005$), an absolute reduction in the risk of death of 6.1%. However, the incidence of serious bleeding was higher in aPC-treated patients (3.5% vs. 2.0%, $p = .06$). aPC infusion was also associated with a reduction in plasma D-dimer concentrations, evidence that aPC attenuated the procoagulant response. aPC also reduced plasma IL-6 concentrations, indicating inhibition of inflammatory responses.

On the basis of these results, aPC therapy is now recommended by the Surviving Sepsis Campaign for adult patients with severe sepsis and organ failure within 24 hours of admission and who do not have increased risk for bleeding (99). The efficacy of aPC has not been demonstrated in patients with severe sepsis but a lower risk of death (i.e., patients with single organ failure or an Acute Physiology and Chronic Health Evaluation [APACHE-2] score of <25) (100). In this study of over 2600 adults the absence of a beneficial treatment effect, coupled with an increased incidence of serious bleeding complications, indicated that aPC should not be used in patients with severe sepsis who are at low risk of death, and the safety of aPC in patients who are at increased risk of bleeding is being assessed in further studies.

Following the report of its benefit in adults at high risk of death, a large phase III randomized, placebo-controlled study of aPC has been performed in children with severe sepsis. This study was stopped following the second planned interim analysis of the data because of safety concerns in young infants and the likelihood that it would not achieve its primary end point of reduction in duration of organ failure. Despite enrolling 477 children with severe sepsis, this study failed to demonstrate any benefit in the primary end point or any of the secondary end points (including 28-day mortality). In addition, there were significant concerns regarding potentially deleterious effects in children under 60 days of age who appeared to have an increased risk of hemorrhagic complications (2).

Despite clear evidence of benefit of aPC in adults with severe sepsis and high risk of death, there is as yet no evidence of benefit in children, and therefore the use of aPC in children is currently not recommended.

Plasminogen Activator Inhibitor and Tissue Plasminogen

The finding of a direct relationship between PAI-1 levels and mortality in meningococcal disease has led to the proposed use of fibrinolytic therapy for meningococcal disease complicated by purpura fulminans (101). There have been anecdotal reports of the successful use of tissue plasminogen activator tissue plasminogen activator (t-PA) in this condition (102). Understandably, there are concerns regarding the potential for catastrophic bleeding in patients with an acquired hemorrhagic diathesis. A review of the use of t-PA as rescue therapy in children with meningococcal disease has demonstrated an unacceptable level of adverse events including fatal intracranial hemorrhage (103).

A study in mice treated with an inhibitor of PAI-1 demonstrated beneficial effects on mortality in LPS-exposed mice (104). This may be a future direction for research as it is likely not to be associated with the hemorrhagic complications of fibrinolytic therapy. Because of the recognized interactions between inflammation and coagulation, manipulation of the coagulation cascade would appear to be an attractive target for new therapies.

Therapies Targeting the Endothelium

Endothelial dysfunction appears to be the central pathologic feature of severe sepsis. This is the main target organ of injury affected by the multiple inflammatory mediators defined above, and the processes causing upregulation of the coagulation and complement systems. Attempts to restore endothelial function by interventions to reduce endothelial cell injury and dysfunction are discussed below.

Platelet-Activating Factor

Platelet-activating factor (PAF) is a phospholipid produced by macrophages, neutrophils, platelets, and endothelial cells. Platelet-activating factor increases cell adhesion, activates endothelial cells, and amplifies release of cytokine mediators. A phase II placebo-controlled study of the PAF receptor antagonist BB-882 was performed in 152 patients with severe infection, which showed that there was no effect on hemodynamic, respiratory, or oxygen transport variables, or mortality (105). However, another study of TCV-309, a different PAF antagonist, in 98 patients with septic shock revealed a substantial reduction in organ dysfunction and morbidity, although there was no reduction in mortality (106). In a further study of a different PAF receptor blocker (BN52021) in 609 patients with severe sepsis, mortality was 50% in the placebo group and 44% in the treatment group ($p = .29$) (107).

Platelet-activating factor acetylhydrolase (PAF-AH) is a member of the phospholipase A_2 family of enzymes. The extracellular form of PAF-AH is a plasma protein that inactivates PAF and other oxidized phospholipids with PAF-like effects (108). The therapeutic rationale for the administration of rPAF-AH in severe sepsis is to increase PAF-AH activity in the presence of generalized inflammation and coagulation. The therapeutic potential for this strategy was supported by the results from a Phase II trial of rPAF-AH in 127 patients with severe sepsis (109). This study showed that 28-day all-cause mortality was 21% in the 1.0 mg/kg rPAF-AH group, 28% in the 5.0 mg/kg rPAF-AH group, and 44% in the placebo group ($p = .07$; 1.0 mg/kg rPAF-AH vs. placebo, $p = .03$). A trend toward reduced multiple organ dysfunction also was observed in the 1.0 mg/kg rPAF-AH group compared with placebo ($p = .11$).

Following this, a phase III study was undertaken in patients with severe sepsis (110); 2522 patients were planned to be enrolled in a prospective, randomized, double-blind, placebo controlled, multicenter trial. Eligible patients were randomized to receive either rPAF-AH 1.0 mg/kg or placebo. The study was terminated after the second planned interim analysis, following the enrollment of 1261 patients (618 placebo and 643 rPAF-AH subjects). The study showed no improvement in 28-day all-cause mortality in the rPAF-AH group compared with placebo (25% for rPAF-AH vs. 24% for placebo; 95% CI, 0.85–1.25; $p = .80$). There were no statistically significant differences between treatment groups in any of the secondary efficacy end points.

One confounding factor from these data was that plasma levels of PAF-AH changed during the course of disease, with higher levels in survivors without organ failure compared to those who died, and higher levels still in those with severe septic shock and multiple organ failure, suggesting that higher levels may not be good, but that dynamic changes may be more important than absolute levels (111).

Neutrophil/Endothelial Cell Interactions

Many of the proinflammatory mediators stimulate adhesion molecule expression on leukocytes, platelets, and endothelial cells. It is likely that the adhesion of activated neutrophils to endothelial cells is implicated in the tissue injury and multiple organ dysfunction that occurs during sepsis (112). Patients with inherited abnormalities of adhesion molecules have recurrent, severe infections typically characterized by a marked leukocytosis, and may develop systemic sepsis and septic shock (113). This highlights the important role these molecules have in host defense. While there is in vitro data suggesting the importance of these interactions in experimental sepsis, the inhibition of adhesion molecules in animal studies of sepsis have shown variable effects (114).

Nitric Oxide

Activation of the inflammatory response results in elaboration of a number of mediators with direct effects on vasomotor tone. Nitric oxide (NO), bradykinin, histamine, and prostacyclin (PGI_2) can all decrease vascular tone and cause vasodilatation and subsequent hypotension.

Nitric oxide is formed by the enzymatic action of NO synthase (NOS) on the guanidino group of the amino acid L-arginine (115). The inducible isoform of NOS (iNOS) is produced in response to endotoxin, platelet-activating factor (PAF), IL-1β, and TNF-α. Glucocorticoids, IL-1ra, PAF antagonists, TNF-α, tyrosine kinase inhibitors, and dihydropyridine calcium-channel blockers inhibit iNOS induction (116).

Nitric oxide is a highly diffusible compound that activates soluble guanylate cyclase in smooth muscle cells. This converts guanosine triphosphate (GTP) to cyclic guanosine monophosphate (cGMP), which relaxes the smooth muscle cell by promoting calcium entry into the sarcoplasmic reticulum (117). It appears that iNOS is the predominant source of excessive NO production responsible for the hypotension and refractory vasodilatation frequently observed in septic shock.

Normally, vasomotor tone is tightly regulated by NO generation from vascular endothelial cells being rapidly inhibited by binding to circulating hemoglobin in red blood cells.

The increased NO resulting from iNOS induction may contribute to the myocardial depression and α-adrenergic hyporesponsiveness associated with sepsis. The NO-induced production of cGMP in cardiac myocytes inhibits the α-adrenergic–stimulated increase in the slow calcium channel and decreases the affinity of calcium for the contractile apparatus. This results in a negative inotropic effect and increases the relaxation phase of the cardiac cycle (118). The implication of NO in the vascular hyporesponsiveness and cardiac depression of sepsis supports the hypothesis that blockage or reduction of NO production will produce clinical benefit in patients with sepsis.

The role of iNOS and cGMP in the vasculopathy of septic shock have been supported by the finding that competitive NOS inhibitors, such as L-N-monomethyl arginine (L-NMMA) and N(G)-nitro-L-arginine methyl ester (L-NAME), act as vasopressors when administered to patients with septic shock (119,120).

There are many animal models of sepsis in which inhibitors of NO production have demonstrated potential benefit as well as potentially harmful effects. It has become clear, however, that nonspecific NOS inhibitors cause detrimental effects secondary to reduced organ perfusion, elevation of pulmonary artery pressure, and increased renal vascular resistance (121,122). This is likely to be due to inhibition of baseline NO production, which is essential for baseline control of organ perfusion under normal circumstances. In addition, there is evidence of increased capillary permeability and intestinal damage associated with L-NMMA after endotoxin challenge, together with a decrease in cardiac index and tissue oxygen delivery (116).

Therefore, animal studies have determined that reduction of NO activity is associated with the potential benefit of improvement of hypotension and vasodilatation, but at the expense of reduction of cardiac output and tissue oxygen delivery and with an increase in pulmonary vascular resistance and subsequent mortality.

Despite these major concerns, several human studies have been carried out. These have shown similar effects to those demonstrated in animal models (120,123). In addition, concerns have been raised over activation of intravascular coagulation (124).

Despite these major concerns, the potential benefits of shock reversal has led to several clinical studies of nitric oxide antagonists in adults with septic shock. A phase II multicentered, randomized, placebo-controlled, safety and efficacy study of the nitric oxide synthase inhibitor 546C88 (N(G)-methyl-L-arginine hydrochloride) was performed in patients with septic shock (125). The predefined primary end point was resolution of shock; 312 patients with septic shock were enrolled in this trial. There was an early increase in systemic and pulmonary vascular tone and oxygen extraction, whereas both cardiac index and oxygen delivery decreased for patients in the 546C88 cohort. Although these parameters subsequently returned toward baseline values, the observed differences between the treatment groups, except for pulmonary vascular resistance and oxygen extraction, persisted throughout the treatment period, despite a reduced requirement for vasopressors in the treatment cohort. These changes were associated with a reduction in plasma nitrate concentrations, which were elevated in both groups before the start of therapy. The conclusion of this study was that this nonselective NOS inhibitor can reduce the elevated plasma nitrate concentrations observed in patients with septic shock. But treatment was also associated with an increase in vascular tone and a reduction in both cardiac index and oxygen delivery. There were no substantive adverse effects demonstrated.

Following this study, an international, randomized, double-blind, placebo-controlled phase III study to assess the safety and efficacy of 546C88 was conducted in adult patients with septic shock (126). The primary end point was survival at day 28. A total of 797 patients with septic shock diagnosed for <24 hours were recruited. The trial was stopped early after review by the independent data safety monitoring board. The 28-day mortality was 59% (259/439) in the 546C88 group and 49% (174/358) in the placebo group ($p < .001$). The overall incidence of adverse events was similar in both groups, although a higher proportion of the events were considered to be possibly attributable to study drug. Most of the adverse events accounting for the disparity between the groups were associated with cardiovascular effects (e.g., decreased cardiac output, pulmonary hypertension, systemic arterial hypertension, and heart failure). The causes of death in the study were consistent with those expected in patients with septic shock, although there was a higher proportion of cardiovascular deaths and a lower incidence of deaths caused by multiple organ failure in the 546C88 group. In this study, the nonselective nitric oxide synthase inhibitor 546C88 increased mortality in patients with septic shock.

The recent development of selective iNOS inhibitors such as S-methylisothiourea (SMT) and transforming growth factor-β (TGF-β), which inhibit iNOS messenger RNA (mRNA), and their application in animal models of septic shock suggest that these agents may offer the benefits of reduced NO production due to iNOS inhibition, without the adverse effects of nonselective NOS inhibition (127,128).

Future Considerations

The most exciting new development in sepsis research in the past years is the discovery of Toll-like receptors (TLRs) as signal-transducing elements detecting multiple antigens, and the rapidly unfolding picture of TLRs as essential players in the innate immune response to infection (129).

On first encounter with a pathogen, the innate immune system can distinguish between different classes of pathogenic bacteria, viruses, and fungi. Additionally, it has become evident that the innate immune response is also vital for activating the slower acting adaptive immune system. The innate immune system can recognize conserved motifs on pathogens that are not seen on higher eukaryotes. These motifs have been referred to as pathogen-associated molecular patterns (PAMPs), whereas their binding partners on immunocompetent cells have been termed pattern-recognition receptors.

Endotoxin interacts with cells via the pattern recognition receptor CD14. Spontaneous binding of endotoxin to CD14 happens at very slow rates. Lipopolysaccharide-CD14 binding is greatly accelerated in the presence of LBP, an acute-phase reactant mainly derived from the liver. CD14 does not have an intracellular domain; cells respond to endotoxin via signaling through TLR4, which needs the presence of a secreted protein, MD-2; TLR2 in turn is essential for signaling the proinflammatory effects of the bacterial lipoproteins, peptidoglycan and zymosan, whereas TLR5 mediates cellular effects induced by bacterial flagellin, and TLR9 mediates effects induced by unmethylated CpG-containing oligonucleotides present in bacterial (but not eukaryotic) DNA. Different members of the TLR family can act together in activating cells in response to pathogens; for example, TLR2 and TLR6 cooperate in detecting certain bacterial components including peptidoglycan (130). The in vivo relevance of induction of an effective innate immune response to infection has been shown with specific-TLR-deficient mice. TLR2-knockout mice are highly susceptible to gram-positive infection, whereas TLR4-knockout mice have reduced resistance to gram-negative infection (131).

Designing methods to neutralize microbial products or block their interaction with specific receptors on immune cells is an attractive concept. Potential targets include LBP, CD14, TLR4, and MD-2 for gram-negative sepsis, and CD14, TLR2, and TLR6 for gram-positive sepsis. Monoclonal antibodies against CD14 have been evaluated in a phase I study (132): 16 healthy subjects received an intravenous injection of LPS (4 ng/kg) preceded by IC14, a recombinant chimeric monoclonal antibody against human CD14. IC14 attenuated LPS-induced clinical symptoms and strongly inhibited LPS-induced proinflammatory cytokine release, while delaying the release of soluble TNF receptor type I and IL-1ra. IC14 also inhibited leukocyte activation, but more modestly reduced endothelial cell activation and the acute-phase response. The capacity of circulating monocytes and granulocytes to phagocytose *E. coli* was only marginally reduced after infusion of IC14. These data provided the first proof that blockade of CD14 is associated with reduced LPS responsiveness in humans in vivo.

A further phase I study was performed in patients with septic shock (133). This study was performed to evaluate the safety, pharmacokinetics, pharmacodynamics, and clinical pharmacology of IC14 in a randomized, double-blind, placebo-controlled, dose-ranging study in 46 patients with severe sepsis. IC14 did not induce antibody formation or increase the incidence of secondary bacterial infection. The pattern of pro- and antiinflammatory cytokines, chemokine, soluble receptor, soluble E-selectin, and acute-phase proteins in response to treatment was highly variable. The results suggested that CD14 blockade with IC14 warrants further clinical investigation to determine its ability to attenuate the proinflammatory response due to infection.

Another interesting mediator is high mobility group (HMG)-1, a protein previously known as DNA-binding protein, which regulates gene transcription and stabilizes nucleosome formation. It has recently been described as a "late" mediator of endotoxin toxicity. Importantly, postponed administration of antibodies against HMG-1 reduced endotoxin-induced lethality, whereas administration of HMG-1 was lethal (134). Furthermore, patients with sepsis have raised concentrations of HMG-1 in their circulation. These first data are promising and warrant further investigation into HMG-1 as a potential therapeutic target.

Macrophage migration inhibitory factor (MIF) is a cytokine that has been shown to be important in innate immunity and sepsis (135). It is constitutively expressed in large amounts by immune, endocrine, and epithelial cells, and is released after exposure to microbial products and proinflammatory cytokines. Macrophage MIF has been shown to regulate innate immune responses to endotoxin and gram-negative bacteria by modulating the expression of TLR4

(136). High levels of macrophage MIF have been detected in patients with severe sepsis and septic shock (137).

Immunoneutralization of macrophage MIF or deletion of the *Mif* gene protects mice against lethal endotoxemia, gram-positive toxic shock syndromes, and experimental bacterial peritonitis. Conversely, mice injected with macrophage MIF together with live bacteria or microbial toxins have increased mortality (137,138). Migration inhibitory factor has been recently described as a predictor of poor outcome in sepsis, and efforts to modulate its production or action may be important as therapeutic modalities for sepsis (139).

Conclusion

The publication of the human genome will lead to massive advances in genomics and proteomics in the coming decade. The possibilities for individualized drug treatment of patients with sepsis, related to their genotype, will become reality. New technology may soon allow bedside testing of patient's genotypes or determination of protein or peptide biomarkers associated with poor outcome, to allow targeted therapy of even the sickest patient.

It is probable that many new agents will be shortly developed based on the unraveling of the host/pathogen interaction. However, until this time we must utilize currently available therapies to the best of our knowledge. Despite huge advances, our treatment of sepsis is still dependent on administration of appropriate antibiotics, intravenous fluid support, and relatively crude methods of organ support. We can only improve upon current treatment of pediatric sepsis *after* there is agreement that properly conducted multicenter clinical trials can and must be carried out in critically ill children in order to test new therapies. To reach this goal, we should model pediatric sepsis trials after the successful clinical trail program that has so greatly improved survival of childhood cancer.

There have only been three large properly controlled phase III studies in children with sepsis, none of which has recruited adequate numbers to definitively determine efficacy. Although these and all the many adult studies except one have failed to demonstrate a significant survival advantage, there is much that can be learned from these unsuccessful studies that is relevant to the design of future sepsis trials. There is no obvious reason why all children with severe sepsis and shock should not be enrolled in a double-blind, placebo-controlled study to evaluate new treatments. These studies should be large enough to minimize random error and avoid type II error (or false-negative results). Definitions for the target population should be explicit, reproducible, and include illness severity scores (8). Protocols for both the use of the investigational agent, and conventional treatment should be standardized. Outcomes should be clinically relevant and predefined, and should include measures of both benefit and harm (8). In addition, the analysis of results should be carried out, both on evaluable patients and on the intent-to-treat population. Finally, a health-economic evaluation of the implications of the introduction of ever-increasingly expensive therapies should be mandatory. Only in this way will we be likely to further influence the unacceptably high mortality rate of severe sepsis in children, with the added advantage of limiting the widespread use of extremely expensive new therapies that have been insufficiently evaluated.

References

1. Booy R, Habibi P, Nadel S, et al. Reduction in case fatality rate from meningococcal disease associated with improved healthcare delivery. Arch Dis Child 2001;85: 386–390.
2. Nadel S, Goldstein B, Williams MW, et al. Drotrecogin alfa (activated) in children with severe sepsis: a multicentre phase III randomised controlled trial. Lancet 2007; 369:836–843.
3. Stiehm ER, Damrosch DS. Factors in the prognosis of meningococcal infection. Review of 63 cases with emphasis on recognition and management of the severely ill patient. J Pediatr 1966;68:457–467.
4. Watson RS, Carcillo JA, Linde-Zwirble WT, Clermont G, Lidicker J, Angus DC. The epidemiology of severe sepsis in children in the United States. Am J Respir Crit Care Med 2003;167:695–701.
5. Goldstein B, Giroir B, Randolph A. International pediatric sepsis consensus conference: definitions for sepsis and organ dysfunction in pediatrics. Pediatr Crit Care Med 2005;6(1):2–8.
6. Beutler B, Poltorak A. Sepsis and evolution of the innate immune response. Crit Care Med 2001;29(7 suppl):S2–6; discussion S6–7.
7. Aird WC. Vascular bed-specific hemostasis: role of endothelium in sepsis pathogenesis. Crit Care Med 2001;29(7 suppl):S28–34; discussion S34–35.
8. Marshall JC, Vincent JL, Fink MP, et al. Measures, markers, and mediators: toward a staging system for clinical sepsis. A report of the Fifth Toronto Sepsis Roundtable, Toronto, Ontario, Canada, October 25–26, 2000. Crit Care Med 2003;31(5): 1560–1567.
9. Bonsu BK, Chb M, Harper MB. Identifying febrile young infants with bacteremia: is the peripheral white blood cell count an accurate screen? Ann Emerg Med 2003;42(2):216–225.
10. Meisner M. Biomarkers of sepsis: clinically useful? Curr Opin Crit Care 2005;11(5):473–480.
11. Stryjewski GR, Nylen ES, Bell MJ, et al. Interleukin-6, interleukin-8, and a rapid and sensitive assay for calcitonin precursors for the determination of bacterial sepsis in febrile neutropenic children. Pediatr Crit Care Med 2005;6(2):129–135.
12. Welch SB, Nadel S. Treatment of meningococcal infection. Arch Dis Child 2003;88:608–614.
13. Han YY, Carcillo JA, Dragotta MA, et al. Early reversal of pediatric-neonatal septic shock by community physicians is associated with improved outcome. Pediatrics 2003;112(4):793–799.
14. Carcillo JA, Fields AI. Clinical practice parameters for hemodynamic support of pediatric and neonatal patients in septic shock. Crit Care Med 2002;30(6): 1365–1378.
15. Lequier LL, Nikaidoh H, Leonard SR, et al. Preoperative and postoperative endotoxemia in children with congenital heart disease. Chest 2000;117(6):1706–1712.

16. Marshall JC, Foster D, Vincent JL, et al. Diagnostic and prognostic implications of endotoxemia in critical illness: results of the MEDIC study. J Infect Dis 2004;190(3):527–534.

17. Braude AI, Douglas H, Davis CE. Treatment and prevention of intravascular coagulation with antiserum to endotoxin. J Infect Dis 1973;128(suppl):157–164.

18. McCabe WR, DeMaria A Jr, Berberich H, Johns MA. Immunization with rough mutants of Salmonella minnesota: protective activity of IgM and IgG antibody to the R595 (Re chemotype) mutant. J Infect Dis 1988;158(2):291–300.

19. Warren HS, Amato SF, Fitting C, et al. Assessment of ability of murine and human anti-lipid A monoclonal antibodies to bind and neutralize lipopolysaccharide. J Exp Med 1993;177(1):89–97.

20. Angus DC, Birmingham MC, Balk RA, et al. E5 murine monoclonal antiendotoxin antibody in gram-negative sepsis: a randomized controlled trial. E5 Study Investigators. JAMA 2000;283:1723–1730.

21. Ziegler EJ, Fisher CJ Jr, Sprung CL, et al. Treatment of gram-negative bacteremia and septic shock with HA-1A human monoclonal antibody against endotoxin. A randomized, double-blind, placebo-controlled trial. The HA-1A Sepsis Study Group. N Engl J Med 1991;324(7):429–436.

22. McCloskey RV, Straube RC, Sanders C, Smith SM, Smith CR. Treatment of septic shock with human monoclonal antibody HA-1A. A randomized, double-blind, placebo-controlled trial. CHESS Trial Study Group. Ann Intern Med 1994;121:1–5.

23. Derkx B, Wittes J, McCloskey R. Randomized, placebo-controlled trial of HA-1A, a human monoclonal antibody to endotoxin, in children with meningococcal septic shock. European Pediatric Meningococcal Septic Shock Trial Study Group. Clin Infect Dis 1999;28:770–777.

24. Chan B, Kalabalikis P, Klein N, Heyderman R, Levin M. Assessment of the effect of candidate anti-inflammatory treatments on the interaction between meningococci and inflammatory cells in vitro in a whole blood model. Biotherapy 1996;9(4):221–228.

25. Beutler B. Endotoxin, toll-like receptor 4, and the afferent limb of innate immunity. Curr Opin Microbiol 2000;3:23–28.

26. Gazzano-Santoro H, Parent JB, Grinna L, et al. High-affinity binding of the bactericidal/permeability-increasing protein and a recombinant amino-terminal fragment to the lipid A region of lipopolysaccharide. Infect Immun 1992;60(11): 4754–4761.

27. Larrick JW, Hirata M, Zheng H, et al. A novel granulocyte-derived peptide with lipopolysaccharide-neutralizing activity. J Immunol 1994;152(1):231–240.

28. Giroir BP, Quint PA, Barton P, et al. Preliminary evaluation of recombinant amino-terminal fragment of human bactericidal/permeability-increasing protein in children with severe meningococcal sepsis. Lancet 1997;350:1439–1443.

29. Levin M, Quint PA, Goldstein B, et al. Recombinant bactericidal/permeability-increasing protein (rBPI21) as adjunctive treatment for children with severe meningococcal sepsis: a randomised trial. rBPI21 Meningococcal Sepsis Study Group (see comment). Lancet 2000;356:961–967.

30. Hellman J, Warren HS. Antiendotoxin strategies. Infect Dis Clin North Am 1999;13(2):371–386, ix.

31. Parker TS, Levine DM, Chang JC, Laxer J, Coffin CC, Rubin AL. Reconstituted high-density lipoprotein neutralizes gram-negative bacterial lipopolysaccharides in human whole blood. Infect Immun 1995;63(1):253–258.

32. Pajkrt D, Doran JE, Koster F, et al. Antiinflammatory effects of reconstituted high-density lipoprotein during human endotoxemia. J Exp Med 1996;184(5): 1601–1608.
33. Wu A, Hinds CJ, Thiemermann C. High-density lipoproteins in sepsis and septic shock: metabolism, actions, and therapeutic applications. Shock 2004;21(3): 210–221.
34. Terblanche M, Almog Y, Rosenson RS, Smith TS, Hackam DG. Statins: panacea for sepsis? Lancet Infect Dis 2006;6(4):242–248.
35. Hackam DG, Mamdani M, Li P, Redelmeier DA. Statins and sepsis in patients with cardiovascular disease: a population-based cohort analysis. Lancet 2006; 367(9508):413–418.
36. Mortensen EM, Restrepo MI, Anzueto A, Pugh J. The effect of prior statin use on 30-day mortality for patients hospitalized with community-acquired pneumonia. Respir Res 2005;6:82.
37. Fernandez R, De Pedro VJ, Artigas A. Statin therapy prior to ICU admission: protection against infection or a severity marker? Intensive Care Med 2006;32(1): 160–164.
38. Aoki H, Kodama M, Tani T, Hanasawa K. Treatment of sepsis by extracorporeal elimination of endotoxin using polymyxin B-immobilized fiber. Am J Surg 1994;167(4):412–417.
39. Gardlund B, Sjolin J, Nilsson A, et al. Plasmapheresis in the treatment of primary septic shock in humans. Scand J Infect Dis 1993;25(6):757–761.
40. Hoffmann JN, Hartl WH, Deppisch R, Faist E, Jochum M, Inthorn D. Hemofiltration in human sepsis: evidence for elimination of immunomodulatory substances. Kidney Int 1995;48(5):1563–1570.
41. Pollack M. Blood exchange and plasmapheresis in sepsis and septic shock. Clin Infect Dis 1992;15(3):431–433.
42. Ronco C, Bellomo R, Homel P, et al. Effects of different doses in continuous venovenous haemofiltration on outcomes of acute renal failure: a prospective randomised trial. Lancet 2000;356(9223):26–30.
43. Reeves JH, Butt WW, Shann F, et al. Continuous plasma filtration in sepsis syndrome. Plasmafiltration in Sepsis Study Group. Crit Care Med 1999;27(10): 2096–2104.
44. van Deuren M, Frieling JT, van der Ven-Jongekrijg J, et al. Plasma patterns of tumor necrosis factor-alpha (TNF) and TNF soluble receptors during acute meningococcal infections and the effect of plasma exchange. Clin Infect Dis 1998;26(4):918–923.
45. Morgera S, Rocktaschel J, Haase M, et al. Intermittent high permeability hemofiltration in septic patients with acute renal failure. Intensive Care Med 2003;29(11):1989–1995.
46. Nemoto H, Nakamoto H, Okada H, et al. Newly developed immobilized polymyxin B fibers improve the survival of patients with sepsis. Blood Purif 2001;19(4):361–368; discussion 368–369.
47. Staubach KH, Boehme M, Zimmermann M, Otto V. A new endotoxin adsorption device in Gram-negative sepsis: use of immobilized albumin with the MATISSE adsorber. Transfus Apher Sci 2003;29(1):93–98.
48. Bengsch S, Boos KS, Nagel D, Seidel D, Inthorn D. Extracorporeal plasma treatment for the removal of endotoxin in patients with sepsis: clinical results of a pilot study. Shock 2005;23(6):494–500.

49. Bone RC, Grodzin CJ, Balk RA. Sepsis: a new hypothesis for pathogenesis of the disease process. Chest 1997;112(1):235–243.

50. Riedemann NC, Guo RF, Ward PA. The enigma of sepsis. J Clin Invest 2003;112(4):460–467.

51. Beutler B, Milsark IW, Cerami AC. Passive immunization against cachectin/tumor necrosis factor protects mice from lethal effect of endotoxin. Science 1985; 229(4716):869–871.

52. Tracey KJ, Fong Y, Hesse DG, et al. Anti-cachectin/TNF monoclonal antibodies prevent septic shock during lethal bacteraemia. Nature 1987;330(6149):662–664.

53. Okusawa S, Gelfand JA, Ikejima T, Connolly RJ, Dinarello CA. Interleukin 1 induces a shock-like state in rabbits. Synergism with tumor necrosis factor and the effect of cyclooxygenase inhibition. J Clin Invest 1988;81(4):1162–1172.

54. Berg DJ, Kuhn R, Rajewsky K, et al. Interleukin-10 is a central regulator of the response to LPS in murine models of endotoxic shock and the Shwartzman reaction but not endotoxin tolerance. J Clin Invest 1995;96(5):2339–2347.

55. Fisher CJ Jr, Agosti JM, Opal SM, et al. Treatment of septic shock with the tumor necrosis factor receptor: Fc fusion protein. The Soluble TNF Receptor Sepsis Study Group. N Engl J Med 1996;334:1697–1702.

56. Marshall JC. Such stuff as dreams are made on: mediator-directed therapy in sepsis. Nat Rev Drug Discov 2003;2:391–405.

57. Panacek EA, Marshall JC, Albertson TE, et al. Efficacy and safety of the monoclonal anti-tumor necrosis factor antibody F(ab')2 fragment afelimomab in patients with severe sepsis and elevated interleukin-6 levels. Crit Care Med 2004;32: 2173–2182.

58. Pathan N, Hemingway CA, Alizadeh AA, et al. Role of interleukin 6 in myocardial dysfunction of meningococcal septic shock. Lancet 2004;363:203–209.

59. Fisher CJ Jr, Dhainaut JF, Opal SM, et al. Recombinant human interleukin 1 receptor antagonist in the treatment of patients with sepsis syndrome. Results from a randomized, double-blind, placebo-controlled trial. Phase III rhIL-1ra Sepsis Syndrome Study Group. JAMA 1994;271:1836–1843.

60. Opal SM, Fisher CJ Jr, Dhainaut JF, et al. Confirmatory interleukin-1 receptor antagonist trial in severe sepsis: a phase III, randomized, double-blind, placebo-controlled, multicenter trial. The Interleukin-1 Receptor Antagonist Sepsis Investigator Group. Crit Care Med 1997;25:1115–1124.

61. van der Poll T, Keogh CV, Buurman WA, Lowry SF. Passive immunization against tumor necrosis factor-alpha impairs host defense during pneumococcal pneumonia in mice. Am J Respir Crit Care Med 1997;155:603–608.

62. Greenberger MJ, Strieter RM, Kunkel SL, Danforth JM, Goodman RE, Standiford TJ. Neutralization of IL-10 increases survival in a murine model of Klebsiella pneumonia. J Immunol 1995;155(2):722–729.

63. Sewnath ME, Olszyna DP, Birjmohun R, ten Kate FJ, Gouma DJ, van Der Poll T. IL-10–deficient mice demonstrate multiple organ failure and increased mortality during Escherichia coli peritonitis despite an accelerated bacterial clearance. J Immunol 2001;166:6323–6331.

64. Marchant A, Deviere J, Byl B, De Groote D, Vincent JL, Goldman M. Interleukin-10 production during septicaemia. Lancet 1994;343:707–708.

65. Munoz C, Carlet J, Fitting C, Misset B, Bleriot JP, Cavaillon JM. Dysregulation of in vitro cytokine production by monocytes during sepsis. J Clin Invest 1991;88:1747–1754.

66. Docke WD, Randow F, Syrbe U, et al. Monocyte deactivation in septic patients: restoration by IFN-gamma treatment. Nat Med 1997;3:678–681.

67. Bilgin K, Yaramis A, Haspolat K, Tas MA, Gunbey S, Derman O. A randomized trial of granulocyte-macrophage colony-stimulating factor in neonates with sepsis and neutropenia. Pediatrics 2001;107:36–41.

68. Kaul R, McGeer A, Norrby-Teglund A, et al. Intravenous immunoglobulin therapy for streptococcal toxic shock syndrome—a comparative observational study. The Canadian Streptococcal Study Group. Clin Infect Dis 1999;28:800–807.

69. Alejandria MM, Lansang MA, Dans LF, Mantaring JB. Intravenous immunoglobulin for treating sepsis and septic shock. Cochrane Database Syst Rev 2001(2): CD001090.

70. Cronin L, Cook DJ, Carlet J, et al. Corticosteroid treatment for sepsis: a critical appraisal and meta-analysis of the literature. Crit Care Med 1995;23:1430–1439.

71. Vincent JL, Sun Q, Dubois MJ. Clinical trials of immunomodulatory therapies in severe sepsis and septic shock. Clin Infect Dis 2002;34:1084–1093.

72. Annane D, Sebille V, Troche G, Raphael JC, Gajdos P, Bellissant E. A 3–level prognostic classification in septic shock based on cortisol levels and cortisol response to corticotropin. JAMA 2000;283:1038–1045.

73. Briegel J, Forst H, Haller M, et al. Stress doses of hydrocortisone reverse hyperdynamic septic shock: a prospective, randomized, double-blind, single-center study. Crit Care Med 1999;27:723–732.

74. Hatherill M, Tibby SM, Hilliard T, Turner C, Murdoch IA. Adrenal insufficiency in septic shock. Arch Dis Child 1999;80:51–55.

75. Riordan FA, Thomson AP, Ratcliffe JM, Sills JA, Diver MJ, Hart CA. Admission cortisol and adrenocorticotrophic hormone levels in children with meningococcal disease: evidence of adrenal insufficiency? Crit Care Med 1999;27:2257–2261.

76. Annane D, Sebille V, Charpentier C, et al. Effect of treatment with low doses of hydrocortisone and fludrocortisone on mortality in patients with septic shock. JAMA 2002;288:862–871.

77. Thys F, Laterre PF. Hydrocortisone in septic shock: too much, too little, too soon? Crit Care Med 2005;33:2683–2684.

78. Kennedy WA, Hoyt MJ, McCracken GH Jr. The role of corticosteroid therapy in children with pneumococcal meningitis. Am J Dis Child 1991;145:1374–1378.

79. Bernard GR, Wheeler AP, Russell JA, et al. The effects of ibuprofen on the physiology and survival of patients with sepsis. The Ibuprofen in Sepsis Study Group. N Engl J Med 1997;336:912–918.

80. Arons MM, Wheeler AP, Bernard GR, et al. Effects of ibuprofen on the physiology and survival of hypothermic sepsis. Ibuprofen in Sepsis Study Group. Crit Care Med 1999;27:699–707.

81. Virdis A, Colucci R, Fornai M, et al. Cyclooxygenase-2 inhibition improves vascular endothelial dysfunction in a rat model of endotoxic shock: role of inducible nitric-oxide synthase and oxidative stress. J Pharmacol Exp Ther 2005; 312:945–953.

82. Haque K, Mohan P. Pentoxifylline for neonatal sepsis. Cochrane Database Syst Rev 2003(4):CD004205.

83. Zeni F, Pain P, Vindimian M, et al. Effects of pentoxifylline on circulating cytokine concentrations and hemodynamics in patients with septic shock: results from a double-blind, randomized, placebo-controlled study. Crit Care Med 1996;24:207–214.

84. Staubach KH, Schroder J, Stuber F, Gehrke K, Traumann E, Zabel P. Effect of pentoxifylline in severe sepsis: results of a randomized, double-blind, placebo-controlled study. Arch Surg 1998;133:94–100.

85. Lauterbach R, Pawlik D, Kowalczyk D, Ksycinski W, Helwich E, Zembala M. Effect of the immunomodulating agent, pentoxifylline, in the treatment of sepsis in prematurely delivered infants: a placebo-controlled, double-blind trial. Crit Care Med 1999;27:807–814.

86. Lauterbach R, Zembala M. Pentoxifylline reduces plasma tumour necrosis factor-alpha concentration in premature infants with sepsis. Eur J Pediatr 1996;155: 404–409.

87. Taylor FB Jr, Chang A, Ruf W, et al. Lethal E. coli septic shock is prevented by blocking tissue factor with monoclonal antibody. Circ Shock 1991;33:127–134.

88. Taylor FB Jr, Chang AC, Peer GT, et al. DEGR-factor Xa blocks disseminated intravascular coagulation initiated by Escherichia coli without preventing shock or organ damage. Blood 1991;78:364–368.

89. Abraham E. Tissue factor inhibition and clinical trial results of tissue factor pathway inhibitor in sepsis. Crit Care Med 2000;28:S31–33.

90. Abraham E, Reinhart K, Opal S, et al. Efficacy and safety of tifacogin (recombinant tissue factor pathway inhibitor) in severe sepsis: a randomized controlled trial. Jama 2003;290:238–247.

91. Dickneite G. Antithrombin III in animal models of sepsis and organ failure. Semin Thromb Hemost 1998;24:61–69.

92. Inthorn D, Hoffmann JN, Hartl WH, Muhlbayer D, Jochum M. Effect of antithrombin III supplementation on inflammatory response in patients with severe sepsis. Shock 1998;10:90–96.

93. Wiedermann CJ, Hoffmann JN, Juers M, et al. High-dose antithrombin III in the treatment of severe sepsis in patients with a high risk of death: efficacy and safety. Crit Care Med 2006;34:285–292.

94. Taylor FB Jr, Chang A, Esmon CT, D'Angelo A, Vigano-D'Angelo S, Blick KE. Protein C prevents the coagulopathic and lethal effects of Escherichia coli infusion in the baboon. J Clin Invest 1987;79:918–925.

95. Taylor FB Jr, Stearns-Kurosawa DJ, Kurosawa S, et al. The endothelial cell protein C receptor aids in host defense against Escherichia coli sepsis. Blood 2000; 95:1680–1686.

96. Faust SN, Levin M, Harrison OB, et al. Dysfunction of endothelial protein C activation in severe meningococcal sepsis. N Engl J Med 2001;345:408–416.

97. Matthay MA. Severe sepsis—a new treatment with both anticoagulant and antiinflammatory properties. N Engl J Med 2001;344:759–762.

98. Bernard GR, Vincent JL, Laterre PF, et al. Efficacy and safety of recombinant human activated protein C for severe sepsis. N Engl J Med 2001;344:699–709.

99. Dellinger RP, Carlet JM, Masur H, et al. Surviving Sepsis Campaign guidelines for management of severe sepsis and septic shock. Crit Care Med 2004;32:858–873.

100. Abraham E, Laterre PF, Garg R, et al. Administration of Drotrecogin Alfa (Activated) in Early Stage Severe Sepsis (ADDRESS) Study Group. Drotrecogin alfa (activated) for adults with severe sepsis and a low risk of death. N Engl J Med 2005;353:1332–1341.

101. Kornelisse RF, Hazelzet JA, Savelkoul HF, et al. The relationship between plasminogen activator inhibitor-1 and proinflammatory and counterinflammatory mediators in children with meningococcal septic shock. J Infect Dis 1996; 173:1148–1156.

102. Aiuto LT, Barone SR, Cohen PS, Boxer RA. Recombinant tissue plasminogen activator restores perfusion in meningococcal purpura fulminans. Crit Care Med 1997;25:1079–1082.

103. Zenz W, Zoehrer B, Levin M, et al. Use of recombinant tissue plasminogen activator in children with meningococcal purpura fulminans: a retrospective study. Crit Care Med 2004;32:1777–1780.

104. Murakami J, Ohtani A, Murata S. Protective effect of T-686, an inhibitor of plasminogen activator inhibitor-1 production, against the lethal effect of lipopolysaccharide in mice. Jpn J Pharmacol 1997;75:291–294.

105. Vincent JL, Spapen H, Bakker J, Webster NR, Curtis L. Phase II multicenter clinical study of the platelet-activating factor receptor antagonist BB-882 in the treatment of sepsis. Crit Care Med 2000;28:638–642.

106. Poeze M, Froon AH, Ramsay G, Buurman WA, Greve JW. Decreased organ failure in patients with severe SIRS and septic shock treated with the platelet-activating factor antagonist TCV-309: a prospective, multicenter, double-blind, randomized phase II trial. Shock 2000;14:421–428.

107. Dhainaut JF, Tenaillon A, Hemmer M, et al. Confirmatory platelet-activating factor receptor antagonist trial in patients with severe gram-negative bacterial sepsis: a phase III, randomized, double-blind, placebo-controlled, multicenter trial. BN 52021 Sepsis Investigator Group. Crit Care Med 1998;26:1963–1971.

108. Tjoelker LW, Wilder C, Eberhardt C, et al. Anti-inflammatory properties of a platelet-activating factor acetylhydrolase. Nature 1995;374(6522):549–553.

109. Schuster DP, Metzler M, Opal S, et al. Recombinant platelet-activating factor acetylhydrolase to prevent acute respiratory distress syndrome and mortality in severe sepsis: Phase IIb, multicenter, randomized, placebo-controlled, clinical trial. Crit Care Med 2003;31:1612–1619.

110. Opal S, Laterre PF, Abraham E, et al. Recombinant human platelet-activating factor acetylhydrolase for treatment of severe sepsis: results of a phase III, multicenter, randomized, double-blind, placebo-controlled, clinical trial. Crit Care Med 2004;32:332–341.

111. Claus RA, Russwurm S, Dohrn B, Bauer M, Losche W. Plasma platelet-activating factor acetylhydrolase activity in critically ill patients. Crit Care Med 2005; 33(6):1416–1419.

112. Parent C, Eichacker PQ. Neutrophil and endothelial cell interactions in sepsis. The role of adhesion molecules. Infect Dis Clin North Am 1999;13:427–447.

113. Hawkins HK, Heffelfinger SC, Anderson DC. Leukocyte adhesion deficiency: clinical and postmortem observations. Pediatr Pathol 1992;12:119–130.

114. Haley M, Parent C, Cui X, et al. Neutrophil inhibition with L-selectin-directed MAb improves or worsens survival dependent on the route but not severity of infection in a rat sepsis model. J Appl Physiol 2005;98:2155–2162.

115. Moncada S, Higgs A. The L-arginine-nitric oxide pathway. N Engl J Med 1993; 329:2002–2012.

116. Cobb JP, Danner RL. Nitric oxide and septic shock. JAMA 1996;275:1192–1196.

117. Murad F. The 1996 Albert Lasker Medical Research Awards. Signal transduction using nitric oxide and cyclic guanosine monophosphate. JAMA 1996;276:1189–1192.

118. Hare JM, Colucci WS. Role of nitric oxide in the regulation of myocardial function. Prog Cardiovasc Dis 1995;38:155–166.

119. Avontuur JA, Boomsma F, van den Meiracker AH, de Jong FH, Bruining HA. Endothelin-1 and blood pressure after inhibition of nitric oxide synthesis in human septic shock. Circulation 1999;99:271–275.

120. Avontuur JA, Tutein Nolthenius RP, Buijk SL, Kanhai KJ, Bruining HA. Effect of L-NAME, an inhibitor of nitric oxide synthesis, on cardiopulmonary function in human septic shock. Chest 1998;113:1640–1646.

121. Cobb JP, Natanson C, Hoffman WD, et al. N omega-amino-L-arginine, an inhibitor of nitric oxide synthase, raises vascular resistance but increases mortality rates in awake canines challenged with endotoxin. J Exp Med 1992;176:1175–1182.

122. Freeman BD, Cobb JP. Nitric oxide synthase as a therapeutic target in sepsis—more questions than answers? Crit Care Med 1998;26:1469–1470.

123. Avontuur JA, Biewenga M, Buijk SL, Kanhai KJ, Bruining HA. Pulmonary hypertension and reduced cardiac output during inhibition of nitric oxide synthesis in human septic shock. Shock 1998;9:451–454.

124. Jourdain M, Tournoys A, Leroy X, et al. Effects of N omega-nitro-L-arginine methyl ester on the endotoxin-induced disseminated intravascular coagulation in porcine septic shock. Crit Care Med 1997;25:452–459.

125. Bakker J, Grover R, McLuckie A, et al. Administration of the nitric oxide synthase inhibitor NG-methyl-L-arginine hydrochloride (546C88) by intravenous infusion for up to 72 hours can promote the resolution of shock in patients with severe sepsis: results of a randomized, double-blind, placebo-controlled multicenter study (study no. 144–002). Crit Care Med 2004;32:1–12.

126. Lopez A, Lorente JA, Steingrub J, et al. Multiple-center, randomized, placebo-controlled, double-blind study of the nitric oxide synthase inhibitor 546C88: effect on survival in patients with septic shock. Crit Care Med 2004;32:21–30.

127. Barth E, Radermacher P, Thiemermann C, Weber S, Georgieff M, Albuszies G. Role of inducible nitric oxide synthase in the reduced responsiveness of the myocardium to catecholamines in a hyperdynamic, murine model of septic shock. Crit Care Med 2006;34:307–313.

128. Rosselet A, Feihl F, Markert M, Gnaegi A, Perret C, Liaudet L. Selective iNOS inhibition is superior to norepinephrine in the treatment of rat endotoxic shock. Am J Respir Crit Care Med 1998;157:162–170.

129. Aderem A, Ulevitch RJ. Toll-like receptors in the induction of the innate immune response. Nature 2000;406(6797):782–787.

130. Ozinsky A, Underhill DM, Fontenot JD, et al. The repertoire for pattern recognition of pathogens by the innate immune system is defined by cooperation between toll-like receptors. Proc Natl Acad Sci U S A 2000;97:13766–13771.

131. Takeuchi O, Hoshino K, Akira S. Cutting edge: TLR2–deficient and MyD88–deficient mice are highly susceptible to Staphylococcus aureus infection. J Immunol 2000;165:5392–5396.

132. Verbon A, Dekkers PE, ten Hove T, et al. IC14, an anti-CD14 antibody, inhibits endotoxin-mediated symptoms and inflammatory responses in humans. J Immunol 2001;166:3599–3605.

133. Reinhart K, Gluck T, Ligtenberg J, et al. CD14 receptor occupancy in severe sepsis: results of a phase I clinical trial with a recombinant chimeric CD14 monoclonal antibody (IC14). Crit Care Med 2004;32:1100–1108.

134. Wang H, Bloom O, Zhang M, et al. HMG-1 as a late mediator of endotoxin lethality in mice. Science 1999;285(5425):248–251.

135. Froidevaux C, Roger T, Martin C, Glauser MP, Calandra T. Macrophage migration inhibitory factor and innate immune responses to bacterial infections. Crit Care Med 2001;29:S13–15.

136. Roger T, David J, Glauser MP, Calandra T. MIF regulates innate immune responses through modulation of Toll-like receptor 4. Nature 2001;414(6866):920–924.
137. Calandra T, Echtenacher B, Roy DL, et al. Protection from septic shock by neutralization of macrophage migration inhibitory factor. Nat Med 2000;6(2):164–170.
138. Bozza M, Satoskar AR, Lin G, et al. Targeted disruption of migration inhibitory factor gene reveals its critical role in sepsis. J Exp Med 1999;189:341–346.
139. Bozza FA, Gomes RN, Japiassu AM, et al. Macrophage migration inhibitory factor levels correlate with fatal outcome in sepsis. Shock 2004;22:309–313.

Index

A

Absolute neutrophil count (ANC), 335
ACE. *See* Angiotensin-converting enzyme
Acinetobacter, 73, 321
Acquired immune deficiency syndrome (AIDS). *See* Human immunodeficiency virus
Acquired immunoparalysis, 338–339
Actinobacillus, 443
Actinomyces, 74
Activated partial thromboplastin time (APTT), 424
Activated protein C (APC), 183, 184, 185
  pathway, 541
  in sepsis, 540–542
Acute disseminated encephalomyelitis (ADEM), 476
Acute epiglottitis, 503–504
  clinical presentation of, 503
  diagnosis of, 503
  etiology of, 503
  treatment, 504
Acute inflammatory demyelinating polyradiculoneuropathy (AIDP), 473
Acute motor-axonal neuropathy (AMAN), 473
Acute motor-sensory axonal neuropathy (AMSAN), 473
Acute paralysis, 472–475
Acute respiratory distress syndrome (ARDS), 265, 419, 493, 525
Acute respiratory infections (ARIs), 487
ADCC. *See* Antibody-dependent cellular cytotoxicity
ADE. *See* Antibody-dependent enhancement
ADEM. *See* Acute disseminated encephalomyelitis
Adenosine triphosphate (ATP), 186
Adenovirus, 449, 470
  vaccine, 157
Adrenal insufficiency, 187, 536
Adrenocorticotropic hormone, 186, 537
Adult respiratory distress syndrome (ARDS), 120
Aedes, 372
Afelimomab, 533
Age, immunity and, 333
AIDP. *See* Acute inflammatory demyelinating polyradiculoneuropathy
AIDS. *See* Human immunodeficiency virus
Airway mucosa, 488
Alternative pathway component defects, 16
AMA-1. *See* Apical membrane antigen 1
AMAN. *See* Acute motor-axonal neuropathy
Amantadine, 220, 420
American Heart Association, 442
Aminoglycoside, 72
Amphotericin B, 105
  in fungal infections, 107
Ampicillin, 72, 504
AMSAN. *See* Acute motor-sensory axonal neuropathy
Anaerobic bacteria, 74
ANC. *See* Absolute neutrophil count

Angiotensin-converting enzyme (ACE)
  in genetic susceptibility, 263–265
  meningococcal disease and, 263–265
  polymorphisms, clinical studies, 264
Anopheles, 372
Antibiotics, 89
  in bronchiolitis, 513
  in diphtheria, 408
  rational use of, 325–326
  in TSS management, 128–129
Antibody deficiency, 24–27
  complications, 27–28
  investigation of, 26–27
  major primary, 25
  treatment, 28–30
Antibody-dependent cellular cytotoxicity
    (ADCC), 4
Antibody-dependent enhancement
    (ADE), 388
Anticoagulant therapies, 538–542
  antithrombin, 539–540
Anticytokine therapies, 531–534
Antiendotoxin, 526–529
Antifungals, 220, 344–345
Antigenic drift, 155, 416
Antiinflammatory therapies, 531–534
Antiretroviral drugs, 361
  starting, 366
Antithrombin III, 256, 539–540
Antiviral agents
  oral, 346
  in PICU, 346
Aorta, coarctation of, 442
APC. *See* Activated protein C
Apical membrane antigen 1 (AMA-1),
    165
Apnea, 515–516
APTT. *See* Activated partial
    thromboplastin time
Arbovirus, 470
ARDS. *See* Acute respiratory distress
    syndrome; Adult respiratory
    distress syndrome
Area spacing, 323
Arg677Trp, 239
ARIs. *See* Acute respiratory infections
Arthropod-borne infections, 371–376
ASD. *See* Atrial septal defect
Aseptic meningitis, 469–471

  clinical features, 469
  diagnosis, 469–470
  medical treatment, 471
  pathogenesis, 469
Aspergillosis, 101–104
  clinical presentation, 101–102
  diagnosis, 102–104
  epidemiology, 101
  invasive, 102
Aspergillus, 18, 22, 79, 101, 109, 218
  isolation of, 102
Aspergillus flavus, 102
Astrovirus, 344
Atovaquone-proguanil (Malarone), 376
ATP. *See* Adenosine triphosphate
Atrial septal defect (ASD), 442
Azathioprine, 48
Azoles, 106

B
Bacille Calmette-Guérin (BCG), 75,
    149–150, 205
Bacteremia, 69
  epidemiology, 197–198
Bacterial disease
  epidemiology of, 199–202
  in PICU, 213–215
    resistance, 213
    staphylococci, 213–214
Bacterial tracheitis, 506–507
  clinical presentation of, 507
Bactericidal/permeability increasing
    protein (BPI), 229, 230–232, 528
  studies on, 231
Bacteroides fragilis, 74, 321
BAL. *See* Bronchoalveolar lavage
B. burgdorferi, 239
B cells, 5–6
BCG. *See* Bacille Calmette-Guérin
Benzodiazepines, 411
Benzylpenicillin, 500
Beta-blockers, 411
Bicuspid aortic valve, 442
Blastomycosis, 104
Bloodstream, nosocomial infections in,
    314–315, 322, 326–327
Bone marrow, 5
  transplant, 36, 49
    patients, 333–334

Bordetella pertussis, 152, 206, 493, 494
Botulism, 474–475
  clinical features of, 474
  diagnosis of, 474
  medical treatment of, 474–475
BPI. *See* Bactericidal/permeability
    increasing protein
Bradykinin, 544
Brain abscess, 478–479
  clinical features, 478
  diagnosis, 479
  medical treatment, 479
British Thoracic Society, 491
Bronchiectasis, 28
Bronchiolitis, 510–516
  admission rates, 511
  antibiotics, 513
  clinical features, 511–512
  complications, 515–516
    apnea, 515–516
    hypotension, 516
  diagnosis, 511–512
  management, 513
  predicting severe, 512–513
  radiology, 512
  virology, 512
Bronchoalveolar lavage (BAL), 103,
    493
Bronchodilators, 513–514
Bruton's disease, 24–25
Budesonide, 506
Burkholderia cepacia, 22, 73
Burns, staphylococcal TSS and, 127

C
C3a, 180, 243
C3b, 243
C5a, 180
cAMP. *See* Cyclic adenosine
    monophosphate
Campylobacter, 198
CA-MRSA. *See* Community-acquired
    methicillin resistant *S. aureus*
Cancer, treatment of, 335–336
Candida, 18, 30, 63, 78, 79, 326, 439
  incidence of, 98
  in neonate, 99–101
    diagnosis, 100–101
    systemic infection, 100

nosocomial infections and, 317–318,
    322–323
  systemic infection, 100
  in utero, 79
Candida albicans, 98
Candida glabrata, 98
Candida parapsilosis, 98
Candida tropicalis, 98
Candidiasis, treatment, 108–109
Candiduria, 100
Capillary leakage
  in dengue, 398
  in sepsis, 181
Cardiac infections, 438
Cardiac surgery, 339
Cardiac troponin T, 451
Cardiobacterium, 443
CARS. *See* Compensatory
    antiinflammatory response
Caspofungin, 109
Catecholamines, 186
CD4, 354
  counts, 354–355
CD5, 10
CD14, 177, 528, 546, 547
  clinical studies on, 234
  in genetic susceptibility, 232–233
CD40 ligand, 6, 26
  deficiency, 39
CD45RA, 11
CD45RO, 11
CD45 staining, 8
CDC. *See* Centers for Disease Control
    and Prevention
Ceftriaxone, 384
Cell-mediated immunity
  defects, 30–37
  tests of, 35
Centers for Disease Control and
    Prevention (CDC), 196, 313, 352
  nosocomial infection definitions of,
    319
Central nervous system (CNS) infection,
    481–484
  initial survey of, 481–483
    airway and breathing, 481–482
    circulation, 482
    glucose, 484
    ICP, 482–483

Central venous catheters (CVCs),
    314–315
Cerebral palsy, 516–517
Cerebrospinal fluid (CSF), 65, 402
  in poliomyelitis, 413
cGMP. *See* Cyclic guanosine
    monophosphate
CHARGE syndrome, 40, 41
CHD. *See* Congenital heart disease
Chemotherapy, 37
  MBL concentrations in, 248–249
Chest radiography, 456, 492, 497
Chest X-ray (CXR), 351
  in PcP, 358
Chickenpox, 48, 84–85
Chikungunya, 390
Chlamydia psittaci, 470
Chlamydia trachomatis, 76, 443, 490
Chloramphenicol, 18
Chlorpromazine, 411
Cholera, vaccine, 157
Chromosome breakage disorders, 42
Chronic granulomatous disease, 21–22
Cidofovir, 82, 346
Cigarette smoke, 488
Ciliary activity, 488
Citrobacter, 72
Classical component deficiencies, 15
Clindamycin, 129
Clonidine, 411
Clostridial, 74
Clostridium botulinum, 474
Clostridium difficile, 320
Clostridium tetani, 161, 409
CMV. *See* Cytomegalovirus
CNS infection. *See* Central nervous
    system infection
Coagulase-negative staphylococci
    (CoNS), 69–70, 216
  mortality from, 70
  resistance of, 70
Coagulation response
  genetic susceptibility and, 256–265
    factor V Leiden in, 257
    PAI-1 and, 257–262
    t-PA and, 257–262
  in sepsis, 182–183
Coartem. *See* Lumefantrine-artemether
Coccidioides immitis, 105

Colchicine, 458
Colloid solutions, 396
Combination antimicrobial therapy, 217
Combined immunodeficiencies, 37–40
  MHC class II deficiency, 37–38
  PNP deficiency, 38–39
Common variable immunodeficiency
    (CVID), 24
  noninfective inflammatory
    complications in, 27–28
Community-acquired methicillin
    resistant *S. aureus* (CA-MRSA),
    69, 214
Compensatory antiinflammatory
    response (CARS), 534
Complement system, 2
  activation pathways, 179, 242
    alternative, 242–243
    classic, 242–243
    lectin, 242–243
  deficiency, 251–252
  disorders, 14–16
    classical, 15–16
    primary, 16
    secondary, 16–17
    tests for, 15
  in genetic susceptibility, 241–249
Computed tomography (CT), 456
  of bronchiectasis, 28
Congenital heart disease (CHD), 441
  cyanotic, 517
CoNS. *See* Coagulase-negative
    staphylococci
Consciousness, impaired, in malaria,
    380–381
  management of, 380–381
Continuous positive airway pressure
    (CPAP), 453, 512
  nasal, 515
Coronaviruses, 421
Corticosteroids, 47, 458
  in sepsis, 536–537
Cortisol, 186, 187
Corynebacterium diphtheriae, 156, 405,
    449
Corynebacterium ulcerans, 406
Coxsackie viruses, 81–82, 449
CPAP. *See* Continuous positive airway
    pressure

C-reactive protein (CRP), 65, 177, 236, 242, 466, 492, 498
Cricothyrotomy, 504
CRM197, 144
Croup, 504–507
  bacterial, 506–507
  incidence of, 505
CRP. *See* C-reactive protein
Cryptococcosis, 105
Cryptococcus neoformans, 105
Cryptosporidium, 37
CSF. *See* Cerebrospinal fluid
CT. *See* Computed tomography
Culex tritaeniorhynchus, 399
Culicis, 372
CVCs. *See* Central venous catheters
CVID. *See* Common variable immunodeficiency
CXR. *See* Chest X-ray
Cyclic adenosine monophosphate (cAMP), 67, 538
Cyclic guanosine monophosphate (cGMP), 544
Cyclosporin A, 44
Cytokines, 7
  deficiencies, 17
  genetic susceptibility and, 265–287
  plasma concentration of, 532
  receptors, 7
  release of, 532
  role of, 523
  in sepsis, 534
Cytomegalovirus (CMV), 31, 36, 82–83, 333, 334, 357, 451
  in PICU, 222
  pneumonitis, 360
  treatment, 360

D
Dalfopristin, 217
Dallas criteria, 451
DCM. *See* Dilated cardiomyopathy
Dehydration, 157–158
Dengue, 386–399
  areas infected with, 387
  clinical manifestations of, 387, 389
  diagnosis of, 392–393
    laboratory, 393
  epidemiology, 386–388

fluid therapy in, 395–397
  laboratory investigations, 393–394
  management, 394–399
    capillary leakage, 398
    fluid overload, 398
    hemorrhagic complications, 397–398
  mild, 390
  outcome, 398–399
  pathogenesis of, 388–388
  severity in, 389
    recognition of, 390
  shock in, 391–392
  transmission of, 386–388
Dengue fever (DF), 386, 388, 390
  laboratory investigations, 393
Dengue hemorrhagic fever (DHF), 388
  cases of, 389
  laboratory investigations, 393–394
  shock in, 391–392
Dengue shock syndrome (DSS), 396–397
Dexamethasone, 506
DF. *See* Dengue fever
DFA. *See* Direct fluorescent antibody
DHF. *See* Dengue hemorrhagic fever
Diarrhea, 30
  infectious, 198–199
DIC. *See* Disseminated intravascular coagulation
DiGeorge syndrome, 40–41
Dilated cardiomyopathy (DCM), 452
Diphtheria, 405–409
  clinical manifestations, 406–407
    acute, 406–407
    late complications, 407
  diagnosis of, 407–408
  faucial, 406
  laryngeal, 407
  management of, 408–409
    antibiotics, 408
    antitoxin dosage, 408
  nasal, 406
  outcome, 409
  pathogenesis, 406
  vaccine, 156–157
Diphtheric myocarditis, 453
Direct fluorescent antibody (DFA), 509
Disseminated intravascular coagulation (DIC), 182, 394, 538
DNAse, 514

Dobutamine, 452
Dopamine, 452
DSS. *See* Dengue shock syndrome
Duke clinical criteria, 445–446
Duncan's syndrome, 39–40

E
Eagle, 129
Early-onset neonatal sepsis (EONS), 59
    presentation of, 63
EBLV. *See* European bat Lyssavirus
Echinocandins, 106
    in PICU, 219–220, 345
ECHO. *See* Enterocytopathogenic human
    orphan
Echocardiography, 450–451, 456
ECMO. *See* Extracorporeal membrane
    oxygenator
EEG. *See* Electroencephalogram
Eikenella corrodens, 443
Electrocardiography, 450, 456
Electroencephalogram (EEG), 378, 403,
    407
Electrolytes, 492
    in malaria, 384
ELISA. *See* Enzyme-linked
    immunosorbent assay
Emboli, 447
Empyema
    parapneumonic, 495–496
    subdural, 479–480
Encephalitis
    acute, 471–472
        clinical findings, 471–472
        diagnosis, 472
        medical treatment, 472
    management, 161
    Murray Valley, 400
    St. Louis, 400
    tick borne, 160
    vaccine, 158–159
Endemic mycosis, 104
Endocarditis, 441–449
    clinical course, 447–449
    clinical manifestations, 443–444
    complications, 447, 448
    diagnosis, 444–446
        Duke criteria for, 445
    epidemiology of, 441–442

fungal, 78
    management, 447–449
    microbiology, 443
    pathogenesis, 442
    surgical treatment of, 448
Endophthalmitis, fungal, 78
Endothelial cell protein C receptor
    (EPCR), 184, 540
Endothelial cells, 543–544
Endothelial dysfunction, 539
    targeting, 542–546
Endotoxins, 528
    removal, 530–531
Enteric gram-negative infections, 71–73
Enteric viruses, diagnosis of, 343
Enterobacter, 71, 72, 440
Enterobacter cloacae, 320
Enterococci, 70–71
Enterococcus, 439
Enterococcus faecalis, 217
Enterocytopathogenic human orphan
    (ECHO), 24
Enterovirus, 81–82
    in PICU, 221–222
    vaccines, 158–159
Enzyme-linked immunosorbent assay
    (ELISA), 15, 393
EONS. *See* Early-onset neonatal sepsis
EPCR. *See* Endothelial cell protein C
    receptor
EPI. *See* Expanded Program of
    Immunization
Epidemiology, infectious disease
    global burden of, 194
    incidence of infectious disease, 195
    preventative strategies, 205–207
    specific microbes, 199–205
        bacterial disease, 199–202
        viral infections, 202–204
    studies on, 195
    syndromes, 195–199
        bacteremia, 197–198
        infectious diarrhea, 198–199
        respiratory illness, 198–199
        sepsis, 195–197
Epinephrine, 514
Epopeptides, 176
Epstein-Barr virus, 39, 44, 342, 451,
    470

Erythrocyte sedimentation rate (ESR), 498
Erythroderma, 32
Erythromycin, 510
Escherichia coli, 71–73, 198, 214, 229, 320, 490
resistance, 72
ESR. See Erythrocyte sedimentation rate
European bat Lyssavirus (EBLV), 160
Exchange transfusion, in malaria, 385
exon 1, 244
EXP1. See Exported antigen 1
Expanded Program of Immunization (EPI), 404
Exported antigen 1 (EXP1), 163
Extracorporeal adsorption apheresis, 531
Extracorporeal membrane oxygenator (ECMO), 452, 453, 515

F
FACS analysis. See Fluorescence-activated cell sorting
Factor V Leiden
clinical studies on, 258
coagulation pathway and, 257
Fax plots, 8
Fcγ receptors, 249–256
allotype distribution, 249–250
classes of, 249
deficiency, 251
in meningococcal disease, 255
polymorphisms, 250
clinical studies on, 252–254
complement deficiency and, 251–252
Fibrin clots, 182
546C88, 545–546
Flavivirus, 386, 399
Flaviviruses, vaccines, 159–160
Flucloxacillin, 18
Fluconazole, 36
in fungal infections, 107
Fluids
in malaria, 384
overload, 398
in pneumonia management, 493–494
therapy, 395
Fluorescence-activated cell sorting (FACS) analysis, 5
Fluorinated pyrimidines, in PICU, 219

Foscarnet, 82
Fungal infections, 77–80, 97–110
clinical manifestations of, 77–78, 99
gastrointestinal, 99
respiratory tract, 99
skin, 99
urinary tract, 99
dissemination of, 78
emerging, 109–110
empirical treatment, 108–109
candidiasis, 108–109
febrile neutropenia, 108
epidemiology of, 98
incidence of, 97–98
outcome of, 79
pathogenesis of, 77
in PICU, 218–220
echinocandins in, 219–220
Polyene macrolides, 218–219
triazoles, 219
prophylaxis, 106–108
amphotericin B, 107
fluconazole, 107
itraconazole, 107
risk factors for, 77–80
therapy for, 80
treatment, 106–109
Fusarium, 109
Fusobacterium, 74

G
G-6-PD. See Glucose-6-phosphate dehydrogenase
G-221C, 245
Ganciclovir, 82
Gastrointestinal infections, 51–53
fungal infections and, 99
Gene therapy, 35, 37
Genetic susceptibility, 225–226
ACE in, 263–265
BPI in, 230–232
CD14 in, 232–233
coagulation response and, 256–265
factor V Leiden in, 257
PAI-1 and, 257–262
t-PA and, 257–262
complement in, 241–249
Fcγ receptors in, 249–256
IFN-γ and, 285

Genetic susceptibility (*cont.*)
  IFN-γ-R1 and, 285–287
  IL-1 and, 273–278
  IL-6 and, 278–280
  IL-10 and, 280–284
  LBP in, 230–232
  MBL in, 241–249
  mendelian inheritance and, 226
  polymorphisms in, 228–229
  studies on, 287
  TAFI and, 262–263
  toll-like receptors in, 233–239
    TLR2, 238–239
    TLR4, 235–238
Genotyping, 289
Giardia lamblia, 24
Gloves, 324
Glucagon, 186
Glucocorticoids, 188, 536
Glucose-6-phosphate dehydrogenase
    (G-6-PD), 22
GLURP, 165
Glutamic acid, 228
Glycopeptide, 22
GM-CSF. *See* Granulocyte-macrophage
    colony-stimulating factor
Gowns, 324
Granulocyte-macrophage colony-
    stimulating factor (GM-CSF),
    535
Group A streptococci, 67
  molecular epidemiology of, 116
  population-based surveys of, 115
  in toxic shock syndrome, 114–115
Group B β-hemolytic streptococcus,
    65–67
  capsular polysaccharide conjugate
    vaccines, 67
  epidemiology of, 201
  presentation of, 66
  risk factors for, 66
  treatment of, 66
  vaccine, 151
Growth hormone, 186, 188
GTP. *See* Guanosine triphosphate
Guanosine triphosphate (GTP), 544
Guillain-Barré syndrome, 407, 413,
    473–474
  clinical features of, 473

  diagnosis of, 474
  medical treatment of, 474

H
HAART. *See* Highly active antiretroviral
    therapy
Haemophilus influenzae, 11, 73, 178,
    197–198, 222, 423, 443, 455, 465
  epidemiology of, 201
  type B vaccine, 143–145
Hand-washing, 324
HBV. *See* Hepatitis B virus
HCV. *See* Hepatitis C virus
HDL. *See* High-density lipoprotein
Heat shock proteins (HSP), 239–241
  families, 241
Heliox, 514
Hemagglutinin, 415, 418
Hemoglobin S, 227–228
Hemophagocytic lymphohistiocytosis
    (HLH), 39, 50
  immunodeficiencies leading to, 42–44
    clinical presentation, 42–44
    treatment of, 44
Hepatitis B virus (HBV), 12, 85–86
Hepatitis C virus (HCV), 85–86
  vertical transmission of, 85–86
Herpes simplex virus (HSV), 83, 340, 472
  manifestations of, 83
  treatment of, 83
  vaccine, 159
HFOV. *See* High-frequency oscillatory
    ventilation
Hib vaccine, 12, 144–145
High-density lipoprotein (HDL), 529
High-frequency oscillatory ventilation
    (HFOV), 515
Highly active antiretroviral therapy
    (HAART), 165
High mobility group (HMG), 547
High-permeability hemofiltration (HP-
    HF), 531
Histamine, 544
Histoplasma capsulatum, 104
Histoplasmosis, 104
HIV. *See* Human immunodeficiency virus
HLA. *See* Human leukocyte antigens
HLH. *See* Hemophagocytic
    lymphohistiocytosis

HMG. *See* High mobility group
Housekeeping, 325
HP-HF. *See* High-permeability
    hemofiltration
HSP. *See* Heat shock proteins
HSV. *See* Herpes simplex virus
Human immunodeficiency virus (HIV),
        46, 50, 86
    antibody tests, 86
    classification of, 352–354
    clinical features of, 350–351
    diagnosis of
        in children, 363
        handling, 362
        in infants, 363–364
        laboratory, 363–364
        respiratory failure, 355–358
    epidemiology of, 204, 350
    immune categories for, 353
    long-term survival with, 365–366
    mother-to-child transmission of, 206
    in older children, 351
    opportunistic infections in, 351
    PEP, 364–365
    PICU admission and, 356
        cross-infection in, 364–365
        nonrespiratory causes, 361–362
    Pneumocystis in, 358–360
    presentation of, 355–358
    progression of, 354–355
    symptom categories for, 352–353
    testing for, 362–363
        age-appropriate, 363
        requesting, 362–363
    treatment
        combination, 365–366
        starting, 365
    vaccine, 165–167
        current strategies, 166–167
        future developments, 167
    vertical transmission of, 86
Human leukocyte antigens (HLA), 6, 189,
        389, 535
Hydrocortisone, 536
Hypercalcemia, 384
Hyperglycemia, 187
Hyper-IgE syndrome, 41
Hyper-IgM syndromes, 26
Hyperkalemia, 384

Hyperpyrexia, 384
Hyponatremia, 394, 402
Hyposplenism, 48–49
Hypotension, 516
Hypothermia, 502
Hypoventilation, in malaria, 377–378
Hypoxemia, 525

I
Iatrogenic immunosuppression, 47–48
ICAM-1. *See* Intercellular adhesion
        molecule-1
ICP. *See* Intracranial pressure
ICU. *See* Intensive care unit
Idiopathic thrombocytopenic purpura,
        49
IFN-γ. *See* Interferon-γ
IFN-γ-R1. *See* Interferon-γ-receptor 1
IgA. *See* Immunoglobulin A
IGF. *See* Insulin-like growth factor
IgG. *See* Immunoglobulin G
IgM. *See* Immunoglobulin M
IL-1. *See* Interleukin-1
IL-6. *See* Interleukin-6
IL-10. *See* Interleukin-10
IL-12. *See* Interleukin-12
Immune system, 1
    innate, 1–4
        defects in, 337
        primary disorders of, 14–23
        susceptibility to infection, 336–338
    sepsis and, 188–189
    specific adaptive, 4–8
        deficiencies, 24–30
Immunity
    age and, 333
    cell-mediated, defects, 30–37
    delayed maturation of, 12–13
        humoral, 13
        hypogammaglobulinemia, 13
    developmental aspects of, 9–12
        after birth, 11–12
        intrauterine infection, 10–11
        neonatal, 10
        prenatal, 9
Immunization
    global, 404, 405
    passive, 154
    schedules, 404

Immunocompromised patients, 332
  severe, 333–336
Immunodeficiency, 13–14. *See also*
    Severe combined
    immunodeficiency
  combined, 37–40
  function tests for, 14
  minor, 336–339
    background, 336
  secondary, 45–49
    causes of, 45
    immunosuppression from
      underlying disease, 45–47
    management of, 49
  severe, 333–336
    bone marrow transplant patients,
      333–334
    solid organ transplants and, 334–335
  syndromic, 40–44
Immunoglobulin
  during fetal life, 9
  replacement therapy, 28–29
    administration of, 29
    in TSS management, 129–131
    VZV, 84
Immunoglobulin A (IgA), 10, 47
  deficiency, 26
  development of, system, 13
Immunoglobulin G (IgG), 9, 10, 26, 29,
    47, 76, 333, 527
Immunoglobulin M (IgM), 5, 10, 76, 527
Immunoparalysis, 338–339, 534–535
Immunosuppression, 44
  in acute myocarditis, 454
  with biologic agents, 48
  from underlying disease, 45–47
Immunosuppressive drugs, 47
Inducible nitric oxide synthase (iNOS),
    544, 545, 546
Infections. *See also* Bacterial disease;
    Cardiac infections; Nosocomial
    infections; Sepsis; Viral infections
  clinical manifestations of, 62–64
  epidemiology of, 59–62
    early *v.* late-onset, 59
    incidence of, 59
    microorganisms causing, 60
    pathogenesis of, 60–61
  focal, 59

  microbiological causes of, 63–64
  fungal, 77–80, 97–110
  global burden of, 194
  innate immune system susceptibility
    to, 336–338
  laboratory diagnosis of, 64–65
    microbiologic, 65
    rapid, 64–65
  protozoal, 87–88
  supportive therapy, 89
  treatment, 88–90
  viral, 80–87
Inflammatory response, in sepsis,
    178–180
Influenza, 80–81
  avian, 156, 415–421
    clinical manifestations of, 418–419
    diagnosis, 419
    epidemiology of, 203, 416–417
    evolution of, 416
    laboratory investigations, 419
    management, 420–421
    outbreaks of, 416–417
    outcome, 420
    pathogenesis of, 417–418
    in PICU, 221
  epidemiology of, 202–203
  intrauterine exposure to, 81
  staphylococcal TSS and, 127
  transmission of, 417
  vaccines, 155–156
Innate immune system, 1–4
  defects in, 337
  primary disorders of, 14–23
    complement, 14–16
  susceptibility to infection, 336–338
iNOS. *See* Inducible nitric oxide
    synthase
Insulin-like growth factor (IGF), 188
Insulin, resistance, 187
Intensive care unit (ICU). *See also*
    Neonatal intensive care unit;
    Pediatric intensive care unit
  gastrointestinal infections, 53
  immunologic approach in, 49–50
  interventions, 52–53
  meningitis, 51
  sepsis, 51
Intensive therapy unit (ITU), 216

Intercellular adhesion molecule-1 (ICAM-1), 21
Interferon-γ (IFN-γ), 529
  genetic susceptibility and, 285
  polymorphisms, clinical studies, 286
Interferon-γ-receptor 1 (IFN-γ-R1), genetic susceptibility and, 285–287
Interleukin-1 (IL-1), 17, 271, 532
  genetic susceptibility and, 273–278
  meningococcal disease and, 277–278
  polymorphisms, 276
    clinical studies, 279
  production of, 281
  sepsis and, 277
Interleukin-6 (IL-6)
  in critically ill patients, 280, 533
  genetic susceptibility and, 278–280
Interleukin-10 (IL-10), 532–533
  community-acquired pneumonia and, 284
  genetic susceptibility and, 280–284
  meningococcal disease and, 284
  polymorphisms, clinical studies, 282–283
  sepsis and, 281–284
Interleukin-12 (IL-12), 3
Intracranial pressure (ICP)
  in CNS infections, 482–483
  in JEV, 403
  in malaria, 381
Intracranial syndromes, 482
Intrauterine growth retardation (IUGR), 86
Intrauterine infection, 10–11
Intravascular catheters, 318
Intravenous immunoglobulin (IVIG), 89, 453
  in sepsis, 535–536
  in TSS management, 129–131
    dosing of, 130–131
    evidence for use of, 130
    rationale for, 130
    trials of, 130
Invasive meningococcal disease, cases of, 147
Invasive pneumococcal disease (IPD), 496
IPD. See Invasive pneumococcal disease

Isolation, 323–324
Isotonic crystalloids, 397
Itraconazole, 23
  in fungal infections, 107
ITU. See Intensive therapy unit
IUGR. See Intrauterine growth retardation
IVIG. See Intravenous immunoglobulin

J
JAK3. See Janus activated kinase 3
JAK5. See Janus activated kinase 5
Janeway lesions, 444
Janus activated kinase 3 (JAK3), 33
Janus activated kinase 5 (JAK5), 226
Japanese encephalitis virus (JEV), 371, 399–404
  clinical manifestations of, 400–402
  diagnosis, 402
  differential diagnosis, 401
  epidemiology, 399–400
  ICP in, 403
  laboratory investigations, 402–403
  management of, 403
  outcome, 403–404
  pathogenesis of, 400
  progression of, 401
JCVI. See Joint Committee on Vaccination and Immunization
JEV. See Japanese encephalitis virus
Joint Committee on Vaccination and Immunization (JCVI), 154

K
Kawasaki disease, 128
Klebsiella, 71, 72, 214, 490
Klebsiella pneumoniae, 320
Kostmann's syndrome, 18
Kybersept, 540

L
Labetalol, 411
β-lactamases, extended, 214
Lactate dehydrogenase (LDH), 498
LAD. See Leukocyte adhesion deficiency
Lariam. See Mefloquine
Laryngitis, 505
Laryngotracheobronchitis, 506
Laryngotracheobronchopneumonia, 506

Late-onset neonatal sepsis (LONS), 59
    presentation of, 63
Layrngotracheitis, 505–506
LBP. *See* Lipopolysaccharide-binding
    protein
LDH. *See* Lactate dehydrogenase
LDL. *See* Low-density lipoprotein
Lectin pathway, 178
Legionella, 423
Leishmania, 289
Lemierre's syndrome, 507–508
Leptospirosis, 470
Leukocyte adhesion deficiency (LAD),
    20–21
Leukocyte function antigen (LFA-1), 20
Leukocyte surface antigens, 5
    important, 6
Leukocytosis, 445, 502
Leukopenia, 419
LFA-1. *See* Leukocyte function antigen
Linezolid, 216
LIP. *See* Lymphoid interstitial
    pneumonitis
Lipopolysaccharide (LPS), 113, 176, 177,
    288, 338
Lipopolysaccharide-binding protein
    (LBP), 177, 229, 230–232, 524, 547
    studies on, 231
Listeria monocytogenes, 71, 89
    early onset, 71
LONS. *See* Late-onset neonatal sepsis
Low-density lipoprotein (LDL), 529
LPS. *See* Lipopolysaccharide
Lumbar puncture, 467, 484
Lumefantrine-artemether (Riamet or
    Coartem), 376
Lung biopsy, 103
Lyme disease, 470
Lymphoid interstitial pneumonitis (LIP),
    351
Lys216Glu, 232
Lyssavirus, 160

M
MAC. *See* Membrane attack complex
Macrophage migration inhibitory factor
    (MIF), 547
    immunoneutralization of, 548
Macrophages, 2–3

Magnesium sulfate, 411
Magnetic resonance imaging (MRI), 401,
    451, 468
Major histocompatibility complex
    (MHC), 7, 36, 117, 266, 529
    deficiency, 37–38
    monocyte, 339
Malaria, 88
    circulation in, 379–380
        shock and, 379
        volume resuscitation, 379–380
    clinical presentation of, 374
    definition of severe, 374–375
    diagnosis of, 375–376
        laboratory investigations, 376
        parasitology, 375–376
        PCR, 376
    emergency treatments, 377–386
        triage, 378
    epidemiology of, 204–205, 371–372
    ICP in, 381
    initial assessment, 377–386
    management of, 376–377
        antimalarial medication, 377
        electrolytes, 384
        exchange transfusion in, 385
        fluids, 384
        general, 383–385
        metabolic derangement, 383–384
        severe falciparum, 376–377
        supportive treatment, 384–385
        uncomplicated, 376
    prognosis, 386
    respiratory patterns in, 377–378
        distress, 378
        hypoventilation, 377–378
    seizure control in, 381–382
    transmission of, 372–373
    unconscious patients with, 380–381
    vaccine, 162–165
        asexual stage, 164–165
        future development of, 165
        pre-erythrocytic, 163–164
        strategies, 164
        transmission blocking, 165
Malarone. *See* Atovaquone-proguanil
Malassezia furfur, 106
Mannan-binding lectin (MBL), 16, 178
    in chemotherapy, 248–249

codon variants, 245
deficiency, 245
in genetic susceptibility, 241–249
plasma concentration of, 244
polymorphisms, 244
    clinical studies on, 246–247
    in pneumococcal disease, 248
SNPs in, 244–245
Mannan-binding protein (MBP), 177
MBL. *See* Mannan-binding lectin
MBL2, 178
MBP. *See* Mannan-binding protein
Measles, epidemiology of, 202
Mediastinitis, 438–441
Mefloquine (Lariam), 376
Membrane attack complex (MAC), 242
Mendelian inheritance, susceptibility
        and, 226–228
Meningitis
    aseptic, 469–471
        clinical features, 469
        diagnosis, 469–470
        medical treatment, 471
        pathogenesis, 469
    management of, 51
    purulent, 465–469
        clinical features, 466
        complications, 467–468
        diagnosis, 466–467
        medical treatment, 468–469
        pathogenesis, 465–466
Meningococcal serogroup C protein,
        146–147
    reduction in, 147
Meningococcal vaccines, 148
Meningococcus
    ACE and, 263–265
    epidemiology of, 199–200
    Fcγ receptors and, 255
    IL-1 and, 277–278
    IL-10 and, 284
    PAI-1 and, 259
    TNF and, 270
Merozoite surface protein (MSP), 165
Metabolic derangement, in malaria,
        383–384
Methicillin-sensitive *S. aureus* (MSSA),
        68–69, 320, 440, 496
    in PICU, 216–217

MHC. *See* Major histocompatibility
        complex
Microsatellites, 227
MIF. *See* Macrophage migration
        inhibitory factor
Mif gene, 548
Miller-Fisher syndrome, 473
Modified vaccinia Ankara (MVA), 164,
        166
MODS. *See* Multiple organ dysfunction
        syndrome
MOFS. *See* Multiple organ failure
        syndrome
Monocytes, 2–3
Mononuclear cells, 281
Moraxella catarrhalis, 12
Mother-to-child transmission, 206
MPO. *See* Myeloperoxidase
MRI. *See* Magnetic resonance imaging
MSP. *See* Merozoite surface protein
MSSA. *See* Methicillin-sensitive *S. aureus*
Mucor, 109
Mucus secretion, 488
Multiple organ dysfunction syndrome
        (MODS), 266
Multiple organ failure syndrome (MOFS),
        176, 196
Murray Valley encephalitis, 400
MVA. *See* Modified vaccinia Ankara
Mycobacterium tuberculosis, 11, 74,
        149–150, 455, 457
    epidemiology of, 201–202
Mycoplasma, 457
Mycoplasma fermentans, 239
Mycoplasma pneumoniae, 423, 470, 472
Mycotic aneurysms, 448
Myeloperoxidase (MPO), 22
Myocardial failure, in sepsis, 181–182
Myocarditis, 449–455
    clinical course, 452–455
    clinicopathologic classification of,
        452
    diagnosis of, 450–451
    diphtheric, 453
    epidemiology of, 449
    immunosuppression in, 454
    infectious causes of, 450
    microbiology, 449
    pathology, 449–450

Myocarditis (*cont.*)
  pathophysiology, 449–450
  sequelae of, 453
Myoglobinuria, 410

N
NADPH. *See* Nicotinamide adenine
    dinucleotide phosphate
National Institute of Child Health and
    Human Development (NICHD),
    60
National Nosocomial Infections
    Surveillance (NNIS), 313, 501
Natural killer (NK) cells, 2–3, 4
NBT. *See* Nitroblue tetrazolium
Necrotizing fasciitis
  diagnosis of, 122–123
  mortality rate of, 122
  streptococcal TSS and, 122–123
Neisseria gonorrhoeae, 178, 180, 288
Neisseria meningitidis, 73, 178, 197–198,
    225, 449, 455
  epidemiology of, 199–200
  vaccine, 145–146
Neonatal intensive care unit (NICU), 59,
    60
  risk factors in, 62
Nephrotic syndrome, 47
Neuraminidase, 415
Neuroendocrine system, sepsis in,
    186–188
Neuromuscular blockade (NMB), 514
Neurosurgical patient, 477–481
Neutropenia, 18
  cyclical, 18–19
  febrile, 108
    duration of, 338
  investigation of, 19
  severe congenital, 18
  Shwachman-Diamond Syndrome-
      associated, 19
  treatment of, 19
Neutrophils, 2–3, 180
  chemotaxis, 20–21
  count, 335
  disorders, 18–19
    neutropenia, 18
  endothelial cell interactions,
      543–544

function disorders, 19–23
  treatment of, 23
function tests, 20
NF. *See* Nuclear factor
NICHD. *See* National Institute of Child
    Health and Human Development
Nicotinamide adenine dinucleotide
    phosphate (NADPH), 22
NICU. *See* Neonatal intensive care unit
NIs. *See* Nosocomial infections
Nitric oxide, 514, 544–546
Nitric oxide synthase (NOS), 544–545
  inhibitors, 545
Nitroblue tetrazolium (NBT), 22, 23
NK cells. *See* Natural killer cells
NMB. *See* Neuromuscular blockade
NNIS. *See* National Nosocomial
    Infections Surveillance
Nod1, 177
Nod2, 177
Nonsteroidal antiinflammatory drugs
    (NSAIDs), 458
  streptococcal toxic shock syndrome
      and, 123–124
  mechanism, 124
NOS. *See* Nitric oxide synthase
Nosocomial infections (NIs), 312,
    338–339
  antimicrobial management, 321–323
  Candida and, 317–318, 322–323
  definitions of, 317–319
    CDC, 319
  diagnosis of, 317–319
  distribution of, 313
  epidemiology, 313–314
  etiologic organisms, 319–321
  preventive measures, 323–327
    antibiotic use, 325–326
    area spacing, 323
    environmental cultures, 325
    gown and gloves, 324
    hand-washing, 324
    housekeeping, 325
    isolation, 323–324
    staffing, 323
    visits, 325
  sites, 314–317
    bloodstream, 314–315, 322, 326–327
    pulmonary, 315

surgical, 316–317
    urinary tract, 316
NSAIDs. *See* Nonsteroidal
    antiinflammatory drugs
Nuclear factor (NF), 17
Nucleoside analogues, 106
Nutrition, 206–207

O

OFI. *See* Organ failure index
Oncologic patients, immunodeficiency
    and, 335–336
Opsonic dysfunction, 245
Organ failure index (OFI), 189
Oseltamivir, 220, 420
Osler nodes, 444
Oxazolidinones, 216

P

PAF. *See* Platelet-activating factor
PAF-AH. *See* Platelet-activating factor
    acetylhydrolase
PAI-1. *See* Plasminogen activator
    inhibitor 1
Palivizumab, 154
PAMPs. *See* Pathogen-associated
    molecular patterns
Panton-Valentine leukocidin (PVL), 214
Paracrine effects, 523
Parainfluenza, vaccine, 157
Paraldehyde, 411
Paramyxoviridae, 153
Parapneumonic effusions, 495–496
    stages of, 496
Parasitemia, 385
Parvovirus, 87, 342, 451
Passive immunization, 154
Patent ductus arteriosus (PDA), 442
Pathogen-associated molecular patterns
    (PAMPs), 176, 182, 229, 546
Pathogen recognition, 178
    in sepsis, 176–177
PCR. *See* Polymerase chain reaction
PCT. *See* Procalcitonin
PDA. *See* Patent ductus arteriosus
Pediatric intensive care unit (PICU), 143,
    196
    bacterial infections in, 213–215
        PRP in, 215

resistance, 213
        staphylococci, 213–214
        VRE in, 215
    CNS infections in, 481–484
    diagnosis in, 339–344
        enteric virus infections, 343
        PCR, 341–342
        respiratory tract infections, 342–343
        techniques, 340–341
        viral load, 341
    fungal infections in, 218–220
        echinocandins in, 219–220, 345
        Polyene macrolides, 218–219
        triazoles in, 219
        voriconazole, 345
    HIV and, 356
        cross-infection prevention, 364–365
        nonrespiratory causes of admission
            in, 361–362
    nosocomial infections in, 313
    resistant infections in, 215–217
        combination antimicrobial therapy,
            217
        extended spectrum γ-lactamases, 217
        MRSA, 216–217
        PRP, 217
        VRE, 217
    treatment in, 344–347
        antifungal agents, 344–345
        antiviral agents, 346
        combined therapy, 344–345
        oral antiviral agents, 346–347
    viral infections in, 220–222
        avian influenza, 221
        CMV, 222
        enteroviruses, 221–222
        influenza, 220–221
Pediatric Prevention Network (PPN),
    313
Pelletier criteria, 444
Penicillin, 129
Penicillin-resistant pneumococci (PRP),
    in PICU, 215
PENTA calculator, 354–355
Pentoxifylline, 538
PEP. *See* Postexposure prophylaxis
Peptidoglycan, 176
Peptococcus, 74
Peptostreptococcus, 74

Pericarditis, 455–458
 anatomy, 455
 complications of, 457
 diagnosis of, 456–457
 epidemiology, 455–456
 microbiology, 455–456
 pathology, 455
 treatment, 457
Peripherally inserted intravenous central
   catheter (PICC), 499
Pertussis, 508–510
 clinical presentation, 508–509
 diagnosis of, 509
 etiology, 508
 prevention, 510
 treatment of, 509–510
 vaccines, 152–153
Petersdorf criteria, 444
PGE₂. See Prostaglandin E₂
Phagocytosis, 21
Phenobarbitone, 411
Physiotherapy, 414
PICC. See Peripherally inserted
   intravenous central catheter
Picornaviridae, 412
PICU. See Pediatric intensive care unit
Plain polysaccharide meningococcal
   vaccine, 146
Plasma, infusion of, 180
Plasminogen activator inhibitor 1
   (PAI-1), 183, 184, 541, 542
 coagulation pathway and, 257–262
 expression of, 185
 meningococcal disease and, 259
 polymorphisms, 259
Plasmodium falciparum, 163, 204, 372,
   374
Plasmodium malariae, 204, 372, 374
Plasmodium ovale, 204, 372, 374
Plasmodium vivax, 204, 372, 374
Platelet-activating factor (PAF), 543
Platelet-activating factor acetylhydrolase
   (PAF-AH), 543
Pneumococcal disease, MBL
   polymorphisms in, 248
Pneumocystis, 28, 37, 42, 47
Pneumocystis carinii, 86, 225, 333, 351
 in HIV, 358–360
Pneumocystis jiroveci, 31, 88

Pneumonia, 50, 488–502
 clinical features of, 491
 community-acquired, 199, 489
   decision tree in investigation of,
     502
   IL-10 and, 284
   TNF and, 270–271, 273
 definition of, 490
 diagnosis of, 317, 497–499
   clinical presentation of, 497
   imaging, 497–498
   investigations, 498
   pleural fluid, 498–499
 drainage, 499
 etiology of, 490
   first year, 490
   after first year, 490
 hospital-acquired, 495
 incidence of, 489
 laboratory investigations, 492–493
 prevention, 494
 radiologic investigations, 491–492
 treatment, 493–494, 499
   fluid management, 493–494
 ventilator-associated, 327, 495,
   500–502
   diagnosis of, 501–502
   epidemiology of, 501
   etiology of, 500–501
PNP. See Purine nucleoside
   phosphorylase
Poliomyelitis, 412–414, 473
 clinical manifestations of, 412–413
 diagnosis, 413
   CSF, 413
 epidemiology of, 203–204
 management of, 413–414
 outcome, 414
 pathogenesis, 412
 prodromal illness in, 413
Poliovirus, 81–82
Polyene macrolides, in PICU, 218–219
Polyenes, 106
Polymerase chain reaction (PCR), 35, 65,
   104, 340, 360. See also Reverse-
   transcriptase PCR
 156S ribosomal, 343–344
 in infection diagnosis, 341–342
 in malaria diagnosis, 376

Polymorphisms, 227, 287
  ACE, clinical studies, 264
  Fcγ receptors, 250
    complement deficiency and, 251–252
  IFN-γ, clinical studies, 286
  IL-1, 276
  IL-6, clinical studies, 279
  IL-10, clinical studies, 282–283
  MBL, 244
    clinical studies on, 246–247
    in pneumococcal disease, 248
  PAI-1, 259
  restriction fragment length, 263
  significance of, 288
  studying, 228–229
  TAFI, 262–263
  TNF, 266
    clinical studies on, 268–269, 274–275
    G-238A, 271
    G-308A, 266–271
    sepsis and, 267–269
Polyribosyl ribitol phosphate (PRP), 11,
    144
Polysaccharides, 11
  conjugate vaccine, 146–147
Postanginal sepsis, 507–508
Postexposure prophylaxis (PEP), HIV, 364
PPN. See Pediatric Prevention Network
Prednisone, 454
Procalcitonin (PCT), 177, 498
Properdin, 243
Prophylaxis. See also Postexposure
        prophylaxis
  fungal infection, 106–109
  TSS, 131–132
Prostaglandin E₂ (PGE₂), 124
Protein C, 183, 256
  deficiency, 185
Protein S, 256
Proteus, 498
Protozoal infections, 87–88
PRP. See Polyribosyl ribitol phosphate
Pseudomonas, 440
Pseudomonas aeruginosa, 18, 73, 320, 321
Pulmonary infections. See also
        Respiratory tract
  nosocomial, 315
Purine nucleoside phosphorylase (PNP),
    deficiency, 38–39

Purulent meningitis
  clinical features, 466
  complications, 467–468
    brain swelling, 467
    obstructive hydrocephalus, 468
    seizures, 467
    SIADH, 467
    subdural effusion, 468
  diagnosis, 466–467
  medical treatment, 468–469
    antimicrobial therapy, 468–469
    chemoprophylaxis, 469
    steroids, 469
  pathogenesis, 465–466
PVL. See Panton-Valentine leukocidin

Q
QRS complex, 450
Quinupristin, 217

R
Rabies immune globulin (RIG), 161
Rabies, vaccines, 160–161
Radiography, 103
Respiratory syncytial virus (RSV), 31,
    80–81, 152, 511
  treatment of, 80–81
  vaccines, 153–154
Respiratory tract
  in children, 487–488
  failure
    causes of, 360–361
    in HIV, 355–358
    in older children, 358
  fungal infections and, 99
  infections, 488
    diagnosis of, 342–343
    epidemiology of, 199
    vaccines, 151–157
  in neonates, 487–488
Restriction fragment length
        polymorphism (RFLP), 263
Reverse-transcriptase PCR (RT-PCR)
  in avian influenza diagnosis, 419
  in bronchiolitis, 512
RFLP. See Restriction fragment length
        polymorphism
Rhabdomyolysis, 410
Rhinosinusitis, 102

Rhizopus, 109
Riamet. *See* Lumefantrine-artemether
Ribavirin, 346
Rickettsia, 457
RIG. *See* Rabies immune globulin
Rimantadine, 220, 420
Rotavirus, 86–87, 198, 344
    vaccine, 158
Roth's spots, 444
RSV. *See* Respiratory syncytial virus
RT-PCR. *See* Reverse-transcriptase PCR
Rubella, 84

S
Salmonella, 3, 11, 47, 72, 198
Salmonella enteritidis, in spinal abscess, 480
Salmonella typhi, vaccine, 150–151, 278
Sanitation, 206–207
SARS. *See* Severe acute respiratory distress syndrome
Scedosporium, 109
SCID. *See* Severe combined immunodeficiency
Secondary immunodeficiency, 45–49
    causes of, 45
    infections and, 46
    management of, 49
Seizures
    in malaria, 381–382
        algorithm for management of, 382
    in purulent meningitis, 467
Sepsis. *See also* Early-onset neonatal sepsis; Late-onset neonatal sepsis
    capillary leakage in, 181
    clinical manifestations of, 62–64
    coagulation response in, 182–183
    cytokines, 534
    diagnosis of, 523–524
    disturbed physiology in, 524
    early *v.* late onset, 59
    epidemiology of, 195–197
    etiology, 521–523
    experimental therapies, 526–530
        antiendotoxin, 526
        antiendotoxin antibodies, 526–527
        statins, 529–530
    genetic differences and, 189–190
    IL-1 and, 277

IL-10 and, 281–284
    immune status and, 188–189
    inflammatory response in, 178–180
    management of, 51
    microbiology of, 65–90
        bacterial causes of, 65–76
    microorganisms causing, 60
    myocardial failure in, 181–182
    in neuroendocrine system, 186–188
    pathogenesis, 287
    pathogen recognition in, 176–177
    pathogens causing, 61, 522
    pathophysiology, 523–524
    postanginal, 507–508
    predisposition for, 189–190
    risk factors for, 89
    shock and, 196–197
    signal transduction, 177
    supportive care, 525
    therapy, 88–90
        activated protein C, 540–542
        anticoagulants, 538–542
        anticytokine, 531–534
        antiinflammatory, 531–534
        antimicrobial, 524–525
        corticosteroids, 536–537
        endothelium-targeting, 542–546
        future considerations, 546–548
        IVIG, 535–536
        pentoxifylline, 538
    TNF polymorphisms and, 267–269
    vasodysregulation in, 181
Sequelae, 517
Serine protease (SERPIN), 257
SERPIN. *See* Serine protease
Serratia, 440
Serratia marcescens, 22, 71, 72
Severe acute respiratory distress syndrome (SARS), 152, 357, 421–425
    clinical manifestations of, 423
    coronavirus, 421
    diagnosis of, 423–424
    epidemiology, 421–422
    incubation period, 422
    laboratory investigations, 424
    management, 424–425
    mortality rate, 425
    outcome, 425

pathogenesis of, 422–423
in PICU, 221
postmortem studies, 422–423
spread of, 425
transmission, 422
Severe combined immunodeficiency
 (SCID), 30–37, 150, 357
 causes of, 33
 investigations, 34–35
 presentation, 30–32
 susceptibility to, 226
 treatment, 36–37
 types of, 33–35
  adenosine deaminase-deficient,
   34
  T- B+ NK+, 34
  T- B+ NK-, 33
  T- B- NK+, 33–34
Shigella, 198
Shock
 definitions of, 522
 in dengue, 391–392
  fluid therapy and, 395–397
  resolution of, 398
 in malaria, 379
Shunt infection
 clinical features, 477
 diagnosis, 477–478
 medical treatment, 478
Shwachman-Diamond Syndrome-
 associated neutropenia, 19
SIADH. *See* Syndrome of inappropriate
 secretion of antidiuretic hormone
Sickle cell disease, 227–228
Signal transducer and activator of
 transcription 3/acute-phase
 response factor (STAT3/APRF),
 278
Signal transduction
 in lymphocytes, 7
 in sepsis, 177
Simian immunodeficiency virus (SIV),
 166
Single nucleotide polymorphisms (SNPs),
 189
 in MBL genes, 244–245
SIRS. *See* Systemic inflammatory
 response syndrome
SIV. *See* Simian immunodeficiency virus

Skin, fungal infections and, 99
S-methylisothiourea (SMT), 546
SMT. *See* S-methylisothiourea
SNPs. *See* Single nucleotide
 polymorphisms
Solid organ transplants,
 immunodeficiency and, 334–335
Specific adaptive immune system, 4–8
 deficiencies of, 24–30
  antibody deficiency, 24–26
  clinical presentation, 24
Spinal abscess, 480
Spinal respiratory paralysis, 414
Splenectomy, 49
Staffing, 323
Staphylococci, TSS, 115–116, 125–127
 burns and, 127
 influenza and, 127
 menstrual, 126
 nonmenstrual, 126–127
 surgical procedures, 127
Staphylococcus aureus, 18, 22, 41, 68–69,
 113, 320, 321, 439, 443, 455, 496
 in spinal abscess, 480
Staphylococcus epidermis, 439, 443
STAT3/APRF. *See* Signal transducer and
 activator of transcription 3/acute-
 phase response factor
Statins, 529–530
 data on, 530
Stegomyia, 386
Stenotrophomonas maltophilia, 73
Sternal wound infections, 438–441
 diagnosis of, 439–441
 epidemiology of, 438–439
 after Ross procedure, 440
 treatment of, 439–441
Steroid therapy, 359
Streptococci, 67–68
 epidemiology of, 200–201
 TSS, 121–125
Streptococcus agalactiae, 67
Streptococcus pneumoniae, 67, 68, 178,
 197–198
 epidemiology of, 200
 genome sequence of, 149
 in pneumonia, 490
 in spinal abscess, 480
 vaccine, 148–149

Streptococcus pyogenes, 67, 113, 321
  vaccine, 151
Streptococcus viridans, 67
  in spinal abscess, 480
Subdural effusion, 468
Subdural empyema, 479–480
Superantigens
  immunologic consequences of, 119
  mechanism of action of, 117–118
  mediated disease, 120
Surfactant treatment, 359, 514–515
Surgical intervention
  cardiac, 339
  in endocarditis, 448
  nosocomial infections and, 316–317
  in TSS management, 128
Surviving Sepsis Campaign, 541
Syndrome of inappropriate secretion of
      antidiuretic hormone (SIADH),
      467
Syndromic immunodeficiencies, 40–44
  chromosome breakage disorders, 42
  DiGeorge syndrome, 40–41
  Wiskott-Aldrich syndrome, 41
Syphilis, 75–76
  maternal, 75
Systemic inflammatory response
      syndrome (SIRS), 46, 178, 245,
      337, 521
  definitions of, 522

T
TAFI. *See* Thrombin-activatable
      fibrinolysis inhibitor
TBE. *See* Tick borne encephalitis
T cell receptors (TCR), 7, 117
T cells
  CD4, 7
  derivation of, 6–7
  stimulation, 118
TCR. *See* T cell receptors
TDT. *See* Terminal deoxynucleotide
      transferase
Terminal deoxynucleotide transferase
      (TDT), 5
Tetanus, 409–412
  clinical manifestations of, 410
  diagnosis, 410
  illnesses similar to, 476–477

  management, 410–411
  outcome, 411–412
  pathogenesis, 409–410
  prevention, 162
  vaccine, 161–162
TF. *See* Tissue factor
TFPI. *See* Tissue factor pathway inhibitor
TGF. *See* Transforming growth factor
Th2. *See* T-helper-2
T-helper-2 (Th2), 34
Thrombin, 182
Thrombin-activatable fibrinolysis
      inhibitor (TAFI), 183, 186
  genetic susceptibility and, 262–263
  plasma levels, 262
  polymorphisms, 262–263
Thrombocytopenia, 394, 397
Thrombomodulin (TM), 184, 540
Thromboplastin, 538
Thrombospondin-related adhesive
      protein (TRAP), 163
Thymus gland, 6
Tick borne encephalitis (TBE), 160
Tissue factor (TF), 183
Tissue factor pathway inhibitor (TFPI),
      538–539
Tissue plasminogen activator (t-PA), 542
  clinical studies on, 260–261
  coagulation pathway and, 257–262
TM. *See* Thrombomodulin
TNF. *See* Tumor necrosis factor
Toll-like receptors, 177, 288, 528, 546–547
  clinical studies on, 240
  complex, 229–230
  defects in, 17–18
  in genetic susceptibility, 233–239
      TLR2, 238–239
      TLR4, 235–238
  signaling, 4
Total parenteral nutrition (TPN), 218, 314
Toxic shock syndrome (TSS), 68, 113–133
  clinical features of, 120–127
      unique, 121
  differential diagnosis, 127–128
  epidemiology, 114–117
      group A streptococci, 114–115
      non-group A streptococcal, 116–117
  management, 128–132
      antibiotic therapy, 128–129

future of, 132–133
  IVIG, 129–131
  secondary prophylaxis, 131–132
  supportive care, 128
  surgical intervention, 128
molecular epidemiology, group A
  streptococci, 115
pathogenesis of, 117–120
  superantigen mechanism of,
    117–119
staphylococcal, 115–116, 125–127
  burns and, 127
  diagnostic criteria for, 125
  influenza and, 127
  menstrual, 126
  nonmenstrual, 126–127
  surgical procedures, 127
streptococcal, 121–125
  diagnostic criteria for, 121
  necrotizing fasciitis and, 122–123
  NSAIDs and, 123–124
  varicella and, 123
superantigens in, 119–120
Toxin-mediated diseases, 113–133
Toxoplasma gondii, 87–88
t-PA. See Tissue plasminogen activator
T. pallidum, 239
TPN. See Total parenteral nutrition
Tracheostomy, 504
Transforming growth factor (TGF), 535,
  546
Transient hypogammaglobulinemia, 13
Transplant
  bone marrow, 36
    patients, 333–334
  solid organ, 334–335
Transthoracic echocardiography (TTE),
  446
TRAP. See Thrombospondin-related
  adhesive protein
T regulatory cells, 46
TREM-1, 177
Triazoles, in PICU, 219
Trimethoprim sulfamethoxazole, 88
Tropical infections, 370–371
  presentation of, 370
Trypanosoma cruzi, 449
TSS. See Toxic shock syndrome
TTE. See Transthoracic echocardiography

Tuberculosis, 74–75, 289
  epidemiology of, 201–202
  postnatal exposure to, 75
  vaccine, 149–150
Tumor necrosis factor (TNF), 17, 183,
  265–275, 526, 532, 533
  community-acquired pneumonia and,
    270–271, 273
  meningococcal disease and, 270
  polymorphisms, 266
    clinical studies on, 268–269, 274–275
    G-238A, 271
    G-308A, 267–271
    sepsis and, 267–269
Tyr387Asp, 243

U
Ultrasonography (US), 497
Unconscious patients, in malaria,
  380–381
Upper airway problems, 517
Urinary tract, 318
  fungal infections and, 99
  infections, nosocomial, 316
US. See Ultrasonography

V
Vaccine. See also Hib vaccine
  adenovirus, 157
  cholera, 157
  common, 144
  diphtheria, 156–157
  encephalitis, 158–159
  enterovirus, 158–159
  flaviviruses, 159–160
  group B γ-hemolytic streptococcus, 151
  haemophilus influenzae type b,
    143–145
  HSV, 159
  influenza, 155–156
  malaria, 162–165
  meningococcal, 148
  Neisseria meningitidis, 145–146
  parainfluenza, 157
  pertussis, 152–153
  plain polysaccharide meningococcal,
    146
  polysaccharide conjugate, 146–147
  preventable diseases, 404–415

Vaccine (*cont.*)
  as preventative strategy, 205–206
  rabies, 160–161
  respiratory tract infections, 151–157
  rotavirus, 158
  RSV, 153–154
  Salmonella typhi, 150–151, 278
  S. pneumoniae, 148–149
  Streptococcus pyogenes, 151
  tetanus, 161–162
  tuberculosis, 149–150
  VZV, 159
VAD. *See* Ventricular assist device
Valacyclovir, 346
Valganciclovir, 82, 346–347
Valine, 228
Vancomycin, 129
Vancomycin-resistant enterococci (VRE),
    70
  in PICU, 215
Variable number of tandem repeats
    (VNTR), 276
Varicella zoster virus (VZV), 84–85
  immunoglobulin, 84
  postnatal exposure to, 84–85
  streptococcal TSS and, 123
  vaccine, 159
Vascular cell adhesion molecule 1
    (VCAM-1), 236
Vascular permeability, 391
Vasodysregulation, 181
Vasopressin, 186
VATS. *See* Video assisted thoracoscopic
    surgery
VCAM-1. *See* Vascular cell adhesion
    molecule 1
Veillonella, 74
Ventricular assist device (VAD), 452
Ventricular septal defect (VSD), 442
Ventriculitis, 477–478
  clinical features, 477
  diagnosis, 477–478
  medical treatment, 478
Ventriculoperitoneal shunts (VPS),
    316
Very low birth weight (VLBW), 196
Video assisted thoracoscopic surgery
    (VATS), 499
Viral infections, 80–87

epidemiology of, 202–204
evolution of, 416
in PICU, 220–222
  avian influenza, 221
  enteroviruses, 221–222
  influenza, 220–221
  SARS, 221
  seasonal, 340
Visits, 325
Vitronectin, 184
VLBW. *See* Very low birth weight
VNTR. *See* Variable number of tandem
    repeats
Volume resuscitation, in malaria,
    379–380
Von Willebrand factor (vWF), 183
Voriconazole, 109
  in fungal infections, 107
  in PICU, 345
VPS. *See* Ventriculoperitoneal shunts
VRE. *See* Vancomycin-resistant
    enterococci
VSD. *See* Ventricular septal defect
vWF. *See* Von Willebrand factor
VZV. *See* Varicella zoster virus

W
West Nile virus, 400
White cell count, 64
WHO. *See* World Health Organization
Whooping cough. *See* Pertussis
Wiskott-Aldrich syndrome, 41
World Health Assembly, 203–204
World Health Organization (WHO), 155,
    384
  Young Infants Study Group, 197–198

X
X-linked agammaglobulinemia, 24
X-linked hyper-immunoglobulin M
    syndrome, 39
X-linked lymphoproliferative disease,
    39–40

Y
Yersinia, 198

Z
Zanamivir, 220, 420